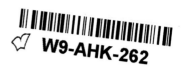

Practical Diagnosis
of
Hematologic Disorders

Authors

Carl R. Kjeldsberg, MD
Professor of Pathology and Medicine
Chairman of Pathology
University of Utah Health Sciences Center
President and CEO, ARUP Inc
Salt Lake City, Utah

Kojo S.J. Elenitoba-Johnson, MD
Assistant Professor of Pathology
University of Utah Health Sciences Center
Director of Molecular Hematopathology
ARUP Inc
Salt Lake City, Utah

Kathryn Foucar, MD
Director, Pathology Services
Professor of Pathology
University of New Mexico School of Medicine
Albuquerque, New Mexico

Jerry Hussong, DDS, MD
Assistant Professor of Pathology
University of Utah Health Sciences Center
Director of Hematologic Flow Cytometry
ARUP Inc
Salt Lake City, Utah

Robert W. McKenna, MD
John Childers Professor and Vice-Chair of Pathology
University of Texas Southwestern Medical Center
Dallas, Texas

Sherrie L. Perkins, MD, PhD
Associate Professor of Pathology
University of Utah Health Sciences Center
Director, Hematopathology
ARUP Inc
Salt Lake City, Utah

LoAnn C. Peterson, MD
Professor of Pathology
Northwestern University Medical School
Chicago, Illinois

Powers Peterson, MD
Department of Pathology
Sentara Norfolk General Hospital
Norfolk, Virginia

George M. Rodgers, MD, PhD
Professor of Medicine and Pathology
University of Utah Health Sciences Center and Veterans Affairs Medical Center
Medical Director, Coagulation Laboratory
ARUP Inc
Salt Lake City, Utah

Practical Diagnosis
of
Hematologic Disorders
Third Edition

Carl R. Kjeldsberg, MD
Editor

ASCP Press
American Society for Clinical Pathology
Chicago, Illinois

Publishing Team
Ted Patla, Philip Rodgers (editorial)
Terri Horning, Erik Tanck, Alan Makinen (production)
Joshua Weikersheimer (publisher)

Notice
Trade names for equipment and supplies described herein are included as suggestions only. In no way does their inclusion constitute an endorsement or preference by the American Society of Clinical Pathologists. The ASCP did not test the equipment, supplies, or procedures, and, therefore, urges all readers to read and follow all manufacturers' instructions and package insert warnings concerning the proper and safe use of products.

Library of Congress Cataloging-in-Publication Data
Practical diagnosis of hematologic disorders / Carl R. Kjeldsberg, editor.—
  3rd ed.
    p. ; cm
  Includes bibliographical references and index.
  ISBN 0-89189-442-X
  1. Blood—Diseases—Diagnosis. I. Kjeldsberg, Carl R., 1938-
  [DNLM: 1. Hematologic Diseases—diagnosis—Handbooks. 2. Hematologic
Diseases—therapy—Handbooks. WH 39 P895 2000]
  RC636.P72 2000
  616. 1'5075-dc21
                                                              99-054756
                                                                   CIP

Printed in Canada

06 05 04 03   5 4 3 2

Dedicated to

Tanya M. Kjeldsberg, DVM

and

Kristina M. Kjeldsberg, MD

*for their
inspiration and motivation*

Contents

Part II   Hemolytic Anemias

Part III   Reactive Disorders of Granulocytes and Monocytes

Part XIII Thrombotic Disorders

Part XIV Anticoagulant Therapy

Part XV Special Techniques

Preface

As in the previous two editions, our goal with the *Practical Diagnosis of Hematologic Disorders* is to provide an up-to-date, concise source of guidelines to the selection, use, and interpretation of laboratory tests, while at the same time providing an overview of the pathogenesis, clinical features, and treatment of the most common hematologic disorders. The entire text has been revised, reworked, rephotographed, or rewritten. Substantial new material has been added, including a chapter on special techniques and posttransplantation-related disorders.

The focus has been on providing practical information. Each chapter is thoughtfully organized and follows a practical format to make finding specific information easy. Each chapter is formatted the same, discussing the relevant physiology, clinical findings, approach to diagnosis, hematologic findings, other laboratory tests, and clinical course and treatment. The book's user-friendly organization makes it easy to find what you want to know about which disease quickly. A handy appendix of reference values for various hematologic parameters is also included.

We hope that this book will continue to interest a broad audience, including medical students, residents and fellows in pathology and medicine, pathologists, hematologists/oncologists, internists, pediatricians, and medical technologists. It should be particularly helpful to those preparing for boards in pathology and internal medicine.

Acknowledgments

I gratefully acknowledge the excellent work and support of my coauthors: M. Kathryn Foucar, MD; Jerry W. Hussong, DDS, MD; Kojo S.J. Elenitoba-Johnson, MD; Robert W. McKenna, MD; Sherrie L. Perkins, MD, PhD; LoAnn C. Peterson, MD; Powers Peterson, MD; and George M. Rodgers, MD, PhD. I also wish to express my sincere appreciation to Joshua Weikersheimer, Publisher of the ASCP Press, for his continued help and guidance with this project. We are indebted to our residents and fellows who continue to teach and inspire us. I also thank Chris Hansen, MD, for his valuable assistance in proofreading chapters in the book.

PART
I

Anemias

1 Diagnosis of Anemia

The bone marrow contains pluripotential stem cells that have the capacity for self-renewal as well as differentiation into mature blood cells. Under the influence of erythropoietin (for the production of RBCs), this primitive stem cell undergoes cellular division and differentiation to form pronormoblasts and normoblasts. This process requires 6 to 7 days and four rounds of cellular division within the bone marrow. During the final step of differentiation the nucleus is extruded to form a reticulocyte, which still contains cytoplasmic RNA. Reticulocytes enter the peripheral circulation, where they appear as faintly blue-gray polychromatophilic cells, persisting for about 24 hours. On the loss of the cytoplasmic RNA, a mature RBC is formed. This RBC remains in the circulation for 120 days before being removed by the spleen and reticuloendothelial system.

1.1 Normal and Pathologic RBCs

The normal RBC is a biconcave disk, 6 to 9 μm in diameter and 1.5 to 2.5 μm thick. In the peripheral smear RBCs are anucleate with a dense outer rim and a clearer center that occupies approximately one third of the diameter of the cell. The cytoplasm is uniformly pink without inclusions. Pathologic RBCs can be larger or smaller than normal RBCs, are often abnormally shaped, and may contain inclusions. Variation in size is referred to as "anisocytosis," and variation in shape is termed "poikilocytosis." **Table 1-1** presents a summary of the morphologic abnormalities in RBCs that may be seen on blood smears, including those associated with specific diseases.

1.2 **Automated Hematology**

In both the office and hospital settings, most patients' blood is evaluated with an electronic blood cell counter. The two principal mechanisms used to analyze samples are voltage pulse-impedance analysis and low- or high-angle light scatter from a coherent or laser light source. In an impedance counter, such as those first developed by Coulter Electronics (Hialeah, Fla), the passage of a particle through an orifice of standard size and volume displaces conductive electrolyte solution within the orifice. If an electric current is applied across the orifice, a change in resistivity and conductivity of the electrolyte solution occurs as the particle passes through it. A detector notes a pulse when the particle passes through the orifice; this pulse is proportional to the volume of the electrolyte solution displaced by the particle. Thus, the counter is capable of counting and sizing particles simultaneously. In a light scatter counter, such as the Technicon H*3 (Technicon, Tarrytown, NY) or Cell-Dyn models (Abbott Diagnostics, Santa Clara, Calif), interruption of the light beam by a particle produces an electronic pulse. The angle of light scatter and the intensity of the light scattered at a particular angle delineates several physical properties of the cell, including cell size, volume, shape, and internal complexity.

With the data obtained, either instrument can generate a histogram of size distribution on the x-axis and relative number of particles on the y-axis. From these data, the RBC number and mean corpuscular volume (MCV) can be determined, and the other indices, such as mean corpuscular hemoglobin concentration (MCHC), can be calculated. Newer instruments also generate an index that provides the degree of dispersion of RBC sizes (anisocytosis) compared with a "normal" size distribution histogram, referred to as a "red cell distribution width" (RDW).

1.3 Evaluation of the Peripheral Smear

Examination of the peripheral smear by a physician who is aware of the patient's clinical condition is extremely useful in evaluating the patient with anemia. Highly skilled laboratory personnel occasionally may overlook subtle changes, such as minimal hypersegmentation of neutrophils in patients with combined folate and iron deficiency (masked macrocytosis) or basophilic stippling in a patient with thalassemia and complicating causes of anemia. These signs may be useful for interpretation by a physician familiar with the patient. Electronically derived red and white blood cell indices, although useful, are simply representations of the mean and overall degree of dispersion of the cell distribution and give little information concerning other parameters, especially the shape of the RBCs (poikilocytosis), the presence or absence of minor populations of abnormal RBCs, and subtle changes in WBCs. Examination of the blood smear for specific shape variations, such as those listed in **Table 1-1**, can provide valuable information to aid in the diagnosis of a patient's underlying disease.

1.4 Anemia

The primary function of the RBC is to deliver oxygen to the tissues. Anemia is defined as a reduction in the total number of RBCs, amount of hemoglobin in the circulation, or circulating RBC mass. This results in impaired oxygen delivery, giving rise to physiologic consequences secondary to tissue hypoxia as well as compensatory mechanisms initiated by the organism to correct anoxia. These signs and symptoms include fatigue, syncope, dyspnea, or impairment of organ function due to decreased oxygen; pallor or postural hypotension due to decreased blood volume; and palpitations, onset of heart murmurs, or congestive heart failure due to increased cardiac output. One should always remember that anemia is not a diagnosis, but a sign of underlying disease. Hence, the workup of a patient with anemia is directed at elucidating the causes for the patient's decreased RBC mass. A thorough history and physical examination are crucial for an intelligent, directed approach to the differential diagnosis of anemia. **Tables 1-2** and **1-3** show important features in a patient's history and physical examination that can yield diagnostic clues as to the cause of

Table 1-1 Pathologic Red Blood Cells in Blood Smears

Red Blood Cell Type	Description
Acanthocyte (spur cell)	Irregularly spiculated cells with projections of varying length and dense center
Basophilic stippling	Punctate basophilic inclusions
Bite cell (degmacyte)	Smooth semicircle taken from one edge
Burr cell (echinocyte), or crenated cell	Cells with short, evenly spaced spicules and preserved central pallor
Cabot's rings	Circular blue threadlike inclusion with dots
Howell-Jolly bodies	Small, discrete basophilic dense inclusions; usually single
Hypochromic cell	Prominent central pallor
Leptocyte	Flat, waferlike, thin, hypochromic cell
Macrocyte	Cells larger than normal (>8.5 μm), well-filled hemoglobin
Microcyte	Cells smaller than normal (<7 μm)
Ovalocyte (elliptocyte)	Elliptically shaped cell
Pappenheimer bodies	Small, dense basophilic granules
Polychromatophilia	Gray or blue hue frequently seen in macrocytes
Rouleaux	Cell aggregates resembling stack of coins
Schistocyte (helmet cell)	Distorted, fragmented cell, two or three pointed ends
Sickle cell (drepanocyte)	Bipolar, spiculated forms, sickle-shaped, pointed at both ends
Spherocyte	Spherical cell with dense appearance and absent central pallor; usually decreased in diameter
Stomatocyte	Mouth- or cuplike deformity
Target cell (codocyte)	Target-like appearance, often hypochromic
Teardrop cell (dacrocyte)	Distorted, drop-shaped cell

Abbreviations: G6PD = glucose-6-phosphate dehydrogenase; DIC = disseminated intravascular coagulation; TTP = thrombotic thrombocytopenic purpura.

Underlying Change	Disease States
Altered cell membrane lipids	Abetalipoproteinemia, parenchymal liver disease, postsplenectomy
Precipitated ribosomes (RNA)	Coarse stippling: lead intoxication, thalassemia; fine stippling: a variety of anemias
Heinz body "pitting" by spleen	G6PD deficiency, drug-induced oxidant hemolysis
May be associated with altered membrane lipids	Usually artifactual: seen in uremia, bleeding ulcers, gastric carcinoma, artifact
Nuclear remnant	Postsplenectomy, hemolytic anemia, megaloblastic anemia
Nuclear remnant	Postsplenectomy, hemolytic anemia, megaloblastic anemia
Diminished hemoglobin synthesis	Iron deficiency anemia, thalassemia, sideroblastic anemia
	Obstructive liver disease, thalassemia
Young cells, abnormal cell maturation	Increased erythropoiesis, oval macrocytes in megaloblastic anemia, round macrocytes in liver disease
	Iron deficiency anemia, thalassemia, sideroblastic anemia
Abnormal cytoskeletal proteins	Hereditary elliptocytosis
Iron-containing mitochondrial remnant or siderosome	Sideroblastic anemia, postsplenectomy
Ribosomal material	Reticulocytosis, premature marrow release of red blood cells
Cell clumping by circulating paraprotein	Paraproteinemia, artifact
Mechanical distortion in microvasculature by fibrin strands, disruption or prosthetic heart valve	Microangiopathic hemolytic anemia (DIC, TTP), prosthetic heart valves, severe burns
Molecular aggregation of hemoglobin S	Sickle cell disorders (not including S trait)
Decreased membrane redundancy	Hereditary spherocytosis, immunohemolytic anemia, transfusion, artifact
Membrane defect with abnormal cation permeability	Hereditary stomatocytosis, immunohemolytic anemia
Increased redundancy of cell membrane	Liver disease, postsplenectomy, thalassemia, hemoglobin C disease, iron deficiency
	Myelofibrosis, myelophthisic anemia

Table 1-2 Patient History in the Diagnosis of Anemia

Historical Information	Possible Causes of Anemia
Age of onset	Inherited or acquired disorder, continuous or recent onset
Duration of illness	Results of previous examinations and blood counts
Prior therapy for anemia	Vitamin B_{12}, iron supplementation, and how long ago
Suddenness or severity of anemia	Symptoms of dyspnea, palpitations, dizziness, fatigue, postural hypotension
Chronic blood loss	Menstrual and pregnancy history, gastrointestinal symptoms, black or bloody stools
Hemolytic episodes	Episode of weakness with icterus and dark urine
Toxic exposures	Drugs, hobbies, and occupational exposures
Dietary history	Alcohol use, unusual diet, prolonged milk ingestion in infants
Family history and racial background	Possible inherited disorder: family members with anemia, gallbladder disease, splenomegaly, splenectomy
Underlying diseases	Uremia, chronic liver disease, hypothyroidism

anemia, hence reducing the number of laboratory tests that need to be performed.

1.4.1 Examination of the Blood

Anemias have been classified under a number of different schema, none of which is completely satisfactory. For practical purposes, an initial morphologic classification of anemia with examination of RBC indices and the peripheral smear is probably most useful. With use of the MCV and the RDW or RBC morphologic index (RCMI), anemias may be classified into six categories (**Table 1-4**). The anemia may be characterized by cell size as microcytic, normocytic, or macrocytic. The absence or presence of anisocytosis (as measured by RDW) further subdivides these three size categories. In general, anemias caused by deficiencies (such as iron, folate, or vitamin B_{12}) tend to have a greater degree of aniso-

Table 1-3 Physical Signs in the Diagnosis of Anemia

Physical Sign	Associated Disease
Skin and mucous membranes	
Pallor	Any anemia
Scleral icterus	Hemolytic anemia
Smooth tongue	Pernicious anemia, severe iron deficiency
Petechiae	Thrombocytopenia and bone marrow replacement or aplastic anemia
Gum hyperplasia	Acute monocytic leukemia
Ulcers	Sickle cell disease
Lymph nodes	
Lymphadenopathy	Infectious mononucleosis, lymphoma, leukemia
Heart	
Cardiac dilatation, tachycardia, loud murmur	Severe anemia
Soft murmurs	Anemia, usually mild
Abdomen	
Splenomegaly	Infectious mononucleosis, leukemia, lymphoma, hypersplenism
Massive splenomegaly	Chronic myelogenous leukemia, myelofibrosis
Hepatosplenomegaly with ascites	Liver disease
Central nervous system	
Subacute combined degeneration of spinal cord	Pernicious anemia (vitamin B_{12} deficiency)
Delayed Achilles tendon reflex	Hypothyroidism

cytosis than anemias caused by genetic defects or primary bone marrow disorders. However, difficulties arise in classification using this scheme, particularly with regard to anemia of chronic disease (ACD).

In addition to pure morphologic criteria, anemias also may be classified by the degree of bone marrow response or peripheral blood reticulocytosis as hyperproliferative, normoproliferative, or hypoproliferative. This often provides insights into the pathogenesis

Table 1-4 Classification of Anemia Based on Red Blood Cell Size and Distribution Width

Cell Size	Normal RDW	High RDW
Microcytosis (MCV <70 μm^3 [70 fL])	Thalassemia minor, anemia of chronic disease, some hemoglobinopathy traits	Iron deficiency, hemoglobin H disease, some anemia of chronic disease, some thalassemia minor, fragmentation hemolysis
Normocytosis	Anemia of chronic disease, hereditary spherocytosis, some hemoglobinopathy traits, acute bleeding	Early or partially treated iron or vitamin deficiency, sickle cell anemia or sickle cell disease
Macrocytosis (MCV >100 μm^3 [100 fL])	Aplastic anemia, some myelodysplasias	Vitamin B_{12} or folate deficiency, autoimmune hemolytic anemia, cold agglutinin disease, some myelodysplasias, liver disease, thyroid disease, alcohol

Abbreviations: RDW = red cell distribution width; MCV = mean corpuscular volume.

of the process. Thus, patients with defects in RBC proliferation or maturation tend to have little or no increase in reticulocytes, reflecting the inability of the bone marrow to increase RBC production in response to the anemia (hypoproliferative). In contrast, patients with anemias caused by decreased survival of the RBCs with a normal bone marrow proliferative response often exhibit increased peripheral blood reticulocytes (normoproliferative or hyperproliferative; **Figure 1-1**). If the degree of reticulocytosis is adequate to replace the loss of RBCs, the anemia is said to be "compensated." If the bone marrow response is inadequate, the anemia will progressively worsen.

Finally, anemias caused by decreased RBC survival are often subdivided by pathogenetic mechanism into those caused by intrinsic or inherited defects and those that are acquired or caused by extrinsic factors. This classification is often useful in understanding the underlying disease process and may facilitate the workup of anemias that arise secondary to extrinsic processes.

1.4.2 Differential Diagnosis of Anemia

Anemia may be either relative (due to increased plasma volume with a normal RBC mass) or absolute (due to a decreased RBC mass). It is important to rule out causes of relative anemia, such as pregnancy or macroglobulinemia, because they represent disturbances in plasma volume rather than decreased RBC mass. Decreased plasma volume, caused by dehydration, may mask a real decrease in circulating RBC mass.

Use of a morphologic classification scheme with RBC index data and the reticulocyte count allows for practical classification of anemias into broad groups. This may facilitate intelligent selection of other laboratory tests to determine the underlying cause of the anemia.

1.4.3 Macrocytic Anemia

Macrocytic anemias (MCV >100 μm^3 [>100 fL]) are less common than normocytic or microcytic anemias. Macrocytic anemias may be subdivided into those with a normal RDW (principally those caused by bone marrow failure, such as aplastic anemia and myelodysplasia), and those with a high RDW (caused by deficiencies of vitamin B_{12} or folic acid or by autoimmune hemolysis or cold agglutinins). However, many exceptions to this general classification scheme exist. For example, a mild degree of macrocytosis (MCV between 102 and 105 μm^3 [102 and 105 fL]) with a normal RDW is relatively common as a direct toxic effect of alcohol. Similarly, some cases of myelodysplasia may have a high RDW.

Further classification of a macrocytic anemia based on the presence or absence of a reticulocyte response is also helpful (*see Figure 1-1*). Hemolytic anemias, blood loss, and partially treated vitamin B_{12} or folic acid deficiencies demonstrate an increased reticulocyte count. Normal to increased reticulocyte counts are more likely to be associated with autoimmune hemolysis, disorders of membrane structural proteins (eg, elliptocytosis), paroxysmal nocturnal hemoglobinuria, and fragmentation hemolysis (**Figure 1-2**). For those patients with a normal or decreased corrected reticulocyte count, disorders associated with decreased bone marrow function—including untreated vitamin deficiency, drugs, toxins, liver and thyroid disease, or primary bone marrow failure—should be suspected. Blood smears that show morphologic features compatible with megaloblastic anemia (oval macrocytes and hyperseg-

Figure 1-1 Classification of macrocytic anemia by reticulocyte count.

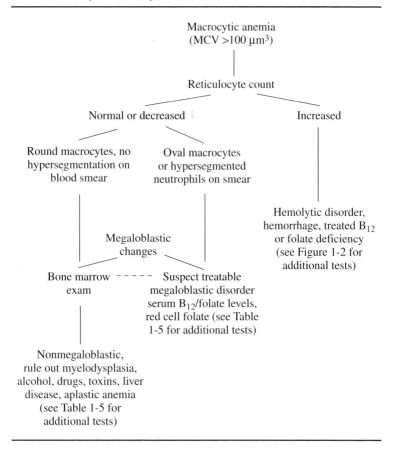

mented neutrophils) may warrant further evaluation with vitamin assays but not bone marrow examination. When megaloblastic changes are present without signs of vitamin B_{12} or folate deficiency, bone marrow examination and additional testing (**Table 1-5**) may be needed. A more extensive consideration of macrocytic anemia is found in Chapter 5.

1.4.4 Microcytic Anemia

The three most common causes of microcytic anemias (MCV $<75 \ \mu m^3$ [<75 fL]) are iron deficiency, thalassemia minor, and

Figure 1-2 Classification of normocytic or megaloblastic
anemias with elevated reticulocyte counts.

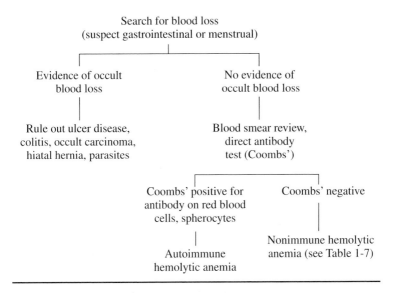

Table 1-5 Ancillary Tests for Macrocytic Anemia Without
Increased Reticulocyte Response

Megaloblastic bone marrow changes present only in erythroid line:
  Thyroid function tests
  Assess iron stores—serum iron, iron-binding capacity, ferritin
  Cytogenetic analysis—evaluate for myelodysplasia

Megaloblastic bone marrow changes present in more than one cell line:
  Dietary and drug history
  Malabsorption studies
  Schilling test if vitamin B_{12} deficiency

ACD (**Figure 1-3**). The RDW is useful in distinguishing thalassemia, which generally (but not invariably) produces elevated RBC counts and lower RDW than would be expected for
the MCV and the degree of anemia. Iron deficiency is almost
always associated with a high RDW. The values seen in ACD are

Figure 1-3 Classification of microcytic anemias.

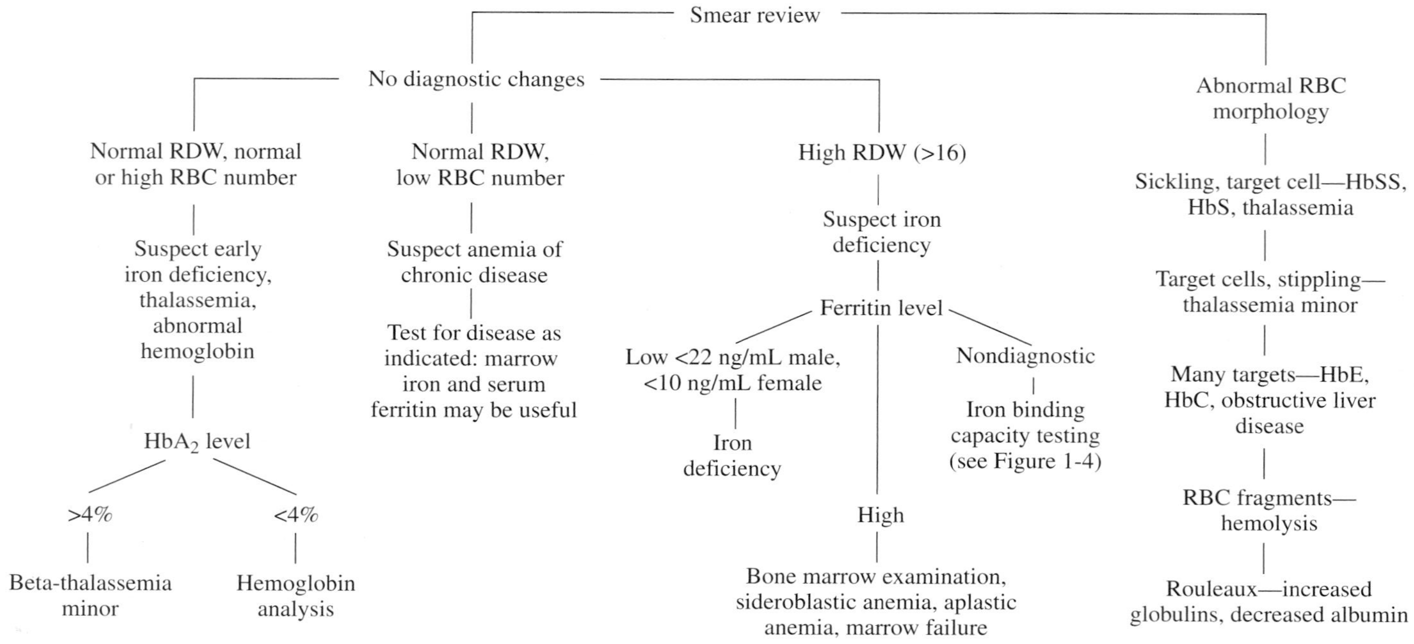

Smear review

— No diagnostic changes

Normal RDW, normal or high RBC number
Suspect early iron deficiency, thalassemia, abnormal hemoglobin

HbA$_2$ level
- >4% — Beta-thalassemia minor
- <4% — Hemoglobin analysis

Normal RDW, low RBC number
Suspect anemia of chronic disease
Test for disease as indicated: marrow iron and serum ferritin may be useful

High RDW (>16)
Suspect iron deficiency

Ferritin level
- Low <22 ng/mL male, <10 ng/mL female — Iron deficiency
- Nondiagnostic — Iron binding capacity testing (see Figure 1-4)
- High — Bone marrow examination, sideroblastic anemia, aplastic anemia, marrow failure

Abnormal RBC morphology
- Sickling, target cell—HbSS, HbS, thalassemia
- Target cells, stippling—thalassemia minor
- Many targets—HbE, HbC, obstructive liver disease
- RBC fragments—hemolysis
- Rouleaux—increased globulins, decreased albumin

extremely variable. Some ACDs may be normocytic, while others, particularly in patients with renal disease, are microcytic. These microcytic processes are associated with normal to high serum ferritin levels. By using serum iron and total iron binding studies, iron deficiency anemia and ACD can usually be distinguished without a bone marrow examination (**Figure 1-4**). A more detailed consideration of microcytic anemias may be found in Chapter 2.

1.4.5 Normocytic, Normochromic Anemia

Patients with normal or hypoproliferative reticulocyte counts and normocytic, normochromic anemias generally require bone marrow evaluation. A peripheral blood smear may provide valuable clues for the differential diagnosis (**Table 1-6**). Patients with normocytic anemia and an elevated reticulocyte count should undergo the same general evaluation as patients with macrocytosis and an elevated reticulocyte count (*see Figure 1-2*). Normocytic, normochromic anemias with elevated reticulocyte counts can be divided into those with positive direct antiglobulin test results (Coombs' test) and those lacking evidence of RBC-bound antibodies. Coombs'-negative hemolytic anemias are heterogeneous. The peripheral blood smear and patient history often suggest possible causes for the anemia (**Table 1-7**). A more detailed discussion of nonhemolytic normocytic anemias may be found in Chapter 3, and the hemolytic anemias are presented in Chapters 6 through 15.

The differential diagnosis of anemia is often tempered or modified by knowledge of other patient data. All algorithmic classification schemes should be qualified by the pragmatic knowledge of the physician in considering the probable causes of anemia in an individual patient or patient population. For example, because 98% or more of the anemias in children under the age of 4 years are caused by iron deficiency, many pediatricians simply treat all children with this type of anemia with iron supplementation and perform workups only for those who fail to respond to this therapy. In many situations, clinical knowledge can suggest several possible causes of anemia. Thus, classification algorithms are suggested pathways for physicians to follow in determining test utilization and should not be considered required routes.

Figure 1-4 Distinguishing iron deficiency versus anemia of chronic disease.

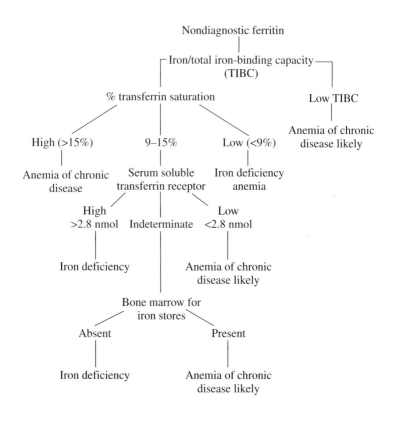

Laboratory Tests

Test 1.1 **The Reticulocyte Count**

Purpose. This test enumerates the number of reticulocytes, indicating bone marrow production of new RBCs.

Principle. Residual RNA in immature RBCs is precipitated and stained with a supravital dye.

Specimen. Venous or capillary blood may be used for this test.

Table 1-6   Normochromic, Normocytic Anemia Without High Reticulocyte Response

Findings on Peripheral Blood Smear	Further Workup
Leukoerythroblastosis	Suspect myelophthisic process—bone marrow examination for space-occupying lesion (metastatic tumor, lymphoma, myelofibrosis) In children suspect infection
Abnormal white blood cells	Suspect leukemia, lymphoma—bone marrow examination
Rouleaux	Suspect myeloma—serum and urine electrophoresis, radiographs to look for lytic lesions, bone marrow examination
No abnormal cells	Suspect anemia of chronic disease or sideroblastic anemia—bone marrow examination; rule out chronic disease processes, ferritin, total iron-binding capacity, and percent transferrin saturation as indicated

Table 1-7 Workup of Coombs'-Negative Anemia

Feature of Anemia	Possible Process	Tests
Episodic anemia	Enzyme deficiency Paroxysmal nocturnal hemoglobinuria	G6PD, other RBC enzymes Sucrose hemolysis, Ham's test, flow cytometry
RBC fragmentation	DIC, TTP, HUS	Coagulation tests, serum haptoglobin levels
Abnormal RBC stippling	Lead poisoning Thalassemia	Lead levels Hemoglobin electrophoresis
Abnormal shapes or increased target cells	Hemoglobinopathy or thalassemia	Hemoglobin analysis
Spherocytes	Hereditary spherocytosis	Osmotic fragility test

Abbreviations: G6PD = glucose-6-phosphate dehydrogenase; DIC = disseminated intravascular coagulation; TTP = thrombotic thrombocytopenic purpura; HUS = hemolytic-uremic syndrome.

Procedure. A blood smear is made, and the RBCs are stained with brilliant cresyl blue or methylene blue. Cells containing stained reticular material are enumerated per 1000 RBCs and expressed as percent reticulocytes (absolute number per 100 RBCs). Many automated hematology analyzers now analyze reticulocyte counts based on staining and light-scatter properties as an optional function of the complete blood count.

Interpretation. Reticulocytes are defined as immature RBCs seen in the peripheral blood that contain at least two dots of stainable reticulin material in their cytoplasm. More immature forms have multiple dots and small networks of skeins of bluish-staining material. Intraobserver variation and uneven distribution of reticulocytes introduce a high analytic variation in manual reticulocyte counting, with interlaboratory coefficients of variation in the 20% range. Duplicate reticulocyte counts or 3-day average values may help to reduce the imprecision of the raw reticulocyte count. Automated reticulocyte counts, owing to larger sample analysis and mechanically defined criteria, tend to be more reproducible.

Effective RBC production is a dynamic process, and the number of reticulocytes should be compared with the number expected to be released in a patient without anemia. This is calculated as 1% of $5 \times 10^6/mm^3$ ($5 \times 10^{12}/L$) RBCs daily for an absolute reticulocyte production of $50 \times 10^3/mm^3$ ($50 \times 10^9/L$). The corrected reticulocyte count takes into account normal RBC proliferation for a specific hematocrit and may be calculated with the following formula:

$$\text{Corrected Reticulocyte Count} = (\text{Percent Observed Reticulocytes} \times \text{Patient's Hematocrit}) \div 45$$

Another complicating factor in reticulocyte count correction is that patients with anemia may release reticulocytes prematurely into the circulation. Reticulocytes are usually present in the blood for 24 hours before they extrude the residual RNA and become erythrocytes. If they are released early from the bone marrow, reticulocytes may persist in peripheral blood for 2 or 3 days. This is most likely to occur when severe anemia causes a marked acceleration in erythropoiesis and release. Some authors have advocated correction of the reticulocyte count for "shift" reticulocytes, called the "reticulocyte production index" (RPI):

$$RPI = [(\text{Percent Reticulocyte} \times \text{Hematocrit Value})$$
$$\div\ 45] \times [1 \div \text{Correction Factor}]$$

The correction factor calculation is shown in **Table 1-8**.

In cases of low erythropoietin (often seen in patients with renal or hepatic disease), application of an RPI correction may mask a failure of bone marrow response, because the shift does not take place fully or at all. In general, RPI values less than 2 indicate failure of bone marrow RBC production or a hypoproliferative anemia. Reticulocyte production indexes of 3 or greater indicate marrow hyperproliferation or an appropriate response.

Test 1.2 **Bone Marrow Examination**

Purpose. Bone marrow examination allows assessment of the cellularity, maturation, and composition of the hematopoietic elements in the bone marrow, as well as evaluation of iron stores. Some infections also may be cultured from the bone marrow.

Principle. The cortical bone is penetrated and a sample of the bone marrow is aspirated. In most cases, a small biopsy specimen of the medullary bone and marrow is obtained. The most common sites for the procedure are the posterior or anterior iliac crest and the sternum.

Specimen. Bone marrow aspiration and biopsy samples.

Procedure. Bone marrow aspiration and biopsy are innocuous procedures when performed by experts. Several sites in the skeleton have been used for bone marrow sampling. Because active hematopoiesis occurs in the long bones of the arms and legs in infants under the age of 8 months, aspiration from the anterior aspect of the tibial tuberosity is useful. For adults, the posterior iliac crest is the recommended site. Patients who are unable to lie on their stomachs may be approached through the anterior iliac crest or sternum. The sternum is aspirated relatively easily, but its structure does not allow biopsy. In elderly patients, sternal bone marrow may be most representative of the patient's hematopoietic status and superior to that of the relatively acellular iliac crest. Sternal aspiration also may be most appropriate for patients who have lesions in the sternum or ribs.

Table 1-8 Correction Factor Calculation

Patient's Hematocrit Value, %	Correction Factor
40-45	1.0
35-39	1.5
25-34	2.0
15-24	2.5
<15	3.0

Processing and interpretation have significant technical variables and require experienced personnel. Bone marrow examination should be limited to situations in which noninvasive procedures do not yield clear answers. **Table 1-9** gives the most common indications for bone marrow examination.

Interpretation. When both a Wright's-stained aspirate preparation and a histologic core needle biopsy are available, optimal evaluation may be performed. The false-negative rate for metastatic carcinoma using aspiration alone is about 25%; for lymphomas it seems to be somewhat higher—30% to 40%—depending on the cell type. Because of the small nature of the biopsy specimen, sampling errors still may be a problem, causing false-negative results. Additional testing, such as iron stains to evaluate iron stores, immunohistochemical staining, flow cytometric analysis, and cytogenetic analysis, may be performed on aspirated bone marrow specimens to provide additional information about the disease process.

1.5 Treatment

Anemia is a symptom rather than a disease, so treatment of anemia is usually aimed at correcting the abnormality that led to it. This may involve identification of a source of blood loss, iron or vitamin supplementation, or discontinuation of a drug that predisposes a patient to hemolysis. The acquired anemias associated with hematopoietic abnormalities, such as myelodysplasia or aplastic anemia, and inherited anemias may require the use of transfusions when symptoms arise due to decreased oxygen delivery to the tis-

Table 1-9 Indications for Bone Marrow Examination
in Anemia

Abnormalities in blood counts and/or peripheral blood smear
    Unexplained cytopenias
    Unexplained leukocytosis or abnormal white blood cells
    Teardrop cells or leukoerythroblastosis
    Rouleaux
    No or low reticulocyte response to anemia

Evaluation of systemic disease
    Unexplained splenomegaly, hepatomegaly, lymphadenopathy
    Tumor staging: solid tumors, lymphomas
    Monitoring of chemotherapy effect
    Fever of unknown origin (with bone marrow cultures)
    Evaluation of trabecular bone in metabolic disease
      (use undecalcified bone)

sues. The benefit of transfusion therapy must be balanced carefully against the risks of disease transmission. Usually transfusions are not required unless the hemoglobin concentration falls below 7 g/dL (70 g/L), unless significant cardiac or pulmonary disease is present and hypoxia would be exacerbated by even modest decreases in oxygen delivery. In addition, long-term transfusion therapy—especially in patients who have hereditary hemochromatosis—exacerbates iron overload and hastens subsequent organ failure. Such patients are unable to decrease gut mucosal iron absorption appropriately when iron loading occurs via transfusion. The frequency of homozygous hereditary hemochromatosis is 0.1% to 0.2%, and many patients have clinically silent disease. Patients with homozygous hemochromatosis may be identified by screening tests for transferrin saturation, which is considered suspicious if greater than 60% saturation is found in a man and greater than 50% in a woman. When follow-up testing of serum ferritin finds levels above normal for a patient's age and gender in addition to elevated transferrin saturation, it strongly suggests that the patient has clinically silent hemochromatosis. In these patients, iron overload due to transfusion therapy may present significant problems.

1.6 References

Carmel R, Cassileth PA. A focused approach to anemia. *Hosp Pract.* 1999;34:71–91.

Desspypris EN. Erythropoiesis. In: Lee GR, Foerster J, Lukens JN, et al, eds. *Wintrobe's Clinical Hematology.* 10th ed. Baltimore, Md: Williams & Wilkins; 1999:169–192.

Lee GR. Anemia: general aspects. In: Lee GR, Foerster J, Lukens JN, et al, eds. *Wintrobe's Clinical Hematology.* 10th ed. Baltimore, Md: Williams & Wilkins; 1999:897–907.

Lee GR. Anemia: a diagnostic strategy. In: Lee GR, Foerster J, Lukens JN, et al, eds. *Wintrobe's Clinical Hematology.* 10th ed. Baltimore, Md: Williams & Wilkins; 1999:908–939.

Perkins SL. Examination of blood and bone marrow. In: Lee GR, Foerster J, Lukens JN, et al, eds. *Wintrobe's Clinical Hematology.* 10th ed. Baltimore, Md: Williams & Wilkins; 1999:9–35.

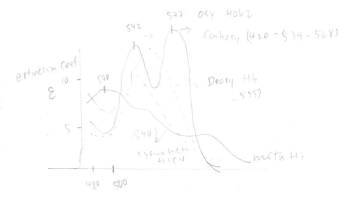

2 Hypochromic Microcytic Anemias

Decreased hemoglobin synthesis gives rise to a hypochromic microcytic anemia. Such a decrease may occur due to deficiencies in either heme or globin chain synthesis. This synthetic defect may arise due to insufficient amounts of iron, abnormal iron metabolism and heme synthesis (due to acquired or hereditary sideroblastic disorders), or secondary to hereditary abnormalities in globin synthesis (such as thalassemias). The most common types of hypochromic anemia are listed in **Table 2-1**.

2.1 Pathophysiology

Hypochromic anemias are characterized by normal cellular proliferation and DNA synthesis but decreased RBC hemoglobin production. The RBC precursors continue to divide, but the lack of hemoglobin leads to formation of hypochromic cells that are smaller than normal (**Image 2-1**). The principal causes of hypochromic anemias include defective synthesis of heme secondary to decreased iron, abnormal iron metabolism or metabolic abnormalities (sideroblastic anemias), and disorders of globin synthesis in the form of thalassemic disorders.

Table 2-1 Causes of Hypochromic Anemia

Disorders of iron metabolism
    Iron deficiency
    Chronic infections or inflammatory states
    Neoplasia
Disorders of heme synthesis
    Sideroblastic anemias
        Hereditary (X-linked or autosomal)
        Acquired idiopathic (myelodysplasia)
        Acquired toxic (lead, drugs, alcohol)
Disorders of globin synthesis
    Thalassemic syndromes
        α-Thalassemia
        β-Thalassemia

The primary cause of defective heme synthesis is iron deficiency. Iron deficiency is the most common cause of anemia and is among the most common of all diseases in humans. The etiology of iron deficiency varies with the age of the patient (**Table 2-2**). In infants and children, a negative iron balance usually occurs because the dietary intake of iron is inadequate to meet the requirements for growth. In adults, iron deficiency is usually the result of pregnancy or blood loss. Because normal daily losses of iron are very small, decreased dietary intake plays only a contributory role in the etiology of the disease. Physicians must identify the underlying cause of iron deficiency to effectively treat the anemia. The first sign of a malignant lesion of the gastrointestinal or genitourinary tract is often occult blood loss and resultant hypochromic, microcytic anemia.

Iron metabolism also may be deranged in many people with chronic inflammatory diseases or malignancies that do not cause overt blood loss. These patients exhibit defective iron cycling between macrophages and developing RBCs, so iron becomes trapped within the macrophage and is unavailable for heme synthesis. This "anemia of chronic disease" (ACD) is often normochromic and normocytic, but also may present as a microcytic, hypochromic anemia. Diagnosis of this entity is discussed further in Chapter 3.

Another group of disorders, sideroblastic anemias, are characterized by abnormal iron metabolism within the RBC itself. In these disorders, iron is sequestered in the developing RBC mito-

Table 2-2 Common Causes of Iron Deficiency Anemia by Age

Infants and children	Inadequate intake Growth spurts with increased iron requirements
Premenopausal women	Menstrual blood loss Pregnancy

Adult men and
  postmenopausal women
	Blood loss due to tumor, peptic ulcer,
	  gastrointestinal or genitourinary bleeding
	Malabsorption
	Inadequate intake

chondria and is unavailable for heme synthesis. The iron swells and distorts the mitochondria. Because the mitochondria in a developing normoblast are found in a perinuclear distribution, iron stains in these disorders show a characteristic pattern of iron around the nucleus, forming a ringed sideroblast (**Image 2-2**). Sideroblastic anemias may be hereditary (either X-linked or autosomal), idiopathic (usually as part of a myelodysplastic disorder), or secondary to a toxic insult (drugs, lead, or alcohol). Hereditary sideroblastic anemias are extremely rare in comparison with acquired forms.

Hereditary disorders of globin synthesis, or thalassemic syndromes, also are very common in Asian, Mediterranean, and black populations. They rival iron deficiency as a cause of microcytic, hypochromic anemia in these groups. Thalassemias are discussed in further detail in Chapter 10.

2.2 Clinical Findings

The clinical findings of hypochromic anemias depend on the severity of the anemia and its underlying cause. Severe anemia is associated with pallor, weakness, dizziness, palpitations, and even dyspnea. Some patients with iron deficiency may have cheilitis or spooning (koilonychia) of the nails. Food cravings for ice, clay (pica), dirt, starch, or pickles also are common.

For a patient with a microcytic, hypochromic anemia, evaluation of clinical features and laboratory testing is required to distinguish between the previously mentioned etiologies. Laboratory test selection is driven by the clinical situation. Thus, new onset of anemia in an elderly person triggers a workup for iron deficiency, ACD, or acquired sideroblastic anemia and is unlikely to be associated with a thalassemic syndrome. Judicious selection of testing allows a definitive diagnosis in a cost-effective manner. Mild to moderate chronic anemia is well tolerated by most patients, particularly those in the younger age groups.

2.3 Diagnostic Approach

Following a clinical history and physical examination, the evaluation of hypochromic anemias may be undertaken as follows:

1. Examination of RBC morphology, indices, and RBC size distribution (**Table 2-3**).
2. Estimation of serum iron levels and total iron-binding capacity, ferritin, or serum transferrin receptor levels. These measurements reflect iron stores and help to distinguish iron deficiency from other causes of microcytic, hypochromic anemia (**Table 2-4**).
3. Measurement of free erythrocyte protoporphyrin. This is of particular value as a screening test for distinguishing iron deficiency from thalassemia minor.
4. Examination of aspirated bone marrow for stainable iron, the most direct assessment of iron stores. Associated dysplasia or demonstration of ringed sideroblasts may reflect a sideroblastic anemia.
5. Hemoglobin electrophoresis, particularly to determine hemoglobin A_2 level, which is increased in most patients with β-thalassemia.
6. Determination of globin chain synthetic ratios, which is often the only means of making a positive diagnosis of mild forms of α-thalassemia.
7. Cytogenetic analysis to document a myelodysplastic syndrome, which shows cytogenetic abnormalities in up to 80% of affected patients. Cytogenetic abnormalities associated with myelodysplasia include complex chromosomal defects, monosomy 7, deletion of 5q, and trisomy 8.
8. Documentation of the hematologic response to iron supplementation therapy, which confirms the diagnosis of iron deficiency.

Table 2-3 Pertinent Findings in Microcytic Hypochromic Anemia

Cause of Anemia	RBC Number	Red Cell Distribution Width	Anisopoiki-locytosis	Basophilic Stippling	Bone Marrow Iron
Iron deficiency	Decreased	Increased	Yes	No	Decreased
Thalassemia minor	Normal or increased	Normal	No	Yes	Increased
Sideroblastic anemias					
Hereditary	Decreased	Variable	Variable	Yes	Increased ringed sidero-blasts
Acquired	Decreased	Dimorphic population	Yes	Yes	Increased ringed sidero-blasts
Chronic disease	Decreased	Variable	Variable	No	Decreased in sidero-cytes; increased in RE cells

RE = reticuloendothelial

2.4 Hematologic Findings

Initial workup of a microcytic, hypochromic anemia usually is aimed at distinguishing iron deficiency anemia from thalassemia. Sideroblastic anemia and ACD also may be considered. Pertinent findings are summarized in **Table 2-3**. Hypochromia, microcytosis, and anisocytosis are usually present in well-developed iron deficiency anemia. However, in early or mild iron deficiency, morphologic abnormalities of the RBCs may be absent. Hypochromia and microcytosis are found uniformly in the thalassemic syndromes, and the reductions in mean corpuscular volume (MCV) and mean corpuscular hemoglobin concentration (MCHC) are generally greater than those observed in the same level of iron deficiency anemia. Microcytosis with significant

Table 2-4 Iron Studies in Hypochromic Anemias

Cause of Hypochromic Anemia	Serum Iron	TIBC	Percent Saturation	Soluble Serum Transferrin Receptor	Bone Marrow Storage Iron
Iron deficiency	Decreased*	Increased*	Decreased*	High	Decreased
Thalassemias	Increased or normal	Decreased or normal	Increased or normal	Variable, may be high	Increased or normal
Sideroblastic anemias	Increased	Decreased or normal	Increased	Variable, may be high	Increased
Chronic disease	Decreased	Decreased	Decreased	Normal	Increased

Abbreviation: TIBC = total iron binding capacity.
*Serum iron and TIBC are occasionally normal in iron deficiency.

elevations of the RBC count to greater than $6 \times 10^6/mm^3$ ($6 \times 10^{12}/L$) are common in thalassemia minor. Basophilic stippling of RBCs is commonly seen in thalassemia but is unusual in iron deficiency anemia. Hypochromia is often present in patients with sideroblastic anemia, but it is not a universal finding. It also occurs in patients with chronic inflammatory or neoplastic disorders and the associated ACD. Characteristically, the variability of RBC size is increased in iron deficiency, but variability is much less than in thalassemia. The size distribution in sideroblastic anemias is variable, but a characteristic dimorphic population of normocytic or microcytic cells and macrocytes is seen in the acquired types.

2.4.1 Blood Cell Measurements
The MCV is decreased in severe iron deficiency anemia and thalassemias. The MCV may be increased in many of the sideroblastic anemias, although microcytosis is more common in the hereditary types. The reticulocyte count may be modestly decreased, normal, or modestly increased. Indices are often normal in patients with hemoglobin levels greater than 10 g/dL (100 g/L). The RBC number is not decreased and may be significantly

increased in patients with thalassemia. RBC number in thalassemias is not proportional to the low hemoglobin level or degree of microcytosis. In contrast, iron deficiency anemia usually shows concordant decreases in RBC number, hemoglobin levels, and MCV, with a characteristic increase in red cell distribution width.

2.4.2 Peripheral Blood Smear Morphology

Hypochromia and microcytosis are present in severe iron deficiency anemia (*see Image 2-1*) but may be lacking in patients with less severe iron depletion. Sideroblastic anemias usually have notable anisocytosis and poikilocytosis in addition to hypochromia. Occasionally, dysplastic features may be noted in WBCs in idiopathic cases. Target cells and basophilic stippling may be prominent in the thalassemias.

2.4.3 Bone Marrow Examination

Bone marrow examination usually is not required for the diagnosis of iron deficiency anemia or thalassemia but is important in documenting a sideroblastic anemia. Erythroid hyperplasia is often present in all of the microcytic anemias but not as prominently as in the hemolytic anemias. The only specific bone marrow findings in microcytic anemias are decreased or absent stainable storage iron in iron deficiency anemia, increased reticuloendothelial iron with decreased sideroblastic iron in ACD, and the presence of ring sideroblasts in sideroblastic anemias (*see Image 2-2*). Iron stores are often increased in thalassemias.

Other Laboratory Tests

Test 2.1 Serum Iron Quantitation and Total Iron-Binding Capacity

Purpose. Serum iron and total iron-binding capacity (TIBC) determinations are particularly useful in distinguishing iron deficiency anemia from other types of hypochromic microcytic anemia. In mild iron deficiency anemia, decreased serum iron levels usually precede changes in RBC morphology or in RBC indices.

Principle. All iron transported in the plasma is bound in the ferric form to the specific iron-binding protein transferrin. Serum iron measures the transferrin-bound iron. Total iron-binding capacity—the iron concentration necessary to saturate the iron-binding sites of transferrin—is a measure of transferrin concentration. Saturation of transferrin is calculated by the following formula:

$$\% \text{ Transferrin Saturation} = [\text{Serum Iron (mol/L)} \div \text{TIBC (μmol/L)}] \times 100$$

Normal mean transferrin saturation is approximately 30%. Unsaturated iron-binding capacity (UIBC) is the difference between TIBC and serum iron.

Specimen. A specimen of blood should be drawn in the morning owing to diurnal variations in serum iron levels. Serum is used for the determination.

Procedure. Serum iron is freed from transferrin by acidification of the serum and is reduced to the ferrous form. After the protein has been precipitated out, the iron in the filtrate is detected spectrophotometrically after reaction with a chromogen such as bathophenanthroline sulfonate. The TIBC is measured by adding iron to the serum and then removing excess unbound iron by magnesium carbonate absorption. The bound iron is then released from transferrin and reduced, and its concentration is measured as in the serum iron test. The TIBC also can be determined by measuring transferrin with immunodiffusion.

Interpretation. The representative normal range of values for serum iron is 60 to 180 μg/dL (12.7 to 35.9 μmol/L); for TIBC, the range is 250 to 410 μg/dL (45.2 to 77.7 μmol/L). The range for percent saturation is 20% to 50%. The serum iron level and percent saturation is low in both iron deficiency anemia and the ACD. Although the value for percent saturation is often reduced to levels below 16% in iron deficiency anemia and is frequently more than 16% in ACD, values for the two conditions overlap. The TIBC is uniformly increased in severe uncomplicated iron deficiency anemia and is decreased or normal in microcytic ACD. In mild iron deficiency anemia, both the serum iron and TIBC may be normal. Serum iron concentration is increased in the siteroblastic anemias and in some cases of thalassemia (*see Table 2-4*).

Notes and Precautions. Serum iron concentrations show wide diurnal variations, with highest levels in the morning. Thus, specimens should be collected in the morning and oral iron therapy should be withdrawn 24 hours before the blood sample is drawn. Iron dextran administration causes plasma iron levels to be elevated for several weeks. A normal plasma iron level and iron-binding capacity do not rule out the diagnosis of iron deficiency when the hemoglobin level of the blood is above 9 g/dL (90 g/L) in women and 11 g/dL (110 g/L) in men.

Test 2.2 **Stainable Bone Marrow Iron**

Purpose. The most direct means for assessing body iron stores is by histochemical examination of aspirated bone marrow for storage iron.

Principle. Iron is stored in reticuloendothelial cells, and iron granules are formed in developing normoblasts. Normoblasts that contain one or more particles of stainable iron are known as "sideroblasts". Iron is stored as ferritin (iron complexed to the apoferritin protein) and hemosiderin (iron-protein complexes with a high iron content and denatured ferritin aggregates). Hemosiderin is the stainable form of storage iron that appears blue when treated with an acid potassium ferricyanide solution used in the Prussian blue reaction.

Specimen. Either sectioned bone marrow aspirate fragments (clot section) or particle smears are used for the assessment of reticuloendothelial iron, but bone marrow aspirate films must be used to detect sideroblasts. Iron staining may be decreased in decalcified sections due to leaching out of iron during the decalcification process.

Procedure. The bone marrow aspirate is stained with the Prussian blue reaction. Heating the staining mixture to 56°C increases its sensitivity. The search for sideroblasts is aided by a counterstain such as basic fuchsin.

Interpretation. Normally, hemosiderin granules are seen in reticuloendothelial cells in every third or fourth oil immersion field. With reduced iron stores, either no or only a few hemosiderin granules are seen in the entire preparation. With increased iron stores, hemosiderin granules are seen in every oil immersion field, often deposited in clumps.

The appraisal of reticuloendothelial iron is extremely helpful in the differential diagnosis of anemia (*see Table 2-4*). Because iron from the breakdown of RBC heme cannot be excreted, it is diverted to the storage compartment. Thus, increased iron is generally present in the marrow of patients with anemia who are not iron deficient. An exception may exist in myeloproliferative disorders in which bone marrow iron stores may be absent without other evidence of iron deficiency, perhaps resulting from impaired storage function. When storage iron is present in the bone marrow, anemia cannot be a result of iron deficiency, unless the patient has recently received parenterally administered iron treatment.

Normally, 20% to 40% of RBC precursors are iron-containing sideroblasts. Although a sideroblast count is not ordinarily necessary for the diagnosis of iron deficiency anemia, it may be useful when an inadequate number of bone marrow particles have been obtained and in patients who have received parenterally administered iron. Decreased bone marrow sideroblasts are seen in iron deficiency anemia, after acute blood loss when reticuloendothelial stores have not yet been depleted, and in ACD. Sideroblastic anemia is characterized by the presence of ring sideroblasts, normoblasts that contain iron granules that surround at least two thirds of the nuclear circumference (*see Image 2-2*).

Notes and Precautions. Some practice is required to distinguish stainable reticuloendothelial iron from artifacts. When a patient has received iron parenterally, either as iron dextran or in the form of blood transfusions, histochemically stainable iron stores may be seen in the bone marrow in the presence of iron deficiency anemia. A well-prepared bone marrow aspirate film is essential for the detection of iron granules in normoblasts, and appropriate positive control slides should be performed simultaneously.

Test 2.3 **Serum Ferritin Quantitation**

Purpose. Small amounts of ferritin or the antigenically equivalent apoferritin normally circulate in the plasma. Estimating serum ferritin levels provides a semiquantitative, less invasive test for iron store determination than the histochemical examination of aspirated bone marrow.

Principle. Ferritin is a storage complex of the protein apoferritin and iron. The largest quantities of ferritin are found in the liver and reticuloendothelial cells. Ordinarily, serum ferritin concentration reflects the amount of stored iron.

Specimen. Serum is used for testing.

Procedure. Reliable estimation of serum ferritin levels has been achieved with a sensitive radioimmune method using a sandwich technique. Ferritin is removed from the serum by solid phase antiferritin antibodies, and radioactively labeled antiferritin antibodies are then permitted to bind to the removed ferritin.

Interpretation. The normal concentration of serum ferritin varies from 10 to 500 ng/mL (10 to 500 µg/L). In iron deficiency anemia, serum ferritin level is diminished, making it a relatively sensitive and reliable indicator. Serum ferritin levels may be low in iron deficiency that is not associated with overt anemia. Elevated ferritin levels are common in iron overload states, including sideroblastic anemia and hemochromatosis. Serum ferritin levels are also elevated in patients with inflammatory diseases and, for poorly understood reasons, in patients with Gaucher's disease.

Notes and Precautions. When iron deficiency and inflammatory disease coexist, serum ferritin levels may be in the normal range.

Test 2.4 Serum Soluble Transferrin Receptor

Purpose. Measurement of serum soluble transferrin receptor levels provides an additional means to quantitate iron deficiency, which is proportional to cell-associated transferrin receptor levels. These levels do not appear to be altered by inflammatory states and may provide a sensitive means to quantitate iron stores when borderline values for iron deficiency are obtained by other testing. Serum soluble transferrin levels are increased in iron deficiency.

Principle. The transferrin receptor is a transmembrane protein that transfers iron from plasma transferrin into the cell. Most transferrin receptors are found in the cell membrane, but a truncated form of the tissue receptor that is complexed with transferrin is found in soluble form in the serum. Transferrin receptor levels reflect iron status, with receptor synthesis being rapidly induced by decreased iron levels. Thus, measurement of the soluble transferrin receptor (which mirrors cellular transferrin receptor levels) provides an additional measurable parameter of iron balance.

Specimen. Serum is used.

Procedure. Serum transferrin receptors are assayed with a sandwich enzyme immunoassay that uses a polyclonal antibody against the serum transferrin receptor protein. Commercially available kits can detect the protein in ranges from 0.85 to 20 mg/L.

Interpretation. Levels of serum soluble transferrin receptors greater than 3.1 mg/L have been used as an indicator of iron deficiency in most studies. This test is best used in combination with other tests of iron status (ferritin, total iron-binding capacity, and serum iron).

Notes and Precautions. Elevated serum soluble transferrin receptor levels have been noted, irrespective of patient iron status, in patients with hematologic malignancies or conditions with increased effective or ineffective hematopoiesis (ie, hemolytic anemias, hemoglobinopathies, or deficiencies of vitamin B_{12} or folate). Normal ranges for pregnant women and pediatric patients are not well established. Blacks and those living at high altitudes may have normal serum soluble transferrin levels 6% higher than upper normal limits. This may be additive (blacks living at high altitudes may have levels up to 12% above upper limits). The observation that serum soluble transferrin receptor levels are not increased in patients with inflammatory disease may be useful in distinguishing iron deficiency from ACD in these patients.

Test 2.5 Free Erythrocyte Protoporphyrin

Purpose. Free erythrocyte protoporphyrin (FEP) levels are elevated in patients with anemias associated with failure of iron incorporation into heme.

Principle. When insufficient iron is available for developing erythroblasts, excess protoporphyrin that was destined to be converted to heme accumulates as FEP. This substance is elevated both in iron deficiency and in conditions associated with an internal block in iron utilization, such as ACD, lead poisoning, and sideroblastic anemias.

Specimen. Whole anticoagulated blood is collected. There is also a spot test for blood specimens collected on filter paper.

Procedure. Free erythrocyte protoporphyrin is extracted from RBCs with ethyl acetate/acetic acid and is quantitated fluorometrically.

Interpretation. Free erythrocyte protoporphyrin is normally less than 100 µg/dL (1.7 µmol/L) packed RBCs. Elevated levels are seen in patients with iron deficiency, chronic disease states associated with decreased transferrin saturation, and acquired idiopathic sideroblastic anemia. Marked elevation of FEP is seen in patients with sideroblastic anemia secondary to lead intoxication with FEP values of about 1000 µg/dL (17 µmol/L) packed RBCs. In patients with microcytic anemias associated with abnormal globin synthesis rather than abnormal heme synthesis (such as thalassemia minor), FEP levels are normal. Because iron deficiency anemia and thalassemia minor are the first and second most common causes of hypochromic microcytic anemia, measurement of FEP may be particularly useful as a screening test to distinguish these two disorders.

2.5 Test Selection

Examination of the peripheral blood smear and RBC indices is essential for determining the etiology of a microcytic anemia. The RBC number, hemoglobin content, MCV, and RDW provide important clues. If iron deficiency is suspected on the basis of a high RDW and low RBC numbers, iron studies such as serum iron, TIBC, serum ferritin, and/or soluble serum transferrin receptor may be ordered. If a thalassemia is suspected on the basis of a high RBC count for the degree of microcytosis and a normal RDW or the presence of target cells, testing can be aimed at determining the hemoglobin A_2 level and possible hemoglobin electrophoresis. If a dimorphic population of RBCs or dysplastic changes are seen in the other blood cells, a bone marrow examination with iron staining for demonstration of ringed sideroblasts is required.

2.6 Course and Treatment

Ultimately, the diagnosis of iron deficiency depends on demonstration of an adequate response to iron therapy. Treatment usually consists of the oral administration of a ferrous iron salt, such as ferrous sulfate, in a dosage providing 0.06 to 0.12 g of iron three times a day. In some circumstances, the parenteral administration of iron dextran may be preferred. Reticulocytosis and a significant rise in blood hemoglobin concentration may occur as early as the third or fourth day after treatment, particularly in children, but is usually seen after 7 or 8 days. The hemoglobin concentration in the blood may not rise significantly until 10 days after treatment begins. Thereafter, complete restoration of the hemoglobin level to normal should be rapid (essentially complete by the sixth week after institution of therapy), regardless of the initial severity of the anemia.

Infection, inflammatory disease, or neoplastic disease may prevent an adequate response, and continued bleeding may blunt the therapeutic effect. The most common cause of failure of iron therapy in patients with a hypochromic microcytic anemia is an incorrect diagnosis. It is important to identify the cause of the iron deficiency (which is almost always blood loss or pregnancy in adults) and to correct it, if possible. Iron deficiency can be an early warning of gastrointestinal or genitourinary tract cancer.

Sideroblastic anemias, other than the acquired idiopathic forms, may respond to treatment with pyridoxine. Many of the drugs that cause toxic sideroblastic anemias are pyridoxine antagonists. If a toxic etiology is suspected, discontinuing the drug or alcohol often leads to rapid improvement in the anemia. Some hereditary sideroblastic anemias are pyridoxine resistant, indicating heterogeneous metabolic abnormalities in affected patients. In both the acquired idiopathic form of the disease and hereditary forms, repeated transfusions may be required to treat severe anemia. Iron overload, due to long-standing transfusion therapy, may become a problem and require chelation therapy. The acquired idiopathic form of the disease is a myelodysplastic syndrome, and small numbers of the patients develop progressive bone marrow failure, cytopenias, or overt acute myelogenous leukemia. However, most patients have stable anemia and associated symptoms over many years.

2.7 References

Bessman JD, Gilmer PR, Gardener FH. Improved classification of anemias by MCV and RDW. *Am J Clin Pathol*. 1983;80:322–329.

Beutler E. Hereditary and acquired sideroblastic anemias. In: Beutler E, Coller BS, Kipps TJ, et al, eds. *Williams Hematology*. 5th ed. New York, NY: McGraw-Hill; 1995:747–751.

Eldinbany MM, Totonchi KF, Joseph NJ, et al. Usefulness of certain red blood cell indices in diagnosing and differentiating thalassemia trait from iron-deficiency anemia. *Am J Pathol*. 1999;111:676–682.

Fairbanks VF, Beutler E. Iron deficiency. In: Beutler E, Lichtman MA, Coller BS, et al, eds. *Hematology*. 5th ed. New York, NY: McGraw-Hill; 1995:490–510.

Guyatt GH, Oxman AD, Ali M, et al. Laboratory diagnosis of iron deficiency anemia. *J Gen Intern Med*. 1992;7:145–153.

Koc S, Harris JW. Sideroblastic anemias: Variations on imprecision in diagnostic criteria, proposal for an extended classification of sideroblastic anemias. *Am J Hematol*. 1998;57:1–6.

Mast AE, Blinder MA, Gronowski AM, et al. Clinical utility of the soluble transferrin receptor and comparison with serum ferritin in several populations. *Clin Chem*. 1998;44:45–51.

North M, Dallalio G, Donath AS, et al. Serum transferrin receptor levels in patients undergoing evaluation of iron stores: correlation with other parameters, and observed versus predicted results. *Clin Lab Haematol*. 1997;19:93–97.

Worwood M. The laboratory assessment of iron status—an update. *Clin Chim Acta*. 1997;259:3–23.

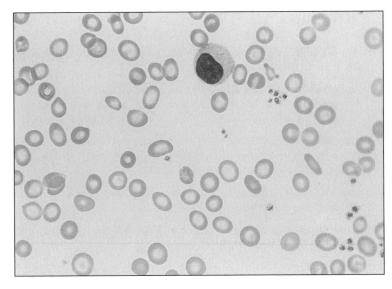

Image 2-1   Iron deficiency anemia. The RBCs are hypochromic and microcytic with notable anisocytosis.

Image 2-2   Ringed sideroblast. Iron stains show a marrow normoblast with coarse iron granules extending completely around the nucleus.

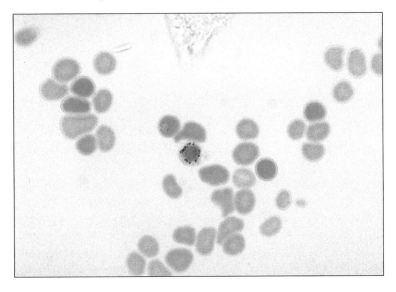

3 Anemia of Chronic Disease and Normochromic, Normocytic Nonhemolytic Anemias

Anemia is the most common hematologic abnormality in patients with chronic diseases. These chronic diseases are highly diverse and include neoplasms, chronic infections, other chronic inflammatory processes, and end organ failure. Despite this heterogeneity of primary disorders, the anemias that occur in these patient populations exhibit many common features; most of these anemias can be attributed to chronic disease, nutritional deficiency, blood loss, or a combination thereof.

3.1 Anemia of Chronic Disease

Anemia of chronic disease (ACD) is defined by a constellation of clinical, morphologic, and laboratory features (**Table 3-1**) and is second only to iron deficiency anemia in incidence. In a tertiary care setting, ACD may be the most frequently encountered type of anemia. Affected patients usually develop normocytic, normochromic anemia that is mild and nonprogressive 1 to 2 months after the onset of chronic disease. This anemia is associated with multiple iron-related abnormalities, including decreased serum iron level, decreased transferrin level, decreased transferrin saturation,

Table 3-1 Characteristics of Anemia of Chronic Disease

Clinical
  Development of anemia 1-2 months after onset of chronic disease

Blood
  Usually normocytic, normochromic anemia with normal mean corpuscular
    volume, mean corpuscular hemoglobin concentration, and red cell
    distribution width
  Inappropriately low reticulocyte count

Iron studies
  Decreased serum/plasma iron
  Decreased transferrin (total iron-binding capacity)
  Decreased transferrin saturation
  Normal to increased ferritin

Bone marrow
  Normal numbers of erythroid precursors
  Decreased sideroblasts (iron-containing precursor cells)
  Increased storage iron

Pathophysiologic mechanisms
  Impaired erythropoiesis, abnormal iron distribution, and mildly decreased
    erythrocyte survival time all linked to sustained production of inhibitory
    cytokines such as TNF-β, IL-1α, and IFNγ,β

Abbreviations: TNF-β = tumor necrosis factor-β; IL-1α = interleukin-1α; IFNγ,β = interferons γ and β.

and normal to increased storage iron (ferritin). The bone marrow examination reveals that erythroid precursors are generally present in normal numbers; erythroid iron is decreased, whereas storage iron is increased.

A variety of inflammatory, infectious, and neoplastic disorders are associated with ACD (**Table 3-2**). Because the etiologies of anemias are considerably more complex in patients with renal failure, endocrine disorders, hepatic failure, and AIDS, these conditions are discussed separately at the end of the chapter, ACD may be a dominant type of anemia in these patients.

3.1.1 Pathophysiology

Three separate pathophysiologic defects together produce ACD: failure of erythropoiesis, lack of iron for hemoglobin synthesis, and decreased RBC survival. The major defect is thought to

Table 3-2 Diseases Commonly Associated With Anemia of Chronic Disease*

Chronic inflammatory disorders
    Rheumatoid arthritis
    Systemic lupus erythematosus
    Sarcoidosis
    Trauma

Chronic infections
    HIV-1 infections
    Other viral infections†
    Tuberculosis
    Pyelonephritis
    Osteomyelitis
    Chronic fungal infections
    Subacute bacterial endocarditis

Neoplasms
    Malignant lymphoma
    Carcinomas
    Chronic leukemias

End organ failure
    Chronic liver disease
    Endocrinopathies

*Patients often have multiple concurrent types of anemia.
†Usually present in patients with underlying immunodeficiency.

be a failure of sufficient erythropoiesis to compensate for mildly decreased RBC survival; erythroid precursors are present in the bone marrow, but presumably in insufficient numbers to compensate for the increased demand for erythrocyte production. The decreased availability of iron for hemoglobin synthesis further aggravates the inadequate erythropoiesis. Sustained overproduction of the inhi-bitory cytokines tumor necrosis factor–β (TNF-β), interleukin-1α (IL-1α), and interferons γ and β (IFNγ, β) are directly or indirectly responsible for the impaired erythropoiesis, abnormal iron distribution, and decreased erythrocyte survival that produces ACD. These inhibitory cytokines exhibit broad multiorgan and multisystem effects. For example, they enhance lactoferrin release by neutrophils; lactoferrin competes with transferrin for binding plasma iron and delivers this iron exclusively to macrophages, reducing available iron for hemoglobin production. Likewise, the modest decrease in erythrocyte survival time is at least partially attributed to fever, mediated by the inhibitory cytokines.

3.1.2 Clinical Findings

Because ACD is generally mild, the patient's symptoms are primarily related to the underlying disease. There are no physical examination findings unique to ACD.

3.1.3 Approach to Diagnosis

In a patient with anemia and a chronic illness, the contribution of ACD to this condition can vary from major to insignificant. Because multifactorial anemia in such a patient population is the rule rather than the exception, the patient's evaluation should identify other concomitant anemia-inducing factors. For example, a patient with a neoplasm may suffer from iron deficiency anemia secondary to chronic blood loss, myelophthisic anemia secondary to bone marrow replacement by tumor, hypoplastic anemia secondary to bone marrow suppression by chemotherapeutic agents, or even microangiopathic hemolytic anemia secondary to drug treatment or mucin production by tumor. **Table 3-3** lists these and other possible factors that may contribute to anemias that occur in patients with neoplasms. During the course of the clinical and hematologic evaluation of the patient, it is often readily apparent that one or more of these additional causes of anemia is present. In clinical practice, the distinction between ACD and iron deficiency anemia is the most frequent diagnostic dilemma.

The laboratory evaluation of patients for ACD usually includes the following steps:

1. Measurement of standard hematologic parameters with reticulocyte count.
2. Evaluation of peripheral blood smear for "clues" suggesting specific types of anemia.
3. Iron studies, including assays of serum iron, transferrin level, percentage of transferrin saturation, and serum ferritin.
4. Appropriate laboratory testing to establish or exclude diagnoses of other types of anemia.
5. Bone marrow aspiration, with iron stains, and biopsy in selected cases that are not clear-cut after routine evaluation.

Table 3-3 Causes of Anemia in Patients With Malignancies

Anemia of chronic disease
Blood loss
Nutritional deficiencies, especially iron
Bone marrow replacement by tumor/fibrosis
Bone marrow suppression by chemotherapy
Chemotherapy-related myelodysplasia
Hypersplenism
Microangiopathic hemolytic anemia secondary to drug treatment
  (eg, mitomycin C)
Microangiopathic hemolytic anemia secondary to intravascular mucin
  released from certain widespread adenocarcinomas
Immune-mediated hemolysis (autoantibody produced by certain
  B-cell neoplasms)

The laboratory approach to the evaluation of these patients must always be correlated with the clinical findings. The approach should be tailored to each case, using clues from the patient's history, disease course, and physical examination to direct the sequence of tests used.

3.1.4 Hematologic Findings

There are no pathognomonic findings in the peripheral blood in patients with ACD. These patients generally have a mild to moderate anemia that is not associated with an appropriate compensatory increase in the reticulocyte count.

Blood Cell Measurements

In ACD, the hemoglobin level ranges from 7.0 to 11.0 g/dL (70 to 110 g/L). The RBCs vary little in size, as indicated by their normal or near-normal red cell distribution width (RDW). The mean corpuscular volume (MCV), mean corpuscular hemoglobin (MCH), and mean corpuscular hemoglobin concentration (MCHC) are generally normal, although the MCV and MCHC may be mildly decreased. Although the reticulocyte count is usually within the normal range, it is decreased when corrected for the degree of anemia. WBC and platelet counts are usually normal;

decreases in these parameters may be attributable to therapy or other factors.

Peripheral Blood Smear Morphology
Erythrocytes are generally normocytic and normochromic without significant anisopoikilocytosis or polychromasia, although they are occasionally mildly hypochromic. There are usually no abnormalities of WBCs or platelets.

Bone Marrow Examination
Erythroid elements in the bone marrow are generally morphologically normal and present in normal numbers. Sideroblasts are decreased, while storage iron is increased substantially. Myeloid and megakaryocytic elements usually are unremarkable. Depending on the underlying chronic disease, a variety of additional bone marrow abnormalities, ranging from granulomas in patients with chronic infections to foci of metastatic tumor in cancer patients, may be detected.

Other Laboratory Tests

Although no single laboratory test is specific for ACD, a well-established laboratory profile includes serum iron, iron transport protein (transferrin, or "iron-binding capacity"), transferrin saturation, and storage iron measurements (serum ferritin).

Test 3.1 **Serum Iron Quantitation**

Purpose. The determination of serum iron, in conjunction with other iron studies described later, is important in distinguishing ACD from other types of anemia that may develop in patients.
Principle, Specimen, Procedure, Notes, and Precautions. See Test 2.1.
Interpretation. A prompt decline in serum iron level is associated with infection and other types of tissue injury. This decrease

precedes the development of anemia, which occurs only if the infection or injury is sustained. A low serum iron level also is seen in iron deficiency anemia.

Test 3.2 Transferrin Measurement (Total Iron-Binding Capacity)

Purpose, Principle, Specimen, Procedure, Notes, and Precautions. See Test 2.1.

Interpretation. Transferrin is characteristically decreased in patients with ACD, in contrast to the substantial elevation of this protein level in patients with iron deficiency anemia. This test, however, is neither specific nor sensitive enough to consistently distinguish between the two types of anemia.

Test 3.3 Transferrin Saturation

Purpose. The percent saturation of transferrin reflects the availability of iron for erythropoiesis and can be calculated by dividing the serum iron level by the transferrin level.

Interpretation. The percent saturation of transferrin is generally decreased in patients with ACD, in whom a range of 10% to 25% saturation is usually found. Although in iron deficiency anemia the percent saturation of transferrin is usually less than 15%, there is some overlap between the percent saturation ranges found in these two disorders.

Test 3.4 Ferritin Quantitation

Purpose. The serum ferritin level is a measure of the patient's total body iron stores.

Principle, Specimen, Procedure, Notes, and Precautions. See Test 2.3.

Interpretation. The serum ferritin level usually is normal or increased in patients with ACD, reflecting their abundant storage iron. The serum ferritin level in patients with iron deficiency anemia generally is markedly decreased.

Notes and Precautions. Because ferritin is an acute phase reactant, it may be elevated spuriously in patients with acute inflammatory processes. Despite this problem, serum ferritin levels are still of value in patients with possible ACD because they can help distinguish such patients from those with iron deficiency anemia. If results of serum ferritin assays are correlated with erythrocyte sedimentation rate, the distinction between ACD and iron deficiency anemia is enhanced.

3.1.5 Ancillary Tests

The free erythrocyte protoporphyrin level is elevated in patients with ACD because the iron available for hemoglobin synthesis is decreased. Measuring free erythrocyte protoporphyrin, however, is not generally done in the initial evaluation for this disorder.

3.1.6 Course and Treatment

Treatment of the underlying disease is of paramount importance in the care of patients with ACD, because eradication or control of the underlying disorder results in improvement of the anemia. Anemia of chronic disease is often mild and usually does not require specific treatment. Transfusion results in temporary improvement but is not recommended unless the patient is symptomatic. Recent evidence suggests that some patients with ACD respond at least partially to recombinant human erythropoietin.

3.2 Anemia With Chronic Renal Disease

The anemia that often occurs in patients with chronic renal disease shares some characteristics with ACD. This anemia generally is normocytic and normochromic, and its severity roughly parallels the severity of the underlying renal disease. As in ACD, multiple factors contribute to the development of anemia in patients with renal disease; however, some important pathophysiologic differences exist between the two disorders. The primary pathophysiologic mechanism for anemia in renal failure patients is decreased erythropoiesis secondary to either decreased or nonfunctional erythropoietin (**Table 3-4**). The bone marrow usually shows erythroid hypoplasia. Azotemia exacerbates the anemia by both

Table 3-4 Causes of Anemia in Patients With Chronic Renal Failure

Hypoproliferation secondary to decreased erythropoietin production (dominant factor)
Hemolysis (decreased erythrocyte survival)
Iron or folate deficiency
Hemorrhage
Chronic infections
Bone marrow suppression from azotemia*
Bone marrow fibrosis from advanced osteitis fibrosa cystica*†
Dilutional anemia from fluid imbalance*

*Rarely a significant contributing factor in anemia of chronic renal failure.
†From secondary hyperparathyroidism.

direct suppression of bone marrow and decreased RBC survival. Other manifestations of the anemia associated with chronic renal disease include burr cells in the blood and decreased serum iron and transferrin levels. Sustained secretion of inhibitory cytokines may be responsible for these iron and transferrin abnormalities.

Several additional factors can exacerbate anemia in these patients. For example, patients may have long-term blood loss because of both platelet and vessel defects secondary to the underlying renal disease. Patients undergoing long-term hemodialysis can readily become folate deficient. Finally, patients with renal disease are prone to fluid overload, which can further decrease the hematocrit value.

The treatment of the underlying renal disease is of primary importance in these patients. Treatment with recombinant human erythropoietin has resulted in amelioration of the anemia in many patients with chronic renal failure.

3.3 Anemia With Chronic Endocrine Disease

Anemia is common in patients with chronic endocrine diseases such as diabetes mellitus and hypothyroidism. The anemia in patients with diabetes is characteristically multifactorial. In addition to ACD, such patients may develop enteropathy, which leads to poor absorption of iron, vitamin B_{12}, and folate. They also may suffer from chronic blood loss and chronic renal insufficiency. The relative contribution of all of these abnormalities to an anemia varies from patient to patient and varies over time in the same patient.

Patients with chronic hypothyroidism also are frequently anemic. The possible factors contributing to an anemia in these patients include decreased oxygen requirements, concurrent pernicious anemia, iron deficiency secondary to menorrhagia, and impaired iron absorption. Treatment of the underlying endocrine disorder is of primary importance, but the anemia generally does not require treatment.

3.4 Anemia Associated With Liver Diseases

The most common liver disease linked to anemia is alcoholism, and anemia is a very common finding in patients with chronic alcoholism. Although this anemia is generally mild to moderate, it can periodically become more severe, corresponding to the patient's alcohol ingestion and the severity of the patient's liver disease. Although anemia in alcoholic patients is at least partially attributable to ACD, many other mechanisms are operative concurrently, including direct toxic effects of alcohol, various nutritional deficiencies, RBC survival defects, abnormal iron metabolism, and hemodilution. The predominant mechanism causing anemia may vary with time, and production, maturation, and survival defects may all play a role in the development of anemia in these patients. The pathogenesis and morphologic features of the various causes of anemia in patients with alcoholism are highlighted in **Table 3-5**.

Alcohol, especially when ingested in large amounts, has a direct toxic effect on hematopoietic elements, resulting in decreased bone marrow cellularity and vacuolization of erythroid precursors. Nutritional deficiencies often found in patients with chronic alcoholism include folate and iron deficiency. Folate deficiency is particularly common in such patients because of decreased ingestion, impaired folate absorption by alcohol, and antagonism of folate function by alcohol. Although typical morphologic features of megaloblastic anemia may be identified in the blood and bone marrow of patients with alcoholism, these changes are often masked by concurrent RBC abnormalities from iron deficiency, hemolysis, or both. Iron stores may be decreased in patients with chronic alcoholism because of both decreased ingestion and chronic gastrointestinal blood loss. Hypochromasia is generally

Table 3-5 Pathogenesis and Morphologic Features of Anemia in Patients With Alcoholism

Mechanism	Morphologic Features	Etiology/Cause
Chronic disease	Normocytic/normochromic anemia	See earlier discussion
Folate deficiency*	Megaloblastic anemia with oval macrocytes and hypersegmented neutrophils	Decreased ingestion, impaired absorption, and antagonistic action of alcohol on folate function
	Macrocytosis may be masked by concurrent iron deficiency	
Iron deficiency†	Hypochromia present but microcytosis often masked by concurrent macrocytosis from hepatic disease	Decreased ingestion of iron and chronic blood loss via gastrointestinal tract
Decreased red blood cell survival	Target cells, spherocytes, sometimes spur cells and microspherocytes	Extracorpuscular ethrocyte defects due to:
		Congestive splenomegaly and portal hypertension
		Lipoprotein abnormalities causing target and spur shapes
		Severe hypophosphatemia
Toxic suppression	Hypocellular bone marrow with vacuolated erythroid precursors	Alcohol toxic to hematopoietic elements
Abnormal iron metabolism	Ring sideroblasts in bone marrow	Complex etiology, not completely known
		Caused in part by decreased functional pyridoxine and inhibition of enzymes involved in hemoglobin synthesis
Hemodilution	None	Portal hypertension associated with fluid overload leading to dilutional anemia

*See Chapter 5 for more details.
†See Chapter 2 for more details.

present, but the microcytosis of iron deficiency may be masked by counteracting macrocytosis caused by liver disease, folate deficiency, acute alcohol ingestion, or a combination of these.

Decreased RBC survival is seen frequently in alcoholic patients with significant hepatic disease. The target cells, spherocytes, spur cells, and microspherocytes that may be identified in the peripheral blood of patients with chronic alcoholism are secondary to extracorpuscular RBC defects caused by congestive splenomegaly, lipoprotein abnormalities in the blood, and severe hypophosphatemia. In addition to iron deficiency, patients with chronic alcoholism may have abnormal iron metabolism manifested by ring sideroblasts in the bone marrow. Although the etiology of this phenomenon is not completely understood, the ring sideroblasts are caused in part by decreased functional pyridoxine and decreased activity of the enzymes involved in hemoglobin synthesis. Finally, portal hypertension is often associated with an increase in plasma volume that leads to dilutional anemia.

It is beyond the scope of this chapter to detail the clinical findings and laboratory features of patients with chronic alcoholism. Details of the laboratory evaluation of patients for possible iron deficiency and folate deficiency can be found in Chapters 2 and 5, respectively. Except for patients with pronounced spur cell formation, marked nutritional deficiency, or gastrointestinal tract bleeding, the anemia associated with chronic alcoholism is generally mild to moderate and does not require treatment. Management of the portal hypertension and congestive splenomegaly is important in ameliorating the RBC survival defects.

3.5 Anemia With AIDS

Cytopenias are common peripheral blood abnormalities in patients with AIDS, and the severity of these cytopenias is roughly correlated with disease status. Consequently, those patients with the most severe cytopenias tend to be those with advanced disease. As with the other disorders presented in this chapter, the anemia in patients with AIDS is multifactorial, although ACD often predominates (**Table 3-6**).

In addition, evidence suggests that HIV-1 may invade bone marrow progenitor cells, resulting in multilineage suppression of hematopoiesis. Likewise, immune aberrations characteristic of this disease may result in defective regulation of hematopoiesis. The anemia in patients with AIDS is frequently exacerbated by

Table 3-6   Causes of Anemia in Patients With AIDS

Anemia of chronic disease
Bone marrow suppression by virus (HIV-1)
Ineffective regulation of hematopoiesis (T-cell/monocyte defects)
Secondary infections and neoplasms
Bone marrow suppression from various drug treatments
Immune mechanisms (autoantibody production)
Sustained parvovirus infection resulting in prolonged red cell aplasia
Iron deficiency, other nutritional deficiencies
Chronic alcoholism, hepatitis, or associated disorders

zidovudine therapy, which is also linked to marked macrocytosis. Bone marrow infiltration by secondary tumors may result in impaired hematopoiesis, and bone marrow suppression also may be the consequence of either various secondary infections or drug treatments required for secondary infections and/or neoplasms. Autoimmune mechanisms may be operative in creating blood cytopenias, although the correlation between Coombs' positivity and hemolytic anemia in patients with AIDS is not clear-cut.

Various nutritional deficiencies can develop in AIDS patients secondary to gastrointestinal blood loss, poor intake, or drugs that act as folate antagonists. One of the secondary infections that patients with AIDS can acquire is parvovirus, which invades erythroid progenitor cells and causes profound red cell aplasia (see Chapter 4). Because patients with AIDS are often unable to mount an immune response to parvovirus, the red cell aplasia is often sustained. Gamma globulin therapy is generally required to ameliorate this secondary viral infection.

3.6 References

Balaban EP, Sheehan RG, Demian SE, et al. Evaluation of bone marrow iron stores in anemia associated with chronic disease: a comparative study of serum and red cell ferritin. *Am J Hematol*. 1993;42:177–181.

Boyd HK, Lappin TRJ. Erythropoietin deficiency in the anaemia of chronic disorders. *Eur J Haematol*. 1991;46:198–201.

Brynes RK, Esplin J. Hematologic manifestations of HIV-1 infection. In: Bick RL, Bennett JM, Brynes RK, eds. *Hematology: Clinical and Laboratory Practice, Vol 1*. St Louis, Mo: Mosby; 1993:619–636.

Foucar K. Anemias. In: Foucar K, ed. *Bone Marrow Pathology*. 2nd ed. Chicago, Ill: ASCP Press. In press.

Foucar K. Bone marrow manifestations of systemic infections. In: Foucar K, ed. *Bone Marrow Pathology*. 2nd ed. Chicago, Ill: ASCP Press. In press.

Girard DE, Kumar KL, McAfee JH. Hematologic effects of acute and chronic alcohol abuse. *Hematol Oncol Clin North Am*. 1987;1:321–334.

Greendyke RM, Sharma K, Gifford FR. Serum levels of erythropoietin and selected other cytokines in patients with anemia of chronic disease. *Am J Clin Pathol*. 1994;101:338–341.

Hocking WG. Hematologic abnormalities in patients with renal diseases. *Hematol Oncol Clin North Am*. 1987;1:229–260.

Keeling DM, Isenberg DA. Haematological manifestations of systemic lupus erythematosus. *Blood Rev*. 1993;7:199–207.

Kontoghiorghes GJ, Weinberg ED. Iron: mammalian defense systems, mechanisms of disease, and chelation therapy approaches. *Blood Rev*. 1995;9:33–45.

Means RT Jr. Pathogenesis of the anemia of chronic disease: a cytokine-mediated anemia. *Stem Cells*. 1995;13:32–37.

Means RT, Dessypris EN. The anemias of chronic disease, renal failure, and endocrine disorders. In: Bick RL, Bennett JM, Brynes RK, eds. *Hematology. Clinical and Laboratory Practice, Vol 1*. St Louis, Mo: Mosby; 1993:419–429.

Means RT Jr, Krantz SB. Progress in understanding the pathogenesis of the anemia of chronic disease. *Blood*. 1992;80:1639–1647.

Moliterno AR, Spivak JL. Anemia of cancer. *Hematol Oncol Clin North Am*. 1996;10:345–363.

Stockman JA III, Ezekowitz RAB. Hematologic manifestations of systemic diseases. In: Nathan DG, Orkin SH, eds. *Nathan and Oski's Hematology of Infancy and Childhood, Vol 2*. 5th ed. Philadelphia, Pa: Saunders; 1998:1841–1891.

4   Aplastic, Hypoplastic, and Miscellaneous Types of Anemia

For clarity, this chapter is divided into three major topics: aplastic and hypoplastic anemias, bone marrow replacement disorders, and congenital dyserythropoietic anemias.

4.1 Aplastic and Hypoplastic Anemias

Both constitutional and acquired disorders of RBC production have been well delineated (**Table 4-1**). These production defects can involve the erythroid lineage (ie, pure red cell aplasia), two cell lines (ie, bicytopenia), or production of all hematopoietic cells (ie, aplastic anemia). The constitutional (hereditary) types of aplastic anemia primarily include Fanconi's anemia, dyskeratosis congenita, and occasional cases of Shwachman-Diamond syndrome. Diamond-Blackfan anemia is the only well-established constitutional pure red cell aplasia (**Table 4-2**). In general, these constitutional disorders are associated with abnormalities in other organ systems, including skeletal and mucocutaneous defects, as well as mental retardation. In addition to the obvious loss of one or more bone marrow lineages, biochemical abnormalities in erythrocytes are characteristic of both Diamond-Blackfan and Fanconi's anemia. These RBC defects include increased fetal hemoglobin, increased

Table 4-1 Types of Constitutional and Acquired Aplastic Anemia and Red Cell Aplasia

Constitutional aplastic anemia	Constitutional red cell aplasia
Fanconi's anemia	Diamond-Blackfan anemia
Dyskeratosis congenita	
Shwachman-Diamond syndrome	
Acquired aplastic anemia	Acquired red cell aplasia
Idiopathic	Transient erythroblastopenia of childhood
Secondary to drugs, toxins, infections, and miscellaneous disorders/conditions	Parvovirus infection* (usually transient)
	Idiopathic pure red cell aplasia
Paroxysmal nocturnal hemoglobinuria (clonal)	Sustained pure red cell aplasia secondary to neoplasms, immune disorders, infections, and drug treatment

*Parvovirus infection may be sustained in an immunocompromised host.

expression of i antigen on the surface membrane, and abnormalities of cytoplasmic enzyme levels. Although Diamond-Blackfan anemia (constitutional red cell aplasia) is generally evident at birth or shortly thereafter, the constitutional aplastic anemias tend to manifest more gradually with the progressive development of trilineage hypoplasia.

Both pure red cell aplasia and aplastic anemia can be acquired, and these acquired hypoplastic disorders are substantially more common than their constitutional counterparts (*see Tables 4-1 and 4-2*). Acquired pure red cell aplasia can be classified as three general types: transient erythroblastopenia of childhood, parvovirus-induced red cell aplasia (usually transient), and acquired (sustained) pure red cell aplasia. Transient erythroblastopenia of childhood is a self-limited disorder that is likely linked to an antecedent viral infection, although a specific cause has not been well documented. Spontaneous recovery occurs, and affected children are otherwise entirely normal. When transient erythroblastopenia occurs in a young child, the chief differential diagnostic consideration is Diamond-Blackfan anemia.

Clinically significant parvovirus infection affects two general categories of patients—those with constitutional anemias associated with decreased erythrocyte survival time and immunocompromised patients who are unable to mount an antibody response to clear the infection. Children and adults who have underlying constitutional RBC survival disorders, such as hereditary spherocytosis or sickle cell anemia, can develop dramatic exacerbation of the underlying anemia secondary to acute parvovirus infection. Because of short-ened RBC survival times, baseline production of erythrocytes great-ly exceeds normal levels in patients with these constitutional hemolytic anemias. Consequently, the hemoglobin and hematocrit levels plummet when RBC production is halted, even temporarily, by parvovirus invasion and destruction of erythroid progenitor cells. Even though thalassemia is both an RBC maturation and an RBC survival disorder, the identical clinical "aplastic crisis" occurs as a consequence of acute parvovirus infection. Viral inclusions within the residual erythroblasts generally can be identified, but the diag-nosis should be confirmed by serologic or molecular studies (**Image 4-1**). Once the patient mounts an immune response to the par-vovirus, the infection is eliminated and erythropoiesis returns to baseline levels. In immunocompromised patients, parvovirus infec-tions are typically sustained with prolonged red cell aplasia; rare reports describe multilineage hypoplasia in this patient population.

In addition to the acquired transient red cell aplasias, both pri-mary and secondary types of acquired (sustained) pure red cell aplasia have been described (**Table 4-3**). Disorders linked to acquired pure red cell aplasia include large granular lymphocytosis of cytotoxic/suppressor T cells, other hematopoietic and non-hematopoietic neoplasms, drug treatments (notably diphenylhy-dantoin), immune disorders, and chronic viral infections.

The causes of acquired aplastic anemia are listed in **Table 4-4** and include drug and toxin exposures, various viral infections, immune aberrations, and radiation. All hematopoietic lineages are either absent or severely attenuated in affected patients (**Image 4-2**).

4.1.1 Pathophysiology

For erythropoiesis to occur, the necessary components include adequate stem cells, which are capable of renewal and differentia-tion; erythropoietin and other growth factors; appropriate immunoregulation of hematopoiesis; and an adequate microenvi-ronment. Deficiencies or defects in all of these components have been suggested in the pathophysiology of the diverse spectrum of congenital and acquired erythropoietic production disorders. Mutations in genes encoding DNA repair proteins are responsible for the generalized DNA repair defects that characterize Fanconi's anemia; similarly, DNA repair defects are postulated to cause dyskeratosis congenita.

Acquired anemias such as transient erythroblastopenia of childhood are probably caused by a self-limited, infection-induced,

Table 4-2 Features of Constitutional and Acquired Aplastic Anemias and Red Cell Aplasia

Type	Clinical Features
Constitutional aplastic anemia	
Fanconi's	Autosomal recessive disease with associated bone, skin, and renal abnormalities
	Mental retardation
	Underlying DNA repair defect
Dyskeratosis congenita	X-linked recessive disorder with skin, nail, and mucosal abnormalities
	Mental retardation
	Likely DNA repair defect
Shwachman-Diamond syndrome	Autosomal recessive; some patients have associated bone abnormalities
Constitutional red cell aplasia	
Diamond-Blackfan anemia	Onset of anemia at birth or early infancy
	Several genetic types
	Short stature, hypertelorism, retardation
	Likely intrinsic progenitor cell defect
Acquired aplastic anemia	Onset at any age
	Most cases idiopathic
	Other cases linked to infections, toxins, drugs, radiation, immune disorders
Acquired red cell aplasia	
Transient erythroblastopenia of childhood	Patient usually more than 1 year old
Parvovirus-induced red cell aplasia	Any age
	Patient typically has either underlying constitutional anemia or immunodeficiency
Acquired sustained pure red cell aplasia	Adolescence through adulthood
	Both idiopathic and secondary types

*Usual features such as increased erythroblasts and intact erythoid maturation noted in occasional immunosuppressed patients

Table 4-2

Blood	Bone Marrow
Thrombocytopenia is typically initial abnormality	Initially normocellular/hypercellular with variable megaloblastic charges
Pancytopenia develops by midchildhood	Eventual aplasia
Decreased reticulocytes	Substantial late development of myelodysplasia or acute myelogenous leukemia
Gradual development of pancytopenia	Initially normocellular/hypercellular Eventual aplasia in one half of patients
Decreased reticulocytes	Reports of late development of acute myelogenous leukemia
Neutropenia predominates	Initial abnormalities are granulocytic
One fourth of cases progress to pancytopenia	Eventual aplasia in one fourth of patients
Decreased reticulocytes	Some patients develop acute myelogenous leukemia
Macrocytic anemia with decreased reticulocytes	Only rare erythroblasts evident Other lineages unremarkable Increased hematogones
Pancytopenia Normal morphology Decreased reticulocytes	Panhypoplasia Variable lymphoid infiltrates
Normocytic, normochromic anemia	Only rare erythroblasts evident Other lineages unremarkable
Decreased reticulocytes	Variable lymphocytosis
Variable RBC morphology depending on underlying chronic anemia	Only erythroblasts evident; these cells may contain intranuclear inclusions* Other lineages usually unremarkable
Decreased reticulocytes	Infection transient in immunocompetent, sustained in immunocompromised patients
Normocytic, normochromic anemia	Only rare erythroblasts evident Other lineages unremarkable
Decreased reticulocytes	

Table 4-3 Types of Acquired Sustained Pure Red Cell Aplasia

Type	Associated Disorders/Conditions
Primary (50% of cases)	Idiopathic
Secondary (50% of cases)	Large granular lymphocytosis T-cell type
	Other hematopoietic neoplasms
	Drug treatments
	Thymoma
	Immune disorders
	Viral infections*

*Not including parvovirus.

immunoregulatory abnormality. Such an abnormality is the likely cause of many other types of acquired pure red cell aplasia and aplastic anemia as well.

The most extensive pathophysiologic studies have been performed on patients with acquired aplastic anemia. Defects described in these patients include deficient or suppressed progenitor cells, humoral and cellular immunoregulatory defects, and microenvironmental abnormalities. The dominant abnormality is destruction of CD34 positive progenitor cells through apoptotic mechanisms stimulated by cytokines released from activated bone marrow cytotoxic T cells. In addition, several viral infections, notably hepatitis and Epstein-Barr viruses, have been linked to aplastic anemia. One theory regarding viral-induced aplasia states that stem cells are directly suppressed or damaged by these infectious agents. Another theory suggests that the viruses initiate an immune response that suppresses hematopoiesis. Finally, many drug treatments and some toxic exposures have been associated with acquired aplastic anemia caused either by a dose-related or an idiosyncratic host response to the drug or by the production of a bone marrow toxic metabolite of the drug. A similar mechanism is proposed for toxic exposures.

4.1.2 Clinical Findings

Depending on its severity, patients with hypoplastic or aplastic anemia may present with weakness, fatigue, or tachycardia. If pancytopenia is present, additional findings can include petechiae and purpura secondary to thrombocytopenia, as well as fever from neutropenia-associated infections. As described earlier, most constitutional types of hypoplastic anemias have associated phenotypic abnormalities, including bony defects, mental retardation, and

Table 4-4 Causes of Acquired Aplastic Anemia

Drugs
    Chloramphenicol
    Phenylbutazone
    Anticonvulsants
    Sulfonamides
    Gold
    Chemotherapy*
Toxins
    Benzene
    Insecticides
    Solvents
Infections
    Hepatitis
    Epstein-Barr virus
    Influenza
    Other infections
Other conditions/exposures
    Radiation exposure
    Immune disorders
    Paroxysmal nocturnal hemoglobinuria†
    Chronic lymphocytic leukemia
    Other neoplasms
    Pregnancy‡

*Predictable transient aplasia is associated with myeloablative chemotherapy.
†Clonal disorder is both a cause and a consequence of aplastic anemia.
‡The epidemiologic association between pregnancy and aplastic anemia has been challenged in recent studies.

skin and nail abnormalities (*see Table 4-2*). Other clinical features such as hepatosplenomegaly and lymphadenopathy are not evident in patients with uncomplicated hypoplastic or aplastic anemias.

4.1.3 Diagnostic Approach

The diagnosis of hypoplastic anemia requires an approach that both identifies the specific type of disorder and excludes bone marrow–effacing diseases, which also can be manifested by blood cytopenias. The approach to diagnosis generally follows these steps:

1. Determine the types and severity of the blood cytopenias.
2. Assess the patient for hepatosplenomegaly and lymphadenopathy on physical examination.
3. Evaluate infants and young children for other manifestations of hereditary hypoplastic disorders, including physical and radiographic defects and family history (*see Table 4-2*).

4. Document bone marrow hypocellularity and rule out an infiltrative or fibrotic process.
5. Use the clinical history and other clinical evidence of chronic hemolytic anemia to assess for a possible parvovirus-related aplastic crisis of an underlying RBC disorder such as hereditary spherocytosis or sickle cell anemia.
6. Evaluate adults with pure red cell aplasia for hematopoietic neoplasms, thymoma, other tumors, drug/toxin exposure, or infection (*see Tables 4-2 and 4-3*).
7. Evaluate patients with acquired aplastic anemia for evidence of neoplasm, immune disorders, toxin/drug exposure, or infection.

4.1.4 Hematologic Findings

In some types of hypoplastic anemia, only erythropoiesis is reduced; in others, all bone marrow cell lines are affected. Therefore, the hematologic manifestations of these conditions can range from isolated anemia to pancytopenia.

Blood Cell Measurements

Patients with hypoplastic anemias generally have a moderate to severe normochromic anemia, which may be normocytic or macrocytic. An elevated mean corpuscular volume (MCV) is characteristic of Diamond-Blackfan anemia and also may be present in some cases of acquired aplastic anemia. Except for patients with hereditary hemolytic anemia and secondary parvovirus-induced red cell aplasia, erythrocytes generally show little anisopoikilocytosis, as evidenced by a normal red cell distribution width (RDW). The reticulocyte count is markedly reduced. In patients with either acquired or constitutional aplastic anemia, thrombocytopenia and neutropenia are present also.

Peripheral Blood Smear Morphology

Erythrocytes, neutrophils, and platelets are generally morphologically unremarkable in the various hypoplastic disorders, except in parvovirus-induced red cell aplasia that occurs in patients with underlying constitutional hemolytic anemias, which are often associated with distinct erythrocyte shape abnormalities.

Bone Marrow Examination

Patients with Diamond-Blackfan anemia, transient erythroblastopenia of childhood, and acquired pure red cell aplasia show a marked decrease in erythroid precursors in the bone marrow with essentially normal granulopoiesis and megakaryocytopoiesis. Erythroid precursors may be totally absent, or only the earliest RBC precursors may be identified. Parvovirus inclusions may be evident in erythroblasts in patients with this type of acquired red cell aplasia (*see Image 4-1*). A lymphocytosis with many hematogones may be present with all types of hypoplastic or aplastic anemias, especially in specimens from young children.

Early in their disease course, patients with Fanconi's anemia may have a normal to hypercellular bone marrow with megaloblastic changes, followed by gradual aplasia. In acquired aplastic anemia and advanced Fanconi's anemia, however, all three cell lines are usually markedly reduced (*see Image 4-2*). There are no specific morphologic abnormalities of the rare residual hematopoietic elements in these patients.

Other Laboratory Tests

Test 4.1 **Fetal Hemoglobin Quantitation**

Purpose. Fetal hemoglobin levels in erythrocytes can be used to distinguish between transient erythroblastopenia of childhood and constitutional disorders such as Diamond-Blackfan and Fanconi's anemias.

Principle, Specimen, Procedure, Notes, and Precautions. See Test 10.6.

Interpretation. Erythrocyte fetal hemoglobin level is characteristically increased in Diamond-Blackfan and Fanconi's anemias but normal in patients with transient erythroblastopenia of childhood. Erythrocyte fetal hemoglobin level also may be increased in some cases of acquired aplastic anemia. Usually, only a small population of erythrocytes contains substantial amounts of fetal hemoglobin; the remainder of erythrocytes contain none.

4.1.5 Ancillary Tests

Because parvovirus infection can be sustained in immunocompromised patients, it is important to assess patients with acquired red cell aplasia for evidence of this infection. Tests include determination of serum IgM and IgG parvovirus titers, molecular tests for parvovirus using specific viral DNA probes, and in situ hybridization studies on bone marrow tissue sections. Other tests that can be used selectively to distinguish among the various types of aplastic and hypoplastic anemias include the RBC i antigen test and cytogenetic studies. Although not available in most laboratories, RBC i antigen can be detected in patients with Diamond-Blackfan and Fanconi's anemia; i antigen is not present on erythrocytes in patients with either transient erythroblastopenia of childhood or other acquired hypoplastic disorders.

In bone marrow cells of patients with Fanconi's anemia, cytogenetic studies generally reveal chromosomal defects, including increased chromosomal breakage; translocations; sister chromatid exchange; and increased sensitivity to diepoxybutane, mitomycin C, and other agents. Karyotypic abnormalities are not usually found in the other types of hypoplastic and aplastic anemias. Family studies may be helpful in identifying inheritance patterns associated with constitutional disorders.

Because erythropoietin level is generally increased in all aplastic and hypoplastic anemias, it is not a useful test in distinguishing between these disorders.

4.1.6 Course and Treatment

The clinical course of hypoplastic and aplastic anemias is diverse. Some patients, such as children with transient erythroblastopenia of childhood, have brief, self-limited episodes of red cell aplasia that require no treatment. Likewise, spontaneous recovery generally occurs in immunocompetent patients with acute parvovirus-induced red cell aplasia, although transfusions may be necessary for exacerbations of the underlying hemolytic anemias.

Children and most adults with constitutional disorders, acquired aplastic anemia, or acquired sustained pure red cell aplasia generally require treatment that may include immune modulation, cytokine therapy, androgens, transfusion, or bone marrow transplantation. In patients with acquired disorders, any antecedent drug treatment should be discontinued, if possible. Suspected toxins should be removed from the patient's environment. In general, blood product transfusions should be reserved for life-threatening situations. Because these transfusions can have a negative effect on the outcome of subsequent bone marrow transplantation, they should be used very judiciously in patients with aplastic anemia who are likely to require such a transplant.

The bone marrow of patients with pure red cell aplasia often responds to corticosteroid therapy. If this fails, other interventions may include plasmapheresis, azathioprine, cyclosporine, anti-thymocyte globulin, or danazol treatment. Human recombinant erythropoietin also may be used to stimulate erythropoiesis. A careful search for underlying causes of acquired (sustained) pure red cell aplasia should be undertaken.

The clinical course of patients with acquired aplastic anemia depends on the severity of the pancytopenia, the patient's age, and the patient's response to treatment. These patients must be monitored carefully for evidence of infection or bleeding. Drugs that have been used successfully to treat some patients with acquired aplastic anemia include antithymocyte globulin, cyclosporine, and human recombinant colony-stimulating factors. Bone marrow transplantation is generally recommended for young patients with severe refractory acquired aplastic anemia.

There is an increased incidence of acute leukemia in patients who recover from any type of bone marrow hypoplastic disorder. Long-term survivors also may develop myelodysplasia or paroxysmal nocturnal hemoglobinuria–like defects. The risk of leukemia is highest in patients with constitutional DNA repair defects such as Fanconi's anemia.

4.2 Bone Marrow Replacement Disorders

Patients with bone marrow replacement disorders suffer from a failure of hematopoiesis because the medullary portion of the bone marrow has been replaced by fibrosis, neoplastic cells, or nonneoplastic cells (**Table 4-5**). Even if the neoplastic cells are of hematopoietic origin, they are incapable of producing normal peripheral blood elements. Therefore, patients with bone marrow replacement disorders generally present with cytopenias ranging from isolated anemia to pancytopenia.

4.2.1 Pathophysiology

Despite the bone marrow's ability to compensate, hematopoiesis fails once a significant portion of the active bone marrow medullary space is replaced by fibrous tissue, tumor, or other abnormal cells. This failure is the primary cause of cytopenias in patients with bone marrow replacement disorders. As described in Chapter 3, however, patients with neoplasms may develop other types of anemia. For example, these patients can suffer from chronic blood loss, anemia of chronic disease, bone marrow suppression

Table 4-5   Causes of Bone Marrow Failure Secondary to Replacement

---

Neoplastic disorders replacing bone marrow parenchyma
  Acute and chronic leukemias
  Malignant lymphoma (Hodgkin's disease and non-Hodgkin's lymphoma)
  Multiple myeloma
  Metastatic carcinoma and sarcoma
Disorders/therapy causing bone marrow fibrosis
  Chronic idiopathic myelofibrosis
  Metabolic bone disorders/endocrine abnormalities
  Following chemotherapy/toxin exposure
Miscellaneous disorders replacing bone marrow parenchyma
  Storage diseases
  Other histiocytic disorders
  Angioimmunoblastic lymphadenopathy
  Mast cell disease

---

by chemotherapy, hypersplenism, and even immune-mediated hemolysis (*see Table 3-3*).

4.2.2 Clinical Findings

The clinical findings in patients with bone marrow replacement disorders are as diverse as the types of disorders themselves. Most patients with significant bone marrow replacement disorders develop symptoms of cytopenia, notably malaise and fatigue secondary to anemia. Manifestations of leukopenia and thrombocytopenia, such as infection or bleeding, also may be present. Patients with acute and chronic leukemias, malignant lymphomas, storage diseases, and chronic idiopathic myelofibrosis often have significant splenomegaly, which can cause left upper quadrant pain and early satiety. Lymphadenopathy also may be present in some of these patients, especially those with lymphomas.

4.2.3 Hematologic Findings

Although most patients with bone marrow replacement disorders have cytopenias, some also have specific morphologic abnormalities that suggest a certain type of replacement disorder.

Blood Cell Measurements

A normocytic, normochromic anemia is the most common cytopenia in patients with bone marrow replacement disorders.

Although these erythrocytes generally show little anisopoikilocytosis, as manifested by a normal RDW, some patients—such as those with chronic idiopathic myelofibrosis—exhibit marked anisopoikilocytosis. The reticulocyte count is typically reduced in these patients, whereas the WBC and platelet counts are more variable and may exhibit changes during the disease course. For example, thrombocytosis may be evident early in the disease course of chronic idiopathic myelofibrosis, but thrombocytopenia is characteristic of advanced bone marrow fibrosis.

Peripheral Blood Smear Morphology
Most secondary bone marrow replacement disorders have no specific morphologic abnormalities of RBCs, WBCs, or platelets. However, patients with primary hematopoietic neoplasms may have pronounced blood abnormalities such as anisopoikilocytosis with teardrop forms, a leukoerythroblastic blood picture, and large platelets. Leukemic or lymphoma cells may be identified in the peripheral blood in patients with these types of replacement disorders. A leukoerythroblastic blood picture also may be seen in patients with bone marrow metastases by other neoplasms.

Bone Marrow Examination
There is a wide spectrum of potential morphologic abnormalities in patients with diverse primary and secondary bone marrow replacement disorders. In some patients, the bone marrow parenchyma is packed with infiltrating tumor cells, whereas in others it is replaced by collagen. In histiocytic disorders, such as storage diseases, the bone marrow may be replaced by distinctive large, benign-appearing macrophages.

Other Laboratory Tests

Because this group of disorders is so diverse, many tests potentially may be used on a selective basis to help establish the diagnosis of specific bone marrow replacement disorders (see Chapters 29 through 38).

4.2.4 Course and Treatment
Fibrotic and benign histiocytic bone marrow replacement disorders tend to exhibit gradually progressive bone marrow infiltra-

tion, while neoplasms generally progress more rapidly. The treatment and disease course vary for each type of replacement disorder.

4.3 Congenital Dyserythropoietic Anemias

Congenital dyserythropoietic anemias (CDAs) are rare disorders initially described in 1951 and characterized by both profound blood and bone marrow morphologic abnormalities of erythroid elements and ineffective erythropoiesis. Other features common to this group of disorders include reticulocytopenia, a mildly elevated indirect bilirubin level, and an elevated lactate dehydrogenase level. An autosomal recessive pattern of inheritance has been determined in some patients with CDA. Patients with CDA generally have a mild to moderate anemia, with marked anisopoikilocytosis (**Image 4-3**).

At least three types of CDA have been described based on specific morphologic features within the bone marrow (**Table 4-6**). In type I, the erythroid elements within the bone marrow show megaloblastic changes with internuclear chromatin bridges. Type II CDA is characterized by binucleated and multinucleated erythroid precursors. In type III CDA, the multinucleation is pronounced with up to 12 nuclei present in some erythroid precursors. Mature erythrocytes are often macrocytic in all types of CDA.

The bone marrow in patients with CDA shows erythroid hyperplasia with asynchronous nuclear-cytoplasmic maturation. Nuclear abnormalities include variations in size and structure as well as shape abnormalities described for the CDA subtypes (*see Image 4-3*). Other nuclear abnormalities, such as lobulation, budding, fragmentation, and karyorrhexis, also have been described. Cytoplasmic abnormalities include vacuolization, basophilic stippling, and excess iron within erythroid precursors.

The pathogenesis of CDA is uncertain, but theories include some primary defect in mitosis or a nuclear or cell membrane defect. Because this type of anemia is mild, affected patients are frequently asymptomatic and do not require treatment.

4.4 References

Alter BP. Arms and the man or hands and the child: congenital anomalies and hematologic syndromes. *J Pediatr Hematol Oncol.* 1997;19:287–291.

Bessler M, Hillmen P. Somatic mutation and clonal selection in the pathogenesis

Table 4-6 Peripheral Blood and Bone Marrow Findings in
Patients With Congenital Dyserythropoietic Anemias

	CDA I	CDA II*	CDA III
Blood			
RBC size	Macrocytic	Normocytic	Normocytic to macrocytic
RBC morphology	Anisopoikilocytosis	Anisopoikilocytosis	Anisopoikilocytosis
Anemia	Mild to moderate	Mild to severe	Mild
Bone marrow			
Erythroid hyperplasia	Prominent	Prominent	Prominent
Erythroid morphology	Megaloblastic; internuclear chromatin bridging; nuclear budding; occasional binucleate forms	Normoblastic; bi- or multinucleated normoblasts; nuclear karyorrhexis	Megaloblastic; "gigantoblasts" (up to 12 nuclei); nuclear karyorrhexis
Other laboratory tests			
Acidified serum test	− (rare +)	+	−
Sugar water test	− (rare +)	−	−
Agglutination by anti-i and anti-I	Slight	+	+ (variable)

*A designation of HEMPAS (hereditary erythroblastic multinuclearity with positive acidified serum [test]) is sometimes applied to patients with CDA II.

and in the control of paroxysmal nocturnal hemoglobinuria. *Semin Hematol.* 1998;35:149–167.

Brown KE, Young NS. Parvovirus B19 in human disease. *Annu Rev Med.* 1997;48:59–67.

D'Andrea AD, Grompe M. Molecular biology of Fanconi anemia: implications for diagnosis and therapy. *Blood.* 1997;90:1725–1736.

Erslev AJ, Soltan A. Pure red-cell aplasia: a review. *Blood Rev.* 1996;10:20–28.

Farhi DC, Luebbers EL, Rosenthal NS. Bone marrow biopsy findings in childhood anemia: prevalence of transient erythroblastopenia of childhood. *Arch Pathol Lab Med.* 1998;122:638–641.

Gillio AP, Verlander PC, Batish SD, et al. Phenotypic consequences of mutations in the Fanconi anemia FAC gene: an International Fanconi Anemia Registry study. *Blood.* 1997;90:105–110.

Guinan EC. Clinical aspects of aplastic anemia. *Hematol Oncol Clin North Am.* 1997;11:1025–1044.

Isildar M, Jimenez JJ, Arimura GK, et al. DNA damage in intact cells induced by bacterial metabolites of chloramphenicol. *Am J Hematol.* 1988;28:40–46.

Kelly JP, Jurgelon JM, Issaragrisil S, et al. An epidemiological study of aplastic anaemia: relationship of drug exposures to clinical features and outcome. *Eur J Haematol Suppl.* 1996;57(suppl):47–52.

Koduri PR. Novel cytomorphology of the giant proerythroblasts of parvovirus B19 infection. *Am J Hematol.* 1998;58:95–99.

Krijanovski OI, Sieff CA. Diamond-Blackfan anemia. *Hematol Oncol Clin North Am.* 1997;11:1061–1077.

Kruyt FA, Youssoufian H. The Fanconi anemia proteins FAA and FAC function in different cellular compartments to protect against cross-linking agent cyto-toxicity. *Blood.* 1998;92:2229–2236.

Liu W, Ittmann M, Liu J, et al. Human parvovirus B19 in bone marrows from adults with acquired immunodeficiency syndrome: a comparative study using in situ hybridization and immunohistochemistry. *Hum Pathol.* 1997;28:760–766.

Oosterkamp HM, Brand A, Kluin-Nelemans JC, et al. Pregnancy and severe aplastic anaemia: causal relation or coincidence? *Br J Haematol.* 1998;103:315–316.

Packman CH. Pathogenesis and management of paroxysmal nocturnal haemoglo-binuria. *Blood Rev.* 1998;12:1–11.

Pont J, Puchhammer-Stockl E, Chott A, et al. Recurrent granulocytic aplasia as clinical presentation of a persistent parvovirus B19 infection. *Br J Haematol.* 1992;80:160–165.

Rosenfeld SJ, Young NS. Viruses and bone marrow failure. *Blood Rev.* 1991;5:71–77.

Shao Z, Chu Y, Zhang Y, et al. Treatment of severe aplastic anemia with an immunosuppressive agent plus recombinant human granulocyte-macrophage colony-stimulating factor and erythropoietin. *Am J Hematol.* 1998;59:185–191.

Stucki A, Leisenring W, Sandmaier BM, et al. Decreased rejection and improved survival of first and second marrow transplants for severe aplastic anemia (a 26-year retrospective analysis). *Blood.* 1998;92:2742–2749.

Wickramasinghe SN. Congenital dyserythropoietic anaemias: clinical features, haematological morphology and new biochemical data. *Blood Rev.* 1998;12:178–200.

Young NS, Maciejewski J. The pathophysiology of acquired aplastic anemia. *N Engl J Med.* 1997;336:1365–1372.

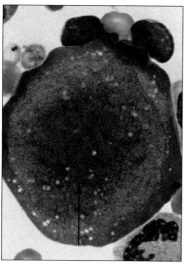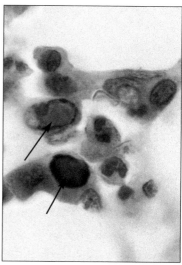

Image 4-1   Composite showing intranuclear parvovirus inclusions (arrows) with erythroid precursors on bone marrow aspirate smears (left) and biopsy sections (right). (Courtesy of Drs P. Ward and C. Sever.) (Left, Wright's; right, H&E)

Image 4-2   Two bone marrow biopsy sections. The contrast between the bone marrow cellularity of aplastic anemia (left) and normal adult bone marrow (right) is striking. (H&E)

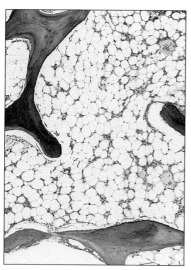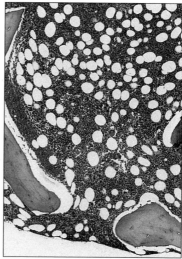

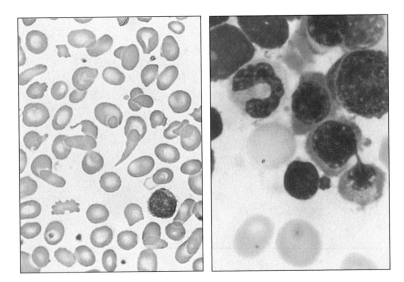

Image 4-3   Blood and bone marrow composite highlighting the dyspoietic features of mature and immature erythroid elements in congenital dyserythropoietic anemia. (Wright's)

5   Megaloblastic Anemias

Megaloblastic anemia occurs when the coenzyme forms of folate and vitamin B_{12} are deficient. The resultant defective DNA synthesis impairs the ability of all proliferating cells to synthesize enough DNA per unit of time to allow for mitosis; as a consequence, more cells are in the DNA synthesis phase of the cell cycle. Because RNA synthesis is not dependent on these coenzymes, an asynchrony between nuclear and cytoplasmic maturation occurs, resulting both in giantism of all proliferating cells and in cell nuclei that appear less mature than the cytoplasm. Ineffective hematopoiesis results from high rates of intramedullary cell death in a setting of bone marrow hypercellularity. Although impaired proliferation of hematopoietic elements is the major clinical manifestation of vitamin B_{12} and folate deficiency, other disorders, especially neuropsychiatric, also can develop and even precede or occur in the absence of hematologic manifestations.

Characteristics of vitamin B_{12} and folate, including dietary sources, recommended daily requirements, normal blood levels, and amounts of stored vitamins, are shown in **Table 5-1**. Vitamin B_{12} circulates in the peripheral blood bound to various proteins. Except in infants, total body stores of vitamin B_{12} are abundant and are sufficient to adequately supply the host for 2 to 5 years. Folate is very heat labile and is destroyed readily in the cooking process.

Table 5-1 Characteristics of Vitamin B_{12} and Folate

	Vitamin B_{12}	Folate
Origin	Synthesized exclusively by bacteria	Synthesized by plants and microorganisms
Dietary source	Meat, fish, dairy products (heat stabile)	Vegetables (especially green leafy) and fruits (heat labile)
Parent compound	Cyanocobalamin	Pteroglutamic acid
Recommended daily requirements (μg)		
Infants	0.3	25-35
Children	0.7-1.4	50-100
Adults	2.0	180-200
Pregnant women	2.2	400
Lactating women	2.6	280
Normal blood levels	150-1000 pg/mL	>3.7 ng/mL (red blood cell: 130-640 ng/mL)
Normal total stores* (major storage site)	3000-5000 mg (liver)	20-70 mg (liver)
Storage duration on deficient diet	2-5 years	3-5 months

*Total stores are much smaller in infants.

Small amounts of folate derivatives circulate largely unbound in the blood; greater concentrations of these derivatives are present intracellularly. Except in infants, total body stores of folate are moderate and are sufficient to maintain normal cellular proliferation for approximately 3 to 5 months. Because of the relatively short time that folate stores will meet host needs, the incidence of folate deficiency secondary to inadequate intake is substantially greater than that of vitamin B_{12} deficiency.

5.1 Pathophysiology

The physiology and biochemistry of vitamin B_{12} and folate are detailed in **Tables 5-2** and **5-3**, respectively. In patients with vitamin B_{12} deficiency, both the megaloblastic anemia and the neurologic complications appear to be secondary to the defective formation of methionine (*see Table 5-3*). The rate-limiting step in DNA

Table 5-2 Physiology of Vitamin B_{12} and Folate

	Vitamin B_{12}	Folate
Compounds in food	Several cobalamin forms	Several polyglutamate forms
Physiology of absorption	Vitamin B_{12} released from food by gastric acid, gastric enzymes, and small bowel enzymes $\rightarrow$ free vitamin B_{12} bound to R-binders primarily; some also binds to IF $\rightarrow$ pancreatic enzymes degrade R-binder– B_{12} complexes $\rightarrow$ released B_{12} is then bound to IF	Polyglutamate deconjugated by conjugase enzymes in bile and small bowel lumen
Site of absorption	Vitamin B_{12}–IF complex adheres to receptors on brush border of ileum (pH and calcium-dependent process)	Deconjugated folate absorbed in jejunum
Physiology of circulation	30% of vitamin B_{12} binds to TCII, which delivers it to liver, bone marrow, and other sites 70% of vitamin B_{12} binds to TCI, TCIII, and R-binders, which deliver it exclusively to liver	Folate circulates unbound in blood as 5-methyl THF
Entry into cells	TCII-B_{12} attaches to specific membrane receptors Vitamin B_{12} transferred across plasma membrane (TCII degraded in this process)	Vitamin B_{12} necessary for folate (THF form) to pass across plasma membranes and be retained in cell
Function	Two active forms, methylcobalamin and 5-deoxyadenosyl cobalamin, which facilitate formation of methionine and succinate, respectively	THF essential for all one-carbon transfer reactions in mammalian cells THF required for both purine and pyrimidine synthesis
Excretion	Bile, urine	Urine, sweat, saliva, feces

Abbreviations: IF = intrinsic factor; TC = transcobalamin; R-binder = found in every tissue in body, named for rapid mobility on electrophoresis; THF = tetrahydrofolate.

Megaloblastic Anemias **73**

Table 5-3 Biochemistry of Vitamin B$_{12}$ and Folate Activity

	Vitamin B$_{12}$	Folate
Biologically active form(s)	Coenzyme B$_{12}$ (5-deoxyadenosyl cobalamin) and methylcobalamin	5-methyl THF
Reactions requiring vitamin B$_{12}$ and/or folate cofactors	I. Homocysteine $\xrightarrow{\text{methylcobalamin}}$ Methionine 5-methyl THF THF Failure in this pathway results in megaloblastosis; reaction also important in central nervous system methylation, and for incorporation of folate into cells II. Methylmalonate $\xrightarrow{\text{Coenzyme B}_{12}}$ Succinate Failure of this reaction not involved in neurologic disease or megaloblastosis	I. Required for both purine and pyrimidine synthesis II. Rate-limiting step in DNA synthesis (pyrimidine synthesis) 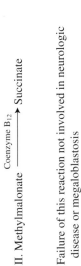 III. Required for methionine synthesis (see I, vitamin B$_{12}$) IV. Folate also essential in amino acid synthesis

Abbreviations: THF = tetrahydrofolate; dUMP = deoxyuridine monophosphate; dTMP = deoxythymidine monophosphate; DHF = dihydrofolate.

Table 5-4 Probable Sequence in Development of Vitamin B_{12} Deficiency

Time Interval After Onset of Intake Failure	Pathologic Abnormality
1-2 years	Vitamin B_{12} level in serum decreased
	Early blood and bone marrow abnormalities, including hypersegmentation and macrocytosis
	Early myelin damage to nerves
2-3 years	Vitamin B_{12} level markedly decreased
	Vitamin B_{12} binders $\leq 10\%$ saturated
	Florid megaloblastosis in blood and bone marrow
	Decreased RBC folate, normal to increased serum folate
	Severe damage to myelin, axonal degeneration

Table 5-5 Sequence in Development of Folate Deficiency

Time Interval After Onset of Intake Failure	Pathologic Abnormality
3 weeks	Decreased serum folate
5-7 weeks	Hypersegmentation of neutrophils in bone marrow and blood
10 weeks	Mild megaloblastic changes in bone marrow
17-18 weeks	Macro-ovalocytes, decreased RBC folate
19-20 weeks	Florid megaloblastosis with anemia

(pyrimidine) synthesis that requires folate is the conversion of deoxyuridine monophosphate to deoxythymidine monophosphate. The sequence of events in the development of vitamin B_{12} and folate deficiency is listed in **Tables 5-4** and **5-5**, respectively. Although folate stores are depleted much more rapidly than vitamin B_{12} stores, the sequence of events in the development of blood and bone marrow abnormalities as deficiency evolves is similar for both. Hypersegmentation of neutrophils appears early in the development of megaloblastic anemia, whereas actual anemia is a late

Table 5-6 Mechanisms of Vitamin B_{12} Deficiency

	Example	Condition/Disorder
Inadequate intake	Dietary deficiency	Strict vegetarianism
Increased requirement	Growth, development	Pregnancy, lactation
Defective absorption	Decreased IF	Pernicious anemia, congenital IF deficiency
	Decreased pancreatic enzymes	Pancreatitis
	Lack of calcium or abnormal pH	Zollinger-Ellison syndrome
	Defective ileal mucosa	Sprue, regional enteritis, surgical resection
	Parasitic or bacterial overgrowth	Tapeworm, blind loop
	Drug interference with absorption	Alcoholism, colchicine treatment, PAS treatment
Defective transport	Decreased TCII	Congenital deficiency of TCII, rare
Disorders of metabolism	Suppression or inhibition of metabolic enzymes	Nitrous oxide administration, enzyme deficiencies
		Inborn errors of metabolism, rare

Abbreviations: IF = intrinsic factor; TC = transcobalamin; PAS = para-amino salicylic acid.

event associated with florid megaloblastic morphologic changes. Damage to myelin in peripheral nerves and eventual axonal degeneration occur progressively throughout the evolution of vitamin B_{12} deficiency.

There are five basic mechanisms leading to vitamin B_{12} deficiency, including inadequate intake, increased requirement, defective absorption, defective transport, and disorders of B_{12} metabolism (**Table 5-6**). By far, the most common mechanism for vitamin B_{12} deficiency is defective absorption. For vitamin B_{12} absorption to occur, there must be normal amounts of intrinsic factor, sufficient pancreatic enzymes to degrade the vitamin B_{12}–R-binder complexes, appropriate calcium and hydrogen ion concentrations to facilitate the transfer of vitamin B_{12} across plasma membranes, an intact ileal mucosal surface, and lack of competing parasites or bacteria for the ingested vitamin B_{12} (*see Table 5-2*). Although abnormalities in any of these components can result in defective absorption, the one most commonly encountered in clinical practice is decreased intrinsic factor in patients with pernicious anemia. Intrinsic factor is secreted by gastric parietal cells stimulated by gastrin and histamine. The antibodies directed against intrinsic factor and parietal cells commonly detected in patients with pernicious anemia may cause the decreased intrinsic factor. Other disorders associated with defective absorption are listed in **Table 5-6**.

Although vitamin B_{12} deficiency may occur secondary to insufficient dietary intake, a stringent diet deficient in all meat, egg, and milk products must be followed for a sustained period. Because vitamin B_{12} stores are so abundant, the increased requirement for this vitamin during pregnancy and lactation is rarely associated with megaloblastic anemia. Vitamin B_{12} deficiency secondary to either transport or metabolic defects is extremely rare and not generally encountered in clinical practice.

The major causes of folate deficiency include dietary deficiency and increased requirement, although defective absorption and disorders of metabolism are occasionally responsible for folate deficiency (**Table 5-7**). Dietary deficiency of folate is common in chronic alcoholics, drug addicts, and patients in low socioeconomic conditions who consume inadequate diets. Excessive cooking destroys folate. Increased folate is required by infants, pregnant and lactating women, and patients with either malignancies or chronic hemolytic anemias. Premature infants have very low folate stores and are highly susceptible to folate deficiency. Disorders and drug treatments associated with defective absorption of folate and abnormal folate metabolism are listed in **Table 5-7**.

5.2 Clinical Findings

Patients with megaloblastic anemia characteristically present with moderate to severe fatigue and malaise of several months' duration. Their skin may be lemon-yellow because of the combined effects of a moderately increased bilirubin level and the marked pallor of the underlying anemia. Because the defective DNA synthesis affects all proliferating cells, such patients experience atrophy of the mucosal surfaces of the tongue, gastrointestinal tract, and vagina. This can cause pain in the mouth and vagina and can lead to secondary malabsorption in the gastrointestinal tract.

Table 5-7 Mechanisms of Folate Deficiency

	Example	Condition/Disorder
Inadequate intake	Dietary deficiency	Alcoholism, drug addiction, poverty
	Inactivation of folate	Overcooking of food
Increased requirement	Growth, development	Pregnancy, lactation, infancy
	States of increased cell turnover	Chronic hemolytic anemias, malignancies
Defective absorption	Defective jejunal mucosa	Sprue, amyloidosis, lymphoma, surgical resection
	Drug-induced malabsorption	Anticonvulsant, antituberculous, oral contraceptive drug therapy, alcoholism
Disorders of metabolism	Suppression or inhibition of metabolic enzymes	Methotrexate, pyrimethamine treatment, alcoholism
		Congenital disorders of folate metabolism, rare

Although the neurologic manifestations of pernicious anemia have been well described, patients with folate deficiency also may rarely develop neuropsychiatric disorders, including irritability, forgetfulness, sleepiness, and depression. Occasionally, patients with folate deficiency manifest peripheral neuropathy similar to that described in patients with vitamin B_{12} deficiency. In pernicious anemia, this peripheral neuropathy is secondary to defective myelin synthesis followed by axonal disruption or degeneration and is insidious in onset, beginning first in peripheral nerves and gradually progressing to involve the posterior and lateral columns of the spinal cord. The clinical manifestations of peripheral nerve involvement include paresthesias, such as numbness and tingling in the hands and feet; decreased vibration sense; and decreased position sense. With progression to spinal cord involvement, the patient may experience ataxia and eventually symmetrical paralysis. If the megaloblastic anemia is untreated, the patient may eventually develop cerebral involvement, which has been called "megaloblastic madness" and is manifested by mental changes, paranoia, and depression.

5.3 Diagnostic Approach

The approach to the diagnosis of megaloblastic anemia includes the following elements:

1. Establishing the presence of a macrocytic anemia
2. Distinguishing between the various causes of macrocytic anemia
3. Determining whether the patient is deficient in vitamin B_{12}, folate, or both vitamins
4. Identifying and treating the underlying disease responsible for the megaloblastic anemia
5. Knowing that neurologic manifestations may predominate in some patients with vitamin B_{12} deficiency in the absence of any hematologic finding

In addition to megaloblastic anemia, peripheral blood macrocytosis may be seen in patients with alcoholism, hypothyroidism, liver disease, reticulocytosis, myelodysplastic disorders, and chemotherapeutic effect. Clinical history and a review of the blood smear help exclude these alternate diagnoses. The clinical history should include questions regarding family history (some rare types of megaloblastic anemia are secondary to hereditary disorders), drug ingestion, intestinal function, diet, occupational exposures, and prior surgical procedures. Evidence of peripheral neuropathy and other neurologic manifestations of vitamin B_{12} or folate deficiency should be assessed by physical examination. Once the diagnosis of megaloblastic anemia has been established, the specific vitamin deficiency causing the anemia must be determined via the laboratory tests discussed in this chapter. Finally, the cause of the vitamin deficiency must be identified and treated appropriately.

5.4 Hematologic Findings

The hematologic findings can be virtually diagnostic in many patients with megaloblastic anemia in whom characteristic abnormalities of erythrocytes and neutrophils can be identified readily. However, in rare cases, the blood of patients with severe vitamin B_{12} deficiency may fail to exhibit substantial erythrocyte or neutrophil abnormalities. In addition, features of megaloblastic anemia may be masked in patients suffering from either concurrent iron deficiency anemia or constitutional microcytic anemia.

5.4.1 Blood Cell Measurements

A patient with megaloblastic anemia typically has a moderate to severe normochromic macrocytic anemia with mean corpuscular volumes (MCVs) ranging from 100 to 150 μm^3 (100 to 150 fL), while the mean corpuscular hemoglobin concentration (MCHC) is normal. Although MCVs at the lower end of this spectrum can be seen in a variety of disorders, a patient with an MCV exceeding 120 μm^3 (120 fL) who is not receiving specific medications such as sulfasalazine is likely to have megaloblastic anemia. Some patients with vitamin B_{12} or folate deficiency have normal MCVs because they also have iron deficiency, inflammatory disorders, or renal failure. Characteristically, the red cell distribution width (RDW) is markedly elevated in megaloblastic anemia because of extreme anisocytosis. Circulating macrocytes are often disrupted, producing minute RBC fragments. The reticulocyte count is very low; in severe cases, the neutrophil and platelet counts also are decreased.

5.4.2 Peripheral Blood Smear Morphology

The peripheral blood smear characteristically contains numerous oval macrocytes as well as schistocytes of various sizes, broken erythrocytes, and spherocytes (**Image 5-1**). RBC fragmentation occurs because of the increased fragility of these large erythrocytes, which probably are damaged during their passage through the spleen. Basophilic stippling and Howell-Jolly bodies also have been seen in RBCs. When the hematocrit value drops below 20% (0.20), nucleated RBCs may be found in the blood. Hypersegmentation of mature neutrophils is a characteristic feature that appears very early in the development of megaloblastic anemia and is a likely reflection of the nuclear maturation defect. Hypersegmentation can be manifested by cells with six or more nuclear lobes or by an elevation in the mean neutrophil lobe count.

5.4.3 Bone Marrow Examination

The bone marrow in patients with megaloblastic anemia is characteristically hypercellular with erythroid and granulocytic hyperplasia. Mitotic activity is abundant, but there is significant intramedullary cell death secondary to the nuclear maturation defect. The proliferating erythroid and myeloid cell lines show megaloblastic changes. In the erythroid elements, the major morphologic manifestation is nuclear-cytoplasmic asynchrony, in which the nuclei are large with finely dispersed chromatin, whereas the cytoplasm is more mature with effective hemoglobinization (*see Image 5-1*). The dominant myeloid abnormality is giantism of bands and metamyelocytes and nuclear hypersegmentation of mature granulocytes. Large megakaryocytes also have been described.

Erythroid megaloblastosis can be masked because of concomitant iron deficiency or other confounding causes of anemia. In patients with such conditions, the peripheral blood and bone marrow erythroid picture may be intermediate between those described for iron deficiency and megaloblastic anemia, although the megaloblastic changes in the granulocytic cell line persist.

Other Laboratory Tests

The primary laboratory tests used in the diagnosis of megaloblastic anemias include measurements of serum vitamin B_{12}, serum folate, and RBC folate. A variety of supplementary tests provide additional sensitivity and specificity in the diagnosis of either vitamin B_{12} or folate deficiency, as well as in determining the likely cause of vitamin B_{12} deficiency, such as pernicious anemia. Some features of primary and ancillary laboratory tests are shown in **Table 5-8**.

Test 5.1 Serum Vitamin B_{12} Quantitation

Purpose. The level of vitamin B_{12} in the blood is a useful measure of the patient's vitamin B_{12} stores.

Principle. Most laboratories currently use a competitive protein binding assay for the determination of serum B_{12} levels. In this assay, a patient's vitamin B_{12} competes with fluorescently labeled B_{12} for a fixed number of binding sites on a solid

Table 5-8 Laboratory Tests for Diagnosis of Megaloblastic
Anemia

Test	Specimen	Procedure
Vitamin B_{12}*	Serum	Competitive protein-binding assay
Folate*	Serum	Competitive protein-binding assay
RBC folate*	Lysed RBCs	Similar to serum folate assay except lysed erythrocytes are used
LDH	Serum/heparinized plasma	LDH catalyzes oxidation of lactate to pyruvate with reduction of NAD to NADH. Absorbance of NADH measured
Iron, IBC	Serum/heparinized plasma	See Chapter 2
IF antibodies	Serum	Competitive protein binding assay
Parietal cell antibodies	Serum	Immunofluorescent test using sections of mouse stomach and appropriate control tissues
Indirect bilirubin	Serum	See Chapter 6
Gastrin	Serum	Competitive protein binding assay
Methylmalonic acid	Serum/plasma/ urine	Gas chromatography-mass spectrometry or high-pressure liquid chromatography
Total homocysteine	Serum/plasma/ urine	Gas chromatography-mass spectrometry or high-pressure liquid chromatography

Abbreviations: IF = intrinsic factor; PA = pernicious anemia; IBC = iron-binding capacity; LDH = lactate dehydrogenase; NAD = nicotinamide adenine dinucleotide; NADH = reduced nicotinamide adenine dinucleotide.

*Test should be performed in all cases of suspected megaloblastic anemia; other tests are helpful in selected clinical settings.

Table 5-8 *Continued*

Interpretation	Notes and Precautions
Decreased in PA and other anemias secondary to vitamin B_{12} deficiency; possible moderate decrease in patient with severe folate deficiency	Low values common in HIV-1 infected patients, may not reflect true deficiency
Decreased in anemias due to folate deficiency; normal or increased in PA	False normal results in some patients with concurrent severe iron deficiency
	Levels fluctuate with diet
	Falsely elevated level with hemolyzed specimen
Because RBCs are metabolically inactive, RBC folate level reflects patient folate status at the time these cells formed; decreased level in folate and vitamin B_{12} deficiency	Because vitamin B_{12} is required for folate to enter cell, level is decreased in either B_{12} or folate deficiency or in combined deficiency
Markedly elevated LDH in megaloblastic anemia due to intramedullary destruction of cells	Hemolysis falsely elevates results
Increased serum iron, storage iron, and IBC in megaloblastic anemias due to decreased iron utilization in erythropoiesis	See Chapter 2
Present in 50% of patients with pernicious anemia	Very specific for PA, present in only 70% of patients
Fluorescence of parietal cells in stomach sections (with negative controls) indicates patient has parietal cell antibodies	Sensitive for PA (positive in 90% of patients) but also found in other disorders
Mildly increased in megaloblastic anemia due to hemolysis of some abnormal RBCs and intramedullary destruction	See Chapter 6
Markedly increased in PA	
Increased in vitamin B_{12} deficiency; normal in folate deficiency	Specialized referral test; highly sensitive and specific; useful in early detection of vitamin B_{12} deficiency
Increased in both vitamin B_{12} and folate deficiency; also increased in some patients with inborn errors of metabolism	Highly sensitive; useful in early detection of deficiency

matrix. The amount of labeled B_{12} that binds is inversely proportional to the patient's vitamin B_{12} levels.

Specimen. Serum is the recommended sample for this test. The specimen must be separated and the test performed within 8 hours of collection; specimen should be frozen if analysis cannot be performed within this time frame.

Procedure. The sample is treated with alkaline potassium cyanide and dithiothreitol to denature B_{12} binding proteins and to convert all forms of vitamin B_{12} to cyanocobalamin. Cyanocobalamin is then immobilized onto a solid substrate by intrinsic factor. A signal is generated using a conjugated monoclonal antibody directed against cyanocobalamin.

Interpretation. Decreased vitamin B_{12} levels are seen in patients with pernicious anemia and all other types of megaloblastic anemia caused by vitamin B_{12} deficiency.

Notes and Precautions. In patients with pernicious anemia and coexisting disease—such as iron deficiency, liver disease, hemoglobinopathy, or myeloproliferative disorders—the vitamin B_{12} level may be normal or even increased. Falsely low levels may be seen in patients with severe folate deficiency, pregnant women, women taking oral contraceptives, and patients with transcobalamin deficiency. Serum vitamin B_{12} levels are often low in patients with HIV-1, although only a small proportion of these patients appear to have a true deficiency. Documentation of a concurrently low RBC folate level enhances the likelihood of true vitamin B_{12} deficiency in this population. Recent dietary supplementation can affect test accuracy.

Test 5.2 **Serum Folate Quantitation**

Purpose. Assays of serum folate, in conjunction with RBC folate, are useful in determining the status of the patient's folate stores.

Principle. Serum folate is currently measured using a competitive protein binding assay analogous to that used for vitamin B_{12}. Using current methodologies, these two assays can be performed simultaneously. The amount of labeled folate that binds to folate binding proteins (FBPs) is inversely proportional to the amount of the patient's folate.

Specimen. Serum is the recommended sample for this test. The specimen must be separated and the test performed within 8 hours of collection; the specimen should be frozen if analysis cannot be performed within this time frame.

Procedure. Multiple analytic platforms exist to measure folate levels. Routine testing has moved from radioactive competitive protein binding assays to chemiluminescence detection technology. In these procedures, the sample is incubated at reaction temperature and the serum specimen combined with either a polyamine solution or a solid substrate containing a folate-binding protein. Both require a subsequent conjugation and binding with a fluorescent substrate. The fluorescent product is measured and is proportional to the concentration of folate in the test sample.

Interpretation. Decreased serum folate levels are detected in patients with megaloblastic anemia secondary to folate deficiency, whereas normal or increased levels of serum folate are found in patients with pernicious anemia.

Notes and Precautions. Because serum folate shows significant fluctuation with diet, a patient can have a normal serum folate level and actually be folate deficient. Folate deficiency also can be masked by a concurrent, more severe iron deficiency in which the serum and RBC folate levels may be within normal limits. The reason for this phenomenon is unknown. Hemolyzed samples give markedly elevated serum folate levels because of the large amounts of folate normally present in erythrocytes.

Test 5.3 **Red Blood Cell Folate Quantitation**

Purpose. RBC folate determination is a more reliable measurement of the status of the patient's folate stores than is serum folate. Because RBCs are metabolically inactive, the RBC folate levels reflect the patient's folate status at the time these cells were produced.

Principle. RBC folate is measured by ion capture assay analogous to that used for measuring serum folate.

Specimen. Whole blood is collected in ethylenediaminetetraacetic acid (EDTA), which can be frozen or processed immediately. RBCs are lysed with ascorbic acid.

Procedure. The procedure for the quantitation of RBC folate is similar to that used for serum folate (see Test 5.2).

Interpretation. Because vitamin B_{12} cofactor is necessary for folate to enter and be retained within RBCs, decreased RBC folate is found in patients with either folate or vitamin B_{12} deficiency. **Table 5-9** compares the serum vitamin B_{12}, serum folate, and RBC folate levels in patients with vitamin B_{12} deficiency, folate deficiency, or both.

5.5 Ancillary Tests

Several additional laboratory tests, including measurements of serum lactate dehydrogenase, bilirubin, serum and storage iron, intrinsic factor antibodies, parietal cell antibodies, gastrin, and deoxyuridine suppression tests can be useful in evaluating patients with megaloblastic anemia. The measurement of metabolites such as methylmalonic acid and total homocysteine are likely to be used more frequently once methodologies are standardized, because of both their high sensitivity in detecting early deficiency and their utility in accurately distinguishing vitamin B_{12} from folate deficiency. The expected values for these tests, along with the reason they are abnormal in megaloblastic anemia, are detailed in Table 5-8.

5.5.1 Parietal Cell and Intrinsic Factor Antibodies

Most patients with pernicious anemia have parietal cell and intrinsic factor antibodies. Although parietal cell antibodies are more sensitive for pernicious anemia, they also are seen fairly frequently in patients with chronic gastritis. Antibodies to intrinsic factor are substantially more specific for pernicious anemia and are present in the majority of patients.

5.5.2 Gastrin Test

Gastrin stimulates parietal cells to secrete intrinsic factor and hydrochloric acid; typically, serum gastrin levels are markedly elevated in patients with pernicious anemia. Recent evidence suggests that some parietal cell antibodies may be directed against the gastrin receptor on these cells, which explains the failure of parietal cells to respond to gastrin. The achlorhydria in gastric juices is secondary to the failure of parietal cells to produce hydrochloric acid; achlorhydria is a further stimulus for gastrin secretion.

Table 5-9   Serum Vitamin B_{12}, Serum Folate, and RBC Folate Levels in Megaloblastic Anemia

Disorder	Serum Vitamin B_{12}	Serum Folate*	RBC Folate
Vitamin B_{12} deficiency	Decreased	Normal or increased	Decreased
Folate deficiency	Normal or mildly decreased	Decreased	Decreased
Deficiency of both vitamin B_{12} and folate	Decreased	Decreased	Decreased

*Fluctuates with changes in dietary folate.

5.5.3 Schilling Test

Although the three-part Schilling test is not used consistently in the initial diagnosis of megaloblastic anemia, it may help to determine the etiology of a megaloblastic anemia in patients with ambiguous results on other tests. The first part of this test measures only the patient's ability to absorb vitamin B_{12}. Intrinsic factor and vitamin B_{12} are given to the patient in the second part of the test; the third part uses antibiotics to destroy bacteria and is designed to detect patients with intestinal bacterial overgrowth disorders. The patient ingests radiolabeled vitamin B_{12}, followed by an injection of a loading dose of unlabeled vitamin B_{12}. A 24-hour urine sample is collected and the amount of radioactivity in this sample is measured. In patients with pernicious anemia, the urinary excretion of labeled vitamin B_{12} is normal only when intrinsic factor is given. Several problems are common in performing the Schilling test. First, the collection of a 24-hour urine sample is cumbersome, and often an incomplete sample is submitted for evaluation. The patient must have normal renal function and normal intestinal mucosa for the test to be valid. In addition, some patients who cannot absorb dietary vitamin B_{12} are able to absorb the crystalline vitamin B_{12} that is used, giving a falsely normal result.

5.5.4 Deoxyuridine Suppression Test

A recently developed test for intranuclear vitamin B_{12} and folate levels, referred to as the "deoxyuridine suppression test", is based on studies of thymidine synthesis. This test of cultured blood lymphocytes, or preferably bone marrow cells, is designed to distinguish between the primary and salvage pathways used in thymidine synthesis. It assesses both vitamin B_{12} and folate levels, because cofactors of both vitamins are required in the primary metabolic pathway of thymidine synthesis. The salvage pathway is favored, however, when a deficiency of either vitamin exists. The primary and salvage pathways can be distinguished by differences in the utilization of a radioactive deoxyuridine substrate. If nucleated blood cells are deficient in either vitamin B_{12} or folate, the salvage pathway is favored, resulting in increased incorporation of radioactive label into cell nuclei. With the addition of the deficient vitamin, the metabolic pathway reverts back to the primary synthetic pathway, and the radioactivity within the nucleus decreases. The nuclei of long-lived cells, such as lymphocytes, can be studied to determine the patient's vitamin B_{12} or folate status at the time these cells were last mitotically active. This information can be useful in selected patients when other test results fail to confirm a vitamin B_{12} or folate deficiency. Recent vitamin or folate therapy does not "mask" this test result, because long-lived cells can be studied.

5.6 Course and Treatment

Correction of the vitamin deficiency by either traditional parenteral injections of vitamin B_{12} or oral doses of folate results in prompt improvement of the patient's hematologic abnormalities, with normalization of the hemogram within 4 to 8 weeks. Recent studies document the efficacy of daily oral vitamin B_{12} therapy in lieu of parenteral therapy. Occasionally, patients with folate deficiency need parenteral therapy until the gastrointestinal tract epithelium has regenerated. Patients with megaloblastic anemia should be evaluated carefully to determine the underlying cause of the vitamin deficiency.

Because the slow development of the anemia allows for some compensation, patients with megaloblastic anemia usually do not require transfusion; however, rare patients may present with cardiovascular decompensation requiring immediate treatment. Transfusion in this clinical situation must be considered carefully owing to the possibility of further cardiac decompensation and death secondary to volume overload. Plasmapheresis with RBC infusions may prevent volume overload. Another cardiac complication that occurs in small numbers of patients receiving treatment for megaloblastic anemia is cardiac arrhythmia, which may result in sudden death. The postulated mechanism for this catastrophic complication is the precipitous decrease in potassium level that occurs following vitamin B_{12} therapy. Patients with megaloblastic anemia undergoing therapy also may develop thrombotic complications because of changes in platelet activity associated with restoration of normal vitamin B_{12} or folate levels in platelets.

Following vitamin therapy, there is a rapid and marked decline in the lactate dehydrogenase and plasma iron levels, as well as a normalization of the serum bilirubin level. The megaloblastic changes in bone marrow erythroid precursors revert to normal within several days of treatment, followed by reversal of the megaloblastic changes within myeloid precursors a few days later. Reticulocytes can be identified in the peripheral blood within 3 to 5 days after treatment is begun, and they generally peak within 7 to 10 days. The height of the reticulocyte count is inversely proportional to the degree of anemia. All peripheral blood parameters return to normal within 1 to 2 months.

In patients with pernicious anemia, the neurologic manifestations of this disorder generally improve substantially with vitamin B_{12} therapy, although they may not resolve entirely. There should be no progression of these neurologic defects, however, while the patient continues to receive vitamin B_{12} therapy. In patients with pernicious anemia, large doses of folate can reduce the hematologic abnormalities, but the neurologic disease still progresses.

Prognosis is good for patients with megaloblastic anemia, provided the vitamin deficiency is adequately treated and the underlying disorder that led to the vitamin deficiency is identified and managed appropriately.

5.7 Acknowledgments

The author is grateful to Anicia Limmany, MT, ASCP, and Michael Crossey, MD, of TriCore References Laboratories for compilation and advice on the laboratory testing methodologies in this chapter.

5.8 **References**

Carmel R. Ethnic and racial factors in cobalamin metabolism and its disorders. *Semin Hematol*. 1999;36:88–100.

Chanarin I, Deacon R, Lumb M, et al. Cobalamin-folate interrelations. *Blood Rev*. 1989;3:211–215.

Green R. Metabolite assays in cobalamin and folate deficiency. *Baillieres Clin Haematol*. 1995;8:533–566.

Green R, Miller JW. Folate deficiency beyond megaloblastic anemia: hyperhomocysteinemia and other manifestations of dysfunctional folate status. *Semin Hematol*. 1999;36:47–64.

Koury MJ, Horne DW, Brown ZA, et al. Apoptosis of late-stage erythroblasts in megaloblastic anemia: association with DNA damage and macrocyte production. *Blood*. 1997;89:4617–4623.

Kuzminski AM, Del Giacco EJ, Allen RH, et al. Effective treatment of cobalamin deficiency with oral cobalamin. *Blood*. 1998;92:1191–1198.

Remacha AF, Cadafalch J. Cobalamin deficiency in patients infected with the human immunodeficiency virus. *Semin Hematol*. 1999;36:75–87.

Rosenblatt DS, Whitehead VM. Cobalamin and folate deficiency: acquired and hereditary disorders in children. *Semin Hematol*. 1999;36:19–34.

Rothenberg SP. Increasing the dietary intake of folate: pros and cons. *Semin Hematol*. 1999;36:65–74.

Toh BH, van Driel IR, Gleeson PA. Pernicious anemia. *N Engl J Med*. 1997;337:1441–1448.

Wickramasinghe SN. The wide spectrum and unresolved issues of megaloblastic anemia. *Semin Hematol*. 1999;36:3–18.

Wickramasinghe SN, Matthews JH. Deoxyuridine suppression: biochemical basis and diagnostic applications. *Blood Rev*. 1988;2:168–177.

Zittoun J, Zittoun R. Modern clinical testing strategies in cobalamin and folate deficiency. *Semin Hematol*. 1999;36:35–46.

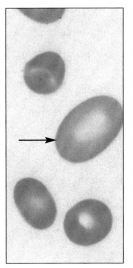 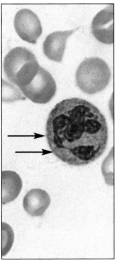 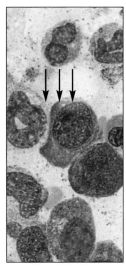

Image 5-1   Composite of blood and bone marrow aspirate smears exhibiting oval macrocytes (one arrow), hypersegmentation of neutrophils (two arrows), and florid megaloblastic erythroid and granulocytic elements (three arrows) in a patient with megaloblastic anemia. (Wright's)

PART II

Hemolytic Anemias

6 Accelerated Erythrocyte Turnover

Hemolysis is characterized by premature removal of circulating RBCs and increased bone marrow production of replacement cells without an overt source of blood loss. This pattern of accelerated erythrocyte turnover is associated with a wide variety of hereditary and acquired hemolytic diseases (**Table 6-1**) that are discussed further in succeeding chapters.

6.1 Pathophysiology

In general, the life span of the RBC comprises three components: the bone marrow production phase, the circulating phase, and final removal of senescent or damaged cells. Establishing a diagnosis of hemolysis requires evaluation of the various phases of the erythrocyte life cycle to demonstrate accelerated RBC turnover.

RBCs arise from a bone marrow stem cell and require approximately 6 days to differentiate from erythroblast to marrow reticulocyte. The daily production of RBCs is estimated at 3×10^9 cells per kilogram of body weight, which normally equals the rate of RBC destruction (1% per day) in a normal situation. Marrow reticulocytes expel their nuclei before passing through marrow sinusoids into the peripheral blood as circulating reticulocytes. Blood reticulocytes shed all remaining reticular network in the circulation over 1 to 2

Table 6-1   Diseases Associated With Accelerated Erythrocyte Turnover

Inherent Defect in Hemolysis	Result
Hereditary disorders	
Membrane defects	Hereditary spherocytosis, hereditary elliptocytosis
Enzyme defects	G6PD deficiency, pyruvate kinase deficiency, glutathione pathway deficiency, other deficiencies of the pentose pathway
Hemoglobin defects	Amino acid substitutions: hemoglobin S, hemoglobin C, etc; decreased production: thalassemia
Acquired or extrinsic disorders	
Infection	Bacterial: *Clostridium perfringens*
	Protozoal: malaria
	Viral: *Mycoplasma,* infectious mononucleosis
	Physiochemical damage: burns, oxidative and nonoxidative
	Mechanical damage: heart valve prosthesis (aortic), ulcerative colitis, hemolytic-uremic syndrome, TTP, DIC
Drugs	G6PD deficiency, immune complexes
Antibody	Alloantibody: incompatible transfusion, fetal-maternal incompatibility
	Autoantibody: idiopathic, secondary to malignant lymphomas, collagen vascular diseases, viral infections, secondary to drugs
Membrane defects	Paroxysmal nocturnal hemoglobinuria

Abbreviations: G6PD = glucose-6-phosphate dehydrogenase; TTP = thrombotic thrombocytopenic purpura; DIC = disseminated intravascular coagulation.

days to become mature erythrocytes. Mature RBCs circulate for about 120 days and are finally removed from the circulation by reticuloendothelial system activity in the spleen, liver, and bone marrow.

A variety of processes may accelerate RBC destruction (*see Table 6-1*). These may generally be divided into intrinsic defects of the RBC (intracorpuscular defects) or or a process external to the cell that affects it (extracorpuscular defects). Intracorpuscular defects include inherited or acquired abnormalities in RBC shape or size, abnormal membrane characteristics, and hemoglobinopathies; extracorpuscular defects include immune or other physiochemical processes that damage RBCs. Hemolysis may be extravascular (mediated by the spleen and other components of the reticuloendothelial system) or intravascular (direct cell lysis). In extravascular hemolysis, the spleen removes marginally damaged RBCs and the liver removes more severely damaged RBCs. Intravascular hemolysis occurs with the most severe cell damage and is associated with mechanical trauma to cells or damage by toxins, thermal damage, or immune mechanisms.

RBC destruction releases cellular contents of heme, globin, and iron. Heme is broken down into biliverdin, reduced to bilirubin by biliverdin reductase in the reticuloendothelial system, conjugated to soluble monoglucuronides and diglucuronides in the liver, and excreted in the feces as urobilin, urobilinogen, and stercobilinogen. Minimal amounts of the soluble urobilinogen are reabsorbed from the portal circulation and excreted in the urine. Iron released from heme is taken up by reticuloendothelial cells and is recycled for bone marrow synthesis of new RBCs or is stored in the reticuloendothelial cells as ferritin or hemosiderin. The globin peptide chains are degraded to component amino acids that return to metabolic pools. Enzymes such as lactate dehydrogenase (LDH), which are normally present within RBCs, also are released with hemolysis. Accelerated RBC turnover results in increased accumulation of all breakdown products, many of which can be measured with relative ease, providing insight into the degree of hemolysis.

When intravascular hemolysis occurs, free hemoglobin is released into the plasma where it is bound by the α_2-globulin haptoglobin. The haptoglobin-hemoglobin complex is then metabolized directly by the reticuloendothelial system. If the binding capacity of haptoglobin is exceeded, free hemoglobin may be seen in the plasma or urine, resulting in hemoglobinemia and hemoglobinuria. Free hemoglobin also may be bound by transferrin and albumin. Oxidation of the ferrous ion of albumin-heme complexes produces the brown pigment, methemalbumin. Increases in free hemoglobin are not as common in extravascular hemolysis, unless vigorous cell destruction occurs.

6.2 Clinical Findings

A detailed and complete history—including drug ingestion, transfusions, medical conditions, operations (such as insertion of heart valves), or a family history of hemolysis or jaundice—is extremely important in determining the cause(s) of accelerated RBC turnover. This historical information helps to narrow the differential diagnosis of hemolysis, facilitating workup and laboratory testing for the patient. Clinical findings depend on the rate of hemolysis and the ability of the bone marrow to compensate for RBC destruction by increased production. If the bone marrow is able to respond to hemolysis so the hematocrit remains normal or near normal, the patient is said to have a well-compensated hemolytic anemia and symptoms may be minimal. However, in severe hemolysis when the bone marrow is unable to match the loss of RBCs, rapid onset of severe anemia may occur. The most common symptoms of anemia are pallor and fatigue. Fever, chills, and headache may be associated with extensive acute hemolytic episodes. If extensive hemolysis occurs, there is increased evidence of hemoglobin catabolism. As normal metabolic pathways are overwhelmed, hemoglobinemia or hemoglobinuria results. With long-standing hemolysis, pigment gallstones may be formed.

Splenomegaly is variable. Chronic hemolysis may not be associated with splenomegaly, whereas acute hemolysis with increased reticuloendothelial activity may be associated with no to moderate splenic enlargement. Hepatomegaly is less common but is usually associated with long-standing hemolysis, reticuloendothelial hyperplasia, and iron deposition. Lymphadenopathy is not characteristic of hemolytic anemia unless there is an underlying lymphoproliferative disorder. Bone pain, secondary to bone marrow erythroid hyperplasia, may be present with long-standing hemolysis.

6.3 Diagnostic Approach

As previously emphasized, a good history and subsequent physical examination of the patient are essential in determining the cause(s) of accelerated RBC turnover. The historical and physical information may then direct laboratory testing in an efficient and cost-effective manner (**Table 6-2**).

If accelerated RBC turnover is suspected, the rate of compensation can be determined by evaluation of bone marrow production, calculation of circulating RBC survival, and measurement of breakdown products of cell destruction. The following approach

Table 6-2   Laboratory Evaluation of Red Blood Cell
                 Production and Breakdown*

Phases of Life Cycle	Laboratory Tests or Findings
Bone marrow production	**Reticulocyte count**, bone marrow cellularity, ^{59}Fe uptake
Red blood cell circulation	**Hemoglobin/hematocrit**, ^{51}Cr red blood cell survival studies
Red blood cell sequestration	^{51}Cr red blood cell sequestration
Red blood cell breakdown	**Haptoglobin, bilirubin, lactate dehydrogenase,** hemoglobinemia, methemalbumin, bone marrow iron
Excretion	**Hemosiderinuria, hemoglobinuria**

*Boldface indicates most useful tests.

provides laboratory information that allows a diagnosis of accelerated RBC turnover to be made:

1. Peripheral blood smear morphology and RBC indices characterize the anemia. An elevated reticulocyte count indicates accelerated release of new RBCs to the peripheral blood, and nucleated RBCs occasionally may be seen.
2. Bone marrow aspiration, including stains for iron, is useful in documenting accelerated marrow erythroid production. When the cause of anemia is clearly hemolysis (eg, in hemoglobinopathies or RBC membrane defects), bone marrow aspiration may be unnecessary.
3. Hemoglobin breakdown products in the plasma and urine can be measured. Because levels of these compounds increase with rapid destruction of RBCs, they may provide a means for monitoring RBC destruction. Tests for these products and their relative usefulness are summarized in **Table 6-3**. In episodes of acute hemolysis, bilirubin (total and fractionated) and plasma or urine hemoglobin are most commonly measured. In less acute or chronic compensated hemolysis, urine hemosiderin may be a more sensitive indicator of long-term occult RBC degradation. Determination of bilirubin in compensated hemolytic anemia is of limited usefulness. Tests for urobilin and fecal and urine urobilinogen are unsatisfactory and unnecessary.
4. Serum haptoglobin is consumed by the binding of free hemo-

Table 6-3 Urine and Serum Pigments in Accelerated Erythrocyte Turnover

Pigment	Normal Range	Comments
Bilirubin, serum	0.5-2.0 mg/dL (8-34 µmol/L)	Limited significance; jaundice seen >3.0 mg/dL (52 µmol/L); fractionation may not be diagnostic in jaundiced patients
Indirect bilirubin, serum	<0.5 mg/dL (8 µmol/L)	Increased early in hemolysis; physiologic evaluation in hereditary conjugation disorders (Crigler-Najjar syndrome, Gilbert's disease)
Hemoglobin, plasma	10 mg/dL (1.6 µmol/L)	Significant above 50 mg/dL (8 µmol/L), cherry-red plasma >150 mg/dL (24 µmol/L), binds to haptoglobin, transferrin, or albumin
Hemoglobin, urine	None present	Appears after haptoglobin saturation, hematuria must be excluded, myoglobinuria gives false-positive result on dipstick test
Methemalbumin, serum	None present	Qualitative determination by haptoglobin electrophoresis or spectrophotometric measurement

globin released from hemolyzed cells. Thus, falls in haptoglobin levels are indicative of hemolysis.

5. Lactate dehydrogenase is released into the plasma as RBCs are rapidly destroyed. Lactate dehydrogenase–1 (LDH_1) is an isoenzyme found predominantly in RBCs and myocardium. Isoenzyme determinations are useful if the source of total LDH elevation is not clearly from RBCs.

6. Radioisotope tracer studies usually are unnecessary and are rarely used unless other laboratory tests fail to document accelerated RBC turnover in the face of strong clinical suspicion. Radioisotope studies are usually limited to chromium 51 (^{51}Cr)–labeled RBC studies, which estimate survival of circulating RBCs and site of cell sequestration and destruction, and to ferrokinetic studies with iron 59 (^{59}Fe), which is incorporated into precursor erythrocytes and evaluates rate of production,

Table 6-4 Common Screening Tests for Causes of Accelerated Erythrocyte Turnover

Inherent Cause of Hemolysis	Test
Hereditary	
Membrane defects	Red blood cell morphologic studies, osmotic fragility
Enzyme defects	G6PD screening, pyruvate kinase screening
Hemoglobin defects	Hemoglobin analysis, Heinz body test, hemoglobin A_2 and hemoglobin F quantitation
Acquired or extrinsic	
Infection	Red blood cell morphologic studies, malarial smears, blood cultures
Physiochemical—burns	Red blood cell morphologic studies—spherocytes
Mechanical—intravascular fibrin, prosthetic valves	Red blood cell morphologic studies—schistocytes
Drugs—enzyme defect	G6PD screening
Drug-induced antibody	Antibody screening with drug-treated cells
Alloantibody or autoantibody	DAT, serum antibody screening, cold agglutinin titer, Donath-Landsteiner test
Membrane defects—PNH	Acid hemolysis test; sucrose lysis test

Abbreviations: G6PD = glucose-6-phosphate dehydrogenase; DAT = direct antiglobulin test; PNH = paroxysmal nocturnal hemoglobinuria.

site of production, rate of RBC release, and site of sequestration.

7. Ancillary screening tests, as summarized in **Table 6-4**, are used to document the cause of accelerated erythrocyte turnover once its presence has been established. These tests are discussed at greater length in subsequent chapters.

6.4 Hematologic Findings

Accelerated RBC destruction or loss stimulates increased bone marrow production. This results in premature release of bone marrow reticulocytes, which appear on Wright's-stained peripheral smears as polychromatophilic macrocytes. Nucleated RBCs also may be seen in prolonged or severe hemolytic anemia. With increased cellular destruction and a competent bone marrow, the reticulocyte count is persistently elevated. Reticulocytosis varies with severity and duration of hemolysis. Bone marrow production may increase fourfold to sixfold, permitting reticulocyte counts as high as 60% to 70%. Chronic hemolysis may deplete bone marrow levels of folic acid, decreasing the ability of the bone marrow to mount a reticulocytosis adequate for the degree of anemia. In acute blood loss, the reticulocytosis is of brief duration and usually less than 5%.

The spleen may be enlarged as a result of increased phagocytic activity. In some patients, particularly those with hereditary intracorpuscular defects, the liver is also enlarged. Depending on the rate of RBC destruction and the ability of the liver to conjugate and excrete the degradation products, variable degrees of jaundice may be present.

6.4.1 Blood Cell Measurements

Anemia can be mild (hemoglobin, 11.5 g/dL [115 g/L]) to severe (hemoglobin, 2 g/dL [20 g/L]). Mean corpuscular volume (MCV) is 80 to 110 μm^3 (80 to 110 fL) because reticulocytes may produce a mild macrocytosis. An MCV greater than 115 μm^3 (115 fL) suggests macrocytic anemia or (rarely) secondary folate depletion. An MCV less than 70 μm^3 (70 fL) in a normochromic anemia suggests hemolysis is due to hemoglobinopathy or paroxysmal nocturnal hemoglobinuria (PNH).

6.4.2 Peripheral Blood Smear Morphology

Morphologic characteristics generally include polychromatophilia, increased macrocytes, and nucleated RBCs in severe cases. The specific appearance of RBCs is variable, depending on the etiology of RBC turnover. Cells associated with specific causes of hemolysis include:

1. Spherocytes—hereditary spherocytosis, autoimmune hemolytic anemia, ABO fetal-maternal incompatibility, burns
2. Target cells—hemoglobinopathies, liver disease, postsplenectomy
3. Cell fragments—hemolytic-uremic syndrome, thrombotic thrombocytopenic purpura (TTP), disseminated intravascular coagulation (DIC), prosthetic valves

6.4.3 Bone Marrow Examination

The bone marrow is hypercellular with marked normoblastic erythroid hyperplasia. Dyssynchronous nuclear and cytoplasmic maturation due to rapid cell turnover may cause mild dyserythropoiesis or megaloblastoid cells without giant metamyelocytes or other stigmata of vitamin deficiency. If folic acid or vitamin B_{12} are relatively depleted by prolonged rapid turnover, a true megaloblastic cell population may appear. Bone marrow exhaustion with resultant aplasia may eventually result. Special staining of particle smears with acid potassium ferricyanide (Prussian blue) shows increased reticuloendothelial iron. If normoblasts contain stainable iron granules, they are often larger than usual and cover the nucleus. Sideroblastic iron is often increased and may form ring sideroblasts when extensive ineffective erythropoiesis is present. Absence of stainable bone marrow iron in the clinical setting of hemolysis suggests PNH or superimposed iron deficiency.

Other Laboratory Tests

Test 6.1 Serum Bilirubin, Total and Fractionated

Purpose. Increases in indirect bilirubin concurrent with clinical jaundice support the diagnosis of hemolysis.

Principle. Hyperbilirubinemia indicates increased RBC destruction, failure of liver conjugation, or blockage of excretory pathways. In hemolysis, an increased bilirubin load is presented to the liver faster than conjugation can proceed so non–water-soluble (indirect) fraction of bilirubin is increased. In liver failure or obstructive jaundice, conjugation results in direct hyperbilirubinemia.

Specimen. Serum specimens, which are stable for days when refrigerated, are used for this test.

Procedure. Bilirubin levels are measured with an internationally standardized test, generally using the Evelyn-Malloy method or a modification. Bilirubin is coupled with a diazo dye, and the color is quantitated spectrophotometrically at 450 nm at 1 minute. The quick-reacting fraction is considered to be direct (or conjugated) bilirubin. The total bilirubin is measured after the addition of alcohol, and the indirect fraction is calculated by subtracting the amount of direct bilirubin from the total.

Inerpretation. Normal ranges for total bilirubin are 0 to 1.5 mg/dL (0 to 25.65 μmol/L) and less than 0.3 mg/dL (5.13 μmol/L) for indirect bilirubin. Total bilirubin levels greater than 2.5 mg/dL (42.75 μmol/L) are usually associated with clinical jaundice. Bilirubin levels depend on the ability of the liver to compensate for increased levels of heme breakdown products. Initially, more than half the bilirubin is in the indirect or unconjugated fraction. If liver function is adequate, after several days the hepatic rate of glucuronide conjugation increases so direct and indirect fractions are nearly equal, and bilirubin fractionation is no longer diagnostic.

Notes and Precautions. In well-compensated hemolytic anemia, levels of total bilirubin may be less than 3 mg/dL (51.3 μmol/L), and no clinical jaundice is seen. Thus, bilirubin levels should not be used to exclude the diagnosis of accelerated RBC turnover.

In hemolytic disease of the newborn, the lipid-soluble, indirect fraction bilirubin is deposited in the striate nucleus of the brain, producing kernicterus. In the newborn, a shift in conjugation from indirect to direct bilirubin usually occurs at 7 to 10 days as liver function matures. Misleading elevations of indirect bilirubin can be seen in hereditary disorders of conjugation (Crigler-Najjar syndrome, Gilbert's disease) and secondary to steroids found in breast milk that interfere with conjugation of bilirubin (breast milk jaundice).

Test 6.2 **Plasma Hemoglobin Quantitation**

Purpose. Increased plasma hemoglobin indicates acute intravascular hemolysis. Quantitation is useful in sera where other pigments (eg, bilirubin) make interpretation of plasma color uncertain.

Principle. Massive RBC injury results in intravascular hemolysis and release of hemoglobin into the plasma. This is detected macroscopically as pink to cherry-red plasma. Free hemoglobin can be quantitated with a modified benzidine reaction that measures oxidation of benzidine by hydrogen peroxide.

Specimen. Five milliliters of blood is collected in heparin or ethylenediaminetetraacetic acid (EDTA). A clot is not a desirable specimen because mechanical hemolysis of RBCs during clot formation does not allow for the most accurate measurement. Blood must be drawn atraumatically, and plasma should be separated within 1 to 2 hours.

Procedure. Visual inspection of the plasma fraction shows a qualitative pink to red tint. Quantification uses a modified benzidine reaction (see "Notes and Precautions") that oxidizes a colorless benzidine dye to violet-blue in the presence of hemoglobin and hydrogen peroxide. The color is measured spectrophotometrically at 515 nm or with a photoelectric colorimeter. Quantitation often requires a reference laboratory.

Interpretation. The normal level of plasma hemoglobin is less than 10 mg/dL (1.6 μmol/L). At low levels, test variability is great, and thus the test is only reliable above 50 mg/dL (8 μmol/L), which is the threshold for visual detection of pink coloration of the plasma. Free hemoglobin levels less than 30 mg/dL (4.8 μmol/L) are technically inaccurate and may be seen with difficult venipuncture, with mechanical destruction of RBCs by Vacutainer® tubes, or during clotting of the specimen. Hemoglobinemia greater than 150 mg/dL (24 μmol/L) results in hemoglobinuria. At levels above 200 mg/dL (32 μmol/L), the plasma becomes clear cherry red.

Notes and Precautions. Benzidine may not be available as a result of federal regulations limiting potentially carcinogenic agents in the environment. Ortholidine (*o*-toluidine) may be substituted. Spectrophotometric results may be falsely high if the serum contains peroxidases or other oxidants that increase the development of color in the benzidine reaction.

Test 6.3 **Serum Haptoglobin Quantitation**

Purpose. Decreased or absent serum haptaglobin indicates hemolysis. Decreased haptoglobin also may be seen in liver failure or (rarely) as a genetic variant.

Principle. Haptoglobin is an α_2-globulin produced in the liver that binds free hemoglobin on a molecule-for-molecule basis. The haptoglobin-hemoglobin complex is metabolized in the reticuloendothelial system, maintaining serum hemoglobin levels below renal thresholds. During intravascular hemolysis, haptoglobin binding is completely saturated. The excess hemoglobin is then bound by other serum proteins (hemopexin, transferrin, and albumin) before spilling into the urine as hemoglobinuria. Absence of haptoglobin implies binding saturation and degradation. Decreased haptoglobin reflects active hemolysis or, alternatively, failure of production due to liver failure. Rare abnormal haptoglobins (such as Hp⁻) are genetic variants that do not bind hemoglobin but are of little clinical significance.

Specimen. Fresh serum is obtained atraumatically. To avoid extraneous hemolysis, serum should not be allowed to remain on RBCs. Testing specimens with macroscopic hemoglobinemia is superfluous.

Procedure. The haptoglobin molecule has separate sites for antibody and hemoglobin binding. Haptoglobin is quantitated with turbidimetric methods using a nephelometer. Antihaptoglobin is added to the patient's serum, forming immune complexes with serum haptoglobin (1:1). These immune complexes scatter light proportionate to their concentration. Most larger hospitals have nephelometers.

Interpretation. The normal range for haptoglobin is 40 to 180 mg/dL (0.4 to 1.8 g/L). Less than 25 mg/dL (0.25 g/L) of haptoglobin is consistent with active hemolysis. Haptoglobin is an acute phase reactant, increasing three to four times in inflammation, infection, or tissue necrosis (eg, pneumonia or myocardial infarction). Such increases may mask changes in haptoglobin levels secondary to hemolysis. Haptoglobin levels greater than 200 mg/dL (2.0 g/L) are consistent with inflammation and not helpful in the diagnosis of hemolysis.

Molecular sites for hemoglobin binding are not the same as those for antibody binding by antihaptoglobin. With radial immunodiffusion testing, elevations of haptoglobin may be falsely interpreted due to measurement of saturated haptoglobin-hemoglobin complexes that have not been removed by the reticuloendothelial system.

Haptoglobin is decreased or absent in patients with liver failure, after recent massive transfusion due to removal of senescent transfused RBCs, and in some abnormally functioning haptoglobin molecules (eg, Hp⁻).

Test 6.4 **Direct Antiglobulin Test (Direct Coombs' Test)**

Purpose. Detection of globulin adsorbed to the patient's RBCs indicates immune mechanisms may be an underlying cause of hemolysis.

Principle. Rabbit antihuman globulin reagent agglutinates human RBCs that are coated with human globulin. Broad-spectrum reagents agglutinate cells coated with IgG, IgM, and/or complement. Monospecific serums agglutinate only RBCs coated with the specific globulin (ie, IgG, IgM, or complement) to which the reagent is directed.

Specimen. Use of the RBCs from EDTA specimens prevents non-specific absorption of complement in specimens. Specimens must be maintained at 37°C until cells and serum have been separated.

Procedure. The patient's RBCs are washed with saline and centrifuged with antiglobulin reagent. Agglutination is graded from 0 to 4+. The adsorbed globulin must be eluted and tested for activity against RBCs before it is classified as an antibody.

Interpretation. Weakly positive results (+/−) usually are not clinically significant and eluates are generally unsuccessful. Strongly positive tests (2 to 4+) due to antibody may not correlate with the degree of hemolysis. Common causes of positive direct antiglobulin tests (DATs) not associated with hemolysis include multiple myeloma, systemic lupus erythematosus (SLE), AIDS, and cephalosporin therapy. A negative DAT result does not exclude hemolysis if RBC destruction has been massive and complete, as in incompatible transfusions.

Notes and Precautions. Refrigeration of blood specimens containing cold agglutinins may cause false-positive results or exaggerated positive results by nonspecific cold adsorption of the agglutinin and complement.

Test 6.5 **Other Serum Pigments**

Principle. For the most part, measurement of methemalbumin is unnecessary for documentation of hemolysis; however, it may be useful in specialized cases. The presence of methemalbumin indicates chronic or continuing hemolysis and may be used as a marker of hemolysis. This is particularly true in patients with hemolysis induced by overconsumption of oxidizing agents. Free hemoglobin dissociates into α and β dimers and binds to plasma proteins, including haptoglobin, transferrin, and albumin. The ferrous iron of hemoglobin bound to albumin oxidizes to ferric iron, forming methemalbumin, which gives a distinctive rusty appearance to serum. Free hemoglobin in the presence of chloride ion produces hematin, which is bound by the protein hemopexin. Tests for methemalbumin are available in reference laboratories. Methemalbumin is not present in a healthy patient and clears within 4 or 5 days of the cessation of hemolysis. Tests for hemopexin are not generally available. Hemopexin has a normal range of 80 to 100 mg/dL (0.8 to 1.0 g/L). Levels less than 40 mg/dL (0.4 g/L) indicate hemolysis.

6.5 Ancillary Tests

6.5.1 Urine Hemoglobin and Hemosiderin

Hemoglobinuria indicates concurrent or recent hemoglobinemia above the renal excretion threshold of 150 mg/dL (1.5 g/L). It usually appears as cloudy, smoky, dark-red, or cola-colored urine. It may be detected qualitatively by peroxidase reaction of o-toluidine or benzidine, which produces a blue color. In the absence of detectable hemoglobin, urine hemosiderin indicates ongoing hemolysis. Even in occult hemolysis, heme is deposited in renal epithelial cells and oxidized to hemosiderin.

In a healthy patient, no urinary hemoglobin or hemosiderin is detectable. Urinary sediments that contain significant numbers of RBCs usually produce some free hemoglobin in hypotonic or alkaline urines. False-positive results may be seen with hematuria or myoglobinuria. Hemosiderin granules must be intracellular to have significance.

6.5.2 Total Lactate Dehydrogenase

Lactate dehydrogenase increases with either normal or pathologic cell destruction as RBC cytoplasmic glycolytic enzymes, including LDH, are released to the plasma. Total LDH is usually measured with spectrophotometric kinetic analysis of the reduced form of nicotinamide adenine dinucleotide (NADH) production. Serum LDH catalyzes the reaction:

$$Lactate + NAD \rightleftharpoons Pyruvate + NADH$$

Because NADH absorbs light at 340 nm, LDH activity can be detected spectrophotometrically by increasing absorbance.

6.6 Laboratory Test Selection

Documentation of accelerated RBC turnover usually may be made on the basis of peripheral blood smear morphology, RBC indices, reticulocyte count, possible bone marrow examination, serum haptoglobin levels, and demonstration of elevation of hemoglobin breakdown products such as serum bilirubin, plasma or urine hemoglobin, or urine hemosiderin. Other tests, such as radioisotopic studies, are rarely required.

Evaluation of the mechanism underlying accelerated RBC turnover may make use of many different laboratory tests, depending on the etiology of the process. By obtaining a good clinical history and physical examination, test selection can be streamlined and directed to document the cause of hemolysis in a cost-efficient and logical manner. Thus, patients with a family history of hemolysis may undergo workup for heritable disorders of the RBC membrane or hemoglobin synthesis, whereas these tests may not be chosen in an elderly patient with acute onset of hemolysis, no family history, and recent onset of generalized lymphadenopathy and splenomegaly.

6.7 References

Erslev AJ, Buetler E. Production of erythrocytes. In: Beutler E, Coller BS, Kipps TJ, et al, eds. *Williams Hematology*. 5th ed. New York, NY: McGraw-Hill; 1995:425–440.

Hillman RS, Finch CA. *Red Cell Manual*. 7th ed. Philadelphia, Pa: FA Davis; 1996.

Lee GR. Hemolytic disorders: general considerations. In: Lee GR, Foerster J, Lukens JN, et al, eds. *Wintrobe's Clinical Hematology*. 10th ed. Baltimore, Md: Williams & Wilkins; 1999:1109–1131.

7 Hereditary Erythrocyte Membrane Defects

Hereditary abnormalities in RBC shape include hereditary spherocytosis and hereditary elliptocytosis (ovalocytosis) These are usually secondary to inheritance of abnormal integral proteins underlying the RBC membrane, which maintain cellular shape, membrane stability, or cellular flexibility. Abnormalities in these proteins may lead to premature hemolysis, as in hereditary spherocytosis, or may have little effect on RBC life span, as in most cases of hereditary elliptocytosis.

7.1 Pathophysiology

The RBC membrane is composed of a lipid bilayer with associated proteins overlying and linked to a protein network, called the "membrane cytoskeleton". This structural configuration gives the RBC enough flexibility to squeeze through capillaries without fragmentation, yet regain a stable biconcave shape in larger vessels without loss of cellular integrity. The membrane cytoskeleton is formed by interactions of a number of proteins, including spectrin, actin, ankyrin, and a protein termed "band 4.1."

Hereditary spherocytosis is the most common type of hereditary hemolytic anemia among individuals of northern European origin, but it occurs in all races throughout the world. It is seen in about 1 in 5000 individuals in the United States. The inheritance is autosomal dominant. Therefore, it is to be expected that one of the patient's parents is affected and that each of the patient's children will have a 50% chance of inheriting the disorder. In this disease, a primary defect in membrane stability is caused by a quantitative decrease in the amount of spectrin or, more rarely, by formation of an abnormal spectrin that does not interact with other proteins within the RBC skeleton. Spherocytes are less flexible than normal RBCs, leading to retention within the spleen. This causes accelerated loss of cellular membrane to form the characteristic spherocytes and premature cellular destruction.

Hereditary elliptocytosis is a heterogeneous group of disorders characterized by the presence of elliptocytes in the peripheral blood smear. These represent RBCs that have failed to regain their normal biconcave shape following passage through the microcirculation. A wide variety of RBC membrane skeletal defects have been associated with hereditary elliptocytosis, including dysfunctional spectrin molecules, decreased spectrin content, and band 4.1 defects or deficiency. Unlike patients with hereditary spherocytosis, 90% of patients with hereditary elliptocytosis do not experience clinically significant hemolysis. Hereditary elliptocytosis is usually inherited as an autosomal dominant trait.

7.2 Clinical Findings

The chronic hemolytic state in hereditary spherocytosis varies widely in severity, ranging from an asymptomatic compensated hemolysis to a moderately severe chronic anemia. The age at which the diagnosis is made usually reflects the severity of the hemolytic process, with the more severe forms of the disease being diagnosed in early childhood. Clinical manifestations usually are first noted in children or adolescents. Typical complaints include mild jaundice and nonspecific manifestations of anemia, such as weakness. Because of an increased bilirubin turnover, patients with this condition have a high incidence of pigment gallstones. Usually, patients can maintain normal hemoglobin levels owing to increased RBC production by the bone marrow. However, infection or other stress may lead to acute anemic episodes due to increased splenic activity (hemolytic crisis) or decreased bone marrow production (aplastic crisis). The most consistently positive physical finding is splenomegaly, which may be marked. Variable degrees of jaundice and scleral icterus are frequently seen. The most consistent and therapeutically important feature of hereditary spherocytosis is the clinical cure by splenectomy of hemolytic anemia. RBC life span after this procedure is restored to normal or near normal.

Hereditary elliptocytosis may present either as a primary cosmetic disorder with little or no hemolysis or, much more rarely, with a moderately severe hemolytic anemia. Patients with the usual form of hereditary elliptocytosis have no anemia or splenomegaly. The hemolytic forms of the disease, composing about 10% of cases, may have splenomegaly and often show spherocytes and fragmented RBCs, in addition to elliptocytes, in the peripheral blood smear.

7.3 Diagnostic Approach

A diagnosis of hereditary spherocytosis should be suspected in patients with chronic hemolytic anemia, especially when spherocytes are seen in the peripheral blood smear. Because of the autosomal dominant inheritance of the disorder, family studies are an important part of the diagnostic evaluation. Sometimes examination of the blood of family members reveals spherocytosis, even when there is no history of anemia, jaundice, or gallstones. This reflects the spectrum of disease observed in hereditary spherocytosis in some affected individuals. On rare occasions, the disorder may arise as a new mutation without a positive family history.

Splenectomy abolishes the hemolysis in hereditary spherocytosis. If significant hemolysis persists after splenectomy in a patient presumed to have hereditary spherocytosis, the presumptive diagnosis is incorrect or not all splenic tissue has been removed. Evaluation of a patient presumed to have hereditary spherocytosis includes the following:

1. Hematologic evaluation, with attention to RBC morphologic characteristics, the mean corpuscular hemoglobin concentration (MCHC), and the reticulocyte count.

2. An osmotic fragility test (see Test 7.1) to confirm the presence of spherocytosis.

3. A direct antiglobulin test (see Test 6.4) to rule out autoimmune hemolytic anemia as a cause for spherocytosis.

4. If the diagnosis is in doubt, estimation of RBC glycolytic or hexose monophosphate shunt enzyme activities (see Chapters 8 and 9).

Elliptocytes are readily identified on the stained blood film (**Image 7-1**). Because this generally represents a benign anomaly, hereditary elliptocytosis should only be considered the cause of anemia when evidence for hemolysis, such as an elevated reticulocyte count, is found.

7.4 Hematologic Findings

7.4.1 Blood Cell Measurements

Hemoglobin levels in patients with hereditary spherocytosis and hemolytic elliptocytosis frequently range between 9 and 12 g/dL (90 and 120 g/L), and the mean corpuscular volume (MCV) is usually in the normal range but may be elevated in the presence of prominent reticulocytosis. The MCHC in hereditary spherocytosis is characteristically elevated to levels as high as 37 g/dL (370 g/L) (normal, 26 to 34 g/dL [260 to 340 g/L]), due to membrane loss without loss of cellular hemoglobin. The reticulocyte count usually ranges between 5% and 15% (0.05 and 0.15). The degree of reticulocytosis in hereditary spherocytosis is characteristically greater than that in other hemolytic anemias with similar hemoglobin levels.

7.4.2 Peripheral Blood Smear Morphology

The central morphologic finding in hereditary spherocytosis is the presence of spherocytes on the peripheral blood film. Spherocytes appear as densely staining RBCs that are slightly smaller than normal with an absence of central pallor (**Image 7-2**). The increased intensity of staining is partially caused by increased cellular thickness due to the spherical shape and the increased MCHC. In mild forms of the disease, spherocytes may not be present in large numbers. The appearance of RBCs varies in different parts of the blood smear. Improper technique in preparing the smear may result in what appear to an inexperienced observer as artifactual spherocytes in portions of the blood smear that are too thin for proper evaluation. Prominent macrocytosis and polychromasia may be present in association with very high reticulocyte counts. Elliptocytosis is diagnosed when most or all of the cells on the smear have an oval shape with a long diameter that is two or more times the short diameter (*see Image 7-1*).

7.4.3 Bone Marrow Examination

The bone marrow characteristically shows normoblastic erythroid hyperplasia when significant hemolysis occurs. During aplastic crises, erythroid precursors are diminished and evidence of viral infection, such as parvovirus B19, may be seen.

Other Laboratory Tests

Test 7.1 Osmotic Fragility Test

Purpose. The osmotic fragility test indirectly measures the presence of spherocytes.

Principle. This test measures the ability of the RBC to swell, a property that reflects the cellular surface-to-volume ratio. In a hypotonic medium, RBCs take up water until the osmotic pressure inside the cell is reduced to that outside the cell. The RBC membrane normally has enough redundancy so the volume of the cell can increase to about 1.8 times the resting volume before reaching the critical hemolytic volume where further entry of water produces lysis. A cell that is spherocytic in the resting state has less membrane redundancy than a normal biconcave cell, so less water can enter before cellular rupture occurs.

Specimen. Blood freshly drawn into heparin or ethylenediaminetetraacetic acid (EDTA) is used. Samples older than 48 hours may show an artifactual shift toward increased fragility.

Procedure. The osmotic fragility test is performed by adding small volumes of blood to a series of tubes containing buffered salt

Table 7-1 Normal Values for Osmotic Fragility Tests

	Lysis (%)	
NaCl (%)	Fresh	Incubated
0.20	97-100	95-100
0.30	97-100	85-100
0.35	90-99	75-100
0.40	50-90	65-100
0.45	5-45	55-95
0.50	0-5	40-85
0.55	0	15-70
0.60	0	0-40
0.65	0	0-10
0.70	0	0-5
0.75	0	0

solutions with an osmolarity equivalent to that of a 0.2% to 0.9% sodium chloride (NaCl) solution. A control tube contains distilled water. After standing at room temperature for 1 hour, the tubes are centrifuged, and the percentage of hemolyzed cells is estimated by measuring the amount of hemoglobin released into the supernatant solution by absorbance at 540 nm.

The tests should be carried out on freshly drawn blood and, if necessary, on blood that has been incubated at 37°C for 24 hours. Incubated osmotic fragility tests are more sensitive for detecting low levels of hemolysis. This may be useful when hereditary spherocytosis is suspected clinically but the levels of hemolysis seen with fresh blood are within normal ranges. However, the increase in sensitivity for detection of osmotic fragility is offset by a loss of specificity in the incubated test.

Interpretation. The normal range of values for the osmotic fragility test is seen in **Table 7-1** and **Figure 7-1**. Increased osmotic fragility is an essential diagnostic feature of hereditary spherocytosis. In mild forms of the disease, however, it is not uncommon to find only a minimal increase in osmotic fragility on freshly drawn blood. Incubated osmotic fragility tests are almost always abnormal in such cases. Decreases in hemolysis

Figure 7-1 Osmotic fragility testing. Osmotic fragility of normal
RBCs and those from a patient with hereditary spherocytosis. Normal areas are shown in the shaded
areas for fresh RBCs (A and B) and for RBCs incubated at 37°C for 24 hours (C and D). The hemolysis
curve for control or normal RBCs is shown in panels
A and C. The hemolysis curve for a patient with
hereditary spherocytosis is represented in panels B
and D.

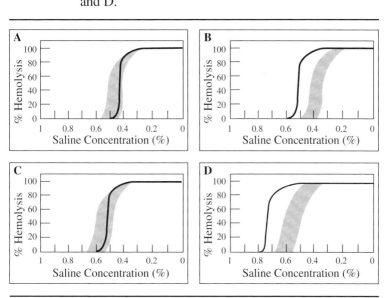

or decreased osmotic fragility are seen in thalassemia, iron
deficiency, and other conditions where there is an increase in
the surface area-to-volume ratio for the RBC.

Notes and Precautions. Because increased osmotic fragility merely reflects the presence of spherocytes, this finding does not
distinguish hereditary spherocytosis from autoimmune
hemolytic disease with spherocytosis, in which the osmotic
fragility of RBCs is also increased, although to a lesser degree.
Reporting osmotic fragility as percent saline concentrations for
beginning and completion of hemolysis is an inadequate representation of test results. Osmotic fragility is best appreciated
when reported graphically (*see Figure 7-1*).

7.5 Course and Treatment

Both hereditary spherocytosis and elliptocytosis are essentially benign disorders. Complications that may occur include the development of cholelithiasis and cholecystitis and the occurrence of aplastic or hemolytic crises, particularly after infection. Splenectomy prolongs RBC survival in hereditary spherocytosis and hemolytic forms of elliptocytosis. However, this may not be required if the bone marrow can compensate for the anemia by increasing RBC production.

7.6 References

Cynober T, Mohandes N, Tchernia G. Red cell abnormalities in hereditary spherocytosis: relevance to understanding of the variable expression of clinical severity. *J Lab Clin Med*. 1996;128:259–269.

Delaunay J. Genetic disorders of the red cell membranes. *FEBS Lett*. 1995;369:34–37.

Hassoun H, Palek J. Hereditary spherocytosis: a review of the clinical and molecular aspects of the disease. *Blood Rev*. 1996;10:129–147.

Palek J, Jarolim P. Hereditary spherocytosis, elliptocytosis and related disorders. In: Beutler E, Coller BS, Kipps TJ, et al, eds. *Williams Hematology*. 5th ed. New York, NY: McGraw-Hill; 1995:536–556.

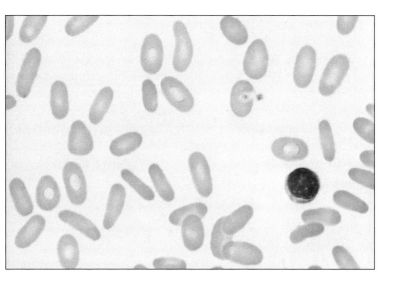

Image 7-1 Elliptocytes.

Image 7-2 Spherocytes apparent as round RBCs without central pallor.

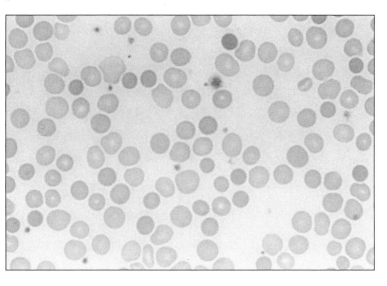

8   Hereditary Erythrocyte Disorders Due to Deficiencies of the Glycolytic Pathway

Mature RBCs have the capacity for a limited number of enzymatic reactions. Thus, the majority of a cell's energy requirements are met by metabolism of glucose to lactate via the glycolytic, or Embden-Meyerhof, pathway. Hereditary deficiencies of some of the glycolytic enzymes have been documented, and several of these deficiencies cause a hereditary nonspherocytic hemolytic anemia (HNSHA), whereas others cause multisystemic disease. Most glycolytic pathway enzymatic deficiencies are rare, with only a few thousand cases documented in the literature. Pyruvate kinase deficiency is the most common and comprises 90% of affected patients.

8.1 Pathophysiology

Glucose is the main metabolic substrate of RBCs. Because the mature erythrocyte does not contain mitochondria, it must depend entirely on anaerobic glycolysis to produce energy. About 90% of glucose metabolism occurs by way of the main glycolytic pathway, in which glucose is metabolized to lactate in a series of enzymatic reactions that give rise to adenosine triphosphate (ATP) and reduced nicotinamide-adenine dinucleotide (NADH) (**Figure 8-1**). There is a net generation of 2 moles of ATP for each mole of glucose that is metabolized. Adenosine triphosphate is essential to the cell, allowing active cationic transport across the cellular membrane and membrane protein phosphorylation. One mole of NADH is generated, which functions in methemoglobin reduction reactions. 2,3-Diphosphoglycerate (2,3-DPG), which alters the hemoglobin oxygen affinity and regulates oxygen delivery to tissues, is another important intermediate formed during glycolysis.

The remaining 10% of glucose is metabolized via the hexose monophosphate (HMP) shunt, bypassing the early steps of the main glycolytic pathway and generating reduced nicotinamide adenine dinucleotide phosphate (NADPH). This coenzyme is required for reduction of glutathione, which is essential to protect hemoglobin and RBC enzymes from oxidative damage (see Chapter 9).

Deficiencies in glycolytic pathway enzymes give rise to hereditary nonspherocytic hemolytic anemia, which is characterized by hemolytic anemia first observed during infancy or childhood that lacks significant numbers of spherocytes, and exhibits normal osmotic fragility. Hereditary nonspherocytic hemolytic anemia may result from a heterogeneous group of disorders. The most important disorders clinically are the glycolytic pathway enzyme deficiencies (**Table 8-1**). Although the exact cause of hemolysis in glycolytic defects is unknown, it is postulated to be secondary to abnormal membrane function and development of irreversible membrane damage. Because reticulocytes retain some mitochondria, they are relatively resistant to hemolysis. Depending on the intracellular levels of ATP, RBC life span may range from near normal to markedly shortened. Other observed causes of HNSHA include the unstable hemoglobins and disorders of the enzymes of the HMP shunt and glutathione metabolism (**Table 8-2**).

8.2 Clinical Findings

Most cases of HNSHA manifest in childhood or infancy with chronic hemolysis, often associated with splenomegaly, some degree of hyperbilirubinemia, and increased reticulocytes. In contrast

Figure 8-1 The glycolytic pathway (Embden-Meyerhof pathway). The enzymes in which a deficiency may lead to a hereditary nonspherocytic hemolytic anemia are underlined.

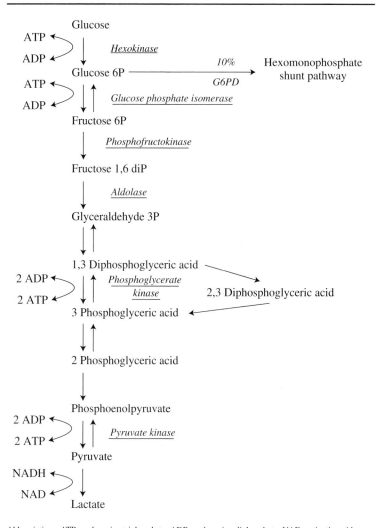

Abbreviations: ATP = adenosine triphosphate; ADP = adenosine diphosphate; NAD = nicotinamide-adenine dinucleotide.

to deficiencies of the HMP shunt, there is no association of anemia with drug ingestion. Patients with phosphoglycerate kinase (PGK) deficiency or aldolase deficiency also may have neurologic manifestations associated with the disease.

Table 8-1   Deficiencies of the Glycolytic Pathway Causing Hemolytic Anemia

Enzyme	Mode of Inheritance	Clinical Manifestation
Hexokinase	AR	Mild to severe HNSHA
Glucose-phosphate isomerase	AR	Moderate to severe HNSHA
Phosphofructokinase	AR	Mild HNSHA, possible myopathy
Aldolase	AR	Mild to moderate HNSHA, possible pyschomotor retardation
Phosphoglycerate kinase	X-linked	Mild to severe HNSHA, retardation, neurologic deficits
Pyruvate kinase	AR	Moderate to severe HNSHA

Abbreviations: AR = autosomal recessive; HNSHA = hereditary nonspherocytic hemolytic anemia.

Most deficiencies of the glycolytic pathway are extremely rare. Pyruvate kinase deficiency, although seen infrequently, is the most prevalent, accounting for about 90% of cases of glycolytic pathway deficiency–associated HNSHA. Pyruvate kinase and most other glycolytic pathway deficiencies are inherited as autosomal recessive traits. Thus, a patient must be homozygous for the trait to be fully expressed. An exception to the autosomal recessive inheritance pattern is PGK deficiency, which is inherited as an X-linked disorder (*see Table 8-1*).

Pyruvate kinase or other glycolytic pathway deficiencies usually are first detected in infancy or later in childhood because of chronic anemia, jaundice, development of pigment gallstones, and slight to moderate splenomegaly due to RBC sequestration. The severity of the anemia and other clinical manifestations is widely variable. Often hemolysis is worsened by infection or other stresses. Severely affected individuals are often jaundiced and anemic at birth, requiring repeated transfusions. Because of increased hematopoietic demand or accelerated hemolysis, infections may give rise to an aplastic crisis or more severe anemia. Individuals affected to a lesser degree may have mild to moderate hemolysis that may or may not require transfusions.

Table 8-2   Defects Associated With Hereditary Nonspherocytic Hemolytic Anemia

---

Enzymatic deficiencies
    Glycolytic pathway: most common
    Hexose monophosphate shunt pathway: rare variants
    Glutathione pathway: rare variants
    Hemoglobinopathies
Unstable hemoglobins

8.3 Diagnostic Approach

In the autosomal recessive forms of HNSHA, the family history is usually negative unless siblings are affected. Biochemical studies of family members, however, reveal the hereditary nature of the disorder by demonstrating subnormal levels of an enzyme, although usually this is not sufficient to cause significant anemia. A child or infant presenting with a chronic hemolytic anemia must first be evaluated for possible nonheritable causes. This usually involves a direct antiglobulin test (Coombs' test; see Test 6.4) to rule out an autoimmune hemolytic process and a sucrose lysis test (see Test 11.1) to rule out paroxysmal nocturnal hemoglobinuria.

If the anemia is thought to be a hereditary process, it is usually next classified as either a nonspherocytic or spherocytic process. This is usually accomplished by evaluation of the peripheral blood smear for spherocytes. An osmotic fragility test (see Test 7.1) will also help rule out hereditary spherocytosis. If the anemia is thought to be an HNSHA, hemoglobin electrophoresis (see Test 10.1) to rule out the hemoglobinopathies and an isopropanol stability test (see Test 10.8) to identify unstable hemoglobins may be performed. Finally, screening tests for deficiencies of specific enzymes such as glucose-6-phosphate dehydrogenase (G6PD; see Tests 9.1 and 9.2) and pyruvate kinase (Test 8.1) may be performed, followed by appropriate quantitative RBC enzyme assays to determine the specific nature of the enzymatic defect.

8.4 Hematologic Findings

There are varying degrees of anemia, with hemoglobin levels ranging from 5 to 12 g/dL (50 to 120 g/L). Reticulocytosis proportional to the severity of the anemia is present (up to 25% or higher) but may be increased to more than 50% after splenectomy. Mean corpuscular volume (MCV) may be moderately increased when reticulocytosis is present. In most cases the morphologic characteristics of the RBCs are unremarkable. Cells are normocytic and normochromic, but when there is extensive hemolysis, reticulocytosis may be macrocytic with polychromatophilia. Rare spicular and densely staining RBCs or nucleated RBCs may be present. Heinz bodies and spherocytes are notably absent. Basophilic stippling of RBCs is prominent in pyrimidine-5´-nucleotidase deficiency.

Other Laboratory Tests

Test 8.1 Fluorescent Screening Test for Pyruvate Kinase Deficiency

Purpose. Fluorescence of NADH acts as a useful screening test for the detection of RBC enzyme deficiencies. In practice, it is often enough to know whether the activity of the enzyme in question is markedly deficient. Slight deviations from normal are unlikely to be of clinical importance.

Principle. Reduced pyridine nucleotides (NADH) fluoresce when illuminated with long-wave ultraviolet light, whereas no fluorescence occurs with oxidized pyridine nucleotides, providing an indicator of enzymatic activity. Screening procedures are available for pyruvate kinase, glucose-phosphate isomerase, NADH diaphorase triosephosphate isomerase, and G6PD (see Chapter 9). Pyruvate kinase screening is the most common screening test for a glycolytic pathway deficiency.

Pyruvate kinase catalyzes the phosphorylation of adenosine diphosphate (ADP) to ATP by phosphoenolpyruvate (PEP). This reaction is coupled with the NADH-dependent conversion of pyruvate to lactate:

$$PEP + ADP \xrightarrow{\text{pyruvate kinase}} Pyruvate + ATP$$

$$Pyruvate + NADH + H^+ \xrightarrow{\text{lactate dehydrogenase}} Lactate + NAD^+$$

Because lactate dehydrogenase (LDH) is present in excess of pyruvate kinase, NAD^+ production is limited by pyruvate kinase levels. Thus, there should be a time-dependent loss of fluorescence as NADH is oxidized to NAD^+ when normal levels of pyruvate kinase activity are present.

Specimen. Whole blood collected in heparin or ethylenediaminetetraacetic acid (EDTA) is suitable for several days at 4°C and for about 1 day at room temperature.

Procedure. The blood sample is centrifuged; the plasma and buffy coat are aspirated. The RBC suspension is lysed by a buffered hypotonic screening mixture. The screening mixture provides PEP, ADP, NADH, and magnesium chloride ($MgCl_2$). It is spotted on filter paper immediately after mixing and every 15 minutes thereafter. After the spots are thoroughly dry, the paper is examined under long-wave ultraviolet light. The patient's sample is compared with that of a healthy control subject.

Interpretation. The first spot should fluoresce brightly. With the normal sample, fluorescence disappears after 15 minutes of incubation. In contrast, in pyruvate kinase–deficient samples, fluorescence fails to disappear even after 45 or 60 minutes of incubation.

Notes and Precautions. False-negative results may be observed if the patient has recently received a transfusion and large numbers of transfused cells containing normal levels of pyruvate kinase are still circulating. There may be little relationship between the severity of hemolysis and the measured level of pyruvate kinase activity to different stabilities of the pyruvate kinase variants or the degree of reticulocytes. Some patients with high reticulocyte counts may have normal screening tests.

Test 8.2 **RBC Enzyme Activity Assays**

Purpose. Quantitative RBC enzyme assays give definitive confirmation of the results of screening tests and allow detection of heterozygotes for possible genetic counseling.

Principle. Most of the quantitative assays of RBC enzyme activity use spectrophotometric techniques that depend on the absorption of light of the reduced pyridine nucleotide, NADPH, or NADH at 340 nm. Reduction results in the formation of NADPH or NADH, with an increase in absorbance at 340 nm, and oxidation results in the formation of NADP or NAD with a decrease in absorbance. The change in absorbance may be used to calculate enzyme activity.

Specimen. Blood is collected in EDTA, heparin, or acid-citrate-dextrose (ACD). Most RBC enzymes are stable for several days at 4°C under these conditions. The blood should not be allowed to freeze, because washed RBCs are used for the enzyme assays, and the stability of RBC enzymes is usually lower in hemolysates than in intact cells.

Procedure. The procedure for each enzyme measurement is different, and all procedures usually require specialized reference laboratories.

Interpretation. Interpretation differs for each enzyme. In general, only very severe enzyme deficiencies cause hemolytic anemia. Even relatively severe deficiencies of some enzymes, such as LDH, glutathione peroxidase, and inosine triphosphate, are without known clinical effect.

Test 8.3 Molecular Identification of Enzyme Defects

Purpose. Molecular analysis provides definitive evidence of an enzymatic defect and may provide information useful in genetic counciling.

Principle. Analysis of DNA sequences may identify the specific molecular defect giving rise to an enzyme deficiency.

Specimen. Bone marrow is collected in heparin, and DNA is isolated for molecular detection of enzyme deficiencies. This methodology is best used for pyruvate kinase defects.

Procedure. DNA is analyzed by Southern blot test and mutational analysis gels to identify functional mutations in the pyruvate kinase gene.

Interpretation. Pyruvate kinase is encoded for two genes that give rise to four distinct isoforms of the enzyme. More than 50 different mutations have been identified as causes of hemolytic anemia. Most are missense mutations that give rise to abnormal proteins. Some nonsense or splicing mutations also have been identified.

Notes and Precautions. The molecular tests for glycolytic pathway enzymopathies are highly specialized and require laboratories that have experience with this testing methodology and interpretation. Many are still considered investigational rather than diagnostic tools.

8.5 Ancillary Tests

Osmotic fragility testing (see Test 7.1) may serve as a useful screen for identifying hereditary spherocytosis and autoimmune hemolytic anemia with spherocytosis, whereas no increase in osmotic fragility is seen in HNSHA. The isopropanol stability test (see Test 10.8) is used to screen for unstable hemoglobins.

8.6 Course and Treatment

The course of nonspherocytic hemolytic anemia varies widely. Severe pyruvate kinase deficiency may require splenectomy early in life; response to such treatment is variable. Other patients have a mild, benign course. Genetic counseling and prenatal diagnosis is possible for most defects.

8.7 References

Baronciani L, Bianchi P, Zanella A. Hematologically important mutations: red cell pyruvate kinase. *Blood Cells Mol Dis*. 1996;22:85–89.

Beutler E. Red cell enzyme defects. *Hematol Pathol*. 1990;4:103–114.

Fairbanks VF, Klee GG. Biochemical aspects of hematology. In: Burtis CA, Ashwood ER, eds. *Tietz Textbook of Clinical Chemistry*. 3rd ed. Philadelphia, Pa: Saunders; 1999:1642–1710.

Glader BE, Lukens JN. Hereditary hemolytic anemias associated with abnormalities of erythrocyte glycolysis and nucleotide metabolism. In: Lee GR, Foerster J, Lukens JN, et al, eds. *Wintrobe's Clinical Hematology*. 10th ed. Baltimore, Md: Williams & Wilkins; 1999:1160–1175.

Jacobasch G, Rapoport SM. Hemolytic anemias due to erythrocyte enzyme deficiencies. *Mol Aspects Med*. 1996;17:143–170.

Lakomek M, Winkler H. Erythrocytic pyruvate kinase and glucose phosphate isomerase deficiency: perturbation of glycolysis by structural defects and functional alterations of defective enzymes and its relation to the clinical severity of chronic hemolytic anemia. *Biophys Chem*. 1997:66:269–284.

Miwa S, Fujji H. Molecular basis of erythroenzymopathies associated with hereditary anemia: tabulation of mutant enzymes. *Am J Hematol*. 1996;51:122–132.

Tanaka KR, Zerez CR. Red cell enzymopathies of the glycolytic pathway. *Semin Hematol*. 1990;27:165–185.

Weatherall DJ. ABC of clinical heamatology: the hereditary anaemias. *Br Med J*. 1997;314:492–496.

9   Hereditary Disorders of the Hexose Monophosphate Shunt: Glucose-6-Phosphate Dehydrogenase Deficiency

About 10% of the RBC glucose is metabolized by the hexose monophosphate (HMP) oxidative shunt. This pathway is essential to protect the cell against oxidative injury and acts to reduce nicotinamide-adenine dinucleotide phosphate (NADP) to NADPH. The latter is an essential reducing agent in circulating RBCs, allowing for detoxification of oxidated metabolic intermediates and maintenance of the RBC membrane. Glucose-6-phosphate dehydrogenase (G6PD) catalyzes the first step of the pathway. Deficiency of this enzyme is the most prevalent inborn metabolic disorder affecting RBCs, afflicting more than 400 million people worldwide, and is an important cause of inheritable hemolytic anemia.

9.1 Pathophysiology

The HMP shunt produces NADPH by a series of enzymatic reactions (**Figure 9-1**). In turn, NADPH is used as a cofactor for glutathione reductase (GR) to regenerate oxidized glutathione (GSSG) into a reduced state. Normally, RBCs make use of reduced glutathione (GSH) to detoxify low levels of oxygen radicals that form

Figure 9-1 Hexose monophosphate shunt.

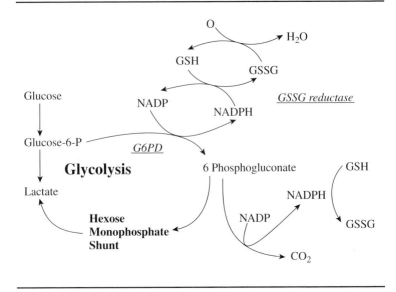

spontaneously or as a result of drug administration, as well as to reduce oxidized sulfhydryl groups of hemoglobin, membrane proteins, or cellular enzymes. RBCs deficient in G6PD are unable to maintain sufficient levels of GSH, thereby impairing the cells' ability to deal with toxic insults or oxidative stress. This leads to integral membrane damage and the accumulation of oxidized cellular products in the form of Heinz bodies. This ultimately leads to premature RBC lysis in the spleen and development of hemolytic anemia. Most patients with G6PD deficiency have episodic anemia induced by infection or drug administration that creates oxidative stress. A minority of patients may have a chronic nonspherocytic hemolytic anemia.

Deficiency of G6PD results from the inheritance of an abnormal G6PD enzyme located on the X chromosome. More than 30 different mutations that give rise to a variety of clinical diseases have been described. Normally, there are two isotypes of G6PD, termed A and B, which can be distinguished by electrophoretic mobility. The B isoform is the most common type of enzyme found in all population groups. The G6PD A isoform, found in about 20% of black men in the United States, migrates more

Table 9-1   Common G6PD Variants

G6PD Variant	Association With Hemolysis	Affected Population
G6PD A	No: normal variant	Blacks
G6PD B	No: normal variant	All
G6PD A$^-$	Yes: moderate	Blacks
G6PD^{MED}	Yes: severe	Whites
G6PD^{CANTON}	Yes: moderate	Asians
G6PD^{IOWA}	Yes: severe, chronic	Sporadic mutation

Abbreviation: G6PD = glucose-6-phosphate dehydrogenase.

rapidly on electrophoretic gels than does the normal B enzyme. However, it has similar enzymatic activity to the B isoform and is not associated with disease. More than 400 other G6PD protein variants have been identified (**Table 9-1**). Up to 11% of U.S. black men have a G6PD variant (G6PD A$^-$) that has the same electrophoretic mobility as G6PD A, but it is unstable, resulting in enzyme loss and ultimate enzyme deficiency as the RBC ages. Thus, older circulating RBCs from individuals with this variant may contain only 5% to 15% of the normal amount of enzymatic activity. G6PD A$^-$ is the most common clinically significant type of abnormal G6PD among the U.S. black population. Other G6PD variants predominate in other racial groups; G6PD Mediterranean (G6PD^{MED}) is found frequently in Sicilians, Greeks, Sephardic Jews, and Arabs. Several other variants, such as G6PD^{CANTON} or G6PD^{MAHIDOL}, are common in Asian populations. The population distribution of G6PD deficiency reflects its probable origins in tropical and subtropical areas and possible increased resistance to malarial infection.

The G6PD gene is encoded on the X chromosome, leading to a sex-linked inheritance pattern. Thus, the effect is fully expressed in affected men, who carry only one X chromosome and inheritance is from the mother. In women, only one of the two X chromosomes in each cell is active. Consequently, women who are heterozygous for G6PD deficiency may have two populations of RBCs: deficient and normal cells. The ratio of deficient to normal cells may vary greatly as a result of the intrinsic variability of X-chromosome inactivation. Some women who are heterozygous for

Table 9-2 Enzyme Deficiencies of Hexose Monophosphate Shunt Pathway Clearly Associated With Hemolytic Anemia

Enzyme Deficiency	Occurrence
G6PD	Common
γ-Glutamylcysteine synthetase	Rare
GSH synthetase	Rare
Glutathione reductase (total deficiency only)	Rare

Abbreviations: G6PD = glucose-6-phosphate dehydrogenase, GSH = reduced glutathione.

the disease appear to be completely healthy, whereas others are fully affected.

Deficiencies of other enzymes in the HMP shunt and glutathione metabolism are comparatively rare (**Table 9-2**). Hereditary RBC GSH deficiency results from a lack of either of two enzymes of GSH synthesis: γ-glutamylcysteine synthetase or GSH synthetase. In some patients, the clinical manifestation of these deficiencies is similar to that of G6PD deficiency; others present with a chronic hemolytic anemia. Dietary deficiencies of flavin adenine dinucleotide (FAD), which is a cofactor for GSSG reductase, may cause a decrease in enzymatic activity that mimics GSSG reductase deficiency but may be remedied by dietary manipulation. Actual GSSG reductase deficiency is rare. Other HMP shunt deficiencies are rarely or never associated with hemolytic anemia.

9.2 Clinical Findings

A G6PD deficiency usually manifests as an episode of acute hemolysis following infection or ingestion of an oxidant drug in an otherwise apparently healthy person. Hemolysis begins acutely in the case of infection or within 1 to 3 days after administration of an oxidant drug (**Table 9-3**), leading to plasma hemoglobinemia (pink to brown plasma), hemoglobinuria (dark or black urine), and jaundice. Rare patients may have a clinical picture of chronic hemolysis or be asymptomatic.

Table 9-3 Drugs Commonly Associated With Hemolysis in Glucose-6-Phosphate Dehydrogenase

Antimalarial agents
    Primaquine
    Quinacrine
Sulfonamides
    Sulfanilamide
    Salicylazosulfapyridine
    Sulfacetamide
Other antibacterial agents
    Nitrofurantoin
    Nitrofurazone
    Para-aminosalicylic acid
    Nalidixic acid
Analgesics
    Acetanilid
Sulfones
    Diaminodiphenyl sulfone
    Thiazolsulfone
Miscellaneous agents
    Dimercaprol
    Naphthalene (mothballs)
    Methylene blue
    Trinitrotoluene (TNT)

In G6PD A$^-$ deficiency, the hemolytic anemia is usually self-limited because the young RBCs produced in response to hemolysis have nearly normal G6PD levels and are relatively resistant to hemolysis. In contrast, other types of G6PD deficiency, such as G6PD^{MED}, where there are decreased levels of the enzyme in all RBCs, may cause severe hemolysis, requiring transfusion therapy. Other stresses that may precipitate acute hemolytic anemia in people who are severely G6PD deficient are the neonatal state and exposure to fava beans. Rare cases presenting as hereditary non-spherocytic hemolytic anemia also are associated with G6PD deficiency (**Table 9-4**). The World Health Organization (WHO) has classified different G6PD variants based on the degree of enzyme deficiency and severity of hemolysis (**Table 9-5**). Only the Class I, II, and III variant groups are clinically significant, with Classes II and III being most common.

Table 9-4   Clinical Features of G6PD Variants

Clinical Feature	G6PD A⁻	G6PD^MED	G6PD^CANTON
Drug-induced hemolysis	Common	Common	Common
Infection-induced hemolysis	Common	Common	Common
Favism	Not seen	Common	Not usually seen
Neonatal icterus	Rare	Observed	Observed
Hereditary nonspherocytic hemolytic anemia	Not seen	Occasionally	Not seen
Degree of hemolysis	Moderate	Severe	Moderate
Chronic hemolysis	Not seen	Not seen	Not seen

Abbreviation: G6PD = glucose-6-phosphate dehydrogenase.

9.3 Diagnostic Approach

The occurrence of episodic hemolysis suggests that a patient may be suffering from hereditary deficiency of one of the HMP enzymes. Patients with the most common type of G6PD deficiency present with acute hemolytic anemia. In such cases, a careful history regarding ingestion of drugs or infections is important. Other causes of episodic anemia include paroxysmal nocturnal hemoglobinuria (see Chapter 11), parasitic infections such as malaria, and unstable hemoglobins (see Chapter 10). When the hemolytic nature of the episodes is less apparent, particularly in cases associated with infection, differential diagnosis includes an aregenerative crisis that may occur in any of the severe hereditary anemias. In neonatal icterus, fetal-maternal Rh or ABO incompatibility must be ruled out (see Chapter 13).

9.4 Hematologic Findings

The severity of the anemia is extremely variable. The hemoglobin concentration in the blood may be near normal or as low as 5 g/dL (50 g/L). Examination of the peripheral blood smear usually does not show a distinctive RBC appearance. Heinz bodies, particles of denatured hemoglobin and membrane proteins, adhere to the

Table 9-5   Clinical Classification of G6PD Deficiency

Class	Enzyme Levels	Clinical Presentation
I	Very severe deficiency (<10% normal)	Chronic hemolytic anemia
II	Severe deficiency	Intermittent hemolysis associated with drugs or infection
III	Moderate deficiency (10%-60% normal)	Intermittent hemolysis associated with drugs or infection
IV	Very mild or no enzyme deficiency	No hemolysis
V	Increased enzyme levels	

Abbreviation: G6PD = glucose-6-phosphate dehydrogenase.

membrane and may be seen initially on supravitally stained preparations used for the enumeration of reticulocytes or with crystal violet staining. They are not seen on Wright- or Giemsa-stained smears. As hemolysis progresses, Heinz bodies disappear, presumably due to splenic removal or hemolysis. Bite cells and RBCs with irregularly contracted hemoglobin on one side (eccentrocytes) may be seen. At the beginning of the hemolytic episode, the reticulocyte count may be normal, but if the episode has been underway for several days, the reticulocyte count is usually elevated according to the degree of anemia. Slight macrocytosis may be seen if reticulocytes are present; otherwise, RBC indices are normocytic and normochromic. The WBC count may be low, normal, or elevated because of granulocytosis.

Other Laboratory Tests

Test 9.1   **Fluorescent Screening Test for G6PD Activity**

Purpose. The fluorescent screening test that detects formation of NADPH, which fluoresces under UV light, is highly reliable for the detection of both severe and mild types of G6PD deficiency in men who are not experiencing an active episode of hemolysis. It is best used as an initial screening mechanism.

Principle. Whole blood or blood hemolysates contain the enzymes of the HMP shunt. In the presence of $NADP^+$, G6PD is oxidized to form 6-phosphogluconate and NADPH. 6-Phosphogluconate dehydrogenase (6-PGD) gives rise to additional NADPH by the following reaction:

$$6\text{-Phosphogluconate} + NADP^+ \xrightarrow{\text{6-PGD}} \text{Ribulose-5-P} + NADPH + H^+$$

When G6PD activity is low, only a small amount of NADPH is formed. In the presence of GSSG, provided in the screening mixture, NADPH is reoxidized in the glutathione reductase reaction to $NADP^+$.

Whereas NAPDH may be detected fluorescently, $NAPD^+$ does not fluoresce. The screening test measures the difference between G6PD and 6-PGD activity (which forms NADPH) and glutathione reductase activity (which consumes NADPH).

Specimen. Blood collected in heparin, ethylenediaminetetraacetic acid (EDTA), acid-citrate-dextrose (ACD), or citrate-phosphate-dextrose (CPD) anticoagulants is satisfactory. Blood stored at 4°C for 1 week, or even spots of blood collected on filter paper and dried, may be used.

Procedure. Whole blood is added to a buffered screening solution containing saponin, glucose-6-phosphate, $NAPD^+$, and GSSG. After incubation for 5 or 10 minutes at room temperature, the mixture is spotted on filter paper, allowed to dry, and observed for NADPH fluorescence under long-wave UV light. In patients with G6PD A$^-$ who have had a recent episode of hemolysis, the test may be modified by centrifuging the blood sample in a microhematocrit tube and using the bottom 10% of the RBC column (representing the reticulocyte-poor, enzyme-deficient cell fraction) for the test.

Interpretation. Normal samples show a bright fluorescence after 5 or 10 minutes of incubation, whereas deficient samples show no fluorescence. No false-positive or false-negative test results are observed. In severe G6PD^{MED} or a similar type deficiency in which even young cells have very low levels of G6PD, a screening test suffices for diagnosis, even in the presence of a severe hemolytic reaction. In patients with

G6PD A⁻ and ongoing or acute hemolysis, however, the remaining young cells and reticulocytes have normal or near-normal G6PD activity, and most of the enzyme-deficient cells may have been removed from the circulation. Diagnosis of G6PD deficiency under these circumstances can be accomplished either by repeating the test in 2 or 3 weeks or by modifying the test using reticulocyte-poor fractions, as previously noted. Heterozygotes may not be detected with the latter method. Recent blood transfusions also may invalidate the results.

Notes and Precautions. Because G6PD is sex-linked, women who are heterozygous for G6PD deficiency have two RBC populations in which some RBCs are grossly deficient and others are normal. Although the deficient cells are susceptible to hemolysis, the enzymatic activity, as measured on hemoly-sates, may be normal, intermediate, or low. The extent of deficiency is a function of the proportion of normal and deficient cells in the particular patient. Special methods for the detection of individual cell G6PD activity may be used to help detect heterozygosity. Leukocytosis ($>12 \times 10^9$ cells/L) may cause spuriously normal results due to leukocyte G6PD activity. In such cases, the use of washed, leukocyte-poor RBCs may be warranted.

Test 9.2 **Quantitative G6PD Assay**

Purpose. In men who are not experiencing hemolysis, the G6PD fluorescent screening test is generally adequate for diagnosis, but quantitative enzyme assays may be useful in identifying deficiencies in patients who have had an episode of hemolysis and women with heterozygous disease.

Principle. Formation of NADPH from NADP⁺ from G6P is measurable by a change in absorbance created by NADPH. The rate of increase of optical density that occurs with the formation of NADPH from NADP⁺ in blood hemolysates is measured at 340 nm in a spectrophotometer.

Specimen. Blood collected in EDTA or ACD solution is satisfactory. The G6PD activity is stable for several weeks at 4°C and for several days at room temperature. The blood should not be allowed to freeze, because enzymatic activity is rapidly lost when RBCs are lysed.

Procedure. The final assay mixture contains 100 mmol/L tris(hydroxymethyl)aminomethane (TRIS) with 0.5 mmol/L EDTA buffer (pH 8.0); 10 mmol/L $MgCl_2$; 0.2 mmol/L NADP; and 0.6 mmol/L G6P. The reaction is started by the addition of the G6P, with water being substituted for G6P in the blank cuvette. The change in fluorescence at 340 nm is used with the hemoglobin concentration to calculate the G6PD activity by the following formula:

$$G6PD = \frac{804 \times \Delta \text{ Absorbance 304 nm/min}}{\text{Hemoglobin concentration (g/100 mL)}}$$

Interpretation. Normal levels of G6PD are 8 to 18 units per gram of hemoglobin. The quantitative assay for G6PD activity may reveal the presence of G6PD deficiency even in patients who have had a recent episode of hemolysis. Because G6PD levels may vary with RBC age, activity should be increased in a patient with reticulocytosis. Normal or slightly lower than normal G6PD activity in such a patient implies that G6PD deficiency is present. Enzyme activity in women with heterozygous disease may be below the normal range.

Notes and Precautions. This assay measures the activity of both G6PD and 6-PGD, because the product of the G6PD reaction, 6-phosphogluconolactone, is converted rapidly to the substrate for the 6-PGD reaction. In practice, this causes no difficulty because no hemolytic anemia has been associated with deficiency of 6-phosphogluconic acid and normal levels of this enzyme do not mask G6PD deficiency. Note the precaution in the diagnosis of heterozygosity discussed under Test 9.1.

Test 9.3 Heinz Body Test

Purpose. Deficiency of G6PD, as well as other rarer enzyme deficiencies, or unstable hemoglobin types are associated with increased numbers of Heinz bodies. This finding supports the diagnosis of drug-induced hemolysis.

Principle. The oxidative pathway of glycolytic RBC enzymes maintains hemoglobin stability. In G6PD deficiency, as well as deficiencies of glutathione synthetic enzymes, or in the presence of unstable hemoglobins, oxidation leads to hemoglobin denaturation. The denatured hemoglobin precipitates, forming Heinz bodies. Normal RBCs can be induced to form Heinz bodies; G6PD-deficient cells produce three or four Heinz bodies per RBC in the presence of oxidant drugs.

Specimen. Fresh whole blood is collected in EDTA.

Procedure. Crystal violet or neutral red is added to a few drops of blood. Wet mount smears are prepared from the mixture after 15 minutes, 30 minutes, or 1 hour of incubation at room temperature. RBCs also can be incubated with phenylhydrazine before preparation of the smears to exaggerate the findings in G6PD deficiency.

Interpretation. Heinz bodies are seen as particles located close to the cellular membrane, ranging in size from 1 to 3 μm. Normal cells may produce a single marginal Heinz body. After phenylhydrazine incubation, G6PD-deficient cells may have three to four Heinz bodies in every cell. If abrupt hemolysis has occurred, the test results may be negative because of hemolysis of the Heinz body–positive cells.

Test 9.4 Reduced Glutathione Determination

Purpose. RBC GSH levels are often decreased in patients with HMP shunt or GSH synthetic pathway deficiencies.

Principle. Almost all RBC nonprotein sulfhydryl groups are in the form of reduced GSH. The dithiol compound, dithio-bis-nitrobenzoic acid (DTNB), is reduced by GSH to form a yellow anion, the optical density of which is readily measured at 412 nm. The absorbance is directly proportional to GSH concentration.

Specimen. Whole blood collected in heparin, EDTA, or ACD solution may be used. The GSH levels remain unaltered for 3 weeks in ACD solution or for 1 day in EDTA or heparin at 4°C.

Procedure. In this procedure, 0.2 mL of whole blood is added to 1.8 mL of distilled water. To lyse the cells, 3 mL of a metaphosphoric acid EDTA–sodium chloride precipitating solution is added, and the mixture is filtered. Then 2 mL of the filtrate is added to 8 mL of 0.3 mol/L Na_2HPO_4 solution, 1 mL of DTNB reagent is added, and the optical density is read at 412 nm.

Interpretation. The normal RBC glutathione concentration is 4.5 to 8.7 μmol/g (47 to 100 mg/dL) of hemoglobin. A severe deficiency of glutathione results from a genetic defect in one of the two enzymes of glutathione synthesis: γ-glutamylcysteine synthetase or glutathione synthetase. Modest reductions of GSH levels and marked instability to challenge by oxidative agents (such as seen with incubation of 1-acetyl 1-2-phenylhydrazine in the incubation mix for 2 hours at 37°C) is found in G6PD-deficient RBCs. Elevated levels of RBC glutathione are found in patients with myeloproliferative disorders and in those with pyrimidine-5´-nucleotidase deficiency.

Notes and Precautions. Virtually all of the protein-free DTNB reducing activity in RBCs is due to glutathione. Because DTNB is reduced readily by other sulfhydryl compounds, such as cysteine, the degree of specificity varies from tissue to tissue.

9.5 Ancillary Tests

In patients with severe glutathione deficiency, it is desirable to measure the activities of γ-glutamylcysteine synthetase and glutathione synthetase. Assay of these enzymes is a relatively difficult radiometric procedure that is best performed by specialized laboratories. Precise identification of the G6PD variants requires electrophoresis, kinetic studies, and other biochemical techniques.

9.6 Course and Treatment

Infants with G6PD deficiency and neonatal icterus may require exchange transfusions. Adult patients with G6PD deficiency should avoid the ingestion of fava beans and oxidative types of drugs. Splenectomy is not usually useful in patients with G6PD deficiency associated with nonspherocytic hemolytic anemia.

9.7　References

Beutler E. G6PD: population genetics and clinical manifestations. *Blood Rev.* 1996;10:45–52.

Fairbanks VF, Klee GG. Biochemical aspects of hematology. In: Burtis CA, Ashwood ER, eds. *Tietz Textbook of Clinical Chemistry*. 3rd ed. Philadelphia, Pa: Saunders; 1999:1642–1710.

Glader BE, Lukens JN. Glucose-6-phosphate dehydrogenase deficiency and related disorders of hexose monophosphate shunt and glutathione metabolism. In: Lee GR, Foerster J, Lukens JN, et al, eds. *Wintrobe's Clinical Hematology*. 10th ed. Baltimore, Md: Williams & Wilkins; 1999:1176–1190.

Mason PJ. New insights into G6PD deficiency. *Br J Haematol*. 1996;94:585–591.

Miwa S, Fujji H. Molecular basis of erythroenzymopathies associated with hereditary hemolytic anemia. *Am J Hematol*. 1998;51:122–132.

Ristoff E, Larsson A. Patients with genetic defects in the gamma-glutamyl cycle. *Chem Biol Interact*. 1998;112:113–121.

10 Disorders of Hemoglobin Synthesis

Hemoglobin is a tetrameric protein composed of four globin poly-peptides complexed with four heme groups. Abnormalities in hemoglobin synthesis are either qualitative (formation of an abnormal hemoglobin molecule at a normal or near-normal rate) or quantitative with a resultant decrease in the amount of hemoglobin synthesized, as in thalassemias.

10.1 Pathophysiology

The normal adult RBC contains predominantly hemoglobin (Hb) A, which is composed of two alpha and two beta globin chains ($\alpha_2\beta_2$). Two other minor hemoglobins found in adults are HbA_2, in which the β chains are replaced by delta chains to form $\alpha_2\delta_2$, and HbF, in which the β chains are replaced by gamma chains ($\alpha_2\gamma_2$) (**Table 10-1**). At birth, HbF is the predominant type of hemoglobin. Within the first year of life, it is largely replaced by HbA to reflect the adult proportions of approximately 97% HbA, 2% HbA_2, and 1% HbF. HbA_{1c} is a minor hemoglobin that is formed by post-translational addition of glucose to the terminal of the HbA beta

Table 10-1 Hemoglobin Types Found in a Healthy Adult

Hemoglobin Type	Globin Chains	% Total Hemoglobin
HbA	$\alpha_2\beta_2$	>95
HbA$_2$	$\alpha_2\delta_2$	≤3.5
HbF	$\alpha_2\gamma_2$	1

chains. HbA_{1c} is found in increased amounts in patients with diabetes mellitus.

Each globin chain (alpha, beta, gamma, and delta) has its own autosomal genetic locus. Qualitative alterations in these globin chains occur via genetic mutations of one of the chains, usually resulting in substitution of a single amino acid. The abnormal hemoglobin chains that are formed may or may not alter the functional characteristics of the hemoglobin. If the hemoglobin structural abnormality gives rise to clinical manifestations, the patient is said to have a "hemoglobinopathy". The most common hemoglobinopathies are beta chain mutations and include HbS, HbC, and HbE (**Table 10-2**). These variants may appear as heterozygous or homozygous defects.

Hemoglobin variants were initially differentiated primarily by their electrophoretic mobility and were assigned as names (ie, HbC, HbE). Later, when an additional hemoglobin variant with the same mobility was discovered, the new variant was distinguished by following the letter previously ascribed to that mobility with the place of discovery of the new variant. Finally, if the exact amino acid structure of a hemoglobin variant was determined, a designation that characterized the amino acid substitution was indicated by a superscript to the involved globin chain (eg, for HbS, $\alpha_2\beta_2^{6\text{-glutamic acid}\rightarrow\text{valine}}$ indicates a mutation changing the glutamic acid at position six in the beta chain to a valine).

When abnormal hemoglobin is synthesized, the clinical manifestations are often determined by the amount of variant present. This is determined by whether the abnormal hemoglobin is inherited as a heterozygous or homozygous state. Homozygous inheritance is associated with more severe manifestations. Sickle cell anemia or sickle cell disease refers to the homozygote for HbS, whereas sickle cell trait is the heterozygous state. The word "disease" is used for homozygote with hemoglobin variants (eg, homozygous HbC disease or HbCC), whereas "trait" refers to the heterozygotes (eg, HbC trait or HbAC). The descriptor "disease" is

Table 10-2 Amino Acid Substitutions in the Beta Chains of Common Hemoglobin Variants

Hemoglobin	Position	Amino Acid Substitution
HbS	6	Glutamic acid → valine
HbC	6	Glutamic acid → lysine
HbE	26	Glutamic acid → lysine

also applied to the HbS heterozygous state in association with other hemoglobin mutations when significant clinical findings are associated with the combination (eg, sickle cell–HbC disease). When letter designations are used for the hemoglobins in heterozygous hemoglobinopathies, the first letter refers to the preponderant hemoglobin found in the RBC. Thus, "HbAS" indicates that the concentration of HbA exceeds that of HbS in the RBCs of that particular heterozygous variant.

Mutations that decrease or prevent the synthesis of one of the globin chains cause quantitative decreases in structurally normal hemoglobin production. This gives rise to thalassemia syndromes. Thalassemias are classified according to the chain affected, the most common being α-thalassemia and β-thalassemia. The α-thalassemias are most commonly caused by the deletion of one or more of the four alpha globin genes. The β-thalassemic disorders are usually due to genetic mutations that affect RNA synthesis, processing, or stability so that decreased levels of normal hemoglobin are formed. β-Thalassemias are classified as either minor (heterozygous) or major (homozygous). Combined disorders involving the structural variants and thalassemias also are seen, the most common being sickle β-thalassemia disease.

10.2 Clinical Findings

10.2.1 Hemoglobin Disorders Caused by Abnormal Globin Chains

Mutations involving the globin protein genes are usually amino acid substitutions. These may produce pronounced changes in the functional properties of hemoglobin, including solubility and oxygen affinity (**Table 10-3**).

Table 10-3   Functional Classification of Abnormal Hemoglobins

Type of Abnormality	Functional Effect	Clinical Disorder	Examples
Qualitative Disorders			
Solubility	Aggregation of hemoglobin	Hemolytic anemia	Hemoglobin S, hemoglobin C
Oxidative susceptibility	Oxidative denaturation	Hemolytic anemia	Unstable hemoglobin
Increased oxygen affinity	Decreased oxygen to tissues	Erythrocytosis	Unstable hemoglobin
Decreased oxygen affinity	Premature oxygen release	Cyanosis/anemia	Unstable hemoglobin
Abnormal heme reduction	Inability to carry oxygen	Cyanosis	Methemoglobin
Quantitative Disorders (Thalassemias)			
Alpha chains	Decreased alpha chains	Range from mild anemia to hydrops fetalis	α-thalassemia
Beta chains	Decreased beta chains	Mild to severe hemolytic anemia	β-thalassemia
Beta and delta chains	Decreased beta and delta chains	Thalassemialike syndrome	δ-β-thalassemia
Combined Disorders			
Abnormal hemoglobin and thalassemia	Decreased chain production with altered solubility	Often milder than homozygous structural disorder	Hemoglobin S thalassemia

The most common clinically significant hemoglobinopathy causing changes in hemoglobin solubility is HbS. The heterozygous sickle trait is generally considered to be an entirely benign disorder, although hematuria may occur on rare occasions. The homozygous disorder, sickle cell anemia, is characterized by moderately severe hemolysis and painful crises resulting from occlusion of blood vessels by the abnormal RBCs, which assume a sickle shape due to hemoglobin polymerization. When the gene for HbS is inherited with the gene for certain other abnormal hemoglobins, particularly for HbC (causing HbSC disease) or β-thalassemia (S-thalassemia), sickle cell diseases similar to sickle cell anemia result even in the heterozygous state. Within the

African American population, the HbS gene has a frequency of approximately 9%; the HbC gene, 3%; and the β-thalassemia gene, 1%. Thus, these mixed disorders are relatively common collectively, affecting approximately 1 in 260 African Americans.

Two other hemoglobinopathies that affect hemoglobin solubility are seen relatively frequently in the heterozygous state: HbD in African Americans and HbE in Asian populations. Both of these conditions result in mild hemolytic anemia in the homozygous state. In HbE disease, the anemia is hypochromic and associated with splenomegaly. Hypochromia is a uniform finding in HbE trait.

The remaining hemoglobinopathies are much less common. Those caused by formation of unstable hemoglobins are usually inherited as autosomal dominant disorders and are characteristically associated with chronic hemolysis. The anemia is often hypochromic. Some unstable hemoglobins are associated with increased oxygen affinity, leading to erythrocytosis and reticulocytosis more severe than that usually observed for the degree of anemia. Other rarely seen hemoglobins have decreased oxygen affinity and produce anemia with cyanosis. A mutant hemoglobin, designated HbM, that is unable to maintain heme iron in the reduced state or to bind oxygen results in hereditary methemoglobinemia. Methemoglobin is brownish, and patients who inherit this type of hemoglobin have cyanosis. HbM is inherited as an autosomal dominant disorder.

10.2.2 Thalassemias

The thalassemic syndromes arise from an impairment in the synthesis of globin chains, leading to a quantitative decrease in the amount of hemoglobin within the cell. Thalassemias are divided into two main categories—α-thalassemia and β-thalassemia—on the basis of which globin chain is affected.

α-Thalassemia is a common disorder in many parts of the world. Severe forms of α-thalassemia are found in Southeast Asia, but milder disease forms are prevalent among those of African descent. Because of gene duplication of the alpha globin chain genetic locus, there are normally four alpha chain genes, with two on each chromosome. α-Thalassemia usually results from the deletion of one or more of these genes. The severity of disease is directly correlated with the number of genes deleted. The spectrum of α-thalassemic syndromes ranges from deletion of one gene (causing no clinical disease) to the deletion of all four genes. The deletion of all four alpha chain genes is fatal. This is a frequent cause of stillbirth in Southeast Asia. The fetal RBC hemoglobin in this situation is composed entirely of gamma chain tetramers, a condition designated "Bart's hemoglobin". Because Bart's hemoglobin avidly binds oxygen, it is unable to release oxygen to the fetal tissues. This results in fetal death from hydrops fetalis, as manifested by severe intrauterine hypoxia, edema, pallor, and hepatosplenomegaly. If one functional alpha chain gene is present, a less severe disorder, called "HbH disease", occurs. At birth, both fetal hemoglobin and Bart's hemoglobin are present. From later infancy to adulthood, as beta globin synthesis replaces fetal hemoglobin, HbH may be detected by hemoglobin electrophoresis. This syndrome is associated with a moderately severe, chronic hemolytic anemia. If two normal alpha chain genes are present, a mild microcytic anemia designated α-"thalassemia minor" or α-"thalassemia trait" is observed. In α-thalassemia minor, no abnormalities are found on hemoglobin electrophoresis, and the diagnosis is often one of exclusion of other causes of anemia. The presence of three normal alpha chains does not result in any clinically detectable abnormality. The characteristics of the α-thalassemias are summarized in **Table 10-4**.

β-Thalassemia is common among those of Mediterranean descent. β-Thalassemia may arise from gene deletion or, more commonly, from point mutations leading to impaired or absent beta chain synthesis. Mutations leading to complete suppression of beta chain synthesis are designated as β^0 variants. Other mutations where diminished synthesis of normal synthesis beta chains occurs are designated as β^+ variants and may result in milder clinical syndromes than the β^0 variants.

As with the α-thalassemias, the degree of disease severity is dependent on the number of abnormal genes inherited. When only one β-thalassemic gene has been inherited (heterozygote), the patient has a benign, hypochromic microcytic anemia designated β-thalassemia minor. This anemia is characterized by microcytosis, with a mean corpuscular volume (MCV) of 60 to 70 μm^3 (60 to 70 fL), a hemoglobin of 10 to 13 g/dL (100 to 130 g/L), and an elevated or normal RBC count. Hemoglobin electrophoresis usually shows increased amounts of HbA_2 due to excess unpaired alpha chains combining with delta chains. Slightly elevated levels of HbF are also present in about 30% of patients with β-thalassemia minor. Often, patients with β-thalassemia minor are mistakenly diagnosed as having iron deficiency, because they have a hypochromic microcytic anemia (see Chapter 2).

Table 10-4   α-Thalassemias

Phenotype	α Globin Output (%)	No. of Functional α Chain Genes and Genotype	Hematologic Findings
Normal	100	4: αα/αα	Normal
Silent carrier	75	3: –α/αα	Normal
α-Thalassemia trait	50	2: –α/–α or – –/αα	Mild microcytic hypochromic anemia
HbH disease	25	1: –α/– –	Hemolytic anemia
Hydrops fetalis	0	0: – –/– –	Stillborn, severe anemia

Abbreviation: – = deleted or absent α chain; – – = both genes on the locus deleted.

When two β-thalassemic genes have been inherited (homozygote), a very serious disorder called β-"thalassemia major" begins in infancy and early childhood. It is characterized by massive hepatosplenomegaly, extreme erythroid hyperplasia in the bone marrow leading to bony deformities, severe hemolytic anemia, and failure to grow or thrive. Hemoglobin electrophoresis shows prominent elevation of the HbF level (ranging from 30% to 100%). At the lower end of the spectrum of HbF values, the fetal hemoglobin is distributed heterogeneously among the RBC population. This allows β-thalassemia major to be distinguished from the benign condition termed "hereditary persistence of fetal hemoglobin" (HPFH), in which a homogeneous distribution is seen.

Another form of thalassemia, called δ-"thalassemia", is associated with suppression of both delta and beta chain synthesis. These disorders are clinically similar to the β-thalassemias. Patients with heterozygous disease present with thalassemia minor, often with prominent elevation of the HbF level. Patients with homozygous disease, however, present with a clinically milder disease than that usually seen in β-thalassemia major. The Lepore syndromes, which are often classified in this category, are caused by a mutant hemoglobin called "Hb Lepore". This hemoglobin results from a crossover mutation leading to a hybrid globin chain consisting of a partial delta chain and a partial beta chain. Hemoglobin Lepore can be detected with electrophoresis or high-performance liquid chromatography (HPLC).

10.3 Diagnostic Approach

Clinical evaluation and family history play a particularly important role in evaluating laboratory data in these disorders. Many of the tests can be performed easily. Evaluation of the hemoglobin disorders proceeds with the following steps (**Figure 10-1**):

1. Hematologic evaluation, with attention to RBC morphology and indices. Supravital stains may be used to detect inclusion bodies (such as HbH).
2. Hemoglobin electrophoresis or HPLC for the detection of globin chain variants with altered electrophoretic mobility. Measurement of HbA_2 also may be determined chromatographically.
3. Tests of hemoglobin solubility as a means of distinguishing HbS from the electrophoretically similar HbD and less frequent variants, if a hemoglobin with an S-like mobility is encountered. Solubility tests and the sickle test also screen for sickle cell trait.
4. Alkali denaturation test or the acid elution test (Kleihauer and Betke method) for fetal hemoglobin evaluation.
5. The isopropanol stability test for detecting unstable hemoglobins.

The following tests may be performed in specialized laboratories, but are rarely required:

6. When indicated, spectrophotometric determinations for methemoglobinemia seen with HbMs and measurement of oxyhemoglobin dissociation or $P_{50}O_2$ for detecting hemoglobins with altered oxygen affinity (see Chapter 12).
7. Globin chain synthetic studies when thalassemia is suspected but cannot be confirmed by simpler methods, and Southern blotting of alpha globin genes when additional genetic data are needed.
8. Detailed structural analysis of globin chains using "fingerprinting" of tryptic digests by means of electrophoresis, chromatography, and amino acid sequencing or nucleic acid analysis.

10.4 Hematologic Findings

The most severe anemia and the most striking morphologic changes are seen in the homozygous disorders. Findings in the

Figure 10-1 Workup of a suspected hemoglobinopathy using high-performance liquid chromatography and electrophoresis.

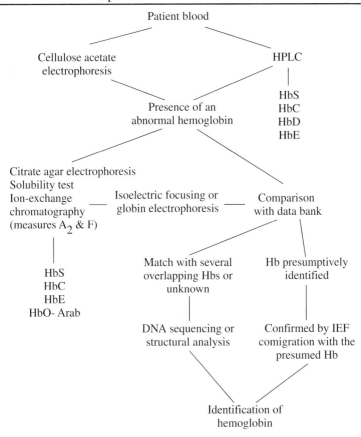

heterozygous states may be normal or show minimal hematologic abnormalities. Hematologic abnormalities may be divided into four classifications: those associated with chronic hemolysis; changes characteristic of a particular disorder; findings seen after splenectomy or (in the case of sickle cell disease) findings related to splenic atrophy; and changes seen with aplastic crisis, which may accompany infections.

10.4.1 Blood Cell Measurement

Anemia may be severe, with hemoglobin levels of 5 to 9 g/dL (50 to 90 g/L) in sickle cell anemia and 2.5 to 6.5 g/dL (25 to 65 g/L) in thalassemia major. Findings in heterozygotes may be normal, as in sickle cell trait, or they may demonstrate mild anemia, as in β-thalassemia minor. Often the thalassemia syndromes are characterized by decreased hemoglobin levels with normal to slightly increased RBC counts and microcytosis out of proportion to the anemia (60 to 70 μm^3 [60 to 75 fL]).

10.4.2 Peripheral Blood Smear Morphology

A wide variety of characteristic RBC changes are associated with the disorders of hemoglobin synthesis and are summarized in **Table 10-5**. **Images 10-1** through **10-3** demonstrate the characteristic morphology seen in β-thalassemia minor, HbC disease, and sickle cell disease, respectively. **Image 10-4** shows the characteristic appearance of Heinz bodies.

10.4.3 Bone Marrow Examination

Erythroid hyperplasia is proportional to the severity of the hemolysis. A prominent increase in iron deposition is often seen.

Other Laboratory Tests

Test 10.1 Hemoglobin Electrophoresis

Purpose. Hemoglobin electrophoresis is the principal procedure used to separate, detect, and identify abnormal hemoglobins. In some laboratories this is supplemented by HPLC analysis (see Test 10.2). There has been recent development of capillary isoelectric focusing methodologies that would allow for fine electrophoretic discrimination on small samples, although this method is not widely available.

Principle. Electrophoresis is the differential movement of charged protein molecules in an electric field. In a basic solution (pH >8) hemoglobins have a negative charge and migrate toward the anode with a mobility proportional to their net negative charges. Because HbS contains valine in place of the glutamic acid of HbA, it has a smaller negative charge and a slower anodal mobility than HbA in an alkaline medium. At an acid pH, hemoglobins are positively charged, and their relative mobilities in relation to the anode are the reverse of that seen in an alkaline medium.

Table 10-5 Red Blood Cell Appearance in Disorders of Hemoglobin Synthesis

Disorder	Morphologic Findings
HbS	Sickle cells
HbC	Target cells, HbC crystals after splenectomy
HbE	Microcytosis, hypochromia, target cells
Unstable Hb	Red blood cell inclusions with supravital dyes
Thalassemia	Microcytosis, target cells, basophilic stippling
Changes due to splenectomy or splenic atrophy	Basophilic stippling, Howell-Jolly bodies, target cells, Pappenheimer bodies, poikilocytosis
Changes associated with hemolysis	Polychromatophilia, fine basophilic stippling, macrocytosis

Specimen. Anticoagulated whole blood or washed RBCs are used for this test.

Procedure. Electrophoresis on cellulose acetate at pH 8.4 to 8.8 is the method of choice for initial electrophoretic testing in the general clinical laboratory (**Figure 10-2**). Patient and control RBCs are hemolyzed and subjected to electrophoresis for 15 to 30 minutes. Hemoglobins A, A_2, F, S, and C are most often included in controls. On completion of electrophoresis, the membrane is stained and the hemoglobins are identified by their relative positions. They can then be quantitated by elution and spectrophotometric assay or by densitometry scanning.

Electrophoresis in citrate agar at pH 6.2 can be used to complement conventional cellulose acetate electrophoresis (*see Interpretation and Figure 10-1*). The procedure is basically the same as that described for cellulose acetate but requires electrophoresis for 45 to 90 minutes.

Interpretations. The electrophoresis patterns of some hemoglobin variants on cellulose acetate are shown in **Figure 10-3**. At an alkaline pH, slow-moving hemoglobins include C, E, A_2, and O; intermediate hemoglobins include D, G, S, and Lepore; hemoglobins A and F are the most anodal. Among the fast-moving hemoglobins are H (**Image 10-5**), I, and Bart's. When a prominent band is found in the HbS region on cellulose acetate electrophoresis at pH 8.6, its identity can be confirmed with electrophoresis on citrate agar at pH 6.2. This separates

Figure 10-2 Comparison of hemoglobin electrophoretic patterns on cellulose acetate and citrate agar gels.

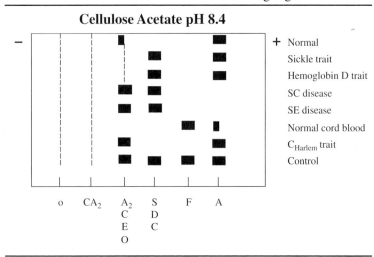

Cellulose Acetate pH 8.4

Normal
Sickle trait
Hemoglobin D trait
SC disease
SE disease
Normal cord blood
C_Harlem trait
Control

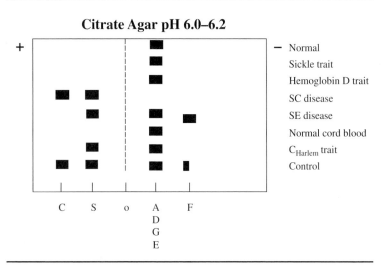

Citrate Agar pH 6.0–6.2

Normal
Sickle trait
Hemoglobin D trait
SC disease
SE disease
Normal cord blood
C_Harlem trait
Control

HbS from HbD and HbG. Citrate agar also differentiates HbC from HbS, HbO, HbE, and HbA$_2$ and provides sharp separation of hemoglobins F and A.

Notes and Precautions. The main limitation of hemoglobin electrophoresis is its inability to detect amino acid substitutions that do not affect charge. Such variants are seen among the unstable hemoglobins and with hemoglobins associated

Figure 10-3 Electrophoretic mobilities of hemoglobins on cellulose acetate (TRIS/EDTA/borate buffer) pH 8.4.

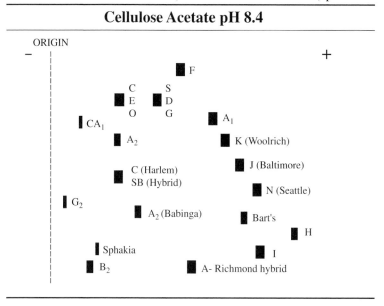

with altered oxygen affinity. As noted previously, different amino acid substitutions may lead to identical changes in elecrophoretic mobility, and these variants cannot be distinguished by electrophoresis.

Test 10.2 **High-Performance Liquid Chromatography Analysis of Hemoglobin**

Purpose. Charge changes in hemoglobin variants allows chromatographic separation of different hemoglobin types based on column retention time, allowing rapid identification and quantification. This technology is approved by the Food and Drug Administration (FDA) for preliminary identification of unusual hemoglobins.

Principle. Differences in charge allow separation of hemoglobin subtypes by column chromatography under high pressure. Hemoglobins are eluted in order of increasing charge, thus giving a unique retention time for each hemoglobin variant. The elution profile and column retention time allow for presumptive identification and qualification of hemoglobin variants.

Specimen. Anticoagulated blood is used.

Procedure. A sample of RBC hemolysate is loaded onto an HPLC nonporous cation-exchange column specific for hemoglobin analysis. The sample is eluted with two phosphate buffers that form an ionic gradient at a rate of 2 mL/min. An analysis of each sample can be run on two programs, which provide complementary data. The short program, which runs in about 6.5 minutes, provides elution profiles that give the retention time and approximate quantification for each hemoglobin variant present. The retention time is compared with known standards and a data bank to provide presumptive identification of the hemoglobin variant. The sample may then be run on a long program (approximately 20 minutes) that provides more accurate retention time data but is not as accurate for quantification.

Interpretation. HPLC is most useful in identification and quantification of hemoglobins A, A_2, F, S, D, and C. More unusual hemoglobins may require long-program analysis, and more than 700 hemoglobin variants have been analyzed and indexed according to elution times. Unusual variants of overlapping elution times may require further analysis by isoelectric focusing, electrophoresis, or globin gene analysis to definitively identify a hemoglobin subtype.

Notes and Precautions. HPLC offers a distinct advantage over classic hemoglobin electrophoresis in that it can more accurately identify and quantitate unusual hemoglobins as well as identify the more unusual variants. Thus, HPLC is a very cost- and time-efficient screening methodology for a suspected hemoglobinopathy. Specialized reference laboratories are usually required for this procedure. Hemoglobin E cannot be separated from HbA_2 by this method, and suspected HbE should be analyzed by standard electrophoresis. Hemoglobin H and Bart's hemoglobin may elute too quickly to be analyzed. Because of overlap, hemoglobins with similar retention times may require further analysis for definitive identification. Although this technology is FDA approved for initial identification of unusual hemoglobins, it is not approved for final identification. Thus, additional testing (such as electrophoresis, solubility testing, or globin chain analysis) is required to support the HPLC identification. The long program does not provide accurate quantification.

Test 10.3 Sickle Cell Test

Purpose. In most cases of sickle cell disease or the heterozygous sickle cell disorders (HbSC disease or the S-thalassemias), a few sickle RBCs are readily seen on the routinely prepared blood smears. In sickle cell trait and some sickle cell disorders with a lesser propensity for sickling, manipulation is required to induce in vitro sickling.

Principle. When RBCs containing HbS are deoxygenated, hemoglobin crystallizes to form the characteristic sickle shape. Deoxygenation can be accomplished by mixing a drop of blood with a reducing agent on a slide.

Specimen. Venous or capillary blood is used.

Procedure. The sickle cell test is performed by mixing the amount of blood that adheres to the end of an applicator stick with a drop of freshly prepared 2% sodium metabisulfite solution and covering the suspension with a cover slip. When sickle hemoglobin is present, cells begin to deform within 10 minutes, assuming crescent and holly leaf shapes. The preparation is observed on the microscope within 30 minutes with high-dry objective.

Interpretation. The test results are positive for sickle cell traits and all sickle cell disorders when HbS is present in a concentration of 25% or greater. Sickling has been described in other relatively rare variants, such as HbC_{Harlem}.

Notes and Precautions. The most frequently encountered technical problem resulting in a false-negative test result is outdated metabisulfite reagent that has lost its reducing power. With HbS disorders, test results may not be positive until an infant is 1 or 2 months of age because of the relatively high percentage of HbF in RBCs during infancy.

Test 10.4 Solubility Test for Hemoglobin S

Purpose. Solubility tests have been used most widely to screen for sickle cell trait and as a means of differentiating HbS from HbD, which are identical on electrophoresis at an alkaline pH.

Principle. The solubility test is based on the relative insolubility of reduced HbS compared with that of other hemoglobin variants and HbA in a high-phosphate buffer solution.

Specimen. Whole blood is used.

Procedure. A solution of 1.24 mol/L potassium dihydrogen phosphate (KH_2PO_4) containing saponin to lyse the RBCs and sodium hydrosulfite (dithionite) to reduce the hemoglobin is used. Blood is added, and the solution is observed for turbidity by reading black lines held behind the test tubes. Commercial kits are available.

Interpretation. Positive test results are indicated by a turbid suspension; the ruled lines behind the test tube cannot be seen. Test results are positive for sickle cell trait and disorders with rare exceptions (eg, HbC_{Harlem}). Results are negative with all other hemoglobins. The differentiation of sickle cell trait from sickle cell disease may not always be clear because it is based on a quantitative difference in turbidity.

Notes and Precautions. In the presence of severe anemia, the blood sample used normally does not contain sufficient HbS to yield turbid solution. With a hemoglobin level less than 7 g/dL (70 g/L), the sample size should be doubled. False-positive results may be seen with lipemic plasma. The solubility test is inadequate as a sole means of screening for genetic counseling because it fails to detect the important carriers of HbC and β-thalassemia. In general, hemoglobin analysis by electrophoresis or HPLC is required for diagnosis of sickle cell disease, and the sickle cell test and solubility test for HbS are most useful as screening tests.

Test 10.5 Alkali Denaturation Test for Fetal Hemoglobin

Purpose. Measurement of fetal hemoglobin helps in the diagnosis and differentiation of thalassemias, double heterozygotes with combined thalassemia and a structural hemoglobin variant, as well as in the diagnosis of HPFH. Because the mobility of HbF is close to that of HbA on routine electrophoresis, measurement of HbF based on electrophoretic techniques has not been reliable.

Principle. Hemoglobin F is relatively more resistant to denaturation by a strong alkali than other hemoglobins.

Specimen. Anticoagulated whole blood is used.

Procedure. Fresh alkali (1.2 N sodium hydroxide) is added to a hemolysate. After 1 minute, denatured hemoglobin is precipitated by the addition of ammonium sulfate. The filtrate contains HbF, which is quantitated spectrophotometrically at 415 nm.

Interpretation. The normal value for HbF is less than 2% (**Table**

Table 10-6 Hemoglobin Analysis in β-Thalassemic Disorders

Classification	Hemoglobin A	Hemoglobin A$_2$	Hemoglobin F
Normal	Normal (97%)	Normal (1.6%-3.5%)	Normal (<1%)
HPFH			Increased (15%-100%)
Heterozygous (thalassemia minor) β-thalassemia	Decreased (>90%)	Increased* (3.5%-8%)	Normal or slightly elevated
Homozygous β$^+$-thalassemia	Present, decreased	Variably increased*	Increased (<100%)
β^0-Thalassemia	Absent	Mildly increased (1.5%-4%)	Increased (nearly 100%)
δ-β-Thalassemia	Absent	Absent	Increased (100%)

Abbreviations: HPFH = hereditary persistence of fetal hemoglobin; β$^+$ = reduced production of beta chains; β^0 = absence of beta chain production.
*Hemoglobin A$_2$ levels may be normal or decreased in patients with coexisting iron deficiency.

10-6). Patients with β-thalassemia minor may have elevated HbF levels of 2% to 5%. Those with less common δ-β-thalassemia minor may show much higher levels. Patients with homozygous β-thalassemia show levels of HbF ranging from 30% to 100%. Levels in patients with HPFH range from 15% to 100%. Elevated HbF levels ranging from 2% to 5% have been reported in a large variety of hematologic conditions, including aplastic anemia, pernicious anemia, hereditary spherocytosis, myelofibrosis, leukemia, and metastatic disease with bone marrow involvement.

Notes and Precautions. The alkali denaturation test is very sensitive at low levels of HbF. At levels greater than 10%, however, the method underestimates HbF, and accurate measurement requires special chromatographic techniques such as HPLC.

Test 10.6 **Quantitation of Hemoglobin A$_2$ With Ion-Exchange Chromatography**

Purpose. Levels of HbA$_2$ are elevated in β-thalassemia minor. Quantitation of HbA$_2$ with routine electrophoresis on cellulose acetate has been uniformly reliable.

Principle. The most accurate and rapid procedure generally available for measuring HbA_2 is chromatography using an anion exchange column to separate HbA_2 from HbA. HPLC also may be used.

Specimen. Anticoagulated whole blood is used.

Procedure. Hemoglobin A_2 is separated from HbA by use of a microcolumn consisting of diethylaminoethyl cellulose (DEAE-cellulose) as the ion exchange resin. The resin is equilibrated with a tris(hydroxymethyl)aminomethane (TRIS) phosphate buffer, and the hemoglobin solution is applied. The more strongly charged HbA adheres to the ion exchange resin. Hemoglobin A_2 passes through and is quantitated spectrophotometrically at 415 nm. Commercial kits with disposable columns are available.

Interpretation. The normal range of values for HbA_2 is 1.6% to 3.5% (*see Table 10-6*). In β-thalassemia, the range is 3.5% to 8%.

Notes and Precautions. A number of hemoglobin variants are copurified under the usual test conditions. These include hemoglobins C, E, O, D, and (to a lesser extent) S. When a HbA_2value greater than 8% is found, the presence of such a variant is likely. Hemoglobin A_2 may be separated and quantitated in the presence of HbS by eluting the two hemoglobins separately, using buffers with different pH for elution. Hemoglobin A_2 levels may not be elevated in the presence of coexisting iron deficiency.

Test 10.7 Acid Elution Test for Fetal Hemoglobin in RBCs

Purpose. The acid elution test is used to differentiate HPFH from other states associated with high fetal hemoglobin levels.

Principle. When hemoglobin is precipitated inside the RBC and fixed with alcohol, the precipitated HbA and most variants can be dissolved in a buffered solution of citric acid and eluted from the cell. Hemoglobin F remains precipitated inside the cell.

Specimen. Whole blood is used.

Procedure. A blood smear is prepared in the usual manner and fixed at 80% ethanol. It is then treated with a citric acid–phosphate buffer (pH 3.3), which elutes HbA from RBCs. The blood film is then stained with eosin, which stains any residual precipitate.

Interpretation. Smears from normal blood show little, if any, staining and appear as ghosts. A heterogeneous distribution of fetal hemoglobin is seen in newborn infants, from fetal-maternal transfusion, and in the thalassemias, with elevated HbF levels. Hereditary persistence of fetal hemoglobin is the only condition in which HbF is evenly distributed among nearly all the RBCs.

Notes and Precautions. The intensity of the staining often differs markedly from one part of the blood film to another, and considerable experience may be required for interpretation. Flow cytometric tests for detection of fetal hemoglobin are currently under development.

Test 10.8 Isopropanol Stability Test

Purpose. The isopropanol stability test is used to detect unstable hemoglobins.

Principle. Unstable hemoglobins have reduced stability when exposed to alcohol denaturation, compared with the stability of normal hemoglobins.

Specimen. Whole blood is used.

Procedure. A hemolysate is added to buffered isopropanol and incubated at 37°C. The preparation is observed for precipitation at 5-minute intervals over 30 minutes.

Interpretation. Unstable hemoglobins generally show turbidity within 5 to 10 minutes, whereas normal hemoglobins should remain clear for 30 minutes. False-positive test results may be obtained with sickle hemoglobin, fetal hemoglobin, and methemoglobin.

Test 10.9 Test for Hemoglobin H Inclusion Bodies

Purpose. Hemoglobin H is unstable and may be difficult to detect on routine electrophoresis. This test allows detection of HbH and may suggest the presence of other unstable hemoglobins.

Principle. Incubation of whole blood with brilliant cresyl blue causes oxidation and precipitation of HbH, resulting in diffuse stippling.

Specimen. Fresh whole blood is used.

Procedure. Three or four drops of whole blood are incubated with 0.5 mL of a 1% solution of brilliant cresyl blue in citrate-saline solution. Blood films are made at 10 minutes, 1 hour, and 4 hours.

Interpretation. The 10-minute slide is a control that shows the number of reticulocytes. Positive cells show a diffusely clumped pattern staining, resembling a golf ball, throughout the cell, with the reticulum staining light blue (*see Image 10-5*). In HbH disease, 50% or more of the cells on the 1-hour slide may be positive. Results with other unstable hemoglobins are variable, with a longer period of incubation usually required for precipitation and fewer cells staining.

10.5 Ancillary Tests

10.5.1 Heinz Bodies

Heinz bodies are particles of denatured hemoglobins attached to the cell membrane (*see Image 10-4*) and are demonstrated with a variety of supravital dyes, such as crystal violet or brilliant cresyl blue. Heinz bodies are found in association with unstable disorders in patients who have undergone splenectomy. They also may be seen during acute drug-induced hemolysis in patients with glucose-6-phosphate dehydrogenase deficiency. Incubation of blood with acetylphenylhydrazine or other reagents that cause hemoglobin oxidative damage results in the formation of Heinz bodies in vitro. The pattern of Heinz body formation when an incubation has been carried out under carefully controlled conditions differs in patients with unstable hemoglobins or oxidative hemolysis and those with normal cells. Testing and interpretation require the services of an experienced laboratory.

10.5.2 Crystal Cells of Hemoglobin C Disease

Crystal cells of HbC disease (*see Image 10.2*) are present in as many as 10% of the circulating cells in affected patients who have undergone splenectomy, but these tetrahedral crystals are rare when a functional spleen is present. Crystal cells may be produced in vitro by hypertonic dehydration of RBCs in a 3% sodium chloride buffer for up to 12 hours.

10.5.3 Globin Chain Analysis

Definitive diagnosis of a hemoglobin variant may require mutation analysis of the specific globin gene by polymerase chain reaction or electrophoretic gene analysis by Southern blot. Analysis is available at specialized laboratories and in the research setting. Often, clinical therapy is not dependent on this type of definitive analysis.

10.6 Course and Treatment

The course and treatment of these hemoglobin synthesis disorders varies greatly, depending on which mutation is present. Sickle cell disorders are characterized by disturbances in the microcirculation because sickle cells are so rigid and do not readily pass through capillaries, leading to microinfarction or vaso-occlusion. This may lead to pain or chronic, relentless organ damage due to infarction. In contrast, the clinical manifestations of HbC disease are minor, related almost entirely to the moderate hemolytic anemia that may be present. The thalassemic syndromes also have a wide range of symptoms and clinical severity. The traits often have mild anemia. In β-thalassemia major, transfusions are required to maintain life. This often leads to iron overload, with attendant cardiac damage, requiring lifelong chelation therapy. Patients with hemoglobin H disease should avoid oxidative drugs, which could precipitate a hemolytic episode. Splenectomy may help to ameliorate the anemia in these patients.

10.7 References

The laboratory diagnosis of haemoglobinopathies. *Br J Haematol.* 1998;101:783–792.

Beutler E. Hemoglobinopathies associated with unstable hemoglobin. In: Beutler E, Litchman MA, Coller BS, et al, eds. *Williams Hematology*. 5th ed. New York, NY: McGraw-Hill; 1995:650–653.

Beutler E. The sickle cell diseases and related disorders. In: Beutler E, Litchman MA, Coller BS, et al, eds. *Williams Hematology*. 5th ed. New York, NY: McGraw-Hill; 1995:616–649.

Lafferty J, Ali MA, Corstairs K, Crawford L. Proficiency testing of hemoglobinopathy techniques in Ontario laboratories. *Am J Clin Pathol.* 1997;107:567–575.

Lukens JN. The thalassemias and related disorders: quantitative disorders of hemoglobin synthesis. In: Lee GR, Foerster J, Lukens JN, et al, eds. *Wintrobe's Clinical Hematology.* 10th ed. Baltimore, Md: Williams & Wilkins; 1999:1405–1447.

Mario N, Baudin B, Aussel C, et al. Capillary isoelectric focusing and high-performance cation-exchange chromatography compared for qualitative and quantitative analysis of hemoglobin variants. *Clin Chem.* 1997;43:2137–2142.

VonHerren F, Thormann W. Capillary electrophoresis in clinical and forensic analysis. *Electrophoresis* 1997;18:2415–2426.

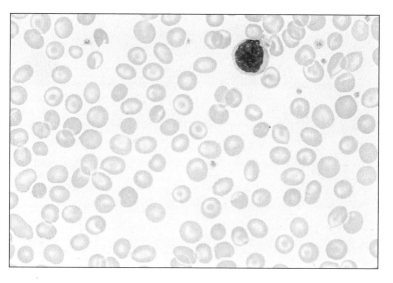

Image 10-1 β-Thalassemia minor. Microcytes and a moderate number of target cells are present.

Image 10-2 Hemoglobin C disease. Many target cells and a hemoglobin C crystal (center) are present.

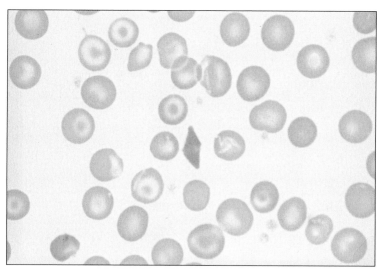

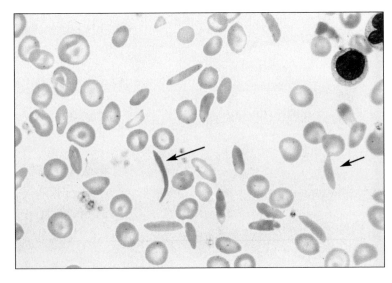

Image 10-3 Sickle cell disease. Several sickle cells (arrows) are seen in addition to target cells and marked anisocytosis.

Image 10-4 Heinz bodies. Supravital staining demonstrates Heinz bodies as coarse, dark dots within the RBCs.

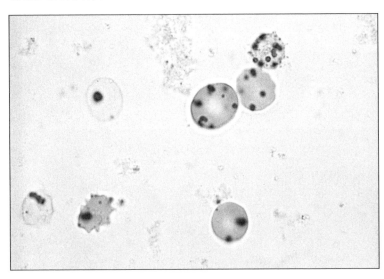

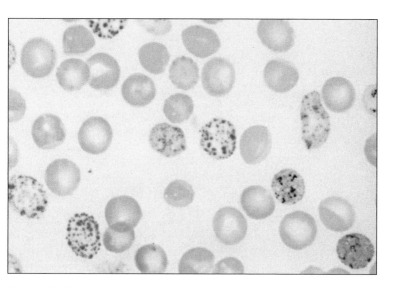

Image 10-5 Hemoglobin H disease. Brilliant cresyl blue staining shows a diffusely clumped staining pattern, demonstrating the presence of denatured unstable hemoglobin.

11 Paroxymal Nocturnal Hemoglobinuria

Paroxysmal nocturnal hemoglobinuria (PNH) is a rare acquired stem cell disorder in which episodic hemolysis characteristically occurs. The hemolysis follows a mutation in the hematopoietic stem cell that causes a partial or complete loss of cell membrane linkage of surface proteins by glycophosphatidylinositol (GPI) anchors. Clinically important proteins affected by this mutation include those regulating activity of the classic complement pathway. Although this defect is seen in all blood cells, the lack of complement regulatory proteins on the RBC result in the episodic hemolysis that clinically characterizes PNH.

11.1 Pathophysiology

PNH is an acquired RBC membrane disorder, arising secondary to a single somatic mutation in the pluripotential hematopoietic stem cell that gives rise to complete or partial deficiency of GPI anchoring of cell surface proteins. The affected gene is phosphatidylinositolglycan A (PIG-A), and reintroduction of this gene into deficient PNH cells corrects the defect in GPI anchor biosynthesis. This mutation may occur spontaneously or in patients with bone marrow injury associated with aplastic anemia or bone marrow hypoplasia.

The GPI anchoring defect causes a deficiency in or lack of at least 19 cell surface proteins. Patients with PNH are deficient in two to three membrane glycoproteins that normally regulate complement activation. Proteins that have been found missing or deficient in affected patients include decay-accelerating factor (DAF or CD55), which regulates the activity of C3 convertase; homologous restriction factor (HRF), which regulates C9 activity and binding; and membrane inhibitor of reactive lysis (MIRL or CD59), which modulates terminal complement-mediated RBC lysis. Deficiency of one or more of these proteins leads to enhanced formation of the membrane complement lytic complex on the cell surface. Thus, although WBCs and platelets are also abnormal, it is the RBC abnormalities that give rise to episodic hemolysis. Hemolysis is sometimes increased at night due to a slight fall in plasma pH that facilitates complement activation.

A peculiar feature of PNH is the variable expression of the abnormal phenotype. This probably reflects genetic mosaicism in which some cells express normal levels of GPI-anchored proteins, others have intermediate expression, and still others are severely deficient. Three different subtypes of PNH cell types have been described based on the relative expression of complement regulatory proteins (**Table 11-1**). It has been suggested that the relative numbers of each class of PNH cells correlate with disease severity and may provide an indicator of disease progression. A patient may have some or all of the PNH type cells present, and the relative numbers of each cell type as well as disease phenotype may shift over time. Although RBCs appear most susceptible to complement-mediated lysis, all hematopoietic cells are affected, which may lead to leukopenia and/or thrombocytopenia in some patients.

11.2 Clinical Findings

PNH is an uncommon disease, with an estimated prevalence of 1 to 10 cases per million. There is a wide spectrum of disease. It usually begins as an insidious onset of anemia. Virtually all patients are anemic, often severely. The classically described pattern of episodic hemolysis—increased at night, causing dark urine after awakening—is frequently not seen. More often, hemolysis occurs

Table 11-1 Types of Cells Observed in PNH

PNH Cell Type	Sensitivity to Complement Lysis	Observed Complement Pathway Defects	GPI Protein Expression	Associated PIG-A Mutations
I	Normal to near normal	Near normal lytic behavior	Near normal to mild deficiency; partial lack of DAF (CD55) and/ or MIRL (CD59)	None
II	Intermediate (10-15 times more sensitive)	Increased C_3 binding to cell; increased C_3/C_5 convertase activity	Partial lack of DAF (CD55) and MIRL (CD59) (DAF deficiency appears most significant)	Missense (partial)
III	Highly sensitive (25 times more sensitive)	Increased binding of C_3 to cell; increased C_3/C_5 convertase activity; increased binding of C_{5b67} complexes; increased C_9 binding	Near total lack of DAF (CD55), MIRL (CD59), HRF	Nonsense, frameshift, deletion or insertion causing gene in-activation

Abbreviations: PNH = paroxysmal nocturnal hemoglobinuria; GPI = glycophasphotidylinositol; PIG-A = phosphatidylinositolgycan A; DAF= decay accelerating factor; MIRL= membrane inhibitor of reactive lysis; HRF= homologous restriction factor.

in an irregular fashion, apparently precipitated by events such as infection, surgery, and transfusions. Hemolysis also may occur chronically. Hemoglobinuria or dark urine may be absent. Chronic urinary iron loss, or hemosiderinuria, is a constant feature and may result in the development of iron deficiency anemia.

Some patients with previous bone marrow aplasia also may develop PNH presenting as a mild anemia with partial deficiencies of GPI-anchored proteins. Often these patients have decreased expression of CD55 and CD59 by flow cytometry, but normal Ham's and sucrose lysis tests. This may represent an early form of PNH and is termed "smoldering PNH." Patients often develop full expression of PNH over time.

Abnormal platelet function in PNH patients is frequently associated with venous thrombosis, which is a major cause of death. Clinically significant thrombosis is seen in about one third of affected patients. Thrombotic events may cause severe episodes of abdominal or back pain or severe refractory headaches. Development of Budd-Chiari syndrome (hepatic vein thrombosis) or cerebral vein thrombosis is common. Thrombophlebitis may occur in the legs or arms and may lead to pulmonary thromboembolism. Arterial thrombosis is rare. Occasionally, patients may experience bleeding due to poor platelet function. Patients are often leukopenic at some stage of the disease, leading to increased susceptibility to infection. In addition, neutrophils show a decrease in leukocyte alkaline phosphatase (LAP) activity. Patients frequently progress to severe cytopenias, requiring transfusions or other therapeutic interventions.

11.3 Diagnostic Approach

Depending on the predominant features of the presenting illness, PNH may need to be differentiated from other causes of chronic hemolytic anemia, pancytopenia, iron deficiency, or hemoglobinuria.

Laboratory evaluation of this disorder is performed using the following steps:

1. Hematologic evaluation with complete blood cell count, peripheral blood morphology, and bone marrow examination is conducted.
2. The sucrose lysis and urine hemosiderin (Rous) tests are used to screen for PNH.
3. The acidified serum (Ham's) test and flow cytometric analysis for decreased expression of the CD55 (DAF) or CD59 (MIRL) proteins are definitive diagnostic tests for PNH.

11.4 Hematologic Findings

11.4.1 Blood Cell Measurements

The degree of anemia associated with PNH varies widely, with hemoglobin levels ranging from less than 6 g/dL (60 g/L) to normal. The mean corpuscular volume (MCV) may be somewhat increased (with prominent reticulocytosis or superimposed folate or vitamin B_{12} deficiency due to chronic hemolysis), or decreased owing to coexistent iron deficiency anemia. Often, the observed reticulocytosis is lower than expected for the degree of anemia. This discrepancy is attributed to the bone marrow stem cell defect.

11.4.2 Peripheral Blood Smear Morphology

No characteristic morphologic changes are seen. Macrocytosis and polychromatophilia may accompany prominent reticulocytosis. Iron deficiency may result in microcytosis and hypochromia. Spherocytes are absent. Variable leukopenia and thrombocytopenia may be seen and is often moderate to severe.

11.4.3 Bone Marrow Examination

Bone marrow cellularity may be decreased or aplastic in some patients, but more often is hypercellular. Normoblastic erythroid hyperplasia is the most frequent finding, with adequate numbers of megakaryocytes and myeloid elements. Some patients may exhibit megaloblastic maturation. Stainable storage iron is usually absent, even when clinical iron deficiency is not present.

Other Laboratory Tests

Test 11.1 Sucrose Lysis Test

Purpose. The sucrose lysis test is the most commonly used screening test for PNH.

Principle. An isotonic sucrose solution of low ionic strength aggregates serum globulins onto the RBC surface. This promotes binding and activation of complement on the RBC membrane. When a small amount of serum (as a source of complement) is added, PNH cells are lysed, whereas normal cells are not.

Specimen. Whole defibrinated blood is used. The blood should be collected in heparin.

Procedure. A small amount of fresh, normal, type-compatible serum is added to the buffered 10% sucrose solution. Washed

RBCs from the patient are added, and the suspension is incubated for 60 minutes at room temperature.

Interpretation. Lysis of greater than 5% of the RBCs, as detected by release of hemoglobin (which imparts a red color to the supernatant) that is detectable by the eye, is compatible with the diagnosis of PNH. Very mild hemolysis, usually amounting to less than 5% of the RBCs, may be found in some megaloblastic anemias and autoimmune hemolytic disease. A definitive diagnosis requires performance of the acidified serum test (Test 11.2) or flow cytometric analysis (Test 11.3).

Notes and Precautions. It was originally suggested that the sucrose lysis test should be carried out using unbuffered sucrose solutions, which may lead to false-negative results. Ethylenediaminetetraacetic acid (EDTA) anticoagulation blocks complement activation and invalidates the test results.

Test 11.2 **Acidified Serum Test**

Purpose. The acidified serum test may be used to make a definitive diagnosis of PNH.

Principle. Complement fixes to RBCs at a slightly acidic pH. Cells from patients with PNH lyse under these conditions, whereas normal RBCs are resistant to lysis.

Specimen. Whole defibrinated blood is used. The blood should be collected in heparin.

Procedure. The test is carried out using type-compatible blood from a healthy control subject and blood from a patient with suspected PNH. RBCs from the patient and control subject are suspended in each of the following serum preparations (from both subjects):

1. Unaltered serum.
2. Serum with a pH adjusted to 6.8 as measured with a pH meter.
3. Serum at pH 6.8 that has been heat activated to 55°C for 3 minutes to destroy complement proteins.
4. Heated serum to which guinea pig complement has been added.

Interpretation. A definitive diagnosis of PNH depends on demonstration of all of the following characteristics of in vitro hemolysis:

1. It occurs with patient cells but not with control cells.
2. It is enhanced by slightly acidifying the serum used.
3. It is abolished by heat inactivating the serum at 55°C to destroy complement proteins.
4. Hemolytic activity is not restored to the heated serum by addition of guinea pig complement.

Some hemolysis may be present in the unaltered serum, but it is generally less than that observed in acidified serum. No hemolysis of control blood cells should occur in any of the tubes.

Notes and Precautions. Ethylenediaminetetraacetic acid anticoagulation of blood may block complement activation. Erroneous test results may be obtained due to underacidification or overacidification of serum. In the original description of the test, the serum pH was not verified with a pH meter because such instruments were not available. Careful adjustment of the serum pH to 6.78 ± 0.1 is necessary if reliable results are to be obtained. The correct performance and interpretation of the test is necessary, and use of a reference laboratory that performs testing on a routine basis may be indicated.

Test 11.3 **Flow Cytometric Analysis for Decreased CD55 and CD59 Expression**

Purpose. Flow cytometric detection of decreased levels of CD55 and/or CD59 allows for a definitive diagnosis of PNH to be made and excludes other causes of hemolysis.

Principle. Deficiency of GPI anchored protein activity leads to decreased expression of proteins linked to the cell surface by GPI anchor. Two proteins, CD55 and CD59, that modulate complement activity are anchored to the RBC surface by this mechanism. Detection of decreased or absent expression of these proteins by flow cytometry analysis provides a sensitive and specific means for diagnosis of PNH.

Specimen. Blood should be collected in a heparin tube.

Procedure. CD59 is present in high levels on the RBC membrane, whereas CD55 is found at lower levels (six to eight times less). The patient's RBCs are stained with either anti-CD59 or anti-CD55 and analyzed by flow cytometry to generate a histogram of protein expression, which is compared with that of normal control cells.

Figure 11-1 Flow cytometric diagnosis of PNH. Flow cytometric histograms from a patient with PNH showing a population of RBCs with decreased expression levels of CD55 (panel A, arrow) and CD59 (panel B, arrow). This patient also has a second population of relatively normal CD55 and CD59 expression in the M1 area, indicating a partial deletion. For comparison, RBC expression of CD55 (panel C) and CD59 (panel D) demonstrating a single population in the M1 area is seen in a normal control.

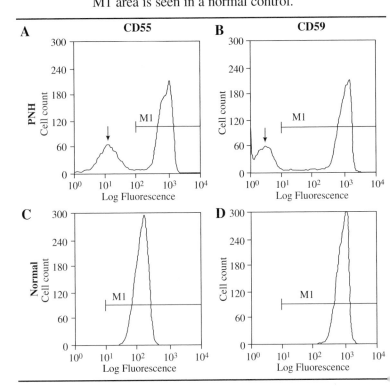

Interpretation. Patients with PNH show decreased or absent expression of CD59 and/or CD55 (ie, decreased or absent fluorescence as seen in **Figure 11-1**). A population of normal cells is also commonly seen in the patient, reflecting phenotypic mosaicism. The degree of deficiency is often associated with the severity of disease.

Notes and Precautions. Blood should be maintained at ambient temperature because refrigeration may cause shedding of antigens and falsely decrease expression of CD59 and CD55. Optimal testing requires blood that is less than 24 hours old, although testing may be performed on samples taken up to 72 hours earlier.

CD59 is expressed at levels six to eight times those of CD55: thus, analysis of CD59 usually demonstrates the clearest pattern of deficiency when compared with normal controls. The number of cells expressing normal, low, or intermediate levels of CD59 may be enumerated. This may provide some insights into disease severity as well as a means for monitoring disease progression. Due to lower levels of expression, CD55 may be more difficult to separate into discrete populations. Flow cytometric analysis also may be performed on granulocytes, but this process is technically more challenging. Flow cytometry is very sensitive and can detect small populations (1% to 5%) of deficient cells, allowing for detection of early (smoldering) PNH or abnormal cell populations after transfusion or recent hemolytic episode.

Test 11.4 **Test for Urine Hemosiderin**

Purpose. Urine hemosiderin is nearly always present in PNH and provides a valuable screening test.

Principle. Even in the absence of discernible hemoglobinuria, chronic low-grade intravascular hemolysis associated with PNH is sufficient to deplete serum haptoglobin. This results in the presence of hemoglobin in the plasma, which is reabsorbed by renal tubules. As the renal tubules become heavily laden with iron, it is excreted in the urine as hemosiderin granules, which are demonstrable with the Prussian blue stain.

Specimen. A random urine specimen is used.

Procedure. The presence of hemosiderin in the urine is demonstrated by adding a drop of a mixture of equal parts of 4% hydrochloric acid and 4% potassium ferricyanide to the sediment of centrifuged urine specimen. The mixture is incubated at room temperature for 10 minutes and agitated frequently.

Interpretation. Hemosiderin appears as blue particles. Although considerable emphasis has been placed on intracellular location of hemosiderin in urine, cells containing hemosiderin may have disintegrated in the urine and free hemosiderin may be the predominant form. Urine from a healthy patient does not contain hemosiderin.

11.5 Ancillary Tests

Quantitative testing of complement sensitivity may give more precise information regarding the size of the complement-sensitive population; however, it is too complex for routine clinical use. RBC acetylcholinesterase activity and leukocyte activity are diminished in PNH. Cytogenetic analysis may show abnormalities, including trisomy 9, loss of chromosome Y, and other deleted or lost chromosomes. No specific cytogenetic pattern has been identified. Molecular analysis documenting PIG-A mutations is definitive but is currently a research tool.

11.6 Course and Treatment

The disease course may be fulminating or chronic. The median survival after diagnosis is 10 to 15 years, with 25% of patients surviving for more than 25 years. The major causes of morbidity and morality are thrombosis, bleeding, and infection. Rarely, acute myelogenous leukemia (1% to 5% of patients) or a myelodysplastic syndrome (5% of patients) may supervene. Thrombotic complications, particularly Budd-Chiari syndrome, may be rapidly fatal. Treatments include symptomatic blood transfusions, androgenic steroids to stimulate hematopoiesis, corticosteroids, thrombolytic or anticoagulant agents, and bone marrow transplant. Allogenic bone marrow transplant is curative. Gene therapies, such as transfection of normal PIG-A or retroviral transfer of CD59, are under investigation. Over a disease course of many years, about one third of patients may have a spontaneous remission or a decrease in disease severity, perhaps reflecting a decreased survival advantage for the abnormal clone.

11.7 References

Fores R, Bautista G, Steegmann JL, et al. De novo smoldering paroxysmal nocturnal hemoglobinuria: a flow cytometric diagnosis. *Haematologica* 1997;82:695–697.

Nishimura J, Smith CA, Phillips KL, et al. Paroxysmal nocturnal hemoglobinuria: molecular pathogenesis and molecular therapeutic approaches. *Hematopathol Mol Hematol*. 1998;11:119–146.

Packman CH. Pathogenesis and management of paroxysmal nocturnal haemoglobinuria. *Blood Rev*. 1998;12:1–11.

Parker CJ, Lee GR. Paroxysmal nocturnal hemoglobinuria. In: Lee GR, Foerster J, Lukens JN, et al, eds. *Wintrobe's Clinical Hematology*. 10th ed. Baltimore, Md: Williams & Wilkins; 1999:1264–1285.

12 Extrinsic Hemolytic Anemia: General Concepts and Transfusion Reactions

In addition to the intrinsic (inherited) hemolytic anemias and the acquired disorder paroxysmal nocturnal hemoglobinuria (PNH), there is a group of hemolytic anemias caused by extrinsic factors such as circulating antibodies and chemical, physical, or infectious agents (**Table 12-1**). Clinically, antibody-mediated hemolysis is the most common. Antibodies can be produced in response to foreign RBC antigens (alloantibody), to self-antigens (autoantibody), or to drugs bound to the RBC membrane. This chapter covers some of the general features of extrinsic hemolytic anemias, as well as alloantibody reactions following incompatible transfusion. Subsequent chapters examine the other types of extrinsic hemolytic anemias.

12.1 Pathophysiology

RBCs contain a large number of cell surface proteins, sugars, and glycoproteins that are immunogenic, thereby providing the basis for modern blood banking (**Table 12-2**). Exposure to a foreign RBC surface component acts as an antigenic stimulus, causing

Table 12-1 Hemolytic Anemia Caused by Extrinsic Factors

Category	Specific Agent
Infectious	Protozoal: malaria, babesiosis Bacterial: cholera, clostridial sepsis Viral

Physicochemical	Burns (full thickness)
	Chemicals:
	    Oxidant type–aromatic (cylic) compounds,
	      chlorates, nitrates, cisplatin
	    Nonoxidant type–copper, arsine, lead
	Drugs: RBC enzyme deficiencies

Antibody-related	Alloantibody: incompatible transfusion, fetal-
	    maternal incompatibility
	Autoantibody: warm-type and cold-type
	    autoantibodies
	Drug-induced antibody: toxic immune
	    complexes (quinidine, quinine); haptens
	    (penicillin); α-methyldopa type

Table 12-2 Most Common Blood Antigens Associated With Clinically Significant Alloantibodies

ABO group antigens
Lewis antigens
Rh antigens including D/d, C/c, E/e
Kidd group antigens
Duffy group antigens
Kell group antigens

production of either IgG or IgM antibodies (**Table 12-3**). IgM is a large molecule (molecular weight, 900,000 d) with 10 antigen-binding sites that allow the linking of several cells or agglutination. IgM tends to bind more readily to cells at lower temperatures (<37°C), hence its association with cold-type immunohemolytic anemia. Complement is activated by IgM binding to the RBC surface, leading to complement-mediated intravascular hemolysis. Clinically important IgM antibodies include the naturally occurring antibodies against RBC antigens that allow recognition of foreign blood types, as well as cold agglutinins that develop following infection or as autoimmune phenomena.

Table 12-3   Properties of Immunoglobulins Acting in
                 Alloimmune Hemolysis

Property	IgM	IgG
Size	900,000 d	160,000 d
Antigen binding sites	10	2
Agglutination	Yes	No
Optimal binding temperature	<37°C	37°C
Common antibodies	A, B blood group antigens	Antigens from previous transfusion or pregnancy
Mechanism of hemolysis	Complement-mediated lysis	Reticuloendothelial cell removal of Ig-coated cells
Type of transfusion reaction	Acute	Delayed

In contrast, IgG is a much smaller molecule (molecular weight, 160,000 d) with only two antigen-binding sites. Thus, IgG tends to coat RBCs but does not cross-link cells or cause agglutination. Clinically important IgG antibodies causing hemolysis include alloantibodies from previous pregnancy or fetal-maternal hemorrhage that cross the placenta and cause hemolytic disease of the newborn, antibodies that were generated from previous transfusions, autoimmune or drug-induced hemolytic reactions, and antibodies found in association with lymphoproliferative or chronic inflammatory disorders. However, most IgG-mediated hemolytic anemias are idiopathic in nature, with no clearly identifiable cause. Hemolysis is secondary to removal of antibody-coated cells by the spleen or cells of the reticuloendothelial system. Large amounts of antibody coating the cells may lead to complement fixation on the cell surface, which increases the rate of cellular destruction by splenic or liver macrophages but does not result in complement-mediated lysis.

Physicochemical injury to RBCs by thermal burns or some chemical agents results in partial loss of RBC membrane and, with formation of microspherocytes, in resultant accelerated splenic removal. Full-thickness (third-degree) burns cause damage to RBCs in the underlying microcirculation. As soon as the damaged cells are removed, hemolysis stops. Infectious agents (eg, malaria, babesiosis) may disrupt the RBC as the parasite proliferates within it. RBC damage also may be secondary to damage to the membrane from an enzyme such as neuraminidase, produced by a microorganism (eg, in cholera).

12.2 Clinical Findings

Destruction of RBCs produces anemia, malaise, fatigue, pallor, and weakness. Jaundice is seen with rapid RBC destruction but may be absent in chronic hemolysis. IgM cold active antibodies may lead to vaso-occlusion secondary to cellular agglutination in fingers and toes where cooling occurs. Hemolysis ranges from mild to severe, and splenomegaly is uncommon. In contrast, IgG antibodies may result in an acute severe anemia or in a chronic unremitting process. Splenomegaly is common, and hepatomegaly may be seen. Lymphadenopathy is rare unless hemolysis is associated with a malignant lymphoma.

Both IgG and IgM alloantibodies act in transfusion reactions. Transfusion reactions vary from intravascular hemolysis to unexplained shortened RBC survival. Acute hemolytic transfusion reactions are usually due to IgM antibodies that recognize transfused RBC incompatibility, causing intravascular hemolysis of donor cells. In most cases, this is due to misidentification of blood samples, because crossmatching procedures should identify most antibodies that cause significant hemolysis. Symptoms associated with acute transfusion reactions include fever, chills, facial flushing, hypotension, nausea, vomiting, hemoglobinemia, and hemoglobinuria with subsequent renal shutdown. Delayed hemolytic reactions occur 3 to 14 days after transfusion in patients who were previously exposed to a blood group antigen via prior transfusion or pregnancy but do not have detectable antibody at the time of crossmatch. This is mediated by a secondary, IgG antibody–type immune response with attendant hemolysis by the reticulo-endothelial system and spleen.

12.3 Diagnostic Approach

A complete history with careful attention to transfusions, drugs, infections, travel, and chronic inflammatory or lymphoproliferative diseases is essential when evaluating an acquired hemolytic process. Infectious diseases, such as bacterial sepsis, that cause hemolysis are generally prostrating illnesses, and clinical findings separate them from immune-mediated hemolysis. Careful examination of the peripheral blood smear and an appropriate travel history can establish the diagnosis of malaria or other intraerythrocytic parasites.

Antibody-mediated hemolysis, in particular transfusion reactions, may occur as an acute process or a delayed process, occurring 3 to 14 days after transfusion. Historical information, such as sources of exposure to RBC products, how recently exposure occurred, and any symptoms associated with the exposure, help to guide the process evaluation. Acute transfusion reactions usually occur owing to errors in identification. Delayed hemolytic reactions occur in patients who have been sensitized to RBC antigens by pregnancy or previous transfusions and have antibody levels too low to detect with pretransfusion screening. The transfusion is usually uneventful, but IgG antibodies are readily induced 3 to 14 days later and become detectable as hemolysis occurs. Workup of suspected antibody-mediated or transfusion reaction hemolysis should include the following steps:

1. Serum antibody screening, which should include serologic techniques and temperature variations to detect both IgG and IgM antibodies.
2. Pretransfusion or posttransfusion antibody identification combined with appropriate antigen typing of the patient's RBCs.
3. Direct antiglobulin test (DAT; see Test 6.4) if the patient has received transfusions in the previous 3 to 6 weeks or if autoimmune hemolysis is suspected.
4. Tests such as plasma/urine hemoglobin, serum haptoglobin, and serum bilirubin to evaluate acute hemolysis. If intravascular hemolysis has occurred, tests to monitor renal function are also performed.

12.4 Hematologic Findings

Often, hematologic tests for transfusion reactions are unrevealing unless transfusions are currently being given. An abrupt fall in hemoglobin up to 14 days after transfusion, a failure to maintain hemoglobin levels after transfusion, or the appearance of jaundice suggests an incompatible transfusion. Prolonged administration of incompatible blood can result in splenomegaly and lead to the mistaken diagnosis of autoimmune hemolytic anemia. Intravascular hemolysis may result from ABO-incompatible transfusion and with a variety of other antibodies, including anti-Kell, anti-Duffy (anti-Fy^a), anti-Kidd (anti-Jk^a or anti-Jk^b), anti-E, anti-C, and anti-S.

12.4.1 Blood Cell Measurements

Variable anemia is present. One unit of packed RBCs should increase the hemoglobin (1.5 g/dL [15 g/L]) or the hematocrit (3% [0.03]) in an adult of average size. Acute hemolysis may be associated with leukocytosis and a left shift. In thermal burns or ABO-incompatible transfusions with marked microspherocytosis, the mean corpuscular volume (MCV) may be decreased as low as 60 to 70 μm^3 (60 to 70 fL).

12.4.2 Peripheral Blood Smear Morphology

Usually, peripheral smear findings are nonspecific. Transfusions that are ABO incompatible and IgG-mediated hemolysis are associated with the formation of microspherocytes. Thermal burns are associated with transient microspherocytosis lasting 24 to 48 hours. Disseminated intravascular coagulation can be associated with RBC fragmentation.

12.4.3 Bone Marrow Examination

Bone marrow examination usually is not helpful. Prolonged transfusions result in an increase in bone marrow iron. Prolonged hemolysis may lead to a compensatory erythroid hyperplasia.

Other Laboratory Tests

Test 12.1 Serum Antibody Screening

Purpose. Serum antibody screening reveals the presence of preformed RBC antibodies.

Principle. When the medium and temperature of reaction is appropriate, antibody to RBC antigens agglutinates or hemolyzes screening cells expressing that specific antigen. These tests are widely available, although the reliability of interpretation is variable.

Specimen. Ten milliliters of serum is obtained fresh to conserve complement, because some antibodies are complement-dependent. If blood must be mailed to a reference laboratory, the serum should be separated from the cells to prevent spurious hemolysis, and both RBCs and serum must be sent for testing. If serum cannot be tested within 48 hours, it should be frozen to conserve complement.

Procedure. The patient's serum is screened with commercially supplied RBC panels in which most of the 18 major antigen groups are represented. Screening cells and serum are incubated at room temperature to detect IgM antibodies and at 37°C, followed by the antiglobulin reaction (indirect Coombs' test), to detect IgG antibodies. IgA antibodies are rarely detected in blood group serology. If antibody is strongly suspected but not detected, laboratories in large hospitals or reference laboratories automatically perform tests at 4°C or they may use enzyme-treated RBCs or low ionic-strength solution (LISS) as the test medium to enhance antibody reaction.

Interpretation. Any degree of hemolysis or agglutination at any stage of the testing is considered positive and graded from 0 to 4+. The antibody must then be identified to assess transfusion hazard and future availability of blood. Results of antibody screening may be negative despite previous reactions to transfusion or incompatible pregnancies, because antibodies may be of such low titer that they are detectable only with enzyme-treated RBCs or with cells homozygous for the antigen. Suspicious histories should be reported to the laboratory so technologists can expand their testing beyond the routine screening procedures. Patients experiencing antigen-incompatible transfusions may have diminished RBC survival or abrupt hemolysis. Antibody is found in 2% to 3% of the previously transfused population, 2% to 3% of those previously pregnant, and less than 1% of all others, for a combined incidence of 5% to 6%.

Test 12.2 **Antibody Identification**

Purpose. Antibody identification assesses the current hazard of transfusion, predicts the reliability of crossmatch procedures, evaluates blood availability (particularly under emergency circumstances), and depicts multiple antibodies.

Principle. The availability and completeness of identification procedures vary in hospital laboratories and may be best handled by a reference laboratory when specimens with positive results from screening are obtained. Depending on the complexity of the identification, results may require 1 to 5 days.

Specimen. Serum separated from the clot and a sample of the patient's RBCs, either from the clot or from a separate anticoagulated (ethylenediaminetetraacetic acid [EDTA]) tube, are used as specimens. If serum cannot be tested within 48 hours, it should be frozen to conserve complement.

Procedure. Serum is tested with commercially available panels of 9 or 10 RBC samples for which all antigens are known. Serum is also tested with the patient's own cells and with samples of cord blood. Serum and cell samples are incubated at room temperature and at 37°C, and followed by the antiglobulin reaction. The presence of agglutination or hemolysis is noted and graded. Variability in the strength of agglutination, the temperature of reaction, or the medium of reaction may indicate the presence of more than one antibody. Once antibody specificity is known, the patient's RBCs are typed for the appropriate antigen.

Interpretation. Alloantibodies agglutinate specific cells of the panel, but not of the patient. The pattern of reactive cell samples is compared with the protocol sheet to determine specificity. The patient's cells should be negative for the particular antigen; if they are not, the antibody specificity is not confirmed and must be reevaluated.

IgG antibodies act at 37°C by indirect antiglobulin, enzyme, or LISS techniques. They usually follow previous transfusion or incompatible pregnancy. Four antibodies–anti-Kell, anti-Fy^a, anti-Jk^a, or anti-Jk^b–are particularly dangerous because they cause intravascular hemolysis and/or disseminated intravascular coagulation. The Kidd antibodies may not be found during antibody screening. However, their titers increase rapidly with incompatible transfusions, causing initiation of intravascular hemolysis as long as 10 days after transfusion when the stimulated antibody titer reaches a critical level. On rare occasions, anti-E or anti-C have caused abrupt intravascular hemolysis. The members of the Rh system (anti-D, anti-C, anti-E, anti-e) follow an immunizing stimulus and destroy cells more slowly by splenic sequestration. IgM antibodies bind complement. Although they may follow incompatible transfusion, they more often appear spontaneously and unpredictably. They include anti-Le^a and anti-Le^b, anti-P1, and anti-M. Many researchers believe that alloantibodies reactive at or below room temperature are not clinically significant. However, if detected, the potential for a transfusion reaction exists.

Once identified, antibodies must be permanently recorded, because titers may decrease over time only to be reinduced with incompatible transfusions. Titers may be so weak that truly incompatible units appear compatible. The most lethal IgM antibodies are anti-A and anti-B, involved in major blood group incompatibility. Such incompatibility is almost always caused by errors in patient identification. These antibodies are not detectable in the usual antibody identification panel, because all the test RBCs are group O.

Test 12.3 Direct Antiglobulin (Coombs') Test

Purpose. The DAT detects antibody coating of circulating RBCs. It does not distinguish alloantibody from autoantibody. After transfusion, in the absence of autoantibody, the coated RBCs should be donor cells, as confirmed by testing RBC antigens.

Principle, Specimen, and Procedure. See Test 6.4.

Interpretation. Positive results may vary from +/– to 4+, depending on the cause. In autoimmune hemolytic anemia, the DAT tends to be high, whereas in transfusion reactions the DAT is usually 1+ or weaker. The donor cells are a minor population in the patient's circulation, giving a characteristic "mixed-field" appearance. Positive test results may be extremely transient. After massive intravascular hemolysis, the DAT may be negative because all the antibody-coated RBCs are lysed. The antibody specificity of the eluate should not match the patient's RBC antigen profile, although in patients transfused with many units or in those with a DAT of 4+, the antigens responsible for hemolysis may be difficult to determine. Retesting after 4 to 5 days while withholding further transfusions may clarify the picture.

Test 12.4 Serum Haptoglobin

Purpose. An absence of haptoglobin indicates hemolysis, liver failure, or rare hereditary variants.

Principle, Specimen, and Procedure. See Test 6.3.

Interpretation. The normal range of haptoglobin is 40 to 180 mg/dL (0.4 to 1.8 g/L). Levels of less than 25 mg/dL (0.25 g/L) are consistent with hemolysis. Haptoglobin levels may be transiently decreased after massive transfusion as a result of destruction of senescent RBCs without hemolysis.

Test 12.5 Plasma Hemoglobin

Principle. IgM antibodies to RBC antigens activate the classic complement pathway, resulting in intravascular hemolysis. IgG antibodies of very high titer also may result in intravascular cell destruction. This releases free hemoglobin into the plasma, which serves as an indicator of hemolysis.

Purpose, Procedure, Specimen, and Interpretation. See Test 6.2.

Test 12.6 Urine Hemoglobin

Purpose. Free plasma hemoglobin levels greater than 150 mg/dL (1.5 g/L) lead to spillover of hemoglobin into the urine. The test for urine hemoglobin confirms intravascular hemolysis, particularly when venous specimens have been technically difficult to obtain or collection is delayed.

Principle. Plasma proteins, haptoglobin, transferrin, and albumin bind free hemoglobin in normal metabolism. When the renal threshold is exceeded, free hemoglobin is detected in the urine. After incompatible transfusion, this is usually a transient occurrence, ending when the incompatible RBCs have been lysed. With other forms of immune-mediated hemolysis, hemoglobinuria may become chronic, reflecting the chronic nature of the hemolytic process.

Specimen. Random urine samples are collected within 2 to 3 hours of the clinical episode.

Procedure. Urine is tested with a dipstick that colorimetrically indicates the presence of hemoglobin.

Interpretation. Normally, no hemoglobin is present in the urine. Significant reactions are 1+ or greater (scale, 0 to 3+). The urine sediment should be examined for RBCs (hematuria), which may give rise to a false-positive test result. Urinary RBCs are not seen with hemolysis but usually result from bladder or prostate surgery and urinary instrumentation. Increased levels of myoglobin in the urine, secondary to muscle damage, also may cause false-positive results. If RBC destruction has occurred slowly over several days, urine hemosiderin may be present without overt hemoglobinuria.

12.5 Course and Treatment

Intravascular hemolysis caused by inadvertent ABO incompatibility activates complement and the coagulation cascade to produce disseminated intravascular coagulation. Hypotension, renal failure, and death may follow. The severity of the reaction is dose-related, so treatment requires early recognition to stop the transfusion. Patient hydration must be maintained to avoid renal failure. Osmotic diuresis with 20% mannitol may aid in clearing plasma hemoglobin. Delayed transfusion reactions produce significant morbidity but less certain mortality. Jaundice and posttransfusion anemia resolve if compatible blood is given. Further transfusion should not be considered until the antibody has been identified and antigen-negative units have been provided.

Hemodialysis may be necessary if renal failure has occurred, and 30% of patients never regain renal function. In delayed or mild hemolytic transfusion reactions, time and transfusion with compatible blood result in resolution of symptoms and an appropriate posttransfusion hemoglobin level. Treatment of catastrophic infectious disease with associated hemolysis involves prompt and intensive treatment of the underlying organism with appropriate intravenous antibiotic therapy. Malaria is treated with chloroquine, primaquine, or other antimalarial agents, and full recovery is common if the patient is treated promptly.

12.6 References

Anstall HB, Blaycock RC. Compatibility testing and pretransfusion screening. In: *Practical Aspects of the Transfusion Service*. Chicago, Ill: ASCP Press; 1996:33–56.

Goodnough LT, Brecher ME, Kanter MH, et al. Transfusion medicine, I: blood transfusion. *N Engl J Med*. 1999;340:438–447.

Jeter EK, Spivey MA. Noninfectious complications of blood transfusion. *Hematol Oncol Clin North Am*. 1995;9:187–201.

Mollison PL, Engelfriet CP, Contreras M, eds. *Blood Transfusion in Clinical Medicine*. 9th ed. Oxford, England: Blackwell; 1993.

Schroeder ML. Principles and practice of transfusion medicine. In: Lee GR, Foerster J, Lukens JN, et al, eds. *Wintrobe's Clinical Hematology*. 10th ed. Baltimore, Md: Williams & Wilkins; 1999:827–834.

13 Extrinsic Hemolytic Anemia: Fetal-Maternal Incompatibility

In fetal-maternal incompatibility or hemolytic disease of the newborn (HDN), the fetus receives antibody passively across the placenta from the mother who has been exposed to foreign antigens through a previous transfusion or has received small transplacental infusions of fetal RBCs during the current or a past pregnancy. Many of the characteristics of HDN are similar to those seen in incompatible transfusions.

13.1 Pathophysiology

HDN develops owing to the transfer across the placenta of specific maternal antibodies against RBC antibodies from the mother to the fetus. The fetus expresses different RBC antigens by virtue of the paternal genetic contribution. Only IgG is capable of crossing the placenta, and the degree of hemolysis is dependent on the amount of antibody as well as the binding avidity of the IgG subtype. Evidence suggests that clinically significant hemolysis correlates with subtype IgG3, whereas IgG1 is not associated with hemolysis.

Antibody-coated RBCs are sequestered in the spleen and liver prior to destruction, causing neonatal hepatosplenomegaly.

Maternal sensitization to fetal RBC antigens is primarily due to fetal-maternal hemorrhage during pregnancy or, more commonly, at the time of delivery when the largest volume of blood exchange may occur. The two major types of fetal-maternal incompatibility are ABO group incompatibility and Rh incompatibility (**Table 13-1**).

Antibodies against ABO-incompatible blood antigens are very common but usually do not cause severe hemolytic disease. This arises in a mother of blood group O with a fetus who is blood group A, B, or AB. It may occur during any pregnancy, even the first, because it is postulated that in addition to RBCs, secreted A or B substance may cross the placenta to induce maternal production of an IgG isotype of anti-A or anti-B in addition to the IgM anti-A and anti-B IgG antibodies normally present. This IgG antibody then crosses the placenta, attaching to the fetal RBCs. Antibody avidity is usually poor, so hemolytic disease is slow to appear, usually 3 to 4 days after delivery.

Rh_0 (anti-D) incompatibility usually appears in pregnancies following the first as a result of fetal-maternal hemorrhage of Rh-positive blood during delivery. This leads to sensitization of an Rh-negative mother to produce antibodies against the locus. This is much less common with the current use of prophylactic anti-Rh immune globulin. Given at each abortion or delivery to Rh-negative women, it prevents immune recognition of D antigen by the mother by masking the immunologic site on any fetal cells that may enter into maternal circulation. In 1% of mothers, sensitization may occur in the first pregnancy (possibly due to placental hemorrhage), but clinical disease in the infant is rare. Occasionally, other antibodies (anti-C, anti-E, and anti-Kell) are involved in fetal-maternal incompatibility. The mechanism is the same as that for anti-D, but these antibodies are less efficient at causing neonatal hemolysis and subsequent jaundice.

13.2 Clinical Findings

Serologic evidence may exist for HDN without clinical evidence of hemolysis, particularly in ABO incompatibility. Destruction of RBCs is primarily caused by reticuloendothelial sequestration of

Table 13-1 Characteristics of Hemolytic Disease of the Newborn

Findings	ABO	Rh_0
Clinical		
Pregnancy associated with disease	Any, including the first	After the first pregnancy
Clinical severity	Unpredictable	More severe with each antigen-positive pregnancy
Prenatal evaluation	None needed	Sequential anti-Rh_0 titers, amniocentesis
Onset of jaundice	3-4 wk after delivery	Intrauterine or immediately after delivery
Treatment*	None; phototherapy or rare exchange therapy	None; early delivery, phototherapy, exchange transfusion, or intrauterine transfusion
Laboratory		
Direct Coombs' test	+/– to 1+	2+ to 4+
Fetal blood group	A, B, or AB	Rh_0 positive
Antibody causing hemolysis	Anti-A or anti-B	Anti-Rh_0 (anti-D)
Maternal blood group	O, A, B	Rh_0 or D^u negative
Maternal antibody screening	Negative	Positive
Peripheral blood (newborn)	Microspherocytes	Not diagnostic

*Treatment options are listed by increasing severity of hemolysis.

IgG-sensitized RBCs. Thus, the fetal liver and spleen are enlarged and jaundice is present in the neonatal period.

In severe Rh-mediated hemolysis (25% of patients), RBC destruction occurs in utero. This leads to severe anemia with high output congestive heart failure and anasarca (hydrops fetalis). Mild disease (50% of patients) may present as a mild hemolytic anemia requiring no therapy, whereas patients with moderate disease (25%) have significant anemia and severe jaundice and are at risk for development of kernicterus. Jaundice is not seen until after birth, when placental transport of bilirubin is lost and the neonatal liver assumes bilirubin metabolism. The immature infant liver is initially unable to conjugate bilirubin rapidly enough in the face of hemolysis, leading to high levels of indirect bilirubin and jaundice. The indirect bilirubin is also deposited in the lenticulostriate nucleus of the brain (kernicterus), which may cause mental retardation, motor spasticity, and death.

13.3 Diagnostic Approach

The type of fetal-maternal incompatibility that produces HDN may be suggested by maternal transfusion and gestational histories. The following tests may be helpful in establishing a diagnosis:

1. Maternal blood group and antibody screening.
2. Newborn blood group.
3. Direct antiglobulin test (DAT; see Tests 6.4 and 13.3) of newborn RBCs and RBC eluates.
4. Examination of a peripheral blood smear from the infant or cord blood for microspherocytes.
5. Serial serum bilirubin tests, if serologic evidence is present for HDN.
6. Tests of the father's blood and the mother's if serologic evidence of HDN is not present, yet the newborn is experiencing hemolysis for undetermined causes and the DAT result is positive. Such testing is expected to exclude unusual incompatibilities between paternal antigens expressed by the child and maternal antibodies.
7. Neutralization studies. Although such studies can be performed to classify the maternal antibody as IgG or IgM, knowledge of which helps to estimate likelihood of placental passage, they are rarely necessary or clinically helpful.

Prenatal studies may anticipate clinical disease in the newborn and may direct prenatal or postnatal management. These studies include sequential titration of anti-D levels in the mother's serum and amniocentesis to determine levels of intrauterine hemolysis.

13.4 Hematologic Findings

There may be a wide spectrum of anemia present, ranging from none to severe. Persistent extramedullary hematopoiesis in an attempt to compensate for hemolysis results in increased circulating nucleated RBCs (erythroblastosis fetalis). HDN caused by ABO and less common RBC antibodies is usually mild. Rh-mediated HDN tends to be progressively more severe with each pregnancy.

13.4.1 Blood Cell Measurements

Levels of hemoglobin in mild anemia are 14 to 16 g/dL (140 to 160 g/L). In moderate anemia, the levels are 10 to 14 g/dL (100 to 140 g/L); and in severe anemia, they are 8 to 10 g/dL (80 to 100 g/L). The reticulocyte count is often greater than 10% (0.10). The WBC count is normal to mildly elevated at 10 to $20 \times 10^3/\mu L$ (10 to $20 \times 10^9/L$). Platelets may be mildly to moderately decreased.

13.4.2 Peripheral Blood Smear Morphology

The peripheral blood smear shows polychromasia, correlating with the increased reticulocyte count, and nucleated RBCs greater than 10 per 100 WBCs (erythroblastosis). Microspherocytes usually indicate ABO hemolytic disease but are not typically prominent. Thrombocytopenia and leukocytosis are common.

Other Laboratory Tests

Test 13.1 Determination of Blood Group

Purpose. Testing of the blood group of the mother, father, and newborn determines whether a fetal-maternal incompatibility exists.

Principle. Maternal and newborn RBC antigens are studied for ABO and Rh_0 expression. Tests can be performed for other antigens if indicated.

Specimen. RBCs from clots or anticoagulated specimens are washed well with saline before testing. Specimens are stable for at least 7 days. Cord RBCs and plasma can be used if the RBCs are washed well to remove contaminants. Infant heel-stick specimens also can be used.

Procedure. Standard typing procedures that detect direct agglutination of RBCs by anti-A, anti-B, and anti-D antibodies are used. All Rh_0-negative cells also are tested for D^u, the partial or gene-suppressed D^u antigen.

Interpretation. In ABO hemolytic disease, the mother's blood is usually group O (ie, negative for A or B antigens) and the infant's blood is group A, B, or AB. Disease also may arise in a group A mother with a group B infant or a group B mother with a group A infant. In Rh hemolytic disease, the mother is Rh negative and the infant is Rh positive. Where the serologic possibility of both ABO and Rh disease is possible (ie, an O-negative mother with an A- or B-positive child), hemolytic disease is more likely caused by ABO incompatibility, because the major blood group incompatibility has usually lysed Rh-incompatible cells throughout the pregnancy. Mothers who are Rh positive are not excluded from having infants with hemolytic disease, because they may be negative for minor antigens in the complex (such as C or E) and their offspring may be positive.

Test 13.2 Maternal Antibody Screening and Identification

Purpose. A positive antibody screen may indicate Rh type of hemolytic disease rather than ABO type, for which screenings are usually negative.

Principle. Maternal serum is screened for antibody, usually early in pregnancy and sporadically thereafter, to detect the presence of IgG or IgM antibodies. Antibody levels are assessed to determine fetal risk and, if necessary, the father's RBC antigens are tested as a predictive measure of fetal expression.

Specimen. Serum less than 48 hours old, obtained at the first obstetric visit, is used. A specimen also should be obtained in the third trimester, and more frequently if the early specimen shows positive results or if an obstetric history of previous hemolytic disease in an infant warrants it.

Procedure. Serum is incubated with test RBCs at room temperature in saline suspension to detect IgM antibodies and by incubation at 37°C followed by antiglobulin reaction to detect IgG antibodies. All antibodies are identified with the same techniques.

Interpretation. In ABO hemolytic disease, only the expected anti-A and/or anti-B antibodies are found in the group O mother, so the antibody screen is negative. In all other types of hemolytic disease, the maternal antibody screen is positive. The antibody must be subclassified to determine its significance to the newborn. Only IgG antibodies cross the placenta, and they must have sufficient affinity to coat the infant's RBCs to produce hemolysis. Common RBC antibodies found in pregnant women are anti-Le^a and anti-Le^b. These antibodies do not produce neonatal disease because they are IgM and cannot cross the placenta, and all infants are Le^a and Le^b negative. Thus, some antibodies are more significant for the mother in a postpartum hemorrhage than for infant HDN.

The current practice of administering Rh immune globulin at 28 weeks of gestation to prevent possible sensitization by the fetus results in a spurious positive maternal antibody screening due to weak anti-D (titer, <1:4). Unlike antibody produced as a consequence of true maternal sensitization, these antibodies do not give a "crisp" pattern of identification.

Test 13.3 Direct Antiglobulin (Coombs') Test in the Newborn

Purpose. The DAT detects antibodies coating the newborn's RBCs.

Principle. Fetal RBCs are coated with passively transmitted maternal IgG antibody specific for RBC antigen.

Specimen. RBCs from either clotted or anticoagulated cord blood can be used. Small capillary specimens from newborn heelsticks are acceptable also. Cord blood samples are stable for at least 1 week and can be tested if clinical symptoms of hemolysis appear.

Procedure. Broad-spectrum antiglobulin reagent is centrifuged with the newborn's RBCs, which have been washed with saline to free them of contaminating substances and serum proteins. Agglutination is graded 0 to 4+. For all tests producing positive results, adsorbed globulin is eluted from the RBC and tested for antibody specificity.

Interpretation. Infant DAT results are +/– to 1+ for ABO hemolytic disease, 2 to 4+ for Rh hemolytic disease, and 2 to 4+ for hemolytic disease caused by other antibodies. The antibody eluted from the neonatal RBCs should match that found in the maternal serum. Antibody found in cord plasma but not on cord RBCs is of doubtful significance, suggesting poor avidity and less likely clinical disease. Antibodies—such as anti-C, anti-E, and anti-Kell—that are adsorbed to fetal RBCs produce a strong DAT but usually minimal hemolysis and jaundice. Improved antiglobulin reagents make false-negative test results less common, and additional saline washing of the cells diminishes false-negative results resulting from neutralization of the Coombs' reagent. On rare occasions, elution of an antiglobulin-negative RBC yields antibody due to concentration of antibodies by the elution process.

Positive DAT results on cord specimens without detectable antibody may indicate adsorption of antibody by Wharton's jelly, but the RBC control is usually positive. The test should be repeated on blood from a heel-stick or venous sample. If results are still positive, private antibody limited to this family should be considered, and maternal serum or infant's plasma should be tested against paternal RBCs for agglutination.

Test 13.4 **Acid Elution (Kleihauer-Betke) Test**

Purpose. Fetal-maternal hemorrhage of even small numbers of Rh-positive fetal RBCs may sensitize an Rh-negative mother, unless she is adequately immunized postpartum with Rh immune globulin. Doses are standardized to compensate for fetal hemorrhage volume of 15 mL of packed RBCs or less. The actual volume of hemorrhage can be calculated by staining a maternal peripheral smear for fetal cells. If the volume of fetal hemorrhage exceeds 15 mL, an increased dosage of Rh immune globulin should be administered. Intrapartum Rh immune globulin is administered at 20 to 28 weeks of gestation, but Kleihauer-stained peripheral smears usually are not useful at this time because the number of potentially positive cells is minimal.

Principle. Fetal hemoglobin is resistant to acid elution, whereas adult hemoglobin is not. A maternal peripheral smear is treated with dilute acid buffer for 10 minutes and then stained. The maternal erythrocyte adult hemoglobin is leached into the buffer, leaving RBC ghosts, whereas the fetal RBCs remain as dense red erythrocytes.

Specimen. Very thin peripheral blood smears fixed in 80% alcohol are prepared from maternal blood collected in ethylenedi-aminetetraacetic acid (EDTA).

Procedure. Dried smears are placed in McIlvaine's buffer (pH 3.2) for 10 minutes, followed by washing in distilled water. The smear is then stained with erythrosin and counterstained with hematoxylin. Two thousand cells are counted and the percentage of densely staining cells with fetal hemoglobin (presumably fetal in origin) is calculated. The percentage can be converted to milliliters by a nomogram, and 300 mg of Rh immune globulin is administered intramuscularly for each 15 mL of packed RBCs calculated. Control smears should be made from cord blood specimens (positive) mixed 1:10 with adult blood (negative), because questionably positive cells are sometimes seen even with the negative control. Test kits are available, so small laboratories may perform this test.

Interpretation. Normal adult cells leak hemoglobin and appear as paler ghosts. Fetal cells are densely pink and refractile. The volume of fetal-maternal hemorrhage is calculated as milliliters of whole blood equal to the percentage of fetal cells multiplied by 50. Hemorrhage in excess of 15 mL packed cell volume requires a proportionate increase in Rh immune globulin administered. Because variability in the amount of acid hemoglobin elution may occur even within the same laboratory, it is important that appropriate controls of fetal (cord) blood and adult blood be done to aid in proper interpretation.

Work is in progress to develop reliable flow cytometric tests to detect fetal cells, using staining for hemoglobin F in permeabilized RBCs. This technology will allow detection of a very small number of fetal cells within a sample.

Notes and Precautions. Adult hemoglobinopathies, such as persistence of fetal hemoglobin, may create a misleading picture. If the volume of fetal cells suggests significant blood loss from an otherwise healthy infant with normal hemoglobin, the possibility of hemoglobinopathy in the mother should be considered.

13.5 Ancillary Tests

Ancillary tests include ultrasonography, which can demonstrate fetal hydrops. Ultrasound localization of the placenta is necessary prior to amniocentesis for measurement of amniotic fluid bilirubin. This is helpful in estimating the rate of RBC destruction and expected degree of fetal anemia. The procedure is undertaken when maternal Rh antibody has been identified and has a significant titer (>1:16 to 1:23 by indirect antiglobin techniques). Depending on the titer, obstetric history, and history of previous hemolytic disease, the first procedure is usually performed at 16 to 18 weeks of gestation. At least two sequential specimens are needed to verify an increase in optical density and to determine whether the differential absorption is increasing, decreasing, or stable, which provides insights into the clinical course of disease. Specimens are obtained every 1 to 2 weeks or, in borderline cases, every few days. If significant hemolysis is suspected based on increased levels of amniotic fluid bilirubin levels, fetal blood sampling or intrauterine transfusion may be required.

Amniotic fluid (5 to 10 mL) is withdrawn and immediately shielded from light, which degrades bilirubin and causes falsely decreased results. The specimen is centrifuged to separate vernix, and the supernatant is scanned in the ultraviolet spectrum from 350 to 700 nm. Bilirubin has a peak absorbance at 450 nm, although the curve is not linear. A tangent is constructed to create a straight line, and the difference in optical density from the tangent to the peak at 450 nm is the change in optical density. An optical density rise at 450 nm is common early in pregnancy, with peak levels at 23 to 24 weeks of gestation, but decreases after 26 weeks if no RBC sensitization is present.

Nomogram zones determined by Liley correlate the spectrophotometric data with week of gestation probability of severe hemolytic disease. This may be verified in severe cases by direct fetal blood sampling via cordocentesis. If the anemia is severe and fetal lungs are markedly immature, intrauterine transfusion is considered. If fetal lung maturation is adequate, early delivery is undertaken, permitting extrauterine exchange transfusion. Intrauterine transfusion has a success rate of approximately 85% unless hydrops is present, in which case the success rate is less than 25%.

13.5.1 Notes

False elevations in absorbance are seen when hemoglobin or meconium contaminate the specimen, because one of several hemoglobin A optical peaks occurs at 450 nm. Amniocentesis interpretation is based on experience with anti-D antibody. There is no guaranteed extrapolation to other antibodies or other causes of hemolysis.

13.6 Course and Treatment

Maternal serum is monitored during pregnancy to detect Rh sensitization and follow its course by changes in antibody titers. High Rh antibody titers (>1:32) require amniocentesis to monitor the progression and severity of anemia in the fetus. Rapid progression of hemolysis may require intrauterine transfusion or early delivery with exchange transfusion to treat severe anemia and hyperbilirubinemia. Mild jaundice after birth is controlled with phototherapy, which oxidizes bilirubin in the infant's skin. ABO sensitization is rarely severe after delivery, often in association with anti-B. No treatment before delivery is necessary, which is also true for most HDN caused by other less common antibodies.

13.7 References

Bowman J. Assays to predict the clinical significance of blood group antibodies. *Semin Perinatol*. 1998;5:412–416.

Bowman JM. Alloimmune hemolytic disease of the fetus and newborn. In: Lee GR, Foerster J, Lukens JN, et al, eds. *Wintrobe's Clinical Hematology*. 10th ed. Baltimore, Md: Williams & Wilkins; 1999:1210–1232.

Davis BH, Olsen S, Biglow NC, et al. Detection of fetal red cells in fetomaternal hemorrhage using a fetal hemoglobin monoclonal antibody by flow cytometry. *Transfusion*. 1998;38:749–756.

Duguid JK. ACP Broadsheet No. 150, March 1997. Antenatal serologic testing and preventing of hemolytic disease of the newborn. *J Clin Pathol*. 1997;50:193–196.

Hadley AG. In vitro assays to predict the severity of hemolytic disease of the newborn. *Transfus Med Rev*. 1995;9:302–313.

Hartwell EA. Use of Rh globulin: ASCP practice parameters. American Society of Clinical Pathologists. *Am J Clin Pathol*. 1998;110:281–292.

Zupanska B. Assays to predict the clinical significance of blood group antibodies. *Curr Opin Hematol*. 1998;5:412–416.

14 Drug-Related Extrinsic Hemolytic Anemia

Drugs produce hemolytic anemia by two different mechanisms: (1) oxidation of hemoglobin in patients with intrinsic defects in hemoglobin synthesis or in enzymes needed to protect the cell from oxidative injury or (2) immune-mediated RBC destruction. The degree of hemolysis can vary from acute intravascular hemolysis to chronic compensated hemolysis with splenic sequestration. In most cases, the hemolytic anemia is reversible when the drug is withdrawn.

14.1 Pathophysiology

14.1.1 Drug-induced Oxidation of Hemoglobin

A number of drugs have been shown to oxidize hemoglobin in RBCs. Normally, this does not present a difficulty because hemoglobin is readily returned to the reduced state. However, in patients with an intrinsic deficiency in the pathways necessary to produce reduced glutathione or in patients with an unstable hemoglobin, oxidation may lead to hemolysis.

Glucose-6-phosphate dehydrogenase (G6PD) deficiency, which was discussed in more detail in Chapter 9, is the most common enzymatic deficiency associated with drug-induced hemolysis. The interaction of an oxidative drug with G6PD-deficient RBCs leads to depletion of glutathione (GSH) and inadequate production of the reduced form of nicotinamide-adenine dinucleotide phosphate (NADPH). The depletion of GSH is followed by irreversible oxidation of hemoglobin. Hemoglobin degradation products polymerize to form Heinz bodies, with resultant membrane damage and reticuloendothelial phagocytosis by the spleen. Young RBCs that have more NADPH are less susceptible to oxidative damage, so as reticulocytosis increases, the effects of low doses of an oxidative drug tend to be self-limited. Drugs that induce hemolysis in patients with G6PD deficiency are listed in **Table 14-1**. Owing to variations in the deficiency phenotype, these drugs do not uniformly cause hemolysis in any person with G6PD deficiency.

Patients with unstable hemoglobins, which were discussed in further detail in Chapter 10, also may be more susceptible to oxidative damage to hemoglobin. An amino acid substitution in either the alpha or beta chain near the attachment site of the heme group to hemoglobin renders the molecule more sensitive to oxidative injury and subsequent denaturation. This leads to the formation of Heinz bodies and hemolysis by reticuloendothelial cell activity.

14.1.2 Drug-induced Immune Hemolysis

Drugs can cause immune-mediated hemolysis by a variety of mechanisms, including adsorption to the RBC membrane as a hapten, formation of toxic immune complexes, or induction of autoantibodies against the RBC membrane (**Table 14-2**). Except for autoantibody-mediated processes, the drug must be present for hemolysis to occur.

Drugs that cause immune hemolysis often have benzene rings activated by hydroxyl (-OH), amine (-NH), or sulfur (-S) groups. The drug must bind to a protein carrier, serum proteins, or RBC membrane to induce antibody production. Furthermore, the antibody produced must have sufficient binding capacity to produce hemolysis. Although by these criteria many drugs are potential causes of hemolysis, most clinically significant cases are caused by penicillin or α-methyldopa.

Drugs such as penicillin and related antibiotics act as haptens by adsorbing to the RBC or binding cell membrane proteins,

Table 14-1   Drugs Commonly Associated With Hemolysis in G6PD

Antimalarial agents
    Primaquine
    Quinacrine
Sulfonamides
    Sulfanilamide
    Salicylazosulfapyridine
    Sulfacetamide
Other antibacterial agents
    Nitrofurantoin
    Nitrofurazone
    Para-aminosalicylic acid
    Nalidixic acid
Analgesics
    Acetanilid
Sulfones
    Diaminodiphenyl sulfone
    Thiazolsulfone
Miscellaneous
    Dimercaprol
    Naphthalene (mothballs)
    Methylene blue
    Trinitrotoluene (TNT)

Abbreviation: G6PD = glucose-6-phosphate dehydrogenase.

forming an antigenic drug-cell complex. The hapten induces IgG antibody to the penicilloyl moiety, common to drugs of this class and cephalosporins. Drug-coated cells are usually destroyed by the reticuloendothelial system, although intravascular hemolysis may occur in rare instances. Immune hemolysis occurs only when all three components—drug, protein (or RBCs), and antibody—are present.

Drug-induced toxic complexes are formed following antibody production after a drug binds to a plasma protein to form an immunogen. The drug-protein complex combines with the resultant antibody, and this antigen-antibody complex may bind to the RBC to cause activation of complement. Although the immune complex may then disassociate from the RBC, the complement cascade continues, causing severe membrane damage and

Table 14-2 Features of Drug-Mediated Immune Hemolysis

Parameter	Drug Absorption, Hapten Formation	Toxic Immune Complex	Warm-Type Autoantibodies
Associated drugs	Penicillin and penicillin-type drugs	Quinine, quinidine, nonsteroidal anti-inflammatory agents	α−methyldopa, procainamide, mefenamic acid
Role of drug	Binds to RBC membrane	Forms antigen-antibody complex that binds to RBC	Unknown
Antibody formed	To drug	To drug	To RBC
Antibody class	IgG	IgM or IgG	IgG
Proteins detected with direct antiglobulin test	IgG, rarely complement	Complement	IgG, rarely complement
Drug needed for hemolysis	Yes	Yes	No
Mechanism of RBC destruction	Splenic sequestration of	Complement-mediated lysis IgG-coated cells clearance of C3b-coated cells	Splenic sequestration and splenic

intravascular hemolysis. Thus, a small amount of drug may induce extensive hemolysis. Drugs associated with this type of reaction include quinidine, quinine, and nonsteroidal anti-inflammatory drugs (NSAIDs).

Finally, some drugs may induce a true warm-type autoimmune hemolytic anemia (AIHA), which persists after removal of the drug. The drug most often associated with this type of reaction is α-methyldopa. The mechanism of antibody production by α-methyldopa is unknown, although drug-induced alterations of the endoplasmic reticulum of plasma cells have been postulated to explain the persistence of antibody production long after the drug has been discontinued. Clinical hemolysis rarely begins after the drug has been withdrawn, but if hemolysis is already present, it may not resolve for several weeks following discontinuation of the drug.

14.2 Clinical Findings

Hemolysis caused by drug interaction with G6PD deficiency or unstable hemoglobins may be an abrupt intravascular event with severe anemia, hemoglobinemia, hemoglobinuria, and jaundice. Anemia occurs 1 to 3 days after exposure to the oxidative drug. If the drug is withdrawn and reticulocytosis begins, the hemolysis abates.

Drug-induced immune hemolysis is usually less clinically severe, although intravascular hemolysis can occur with all categories of drug-related hemolysis. Hepatosplenomegaly and lymphadenopathy are not associated with drug-induced hemolytic anemia.

14.3 Diagnostic Approach

Proper diagnostic evaluation requires an awareness of drugs associated with hemolysis and a high index of suspicion in a patient who is currently receiving or has recently received such drugs and who has unexplained anemia. Evaluation proceeds with the following steps:

1. Hematologic findings show a normochromic anemia that may be actively hemolytic. Bone marrow aspiration is usually not needed.
2. Test results for Heinz bodies may be positive in patients with G6PD deficiency or unstable hemoglobins.
3. The direct antiglobulin test (DAT) result is positive in immunohemolytic processes, although to a variable degree depending on the mechanism of drug action.
4. Serum antibody screening tests with standard reagent RBCs are usually negative.
5. Special testing of eluates from Coombs'-positive RBCs in parallel with serum against specific drug-treated RBCs is performed.

14.4 Hematologic Findings

The anemia may be severe or mild to moderate if well compensated by bone marrow activity. The degree of anemia may also vary, depending on the drug mechanism of action, dosage, and the type of antibody evoked. A reactive leukocytosis may appear. In G6PD deficiency and unstable hemoglobins, hemolysis begins as Heinz bodies appear. As the hemolysis persists, Heinz antibodies are removed in the spleen and tend to disappear.

14.4.1 Blood Cell Measurements

Hemoglobin can be markedly decreased to 3 g/dL (30g/L) in severe hemolysis. Elevations in mean corpuscular volume (MCV) to 105 to 110 μm^3 (105 to 110 fL) reflect reticulocytosis. The WBC count is often elevated to 10 to 20 × 10^3/μL (10 to 20 × 10^9/L), and a left shift to the myelocyte stage may be seen.

14.4.2 Peripheral Blood Smear Morphology

Nucleated RBCs and polychromasia are general findings. Spherocytes may be seen with α-methyldopa–type AIHAs. Bite cells may be seen when Heinz bodies have been extracted by the spleen. Heinz bodies are not visualized on Wright-stained smears, but are seen with crystal violet stains.

14.4.3 Bone Marrow Examination

The bone marrow is often hypercellular with normoblastic erythroid hyperplasia and increased iron stores.

Other Laboratory Tests

When immune hemolysis is suspected, whole blood is obtained fresh and allowed to clot at 37°C before the serum is separated. Freezing serum samples should be avoided because this frequently disrupts immune complexes. The RBCs for testing can be obtained from the clot or from a separately collected ethylenediaminetetraacetic acid (EDTA) specimen, which prevents nonspecific adsorption of complement. Specimens for evaluation in G6PD deficiency may be collected in EDTA.

Test 14.1 **Direct Antiglobulin (Coombs') Test**

Purpose. The DAT must show positive results for drug-induced immune-mediated hemolysis to be considered seriously. Adsorbed globulin may be IgG, IgM, or complement.

Principle, Specimen, and Procedure. See Test 6.4.

Interpretation. No matter what the mechanism of action, all antibody types have common antibody globulin and/or complement attached to the RBC detectable with this test. Without a positive result on the DAT, drug-related immune hemolytic anemia is unlikely. The DAT in G6PD-mediated drug hemolysis is negative. Often the result in drug-induced hemolytic anemias is weakly positive, and use of RBC eluates may be necessary for antibody detection. The adsorbed globulin, once detected, is eluted and tested in parallel with the patient's serum against drug-treated RBCs and untreated RBCs. The effects of neutralization of the eluate with the suspected drug are studied as well. Findings for each category of drug-induced immune hemolysis are summarized in **Table 14-2**.

Test 14.2 **Serum Antibody Tests and Tests With Drug-Treated RBCs**

Purpose. Agglutination of drug-treated cells by patient serum is consistent with drug-immune hemolysis but is not as diagnostic as identifying the globulin actually adsorbed to the RBC. For α-methyldopa, reactions are positive with untreated patient RBCs, defining the antibody as autoantibody.

Principle. In general, the organic drug binds with a serum protein or the RBC membrane to produce an immunogenic complex. Antibody production, strength, and avidity vary with the drug and the patient, as well as with the duration and route of exposure to the drug. Avidity of the drug (drug adsorption type) or complexes of drug and antibody that fix complement (immune complex type) for binding to the RBC membrane is the final common pathway to hemolysis. Some drugs, acting by an unknown mechanism, induce production of a true warm-type AIHA. Ease of demonstration of the drug-related antibody varies with the mechanism of action.

Procedure. Tests for the following are available in reference laboratories and most sophisticated hospital blood banks:

1. Drug adsorption. RBCs pretreated with weak dilutions of penicillin drugs can be refrigerated for 2 to 3 weeks for future testing. Treated cells are positive with either direct (IgM) or indirect (IgG) antibody testing. Antibody can be titered against drug-treated cells or neutralized by the appropriate drug.

2. Toxic immune complexes. This is done when DAT shows complement coating the cells. The patient's blood is either pretreated with the drug or drug is added at the time of the test with patient serum and fresh complement. A DAT is performed. Concentrations of drugs and serum samples are varied to achieve optimal antigen-antibody concentration. Drug neutralization is not demonstrable.

3. True warm-type AIHA. The DAT shows agglutination of RBCs without the drug being present, demonstrating that autoantibodies are present. Weak autoantibodies may require enzyme-treated RBCs for demonstration.

Interpretation.

1. Drug adsorption (penicillins). This type of antibody is common and easily demonstrated. Only IgG antibodies produce significant hemolysis. The antibody may react with one or more penicillin congeners, varying between patients. Cross-reactions with cephalothin-treated cells occur as a result of similarities in chemical structure. Antibody titers do not correlate well with clinical hemolysis. The DAT is positive (2 to 4+) with anti-IgG reagents. Weakly positive (±) DAT results usually are not associated with clinical hemolysis. The appearance of a positive DAT is dose and time related, usually requiring intravenous antibiotic administration of 10 to 20 million units daily for at least 10 days. Patient RBC eluates and the serum react only when the drug is present on the RBC membrane, and reactivity is neutralized by high levels of the drug or any cross-reacting drugs, such as methicillin, ampicillin, and oxacillin. Serum antibody alone is not diagnostic because much of the population has IgM antibodies from dietary exposure. Atopic reactions (urticaria, asthma, etc) are unrelated and are caused by IgE antibody.

2. Toxic immune complexes (quinine-quinidine). Negative test results do not exclude the diagnosis of hemolysis because many unknown variables exist. However, this is one of the least common causes of hemolytic anemia in general and of drug-associated immune hemolysis in particular. The DAT

result is usually positive, generally because of complement. This can, on rare occasions, provoke intravascular hemolysis not seen in other types of drug-immune hemolytic anemia. If hemolysis has occurred, results of the DAT may be negative. RBC eluates, because they usually contain insignificant amounts of antibody globulin, may not react with drug-treated RBCs.

3. True warm AIHA (α-methyldopa). This group is very common and, because antibodies may persist after the drug is withdrawn, its presence is unsuspected until blood is cross-matched for transfusion. The positive DAT results vary from weakly positive to 4+. Formation of autoantibodies is common, and they are found in 10% of patients receiving 1 g/d of the drug for longer than 3 months. The direct antiglobulin result becomes progressively stronger followed by the appearance of serum antibody. Despite the serologic evidence, only 1% of patients taking α-methyldopa actually experience hemolysis. These patients should be monitored with a DAT every 3 to 6 months. Withdrawal of the drug reverses the process, with subsequent decreases in serum antibody followed by disappearance of positive DAT results. The presence of antibody and its specificity determines risk with transfusion. Without serum antibodies, transfusion risk is negligible. With serum antibody in a patient with active hemolysis, RBC survival is decreased, as it is for patients with any warm hemolytic anemia.

Test 14.3 RBC Glucose-6-Phosphate Dehydrogenase Assay

Purpose. A deficiency of G6PD in a patient with acute hemolysis supports a diagnosis of drug-related hemolysis.

Principle, Specimen, and Procedure. See Test 9.2. Screening tests are available using prepared reagents and fluorometry. These may be followed by quantitative assays.

Interpretation. The normal range is 2.2 to 5.0 IU/g hemoglobin. Young RBCs have proportionately more G6PD, so marked reticulocytosis may spuriously elevate the level. Low-normal G6PD levels in the presence of reticulocytosis should be viewed with suspicion and the patient retested in 4 to 6 weeks after likely drugs have been withdrawn and the hemolytic process has resolved. Similarly, if transfusions have been given, retesting must wait for 6 to 8 weeks. Hypochromic anemias may appear to have increased G6PD. Screening tests may miss heterozygote G6PD-deficient RBCs, so quantitative assays may be necessary.

Test 14.4 **Heinz Body Test**

Purpose. Deficiency of G6PD, as well as other rarer enzymes, or unstable hemoglobin is associated with increased numbers of Heinz bodies. This finding is supportive of the diagnosis of drug-induced hemolysis.

Principle. The oxidative pathway of glycolytic RBC enzymes maintains hemoglobin stability. In G6PD deficiency, as well as deficiencies of glutathione synthetic enzymes, or unstable hemoglobins, oxidation leads to hemoglobin denaturation. The denaturation hemoglobin precipitates, forming Heinz bodies. Normal RBCs can be induced to form Heinz bodies; G6PD-deficient cells produce three or four Heinz bodies per RBC in the presence of oxidative drugs.

Specimen. Fresh whole blood is collected in EDTA.

Procedure. Crystal violet or neutral red is added to a few drops of blood. Wet mount smears are prepared from the mixture after 15 minutes, 30 minutes, or 1 hour of incubation at room temperature. RBCs also can be incubated with phenylhydrazine before preparation of the smears to exaggerate the findings in G6PD deficiency.

Interpretation. Heinz bodies are seen as particles located close to the cellular membrane, ranging in size from 1 to 3 µm. Normal cells may produce a single marginal Heinz body. After phenylhydrazine incubation, G6PD-deficient cells may have three to four Heinz bodies in every cell. If abrupt hemolysis has occurred, the test results may be negative because of hemolysis of the Heinz body–positive cells.

14.5 Course and Treatment

Immune hemolysis due to drugs is usually mild, although rare cases of severe hemolysis have been reported. All suspicious drugs should be discontinued immediately until the cause of hemolysis is determined. If severe intravascular hemolysis has occurred, the patient can be supported with transfusion. In all cases, except for cases where a true warm-type autoantibody has been generated, the antibody is dependent on the presence of the drug, and transfusion is tolerated as soon as the drug is cleared from the circulation. With warm-type autoantibodies, such as those seen with α-methyldopa, antibody persists in the absence of the drug. If the DAT result is positive but there is no detectable serum antibody, transfused RBCs survive normally. However, in the rare patient with acute severe warm-type AIHA, transfused cells have a markedly decreased survival rate. Therefore, the risk of death from anemia must be weighed against hemolytic complications of transfusion.

Drugs chemically similar to the inciting drug cannot be used again in the patient, because the drug-induced antibody persists for life. When α-methyldopa or procainamide-type drugs incite a warm-type AIHA, it may be difficult to determine whether the hemolysis is caused by unrelated autoimmune disease or by the drug. Active hemolysis of the methyldopa type usually resolves with steroid therapy within 1 to 2 weeks. Steroids can then be tapered without relapse, although the positive DAT result may persist for up to 2 years. If clinical hemolysis is not present, the serologic findings should be allowed to reverse without steroid therapy. Drug-induced hemolysis in G6PD deficiency is often self-limited as reticulocytes with greater concentrations of enzyme are produced. Drug-induced hemolysis may vary from mild to severe, depending on the subtype of disease and the oxidative stress (see Chapter 9).

14.6 References

Beutler E. Glucose-6-phosphate dehydrogenase deficiency. In: Beutler E, Coller BS, Kipps TJ, et al, eds. *Williams Hematology*. 5th ed. New York, NY: McGraw-Hill; 1995:564–580.

Packman CH, Leddy JP. Drug-related immune hemolytic anemia. In: Beutler E, Coller BS, Kipps TJ, et al, eds. *Williams Hematology*. 5th ed. New York, NY: McGraw-Hill; 1995:691–696.

Petz LD. Drug-induced autoimmune hemolytic anemia. *Transfus Med Rev*. 1993;7:242–254.

15 Autoimmune Hemolytic Anemia

Autoimmune hemolytic anemia (AIHA) is caused by antibodies against a person's own RBC antigens, leading to premature lysis and shortened RBC life span. There are two major subcategories of AIHA, classified by the temperature at which the autoantibody best associates with the RBC. Antibodies that are most active at 37°C give rise to warm-type AIHA and clinical syndromes that differ from those that are most active at 4°C (cold-type AIHA). The clinical and laboratory characteristics of each type of AIHA are summarized in **Tables 15-1** and **15-2**.

15.1 Pathophysiology

It is unknown why autoantibodies against RBCs are formed, although a derangement in normal immune function must occur that allows recognition of self-antigens as immunogenic. RBC autoantibodies may be formed in association with immune or neoplastic disorders, during the ingestion of certain drugs, following infection, or as an idiopathic process. Autoimmune hemolytic anemia can appear at any age, including infancy, although it is more

Table 15-1   Clinical Characteristics of Autoimmune Hemolytic Anemias

Clinical Findings	Warm Type (70%)	Cold Type (30%)
Onset	Abrupt	Insidious
Jaundice	Usually present	Often absent
Splenomegaly	Yes	Absent
Age	All ages	All ages
Sex	Slightly more women	Women predominate
Origin of autoantibody		
Idiopathic	50%-60%	30%-40%
Drug-induced	25%-30%	1%-5%
Lymphoproliferative disorder	10%-15%	15%-20%
Viral or mycoplasma	0%	25%-35%
Other (inflammatory diseases, other malignancies)	5%-10%	5%-10%

frequent in older age groups. In general, RBC lysis occurs following cell membrane binding of IgG or IgM autoantibodies with or without subsequent complement fixation.

Warm-type AIHA is the most common, making up about 70% of AIHA cases. It is associated with IgG autoantibodies in about 90% of cases. These antibodies coat the RBC, leading to increased recognition and subsequent interaction with splenic macrophages, thus enhancing phagocytosis of the RBC membrane. This results in formation of spherocytes and shortened RBC survival by extravascular hemolysis. If the RBC is heavily coated with IgG, complement also binds to the cell membrane. This usually does not lead to complement-mediated cellular lysis, but the presence of C3 on the cell surface markedly enhances macrophage binding efficiency and increases reticuloendothelial-mediated destruction in the liver and spleen. In addition, any process that increases the activity of the mononuclear phagocytic system, such as infection, may further increase hemolytic activity.

Cold-type AIHA is caused primarily by IgM autoantibodies called "cold agglutinins". Because of the 10 antigen binding sites present on each IgM molecule, they tend to agglutinate RBCs at low temperatures (optimally at <16°C, but also at temperatures between 25°C and 31°C) such as are found in peripheral areas of

Table 15-2 Laboratory Characterization of Autoimmune Hemolytic Anemias

Laboratory Parameter	Warm Type	Cold Type
Usual immunoglobulin type	IgG	IgM
Direct antibody test	2+-4+	2+-4+
Monospecific sera		
Anti-IgG only	1+	0
Anti-IgG+ anti-Cl	1+	0
Anti-Cl only	Rare	1+
Complement activation	Little or none	Yes
Serum complement levels	Normal or decreased	Decreased
Osmotic fragility	Increased	Normal
Peripheral blood findings	Spherocytes, nucleated RBCs	RBC agglutination

the circulation. The agglutinated cells are more susceptible to trauma and mechanical hemolysis. If the antibody is active at temperatures approaching 37°C, it fixes and activates the classic complement cascade on the RBC surface, leading either to intravascular complement-mediated cellular lysis or increased extravascular macrophage-mediated hemolysis in the spleen and liver. In some patients, complement activation proceeds to C3d and stops. Because macrophages have no receptors for this complement component, the cell escapes hemolysis in the spleen. This effect is seen in chromium 51 (^{51}Cr) survival studies when an initial episode of abrupt cell destruction is followed by a slower second phase, in which cell survival times may approach normal.

Some patients with warm-type AIHA also have cold agglutinins, giving rise to a mixed picture. In most cases the cold agglutinin does not function in hemolysis, although rare patients demonstrate active cold agglutinin disease (CAD). This is most often seen in patients with lymphoproliferative disorders or autoimmune diseases. The laboratory features are also mixed.

Autoimmune hemolytic anemia also may be divided by pathogenetic mechanism into either primary (idiopathic) or secondary types. The primary type usually develops in older individuals with no evidence of underlying disease, constituting about 30% to 60% of patients with AIHA. The remaining cases are secondary to an underlying disease, drug use, or infection (**Table 15-3**). In some

Table 15-3 Diseases Associated With Autoimmune Hemolytic Anemia

Disease	Antibody Specificity	
	Warm Antibody	Cold Antibody
Malignancy		
Chronic lymphocytic leukemia	Anti-Rh, LW, Wright[b]	Anti-I
Non-Hodgkin's lymphoma	Anti-u, En[a]	Anti-I
Hodgkin's disease	Anti-Rh	Anti-I
Carcinoma (ovary, thymus, gastrointestinal)	Variable	NA
Inflammatory Disease		
SLE, rheumatoid arthritis, ulcerative colitis	Anti-Rh, LW, Wright[b]	Anti-I, anti-i
Infection		
Mycoplasma	NA	Anti-I
Epstein-Barr virus	NA	Anti-i
Clostridium, Escherichia coli	Anti-T	NA
AIDS	Variable	Anti-I
Drugs		
Methyldopa	Anti-Rh	NA
L-dopa	Anti-Rh	NA

Abbreviations: SLE = systemic lupus erythematosus; NA = not applicable.

cases, the hemolytic anemia may precede the associated disease by several years, necessitating persistent, careful screening for these disorders. Warm-type AIHA secondary to drug use was discussed further in Chapter 14.

15.2 Clinical Findings

The clinical history often suggests the underlying cause of AIHA. Warm-type AIHA is of abrupt onset, with jaundice and spleno-megaly, and anemia may be severe. Cold-type AIHA also may present as an acute onset of anemia. It may occur following an infection such as *Mycoplasma* pneumonia, infectious mononucleosis, or cytomegalovirus (CMV), or it may be found in association with a lymphoproliferative malignancy. The anemia may range from mild to severe, and intravascular hemolysis may occur. Alternatively, cold-type AIHA may have an insidious onset, with minimal symptoms until severe anemia develops. Cold-type AIHA usually is not associated with jaundice or splenomegaly despite marked anemia.

Most people have low, clinically insignificant, or physiologic titers of cold agglutinins ($\leq 1:32$) that bind to RBCs only at temperatures well below those found even in exposed extremities. When increased production of the IgM leads to higher titers ($\geq 1:256$), the temperature of cellular agglutination rises to approximately 37°C, resulting in complement fixation and a positive direct antiglobulin (Coombs') test (DAT; see Test 6.4). Cold-type AIHA is often subdivided into three clinically distinct disease categories: acute postinfectious, chronic idiopathic, and CAD (**Table 15-4**). All three disease types produce similar cold agglutinin–type antibodies, but clinical features vary with titer. Acute postinfectious cold-type AIHA is usually seen in younger patients and has an acute, often self-limited course, following mycoplasmal pneumonia, CMV, or Epstein-Barr virus (EBV). In contrast, chronic idiopathic disease and CAD usually occur insidiously in older patients. Chronic idiopathic disease is usually seen in elderly women, whereas CAD is usually associated with an underlying lymphoproliferative malignancy (usually large cell non-Hodgkin's lymphoma).

Paroxysmal cold hemoglobinuria (PCH) is clinically closely related to cold-type AIHA. It is due to acquisition of an IgG antibody called the "Donath-Landsteiner hemolysin". This antibody has a characteristic biphasic mode of action, first adsorbing to RBCs at low temperatures and then causing intravascular hemolysis and hemoglobinuria as the temperature rises to 37°C. It is important to diagnose PCH because it is usually self-limited and treated by keeping the patient warm.

15.3 Diagnostic Approach

A good clinical history of the hemolytic episode and any other accompanying problems (such as recent infection), combined with pertinent clinical findings (such as the presence of splenomegaly), provide important diagnostic clues to the cause of the AIHA and

Table 15-4   Characteristics of Cold Agglutinin–Associated Disease

Clinical Parameter	Physiologic	Acute Postinfectious	Chronic Idiopathic	CAD
Age	Any	Young	Older	Older
Onset	Asymptomatic	Acute, 10-14 days	Insidious	Insidious
Splenomegaly	No	Frequent	No	With lymphoma
Titer	≤1:32	≥1:64	≥1:256*	>1:10,000*
Specificity	Anti-I	Anti-I, anti-i	Anti-I, anti-i	Anti-I
DAT results	Negative	+(G,M,C3)	+(C3)	+(C3)
Intravascular hemolysis	No	40%	No	Rare

Abbreviations: CAD = cold agglutinin disease; DAT = direct antiglobulin test.
*Representative range for titer.

facilitate the workup. Evaluation of the hemolysis proceeds with the following steps:

1. Hematologic analysis shows a normochromic normocytic anemia, which may be hemolytic in nature as evidenced by polychromasia, macrocytosis, and the presence of microspherocytes, nucleated RBCs, or RBC agglutination. Bone marrow examination usually is not required.

2. Results of DAT or other methods of serum antibody detection should be positive and can identify the adsorbed globulins, allowing categorization of the process as a warm-type, cold-type, or mixed AIHA. If the DAT results are negative, immune hemolysis cannot be proven.

3. If a cold-type AIHA is suspected, further testing may include cold agglutinin titers, the Donath-Landsteiner test to exclude PCH, antibody titers for viruses or *Mycoplasma*, or search for an occult lymphoma or lymphoproliferative disorder in elderly patients to further characterize the type of hemolytic disease.

4. If a warm-type AIHA is suspected, further workup to identify an underlying cause, such as autoimmune disorders, malignancy, lymphoma, or other lymphoproliferative disorder, is required. Possible drug-induced causes should be considered, and use of pertinent drugs discontinued.

15.4 Hematologic Findings

15.4.1 Blood Cell Measurements

Anemia may be severe (hemoglobin level, <3 g/dL [<30 g/L]) with normochromic normocytic indices. There is variable reticulocytosis, but the reticulocyte count is usually increased. In acute hemolysis, a nonspecific stress granulocytosis with a left shift may be present. The leukocytosis can reach leukemoid proportions (>50 × 10^3/mm^3 [>50 × 10^9/L]).

15.4.2 Peripheral Blood Smear Morphology

Nucleated RBCs, marked polychromasia, poikilocytosis, and anisocytosis are usually evident. In warm-type AIHA, microspherocytes are present, resulting from partial ingestion of antibody-coated RBC membrane by the mononuclear phagocytic system. Cold-type AIHA may have similar morphologic changes if it is acutely postinfectious, but the more chronic disease states may have few RBC changes. IgM cross-linking of cells may cause RBC aggregation in the peripheral smear (**Image 15-1**).

15.4.3 Bone Marrow Examination

Bone marrow examination usually is not required. If performed, it demonstrates a hypercellular marrow with marked normoblastic erythroid hyperplasia. Usually marrow iron is markedly increased, reflecting the accelerated erythroid turnover. Prolonged severe hemolysis may result in relative deficiencies of folic acid or vitamin B$_{12}$, causing superimposed megaloblastic maturation. Occasionally, bone marrow examination may reveal an underlying lymphoproliferative disorder associated with autoantibody production.

Other Laboratory Tests

Complete evaluation of a hemolytic process suspected to be AIHA by the following tests requires 15 to 20 mL of blood that is obtained and maintained at 37°C until clotted. The serum is promptly removed from the cells and frozen to preserve complement. An ethylenediaminetetraacetic acid (EDTA) specimen is also obtained. The EDTA blocks nonspecific adsorption of complement, which allows a more accurate assessment of DAT results. The majority of tests performed are aimed at demonstrating the presence of autoantibody and characterizing it. Other testing may be aimed at determining an underlying etiology, such as infection or malignancy, for the process or to rule out other non–immune-mediated causes of hemolysis.

Test 15.1 **Direct Antiglobulin (Coombs') Test**

Purpose. The DAT depicts globulin adsorbed to the patient's RBCs and identifies the immunoglobulin class.

Principle and Procedure. See Test 6.4.

Interpretation. A clinically significant DAT result is positive (1 to 4+) with broad-spectrum reagents. Monospecific reagents identify the adsorbed globulin type. In warm-type AIHA, monospecific reagents for IgG or IgG and complement are positive. Monospecific reagents in cold-type AIHA show only complement, because IgM antibody quickly separates from RBCs collected at 37°C. C3d is believed to be a clinically significant fraction in AIHA, because it indicates prior absorption of C3 to the RBC membrane. Very weak complement reactions (+/–) are not significant, but weak anti-IgG reactions may occasionally be clinically important.

    Very rarely, AIHA is present without a positive DAT result, requiring ultrasensitive methods or radioisotopic analysis to detect antibody molecules on the RBCs. These tests are not generally available and require the services of a reference laboratory.

Test 15.2 **Serum Antibody Detection**

Purpose. These tests detect serum antibody that coats RBCs under the test conditions, identify its blood group specificity, and characterize the temperature of reactivity.

Principle. An indirect Coombs' test—or its modifications—depicts serum antibody binding to RBCs following incubation of test cells with the patient's serum. This is followed by washing and addition of direct antibody reagents to detect cell-bound complement and/or immunoglobulin. Enzymatic treatment of cells (by ficain, papain, bromelain, or trypsin) may increase the detection of very low levels of antibody. Alternatively, direct agglutination of saline-suspended cells also depicts serum RBC antibodies. If screening tests show positive results, the antibody is identified (see Test 12.2).

Procedure. The patient's serum and RBC mixtures are tested at 37°C and at 4°C. In addition to panels of reagent RBCs, the patient's own cells and specimens of cord blood are included. The presence of agglutination or hemolysis is significant and is graded 0 to 4+ (see Test 12.1).

Interpretation. Warm autoantibodies agglutinate test cells by indirect antiglobulin tests and enzyme techniques strongly at 37°C, with no increase at 4°C. These are usually an IgG subtype. Specific antibody is found in 30% of cases and is usually related to the Rh loci (e, C, D, and c), although the appearance of narrow specificity may reflect differences only in titers of antibody components. In the remaining cases, the antibody is directed at some primitive precursor of the Rh system or of the Wright system, and all cells are agglutinated except for very rare test cells used at reference laboratories, such as Rh null cells.

Because antibodies from previous transfusions may be present concurrent with autoantibodies, specificity should be determined. Although transfusions should be avoided, antibody specificity may help in selecting blood that is least incompatible if life-saving transfusion is needed. With steroids, serum antibodies may change specificity or disappear, although the positive DAT result often persists. The presence of serum antibody correlates more strongly with active AIHA.

Cold autoantibodies are usually IgM and show strong reactivity at 4°C and weaker reactivity at 37°C. Sometimes this differential reactivity is more apparent with diluted serum, in saline-washed suspensions, or in enzyme-treated cells. The antibodies may be hemolytic in vitro. Specificity is usually anti-I (reactive with all normal adult cells but not with cord blood RBCs). Anti-i specificity (stronger reactions with cord RBCs than with adult cells) is seen in rare patients with AIHA associated with infectious mononucleosis. Cold autoantibodies should be titered, as hemolytic pattern is often associated with antibody levels. To determine whether antibodies are autoantibodies, the patient's RBC antigens must be tested and typed for the Rh and I systems.

Test 15.3 **RBC Eluates**

Purpose. The globin fraction is eluted off the RBC membrane to determine whether the globulin depicted by the DAT is antibody and to determine the blood group specificity of the globulin.

Principle. RBC antibody-antigen bonds are disrupted by heat or by destroying the RBC membrane, thereby releasing bound antibody so it can be analyzed further.

Procedure. The test is usually performed by a blood bank or reference laboratory. When the DAT result is positive, heating the RBCs at 56°C or chemically destroying them with cold organic solvents elutes the adsorbed antibody, which can be tested in parallel with the serum.

Interpretation. In warm-type AIHA, the eluate antibody is the same as that identified in the serum. After recent incompatible transfusion in the absence of AIHA, the DAT may yield positive results due to the presence of autoantibody-coated donor cells. Antigen typing of RBCs in such cases often shows a mixed field of donor RBCs and patient cells. After incompatible transfusion in the presence of AIHA, specificity of eluate and serum antibody may not be clarified until transfused cells have been cleared, which usually requires several days. An eluate that does not react with RBCs suggests nonspecific globulin adsorption, such as that seen in patients with myeloma or recent cephalothin therapy. In cold-type AIHA antibody, material is not elutable and there is no reaction with RBCs.

Test 15.4 **Cold Agglutinin Titer**

Purpose. The presence of increased cold agglutinins usually establishes that the AIHA is of the cold antibody type. Titers may indicate underlying disease subtype and serve as a means to follow disease status.

Principle. Cold agglutinins usually have anti-I specificity and agglutinate saline suspensions of adult RBCs that have the I antigen on the membrane. Rare cold agglutinins with anti-i specificity do not agglutinate adult RBCs at the same titer but can be titered with cord blood specimens.

Procedure. The patient's serum is titrated by small-volume serial dilutions (1:4, 1:8, 1:16, 1:32, etc) and incubated for 2 hours at

4°C with a standard suspension of RBCs from the patient or a group O donor (to avoid ABO blood group incompatibility). Cell-serum suspensions are evaluated for agglutination, and the titer is established as the highest serum dilution producing detectable agglutination.

Interpretation. A low titer of cold agglutinins is considered physiologic and is not pathologic. Clinical significance is associated with titers greater than 1:64 (**Table 15-4**). With an increase in titer, the temperature of RBC agglutination often rises toward 37°C, and antibody with complement fixes on the patient's RBCs, as demonstrated by a positive DAT result. Physiologic cold agglutinins have titers of 1:32 or less. Titers of 1:64 or more are seen after recent respiratory viral infections. Viral pneumonia is associated with titers of 1:128 to 1:8000. Titers of 1:256 or more are observed in cold-type AIHA in elderly women. In chronic CAD, titers are often 1:50,000 or higher. Progress of cold-type AIHA can be followed up by repeating titers weekly in viral pneumonia or idiopathic disease and monthly in CAD, particularly in diseases associated with a lymphoproliferative process.

Test 15.5 **Donath-Landsteiner Test**

Purpose. The Donath-Landsteiner test facilitates diagnosis of PCH, allowing it to be distinguished from cold-type AIHA. PCH is usually a self-limited disease that is treated conservatively by keeping the patient warm.

Principle. This test reproduces in vitro the biphasic reaction that characterizes PCH. The Donath-Landsteiner hemolysin is a complement-dependent IgG antibody that agglutinates cells at 4°C and lyses them at warmer temperatures (usually 37°C). Other hemolysins may react at a single temperature, 4°C or 37°C, but are not biphasic. The Donath-Landsteiner hemolysin does not lyse cells with reverse incubations of 37°C to 4°C.

Procedure. The patient's serum is incubated with test RBCs at 4°C for 30 minutes and then at 37°C for 30 minutes and observed for hemolysis, which is usually marked (3 to 4+). If biphasic hemolysis is present, it is tested against panels of reagent RBCs to determine blood group specificity, which is often in the P or I system.

Interpretation. A biphasic hemolysin is diagnostic of PCH, which occasionally may clinically mimic cold-type AIHA. If intravascular hemolysis has recently occurred, the DAT results may be negative. PCH often occurs following a viral infection but can also be seen with congenital syphilis, so follow-up serologic testing should be performed.

Test 15.6 Ham's Test for Acid Hemolysis

Purpose. A Ham's test is performed to exclude paroxysmal nocturnal hemoglobinuria, which is caused by an acquired clonal defect of the RBC membrane rather than an antibody-mediated process. Whenever antibody hemolysis is suspected, PNH should be considered and excluded.

Principle, Specimen, and Procedure. See Test 11.2.

Interpretation. False-positive hemolysis results are seen if the acidified sera contains a cold agglutinin. True-positive results occur only with human (not guinea pig) complement. The acid hemolysis test can be confirmed with sucrose lysis.

Test 15.7 Serum Complement Measurement

Purpose. A decrease in serum complement is often associated with IgM antibodies and cold-type AIHA. It may be decreased in some patients with warm-type AIHA.

Principle. Sheep RBCs are lysed in the presence of rabbit anti-sheep antibody if complement from the patient's serum is present. The reaction can be used to quantitate complement.

Specimen. Fresh serum is separated from RBCs and frozen immediately.

Procedure. Serum complement is measured spectrophotometrically by lysis of 50% of an RBC suspension in 1 hour. This is achieved by 50 to 100 U of complement in most laboratories, but normal ranges must be determined for each laboratory.

Interpretation. Serum complement is decreased in cold AIHA due to complement binding by antibodies. Levels also may be decreased in warm AIHA when complement is fixed to the cell membrane. Lytic complement tests are not easily performed and often require the services of reference laboratories.

Test 15.8 Serum Haptoglobin Quantitation

Purpose. Haptoglobin is decreased or absent in hemolysis, liver failure, and rare genetic variants. A low serum haptoglobin level indicates that hemolysis may be present if liver function is normal.

Principle, Specimen, and Procedure. See Test 6.3.

Interpretation. Normal values are usually 40 to 80 mg/dL (0.4 to 0.8 g/L). With active hemolysis, values of less than 10 mg/dL (0.1 g/L) are seen. In cold-type AIHA secondary to viral or *My-coplasma* pneumonia, haptoglobin may be increased as an acute reactant protein, obscuring expected decreases with hemolysis.

Test 15.9 Osmotic Fragility Test

Purpose. This test detects spherocytes, which are more sensitive to osmotic lysis than are normal RBCs.

Principle, Specimen, and Procedure. See Test 7.1.

Interpretation. Hemolysis increases with the presence of spherocytosis, often seen in warm-type AIHA. Review of the peripheral smear should show spherocytes, and it is usually unnecessary to confirm this morphologic finding by osmotic fragility testing.

Test 15.10 Antibody Titers for *Mycoplasma* and Viruses

Purpose. Testing for *Mycoplasma* and virus antibody titers identifies (often in retrospect) possible infectious agents as the cause of cold-type AIHA.

Principle. These antibodies require acute and convalescent phase sera obtained 7 to 10 days apart to show a rise in titer of antibody for specific organisms.

Procedure. The tests are usually performed at county or state reference laboratories, which require acute and convalescent specimens to be submitted. The agent suspected should be specified. The most common etiologic agents of interest are *Mycoplasma* and, less frequently, EBV or CMV.

Interpretation. A three-dilution rise in titer is required for the test to aid diagnosis, because previous exposure to these viruses is fairly common. IgM antibody suggests recent infection.

Test 15.11 **Antinuclear Antibody Test**

Purpose. Antinuclear antibody testing by indirect immunofluorescence should be ordered when warm-type AIHA is diagnosed, particularly in young women, to determine whether systemic lupus erythematosus (SLE) or another collagen vascular disease is the underlying cause. The hemolysis frequently precedes diagnosis of SLE by months or even years.

Principle. The patient's serum contains autoantibody to nuclear material. If antinuclear antibodies are present, they bind to the cell nuclei and can be depicted with fluorescence.

Procedure. The patient's serum is incubated with a source of nuclear antigen (eg, tissue culture cells, rat kidney, human granulocytes). The antigen-antibody combination is demonstrated by an antiglobulin reagent tagged with a fluorescent dye. The patient's serum can then be titered.

Interpretation. Titers greater than 1:20 are suspicious in most laboratories, and titers of 1:80 or greater are considered diagnostic of collagen vascular disease. Suspicious positive test results may be seen in up to 3% of older individuals. High antinuclear antibody titers in the elderly in the proper clinical setting suggest drug-induced AIHA of the methyldopa type (see Chapter 14).

Test 15.12 **Evaluation of Occult Lymphoma**

Warm-type AIHA may precede lymphoma by years. Similarly, AIHA may be the only recognizable clinical sign in concomitant unsuspected lymphoma.

Physical examination and radiologic evaluation of all lymph node areas, liver, and spleen may help detect an unsuspected lymphoma. A biopsy should be performed when adenopathy or hepatosplenomegaly is found.

15.5 Course and Treatment

Warm-type AIHA usually responds in 7 to 10 days to high-dose corticosteroid therapy, which suppresses antibody production and inhibits macrophage activity. In steroid-resistant cases, immunosuppressive medication or splenectomy to decrease reticuloendothelial activity is usually successful.

Little effective therapy is available for cold-type AIHA, which does not respond to steroids, immunosuppressive drugs, or splenectomy. Postinfectious cold-type AIHA is usually self-limited, but in some severe cases plasmapheresis may help to decrease antibody levels. In CAD associated with a lymphoproliferative disorder, treatment of the underlying disease often results in improvement of cold agglutinin titers. Chronic idiopathic cold-type AIHA seen in elderly women waxes and wanes, possibly in relation to infections or other stresses.

PCH is usually treated by keeping the patient warm. It is self-limited, responding to recovery from the underlying infection. Aggressive therapy should therefore be avoided.

Transfusions should generally be avoided in patients with either warm- or cold-type AIHA to minimize formation of further alloantibodies, which can complicate crossmatching. In addition, transfusion may increase autoantibody titers and avidity for RBCs, accelerating hemolysis. RBC survival is less than 1 week in warm-type AIHA and may be minutes or hours in cold-type AIHA, making transfusions of limited usefulness unless symptoms of impending stroke or myocardial infarction are present.

15.6 References

Garratty G. Autoimmune hemolytic anemia. In: Garratty G, ed. *Immunobiology of Transfusion Medicine*. New York, NY: Marcel Dekker, 1994.

Hashimoto C. Autoimmune hemolytic anemia. *Clin Rev Allergy Immunol.* 1998;16:285–295.

Sokol RJ, Booker DJ, Stamps R. ACP Broadsheet No 145. Investigation of patients with autoimmune haemolytic anemia and provision of blood for transfusion. *J Clin Pathol.* 1995;48:602-610.

Telen MJ, Rao N. Recent advances in immunohematology. *Curr Opin Hematol.* 1994;1:143–150.

Thomas AT. Autoimmune hemolytic anemias. In: Lee GR, Foerster J, Lukens JN, et al, eds. *Wintrobe's Clinical Hematology.* 10th ed. Baltimore, Md: Williams & Wilkins; 1999:1233–1263.

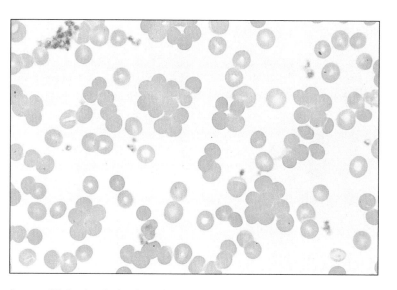

Image 15-1 Agglutination of RBCs in a patient with cold agglutinin disease.

PART III

Reactive Disorders of Granulocytes and Monocytes

16 Neutrophilia

The normal range for absolute neutrophil count shows significant age variation. For example, a brisk neutrophilia, often exceeding 30 × 10³/mm³ (30 × 10⁹/L), is typical at birth. Shortly after birth, the absolute neutrophil count plummets and lymphocytes predominate by 2 weeks of age. The normal range for absolute neutrophil count in infants is approximately 2.5 to 7.0 × 10³/mm³ (2.5 to 7.0 × 10⁹/L), whereas the normal range for children and adults is approximately 1.5 to 7.0 × 10³/mm³ (1.5 to 7.0 × 10⁹/L). These normal ranges reflect only the circulating pool of neutrophils; an equal number of neutrophils are attached to the vascular endothelium, or marginated pool.

Beyond the neonatal period, neutrophilia is defined as an absolute neutrophil count that exceeds 10 × 10³/mm³ (10 × 10⁹/L). The causes of reactive neutrophilia are listed in **Table 16-1** and include a broad spectrum of disorders, ranging from infections to metabolic defects; bacterial infections are the predominant cause of neutrophilia in clinical practice. Other causes of reactive neutrophilia include therapeutic or endogenous drugs/hormones, acute stress, acute tissue necrosis, and other infectious/inflammatory processes (**Images 16-1** and **16-2**). A recently identified cause of nonneoplastic neutrophilia is Hantavirus pulmonary syndrome; in addition to a nontoxic neutrophilia with left shift, thrombocytope-

Table 16-1   Reactive Neutrophilias

Infections
  Primarily in bacterial infections
  Less common in viral, mycobacterial, leptospiral, or toxoplasmal infections
  Hantavirus pulmonary syndrome*
Drugs, hormones
  Excess CSF (therapeutic, CSF-producing tumors)
  Epinephrine (therapeutic or endogenous production)
  Corticosteroids (therapeutic or endogenous production)
  Lithium
  Poisons/toxins/venoms
Tissue necrosis
  Burns
  Trauma
  Infarct
  Acute gout
Inflammatory disorders
  Collagen vascular disorders
  Other autoimmune disorders
Miscellaneous
  Stress/severe exercise
  Pregnancy
  Smoking
  Acute hemorrhage/hemolysis
  Postsplenectomy
Metabolic
  Ketoacidosis
  Uremia
  Eclampsia
Constitutional (very rare)†
  Hereditary neutrophilia
  Familial cold urticaria
  Leukocyte adhesion deficiency

Abbreviation: CSF = colony-stimulating factor.
*Neutrophilia secondary to acute, severe respiratory distress; neutrophils lack toxic changes.
†These disorders are rarely encountered in clinical practice.

nia, hemoconcentration, and circulating immunoblasts are evident in patients with florid disease (**Images 16-3** and **16-4**). Constitutional neutrophilia is exceedingly rare and is generally linked to neutrophil migration defects (see Chapter 21).

   Absolute neutrophilia also is a feature of a variety of hematopoietic neoplasms, especially chronic myeloproliferative disorders. In affected patients the neutrophils are part of the neoplastic process. Because chronic myeloproliferative disorders represent clonal stem cell defects, the mature RBCs, WBCs, and platelets within the peripheral blood are all derived from the neoplastic clone. A variety of blood features and several specialized blood studies are useful in separating these clonal disorders from nonneoplastic neutrophilias (discussed later in this chapter).

16.1 Pathophysiology

For granulopoiesis to occur, the bone marrow must contain sufficient stem cells and progenitor cells, an adequate microenvironment for hematopoiesis, and sufficient regulatory factors. Granulopoiesis is a precisely regulated system of cell proliferation and maturation; regulation is largely achieved by factors produced within the bone marrow microenvironment. The most well-characterized of these regulatory factors is a family of glycoproteins called colony-stimulating factors (CSFs). By binding to an appropriate surface receptor on progenitor cells, these regulatory proteins stimulate production of granulocytes (granulocyte CSF [G-CSF]), monocytes (monocyte CSF [M-CSF]), or both (granulocyte-monocyte CSF [GM-CSF]). Colony-stimulating factors also induce a hyperfunctional state in mature neutrophils and monocytes, cells that also express CSF receptors. The hyperfunctional state of these mature cells is linked to morphologic changes such as toxic granulation, Döhle's bodies, and prominent cytoplasmic vacuolization (*see Image 16-1*). CSFs are produced by a variety of cells within the bone marrow microenvironment, including monocytes/macrophages and T lymphocytes.

Although specific stages of granulocyte maturation have been defined, this process is a biologic continuum characterized by both a progressive decrease in nuclear size with eventual segmentation and a progressive increase in cytoplasmic granularity. The arbitrarily defined stages of granulopoiesis consist of myeloblasts, promyelocytes, myelocytes, metamyelocytes, band neutrophils, and segmented neutrophils. Myeloblasts, promyelocytes, and myelocytes are capable of mitotic division, but metamyelocytes, band neutrophils, and segmented neutrophils have lost this capability. Primary granules are initially recognized in "late" myeloblasts and promyelocytes. These lysosomal granules contain numerous cytolytic enzymes, the most notable of which is myeloperoxidase.

Secondary granules are first apparent at the myelocyte stage of maturation, and they eventually outnumber primary granules, giving the cytoplasm a homogeneous pink blush. Like primary granules, secondary lysosomal granules contain numerous cytolytic enzymes. The most commonly evaluated secondary granule enzyme is leukocyte (neutrophil) alkaline phosphatase. A third type of granule subset, the gelatinase granule, has recently been identified in band and segmented neutrophils.

The time required for granulopoiesis is highly variable, ranging from 1 to 3 weeks. Once neutrophils are released into the peripheral blood, they circulate for only a few hours before egressing to tissues. Homeostatic rates of neutrophil production exceed 1 to 2×10^9 neutrophils per kilogram per day.

Baseline granulopoiesis can be stimulated in many infectious and inflammatory conditions (**Table 16-2**). The primary mechanisms for neutrophilia include demargination of the marginated pool, release of the bone marrow maturation-storage compartment, and increased neutrophil production. Demargination of neutrophils is caused by epinephrine release and can occur within minutes. Because the circulating and marginating pools are approximately equal, this mechanism is predicted to approximately double the absolute neutrophil count. Greater increases in the absolute neutrophil count result from release of the bone marrow maturation-storage compartment, a phenomenon induced by corticosteroids, acute infections, and acute inflammation. In addition to a substantial absolute neutrophilia, a left shift with circulating band neutrophils, metamyelocytes, and even myelocytes is a predictable finding in patients in whom mobilization of the bone marrow maturation-storage compartment has occurred.

For a neutrophilia to be sustained, increased bone marrow production must occur. This is the slowest mechanism of neutrophilia, but results in significant sustained neutrophilia. This process is mediated by CSFs; conditions linked to sustained increased CSF production include chronic infections, chronic inflammation, CSF-producing tumors, and therapy with recombinant human CSF.

16.2 Clinical Findings

The clinical findings in patients with reactive neutrophilia are diverse, depending on the underlying disorder. Fever is a hallmark

Table 16-2 Mechanisms Causing Nonneoplastic Neutrophilia

Mechanism	Time Course	Causes
Demargination*	Minutes	Epinephrine release, acute stress, exercise
Mobilization of maturation-storage compartment	Hours	Corticosteroids, infection, inflammation
Increased production	Days	Sustained infection, chronic inflammation, CSF-producing tumors, CSF therapy, lithium therapy

Abbreviation: CSF = colony stimulating factor.
*Detachment of marginated neutrophils from the endothelium into the circulating pool.

of acute infection, but various other signs and symptoms are linked to the specific site of infection. Patients in whom the neutrophilia is part of a bone marrow neoplasm (eg, patients with chronic myeloproliferative disorders) generally present with symptoms of fatigue and malaise. Fever is not present unless these patients have developed a secondary infection. Splenomegaly and variable hepatomegaly are common clinical findings in patients with chronic myeloproliferative disorders. Striking leukocytosis (>500,000/mm^3) in CML can be associated with neurologic findings secondary to altered cerebral microcirculation.

16.3 Diagnostic Approach

The evaluation of a patient with an increased absolute neutrophil count must include both the distinction between a reactive and neoplastic process and the determination of the likely cause of a reactive neutrophilia. The distinction between a reactive neutrophilia and a chronic myeloproliferative disorder, notably chronic myelogenous leukemia (CML), is based on the assimilation of a variety of clinical, hematologic, morphologic, and chemical parameters (**Tables 16-3** through **16-5**). In general, pronounced toxic changes, a limited left shift, and normal absolute basophil count indicate a reactive neutrophilia, whereas CML is characterized by a strikingly elevated nontoxic leukocytosis with left shift, including

Table 16-3 Morphologic Features of Reactive Neutrophilia

Blood	Comments
Leukocytosis	Usually $<30 \times 10^3/mm^3$ ($<30 \times 10^9/L$); higher WBC count in young children
	Rarely exceeds $50 \times 10^3/mm^3$ ($50 \times 10^9/L$) except in patients receiving CSF therapy (or with CSF-producing tumor)
Left shift	Bands and metamyelocytes typical; may also see myelocytes
	In neonates with sepsis may see circulating myeloblasts along with other granulocytic elements
Döhle bodies	Retained portion of cytoplasm from more immature state of maturation
Toxic granulation	Etiology controversial; either retained primary granules or altered uptake of stain by secondary granules
Cytoplasmic vacuoles	Prominent neutrophil vacuoles correlate with sepsis
Other lineages	Thrombocytosis common; if DIC develops, thrombocytopenia is found
	Eosinophilia or monocytosis may accompany neutrophilia
	Basophilia not present

Abbreviations: CSF = colony-stimulating factor; DIC = disseminated intravascular coagulation.

blasts, abnormalities in other lineages, and prominent absolute basophilia.

The following approach to diagnosis should be considered:

1. Assess the complete blood count with differential.
2. Evaluate the morphology for toxic changes and for evidence of multilineage abnormalities.
3. Conduct appropriate microbacterial studies to evaluate for a possible infection.
4. Integrate the blood findings with clinical features and chemical analyses.
5. Examine bone marrow or perform cytogenetic/molecular evaluation in selected patients with whom a neoplastic disorder is the primary diagnostic consideration.

Table 16-4 Morphologic Features of Blood in Patients Receiving Recombinant Growth Factor Therapy*

Marked leukocytosis with increase in neutrophils (increase in monocytes, with variable increase in eosinophils, lymphocytes, and sometimes basophils in patients receiving GM-CSF)

Prominent toxic changes in mature and immature granulocytes

Left shift with circulating blasts (usually low percentage) and erythroblasts (occasional)

Nuclear-cytoplasmic asynchrony†

Nuclear segmentation defects†

Transient increase in blasts prior to neutrophil recovery may mimic leukemia

Rare binucleate (tetraploid) neutrophils present (G-CSF)

Circulating myeloid cytoplasmic fragments

Abbreviations: GM-CSF = granulocyte-monocyte colony-stimulating factor; G-CSF = granulocyte colony-stimulating factor.
*Therapy may be recombinant human GM-CSF or recombinant human G-CSF.
†Generally seen in patients receiving concomitant chemotherapy

Table 16-5 Comparison of Reactive Neutrophilia With Chronic Myelogenous Leukemia (CML)

Parameter	Reactive Neutrophilia	CML
WBC	Usually <30 × 10³/mm³ (<30 × 10⁹/L)	Usually >50 × 10³/mm³ (>50 × 10⁹/L)
Toxic neutrophils	Present	Usually absent*
Left shift	Includes myelocytes	Includes blasts
Basophilia	Absent	Present
Platelet count	Variable, decreased with sepsis	Increased
Platelet morphology	Unremarkable	Abnormal, variable micromegakaryocytes
Nucleated erythroid cells in blood	Absent	Present
Splenomegaly	Absent	Present
Fever	Usually present	Usually absent
Uric acid	Normal	Increased
LAP	Increased	Low*
Karyotype	Normal	Philadelphia chromosome; (9;22) (q34;q11)
Molecular	Normal	BCR/ABL gene rearrangement

Abbreviation: LAP=leukocyte alkaline phosphatase.
*Except in patients with secondary infection.

16.4 Hematologic Findings

16.4.1 Blood Cell Measurements

In a reactive neutrophilia the WBC count rarely exceeds $30 \times 10^3/mm^3$ ($30 \times 10^9/L$). In exceptional patients, including either young children with infection or patients receiving recombinant human CSF therapy, the WBC count may exceed $50 \times 10^3/mm^3$ ($50 \times 10^9/L$). A neoplastic disorder should be strongly considered when the WBC count exceeds $100 \times 10^3/mm^3$ ($100 \times 10^9/L$), except in the circumstance of pharmacologic doses of recombinant CSF (*see Table 16-5*).

Depending on the underlying disorder, the hemoglobin, hematocrit, and platelet values are highly variable in patients with reactive neutrophilia. For example, if an infectious or inflammatory condition is long-standing, an anemia of chronic disease may have developed (see Chapter 3). In patients with severe infections and secondary disseminated intravascular coagulation, RBC fragmentation and thrombocytopenia may be evident. Thrombocytosis, however, accompanies many cases of reactive neutrophilia that are secondary to acute stress.

16.4.2 Peripheral Blood Smear Morphology

The morphologic features of reactive neutrophilia are listed in **Table 16-3**. Although highly variable, the WBC count usually does not exceed $30 \times 10^3/mm^3$ ($30 \times 10^9/L$); exceptions do occur, especially in patients receiving CSF therapy (*see Table 16-4*). In addition to an increase in mature neutrophils, a left shift including bands and metamyelocytes is typical in patients with a marked reactive neutrophilia. In septic newborns, circulating blasts and promyelocytes also may be evident. However, circulating blasts are not a typical feature of reactive neutrophilia in adults, except in those receiving recombinant human CSF. Toxic changes within the cytoplasm of reactive neutrophils include Döhle bodies; toxic granulation; and, when sepsis is present, prominent cytoplasmic vacuoles. In exceptional cases of sepsis, intra- and extracellular bacteria or fungi may be identified on the peripheral smear, usually a grave finding. Some cases of reactive neutrophilia are characterized by nuclear hyposegmentation (pseudo–Pelger–Huët change). The absolute neutrophilia may be accompanied by eosinophilia or monocytosis in a variety of infectious and inflammatory processes. Notably, basophilia is not a feature of a reactive neutrophilia.

One area of particular controversy is the utility of the band count in evaluating a patient for possible bacterial infection. Despite the reliance of clinicians, especially neonatologists and pediatricians, on the band count, both the accuracy of band counts and their sensitivity in predicting infection has been challenged in recent years. In several studies, the factors found most sensitive in predicting bacterial infection include WBCs, absolute neutrophil count, and the presence of immature myeloid elements such as myelocytes and promyelocytes.

In patients with chronic myeloproliferative disorders, toxic changes are absent unless a concurrent acute infection is present, the left shift includes blasts, and basophilia is common. Numerical and morphologic abnormalities of platelets and RBCs are common, and both circulating erythroid and megakaryocytic precursors may be evident (*see Table 16-5*).

16.4.3 Bone Marrow Examination

In a straightforward reactive neutrophilia, bone marrow examination is generally unnecessary. In patients with a sustained reactive neutrophilia, the predicted bone marrow findings include a granulocytic hyperplasia. However, bone marrow examination may be warranted for culture or to exclude a possible neoplastic process.

Other Laboratory Tests

Test 16.1 **Leukocyte (Neutrophil) Alkaline Phosphatase**

Purpose. The leukocyte alkaline phosphatase (LAP) test provides evidence in differentiating CML from leukemoid reactions, although more precise diagnostic tests such as molecular/cytogenetic analyses have supplanted the routine use of this test in clinical practice (see Test 32.1).

Principle. LAP is an enzyme present within the secondary (specific) granules of maturing neutrophils from the myelocyte stage onward. Stimulated neutrophils contain increased amounts of LAP. Therefore, the test helps distinguish reactive neutrophilia (increased LAP) from the abnormally maturing clonal granulocytes of CML (decreased LAP).

Procedure. LAP is usually determined semiquantitatively by specific cytochemical staining of peripheral blood smears. The LAP present in the neutrophils hydrolyzes a substrate that is then coupled to a dye, forming brown-to-black particles in the cytoplasm of these cells at the enzyme sites. The smears are then counterstained, examined microscopically, and 200 segmented or band neutrophils are counted and graded 0 to 4+ by evaluating the number of cytoplasmic particles. The LAP score is calculated by adding the products of the number of cells multiplied by the grades, as shown in the following example. The range of normal scores is 13 to 130, although there may be slight variation in each laboratory. Recently a quantitative flow cytometric technique to measure LAP has been developed, but this method is not commonly used in clinical practice.

No. Cells × Grade	Score
10 × 0	0
30 × 1	30
30 × 2	60
20 × 3	60
10 × 4	40
100 cells	190 LAP score

Specimen. Freshly prepared patient and control blood smears are obtained from finger-stick capillary blood. Blood smears should be dried at least 1 hour before fixation. If not stained immediately, fixed slides may be stored overnight in a freezer without significant loss of enzyme activity.

Interpretation. The general LAP scores in reactive conditions, pregnancy, and chronic myeloproliferative disorders are listed in **Table 16-6**. The LAP score may be increased in CML patients with secondary infections. A rising LAP score also characterizes some cases of CML in early blast crisis.

Notes and Precautions. Improperly stored smears lose enzymatic activity and give falsely low LAP scores. Ethylenediaminetetraacetic acid (EDTA) anticoagulant inhibits this reaction.

Table 16-6   Leukocyte Alkaline Phosphatase Scores

Low score
    CML (very low score)
    Other hematopoietic neoplasms, especially myelodysplasia
    Rare infections
    Paroxysmal nocturnal hemoglobinuria
High score
    Infections
    Chronic myeloproliferative disorders (not CML)
    Inflammatory processes/some nonhematopoietic neoplasms
    Pregnancy
    Stress
    Oral contraceptives
    Drug treatments (lithium, corticosteroids, estrogen, colony-stimulating
      factor)
Severe aplastic anemia

Abbreviation: CML = chronic myelogenous leukemia.

16.5 Ancillary Tests

A variety of other laboratory tests may be used to evaluate selected patients with neutrophilia. For example, serologic tests for collagen vascular disorders, uric acid levels, and gallium scans may be warranted for specific clinical indications. Either routine cytogenetic studies or molecular analyses for BCR/ABL gene rearrangements are essential in establishing the diagnosis of chronic myelogenous leukemia. In addition, clonal cytogenetic abnormalities are identified in approximately one third of patients with other chronic myeloproliferative disorders.

16.6 Course and Treatment

The course and treatment of neutrophilia depends on the underlying disease process.

16.7 References

Ardron MJ, Westengard JC, Dutcher TF. Band neutrophil counts are unnecessary for the diagnosis of infection in patients with normal total leukocyte counts. *Am J Clin Pathol.* 1994;102:646–649.

Armitage JO. Emerging applications of recombinant human granulocyte-macrophage colony-stimulating factor. *Blood.* 1998;92:4491–4508.

Bakken JS, Krueth J, Wilson-Nordskog C, et al. Clinical and laboratory characteristics of human granulocytic ehrlichiosis. *JAMA.* 1996;275:199–205.

Borregaard N, Sehested M, Nielsen BS, et al. Biosynthesis of granule proteins in normal human bone marrow cells: gelatinase is a marker of terminal neutrophil differentiation. *Blood.* 1995;85:812–817.

Dinauer MC. The phagocyte system and disorders of granulopoiesis and granulocyte function. In: Nathan DG, Orkin SH, eds. *Nathan and Oski's Hematology of Infancy and Childhood,* Vol 1. 15th ed. Philadelphia, Pa: Saunders; 1998:889–967.

Foucar K. Constitutional and reactive myeloid disorders. In: Foucar K, ed. *Bone Marrow Pathology.* 2nd ed. Chicago, Ill: ASCP Press. In press.

Gombos MM, Bienkowski RS, Gochman RF, et al. The absolute neutrophil count: is it the best indicator for occult bacteremia in infants? *Am J Clin Pathol.* 1998;109:221–225.

Gullberg U, Andersson E, Garwicz D, et al. Biosynthesis, processing and sorting of neutrophil proteins: insight into neutrophil granule development. *Eur J Haematol.* 1997;58:137–153.

Meyerson HJ, Farhi DC, Rosenthal NS. Transient increase in blasts mimicking acute leukemia and progressing myelodysplasia in patients receiving growth factor. *Am J Clin Pathol.* 1998;109:675–681.

Nolte KB, Feddersen RM, Foucar K, et al. Hantavirus pulmonary syndrome in the United States: a pathological description of a disease caused by a new agent. *Hum Pathol.* 1995;26:110–120.

Parry H, Cohen S, Schlarb JE, et al. Smoking, alcohol consumption, and leukocyte counts. *Am J Clin Pathol.* 1997;107:64–67.

Peterson L, Foucar K. Granulocytosis and granulocytopenia. In: Bick RL, ed. *Hematology: Clinical and Laboratory Practice.* St Louis, Mo: Mosby; 1993:1137–1154.

Rambaldi A, Masuhara K, Borleri GM, et al. Flow cytometry of leucocyte alkaline phosphatase in normal and pathologic leucocytes. *Br J Haematol.* 1997;96:815–822.

Schmitz LL, Litz CE, Brunning RD. Morphologic and quantitative alterations in hematopoietic cells associated with growth factor therapy: review of the literature. *Hematol Pathol.* 1994;8:55–73.

Shibano M, Machii T, Nishimori Y, et al. Assessment of alkaline phosphatase on the surface membrane of neutrophils by immunofluorescence. *Am J Hematol.* 1999;60:12–18.

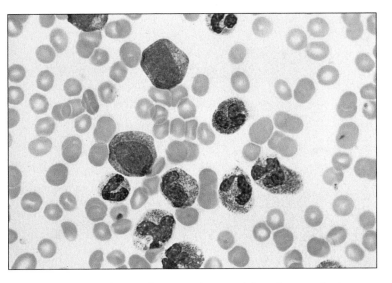

Image 16-1 Blood smear from a patient receiving pharmacologic doses of recombinant human granulocyte colony-stimulating factor. A striking leukocytosis with pronounced toxic changes and left shift is evident. (Wright's)

Image 16-2 Blood smear from a patient with human granulocytic ehrlichiosis. Both toxic neutrophilia and intracytoplasmic morulae are present. (Courtesy of Dr P. Ward.) (Wright's-Giemsa)

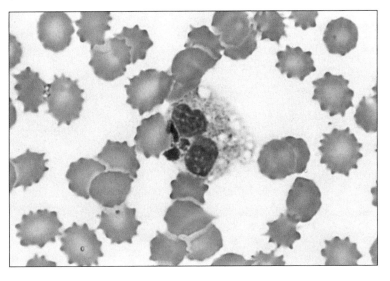

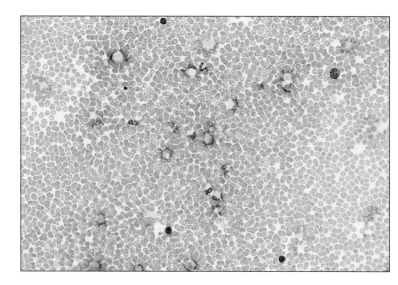

Image 16-3 Peripheral blood smear highlighting the constellation of features that characterize florid Hantavirus pulmonary syndrome: thrombocytopenia, neutrophilia with left shift, hemoconcentration secondary to plasma leakage into lungs, and circulating immunoblasts. (Wright's)

Image 16-4 Blood smears from two patients with florid Hantavirus pulmonary syndrome. Nontoxic neutrophilia, left shift to promyelocytes, and circulating immunoblasts with basophilic cytoplasm are evident; note thrombocytopenia. (Wright's)

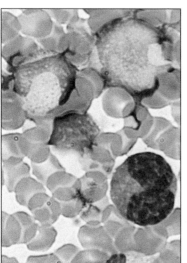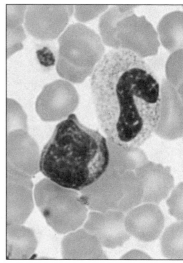

17 Eosinophilia

Eosinophils are normally present in the blood in low numbers, and there are no age-related variations in normal absolute eosinophil counts. Eosinophilia is defined as an absolute eosinophil count exceeding $0.6 \times 10^3/mm^3$ ($0.6 \times 10^9/L$). In an ambulatory setting, eosinophilia is detected in fewer than 1% of adult and pediatric patients by screening complete blood count (CBC), although a higher incidence would be expected in geographic regions in which parasitic infections are common. Causes of reactive eosinophilia are summarized in **Table 17-1**; the most common causes are drug treatments, allergies, or parasitic infections. Parasites must invade tissues to produce eosinophilia. More recently identified causes of reactive eosinophilia include an eosinophilia-myalgia syndrome secondary to L-tryptophan ingestion; therapy with pharmacologic doses of recombinant human interleukins is also associated with a brisk, reactive eosinophilia.

In addition, various nonhematopoietic neoplasms can be associated with either reactive peripheral blood eosinophilia or eosinophilic infiltrates within the neoplasm itself. Both tumor-associated blood eosinophilia and tumor-associated tissue eosinophilia are linked to factors produced by the tumor cells that induce eosinophil production. Tumor-associated blood eosinophilia is generally associated with more advanced disease and a worse prognosis overall.

Table 17-1 Causes of Reactive Eosinophilia*

Allergic and hypersensitivity reactions
Drug allergies
Cytokine therapy (recombinant human interleukins)
Cutaneous disorders
Connective tissue diseases/collagen vascular diseases
Parasitic infections
Neoplasms (carcinoma, lymphoma, Hodgkin's disease, acute lymphoblastic leukemia)[†]
Immunodeficiency disorders
Sarcoidosis

*In a substantial proportion of ambulatory patients the cause of the eosinophilia is not determined.
[†]Increased eosinophil production secondary to cytokines released by neoplastic cells; eosinophils are not neoplastic.

In these patients, the sustained blood eosinophilia with subsequent degranulation can result in tissue damage, further compromising the overall debilitated condition of the patient.

Finally, increased blood eosinophils can be a feature of a variety of hematopoietic neoplasms, including chronic myeloproliferative disorders and certain acute leukemias (**Table 17-2**). In patients with these conditions, the eosinophils are part of the neoplastic clone and often exhibit prominent morphologic abnormalities.

17.1 Pathophysiology

Although eosinophils are derived from the same progenitor cells that give rise to other granulocytic elements within the bone marrow, eosinophil production is influenced by the synergistic action of interleukin-1, interleukin-3, and interleukin-5 produced in the bone marrow microenvironment. Like other regulatory factors, these interleukins not only stimulate production of eosinophils but also enhance functional activity of mature eosinophils, most notably by interleukin-5. Although the distinctive granule used to identify the eosinophil is a secondary granule, the stages of eosinophil maturation are presumed to parallel other granulocytic cells and include myeloblasts, promyelocytes, eosinophilic myelocytes, eosinophilic metamyelocytes, and mature eosinophils. These

Table 17-2   Hematopoietic Neoplasms Demonstrating Clonal Mature Blood Eosinophilia

Chronic myeloproliferative disorders
    Chronic myelogenous leukemia
    Chronic eosinophilic leukemia
    Systemic mast cell disease*
    Other chronic hematopoietic neoplasms
Acute leukemias
    Acute myelomonocytic leukemia with eosinophilia (variable blood
      eosinophilia)
    Other myeloid leukemias
    Acute lymphoblastic leukemia with eosinophilia*

*Evidence regarding whether the eosinophils are part of a neoplastic clone is controversial. Eosinophils may be reactive, nonclonal.

---

mature eosinophils characteristically have bilobed nuclei and contain abundant large, refractile eosinophilic granules.

Eosinophils are present in low numbers in the peripheral blood, and normal eosinophil function is dependent on migration to solid tissue; eosinophil recruitment into tissue is mediated by chemokines such as eotaxin. Eosinophils demonstrate two main functions: (1) modulation of immediate hypersensitivity reactions and (2) destruction of parasites. Release of eosinophil secondary granules plays a key role in both of these functions. These secondary granules contain major basic protein, peroxidase, arylsulfatase, histamine oxidase, and eosinophil cationic protein. In addition, the surface membranes of eosinophils express Fc receptors for IgE, IgG, and certain complement components.

17.2 Clinical Findings

The cause of eosinophilia may be either clinically obvious or obscure. In outpatient settings the cause of isolated mild eosinophilia often is not determined. For patients with sustained eosinophilia, the clinical features of the diverse disorders that cause eosinophilia must be considered, along with the fact that the eosinophilia itself can produce distinctive clinical manifestations.

A sustained peripheral blood eosinophilia can result in endothelial and endomyocardial damage from intravascular degranulation of these cells. The potent cytolytic enzymes contained within eosinophil secondary granules damage endothelial cells throughout the body. As a consequence, either thrombosis or endomyocardial fibrosis may result. Although both neoplastic and reactive eosinophils can be associated with this type of tissue damage, it is far more common in patients with neoplastic eosinophilic disorders such as chronic eosinophilic leukemia or other chronic myeloproliferative disorders with a prominent eosinophilic component. Patients with these chronic myeloproliferative disorders may also exhibit organomegaly, pulmonary infiltrates, and central nervous system disease, in addition to the more common thrombotic and cardiac disorders.

Eosinophilia-myalgia syndrome was identified fairly recently as a cause of peripheral blood eosinophilia, linked to L-tryptophan ingestion (**Image 17-1**). Affected patients were usually women who presented with severe myalgia and arthralgia; fatigue; peripheral blood eo-sinophilia; and, less frequently, respiratory disorders, skin changes, and neuropathy. Following an isolated outbreak of cases, eosinophilia-myalgia syndrome was linked to L-tryptophan produced by a single Japanese manufacturer and was thought to have been caused by a toxic contaminant introduced in the manufacturing process.

17.3 Diagnostic Approach

In any patient with a sustained eosinophilia, it is important to distinguish a reactive (secondary) process from a chronic myeloproliferative disorder or other neoplasm with an eosinophilic component. Once an eosinophilia is confirmed as reactive, an attempt should be made to determine the underlying cause, especially if the absolute eosinophilia is substantial and sustained.

The following approach to diagnosis should be considered:

1. Perform a clinical evaluation and assess the patient's history of drug treatments.
2. Evaluate for possible parasitic infection, including any history of travel to foreign countries.

3. Perform appropriate laboratory tests for possible parasitic infection if clinically warranted.
4. Perform a physical examination for evidence of organomegaly or pulmonary infiltrates.
5. A chest radiograph or lung biopsy may be warranted in patients with possible pulmonary infiltrates.
6. Evaluate the patient for neoplasms associated with blood eosinophilia as a consequence of cytokine production by the tumor.
7. Assess for a possible chronic myeloproliferative disorder, systemic mast cell disease, or other clonal disorder with blood eosinophilia.

17.4 Hematologic Findings

17.4.1 Blood Cell Measurements

Eosinophilia is present when the absolute eosinophil count exceeds $0.6 \times 10^3/mm^3$ ($0.6 \times 10^9/L$). Eosinophils have a diurnal variation, highest in the morning and decreasing in the afternoon.

17.4.2 Blood Morphology

The morphology of circulating eosinophils is of only moderate help in distinguishing reactive from clonal eosinophil disorders, because eosinophil dyspoiesis such as hypogranularity and nuclear segmentation defects can be seen in both clonal and nonclonal populations. In particular, hypodense eosinophil morphology has been linked to sustained interleukin production, a mediator of secondary eosinophilia. In general, the combination of severe eosinophil dyspoiesis *plus* abnormalities or dyspoiesis in other lineages favors a neoplastic process that should be confirmed by cytogenetic/molecular studies (**Image 17-2**). Hypersegmented (trilobed), hypogranular, degranulated, or vacuolated eosinophils are especially prominent in chronic myeloproliferative disorders formerly termed "idiopathic hypereosinophilic syndromes," a clinical designation that is no longer recommended if clonality of the disorder can be established.

17.4.3 Bone Marrow Examination

Bone marrow examination generally is not required in patients with straightforward reactive eosinophilia unless indicated for other reasons such as tumor staging. However, both bone marrow examination and cytogenetic studies are valuable in patients with a possible myeloproliferative disorder or other neoplasm in which the eosinophils are likely to be part of a clonal process.

17.5 Ancillary Tests

1. In an ambulatory setting the detection of an isolated mild eosinophilia is generally not associated with a serious illness; consequently an extensive medical workup may not be necessary in otherwise healthy patients without distinctive clinical abnormalities or additional CBC abnormalities.
2. If a parasitic infection is suspected, both stool examination for ova and parasites and serologic tests for parasites may be warranted.
3. Even though cytogenetic/molecular studies are required for confirmation, aberrant periodic acid–Schiff (PAS) or chloroacetate esterase positivity is a feature of neoplastic mature eosinophils that is not generally noted in reactive eosinophils.
4. Fluorescence in situ hybridization (FISH), cytogenetic, or molecular analyses may be useful both in establishing the diagnosis of a clonal hematopoietic disorder and in establishing the clonality of the eosinophils specifically. Fluorescence in situ hybridization can be applied to smear preparations in which eosinophil identification is readily apparent, whereas assessment of eosinophil clonality by either molecular or cytogenetic techniques requires a purified eosinophil population.
5. Measurement of serum interleukin-5 levels may be useful in selected patients with presumed secondary eosinophilia.
6. Although nonspecific, the determination of serum IgE levels may be useful in selected situations.
7. Nasal smears or sputum cytology for eosinophils may be useful in selected patients. Nasal eosinophilia is common in allergic rhinitis, and abundant eosinophils in sputum may be evident in patients with Löffler's pneumonia. Charcot-Leyden crystals may be present.

8. A chest radiograph is useful to evaluate for either Löffler's pneumonia or sarcoidosis.
9. Biopsy of the gastrocnemius muscle, diagnostic in most cases of trichinosis, is used only in severely ill patients in whom the diagnosis is in doubt.
10. Serologic tests for collagen vascular disorders may be helpful in selected patients.

17.6 Course and Treatment

Treatment of reactive eosinophilia depends on the underlying cause. An eosinophilia that is a manifestation of a chronic myelo-proliferative disorder often requires therapy to arrest the progressive endothelial cell damage with associated subendocardial fibrosis that results from sustained intravascular eosinophil degranulation.

17.7 References

Belongia EA, Hedberg CW, Gleich GJ, et al. An investigation of the cause of the eosinophilia-myalgia syndrome associated with tryptophan use. *N Engl J Med.* 1990;323:357–365.

Brigden M, Graydon C. Eosinophilia detected by automated blood cell counting in ambulatory North American outpatients: incidence and clinical significance. *Arch Pathol Lab Med.* 1997;121:963–967.

de Andres B, Rakasz E, Hagen M, et al. Lack of Fc-epsilon receptors on murine eosinophils: implications for the functional significance of elevated IgE and eosinophils in parasitic infections. *Blood.* 1997;89:3826–3836.

Dinauer MC. The phagocyte system and disorders of granulopoiesis and granulocyte function. In: Nathan DG, Orkin SH, eds. *Nathan and Oski's Hematology of Infancy and Childhood, Vol 1.* 5th ed. Philadelphia, Pa: Saunders; 1998:889–967.

Enokihara H, Kajitani H, Nagashima S, et al. Interleukin 5 activity in sera from patients with eosinophilia. *Br J Haematol.* 1990;75:458–462.

Hirshberg B, Kramer MR, Lotem M, et al. Chronic eosinophilic pneumonia associated with cutaneous T-cell lymphoma. *Am J Hematol.* 1999;60:143–147.

Kamb ML, Murphy JJ, Jones JL, et al. Eosinophilia-myalgia syndrome in L-tryptophan-exposed patients. *JAMA.* 1992;267:77–82.

Koike T, Enokihara H, Arimura H, et al. Serum concentrations of IL-5, GM-CSF, and IL-3 and the production by lymphocytes in various eosinophilia. *Am J Hematol.* 1995;50:98–102.

Navarro-Roman L, Medeiros LJ, Kingma DW, et al. Malignant lymphomas of B-cell lineage with marked tissue eosinophilia: a report of five cases. *Am J Surg Pathol.* 1994;18:347–356.

Palframan RT, Collins PD, Williams TJ, et al. Eotaxin induces a rapid release of eosinophils and their progenitors from the bone marrow. *Blood.* 1998;91:2240–2248.

Rothenberg ME, Owen WF Jr, Silberstein DS, et al. Human eosinophils have prolonged survival, enhanced functional properties, and become hypodense when exposed to human interleukin 3. *J Clin Invest.* 1988;81:1986–1992.

Sanderson CJ. Interleukin-5, eosinophils, and disease. *Blood.* 1992;79:3101–3109.

Sasano H, Virmani R, Patterson RH, et al. Eosinophilic products lead to myocardial damage. *Hum Pathol.* 1989;20:850–857.

Slutsker L, Hoesly FC, Miller L, et al. Eosinophilia-myalgia syndrome associated with exposure to tryptophan from a single manufacturer. *JAMA.* 1990;264:213–217.

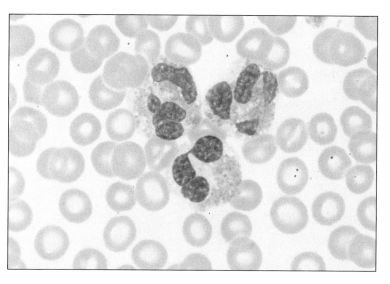

Image 17-1 Peripheral blood from a patient receiving recombinant interleukin therapy. A marked absolute eosinophilia is evident. (Wright's)

Image 17-2 Peripheral blood smear from a patient with chronic eosinophilic leukemia. A striking eosinophilia with dyspoietic changes is noted. (Wright's)

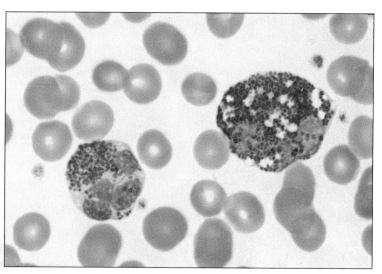

18 Basophilia

Basophils are normally the least numerous granulated cells within the peripheral blood. These cells generally account for less than 2% of WBCs, and the absolute basophil count is characteristically less than $0.1 \times 10^3/mm^3$ ($0.1 \times 10^9/L$). There are no established age-related variations in absolute basophil count.

Basophilia is defined as an absolute basophil count that exceeds $0.2 \times 10^3/mm^3$ ($0.2 \times 10^9/L$). Reactive basophilia is an uncommon blood finding, and the absolute basophil counts are generally only moderately increased in these cases. Conditions occasionally associated with reactive basophilia include allergic disorders and hypersensitivity reactions; inflammatory disorders such as ulcerative colitis and rheumatoid arthritis; chronic renal disease; and infections, including influenza, chicken pox, and, historically, smallpox (**Table 18-1**). The absolute basophil count also may be modestly increased following radiation exposure.

In contrast, neoplastic disorders with a substantial mature basophilic component are encountered much more frequently in clinical practice than are reactive basophilias. The absolute basophil count is substantially higher in patients with these neoplastic conditions. Chronic myeloproliferative disorders, especially chronic myelogenous leukemia (CML), are the most common malignancies in which an absolute basophilia is present. Even

Table 18-1 Causes of Reactive Basophilia

Allergic or hypersensitivity reactions
Inflammatory disorders (collagen vascular disease)
Endocrinopathy
Renal disease
Rare infections
Irradiation
Rare carcinomas
Medications (estrogen, antithyroid agents)

though the percentage of basophils is generally less than 10% of the WBCs in patients with CML, because of the marked leukocytosis, the absolute basophil count is strikingly elevated. A rising absolute basophil count can precede overt blast crisis in some CML patients. Basophilia is a consistent feature in the blood of patients with CML, whereas only about one third of patients with other chronic myeloproliferative disorders demonstrate this characteristic. Various acute leukemias also can exhibit a basophilic component, but these cells are generally very immature, requiring special studies for their identification. Rarely, a more mature basophilia is noted in acute myeloid leukemias.

18.1 Pathophysiology

Although the mechanisms responsible for basophil production have not been completely delineated, regulatory factors currently thought to play a role in this process include interleukin-3, granulocyte-monocyte colony-stimulating factor (GM-CSF), interleukin-4, and interleukin-5. Even though the earliest stages of maturation are not distinguishable from other myeloid lineages, the proposed stages of basophil maturation include myeloblast, promyelocyte, basophilic myelocyte, basophilic metamyelocyte, and mature basophil. Basophils are recognized in the peripheral blood and bone marrow by their distinctive secondary granule, which is large, deeply basophilic, and often obscures the segmented nucleus. These secondary granules contain numerous proteins that are essential for basophil function. These proteins include heparin, histamine, eosinophil chemotactic factor, arylsulfatase A, and slow-reacting substance of anaphylaxis, as well as many other substances.

Basophils appear to be closely related to tissue mast cells. Despite the differences in immunophenotype and morphology between basophils and mast cells, the granule contents of these two cells are remarkably similar. Likewise, both basophils and mast cells function in immediate hypersensitivity reactions via granule release. Basophil degranulation occurs in response to the binding of IgE antibodies to Fc receptors on the cell membrane.

18.2 Clinical Findings

The clinical findings in patients with reactive basophilia are quite variable, reflecting the spectrum of disorders associated with this blood abnormality. Some patients with allergic and hypersensitivity reactions may have urticaria, whereas patients with collagen vascular disorders, endocrinopathy, or renal disease exhibit diverse symptomatology and clinical findings.

The clinical features of patients with neoplastic mature basophilia are more distinctive. As described earlier, a striking mature basophilia is typical of CML, and affected patients frequently have marked splenomegaly at presentation. These patients also may complain of malaise, fatigue, and left upper quadrant pain. Hepatomegaly is variable but present in a substantial number of CML patients (see Chapter 32).

18.3 Diagnostic Approach

Reactive basophilias must be distinguished from chronic myeloproliferative disorders with a mature basophilic component. A variety of clinical and hematologic parameters are useful in making this distinction.

The following approach to diagnosis should be considered:

1. Perform a complete blood count with differential.
2. Determine the absolute basophil count and assess the morphology of basophils.

3. Evaluate other lineages for evidence of a chronic myeloproliferative disorder. For example, in patients with CML, a marked
leukocytosis with left shift to myeloblasts is characteristic. In
addition to an absolute basophilia, eosinophilia is also common. Likewise, most CML patients demonstrate a marked,
atypical thrombocytosis.
4. Correlate findings with clinical features and assess for
splenomegaly.
5. Evaluate the chemical indicators of increased cell turnover,
such as uric acid.

18.4 Hematologic Findings

18.4.1 Blood Cell Measurements

Basophils are noteworthy when the absolute basophil count
exceeds $0.2 \times 10^3/mm^3$ ($0.2 \times 10^9/L$). Most reactive basophilias are
characterized by a modest increase in basophils, whereas in neoplastic disorders the absolute basophil count is often strikingly
increased. Except for anemia (usually anemia of chronic disease),
other peripheral blood abnormalities are not generally present in
patients with reactive basophilia.

18.4.2 Blood Morphology

Basophils are morphologically unremarkable in reactive basophilia. In contrast, a variety of morphologic abnormalities, including degranulation of basophils, may be present in the blood of
patients with chronic myeloproliferative disorders (see Chapters 29
through 32).

18.4.3 Bone Marrow Examination

Bone marrow examination is not generally required in the
evaluation of patients with a reactive basophilia. In contrast, bone
marrow examination with cytogenetic studies is often essential in
establishing the diagnosis of various chronic myeloproliferative
disorders.

18.5 Course and Treatment

In patients with reactive (secondary) basophilia, both the clinical course and appropriate therapy are determined by the underlying disorder. In general, the increase in basophils within the peripheral blood is not associated with any specific disease manifestations. The treatment of chronic myeloproliferative disorders such as CML is usually directed toward disease eradication (see Chapter 32).

18.6 References

Ademokun AJ, Irving JA, Maung ZT, et al. Basophilia, t(15;17) translocation and atypical AML. *Leukemia.* 1995;9:225–226.

Costa JJ, Weller PF, Galli SJ. The cells of the allergic response: mast cells, basophils, and eosinophils. *JAMA.* 1997;278:1815–1822.

Denburg JA. Basophil and mast cell lineages in vitro and in vivo. *Blood.* 1992;79:846–860.

Denburg JA, Silver JE, Abrams JS. Interleukin-5 is a human basophilopoietin: induction of histamine content and basophilic differentiation of HL-60 cells and of peripheral blood basophil-eosinophil progenitors. *Blood.* 1991;77:1462–1468.

Dinauer MC. The phagocyte system and disorders of granulopoiesis and granulocyte function. In: Nathan DG, Orkin SH, eds. *Nathan and Oski's Hematology of Infancy and Childhood, Vol 1.* 5th ed. Philadelphia, Pa: Saunders; 1998:889–967.

Jandl JH. Granulocytes. In: Jandl JH, ed. *Blood: Textbook of Hematology.* 2nd ed. Boston, Mass: Little, Brown; 1996:615–649.

Stockman JA III, Ezekowitz RAB. Hematologic manifestations of systemic diseases. In: Nathan DG, Orkin SH, eds. *Nathan and Oski's Hematology of Infancy and Childhood, Vol 2.* 5th ed. Philadelphia, Pa: Saunders; 1998:1841–1891.

19 Monocytosis

Although generally present in low numbers, monocytes and related cell types are ubiquitous inhabitants of all organ systems in the body. Monocytes generally compose only 2% to 9% of WBCs, with an absolute count of 0.1 to 0.9×10^3/mm^3 (0.1 to 0.9×10^9/L). Slightly higher numbers of monocytes may be identified within the blood of normal infants. However, there are no striking age-related variations in normal absolute monocyte count.

Monocytosis is defined as an absolute monocyte count that exceeds 1.0×10^3/mm^3 (1.0×10^9/L) in adults and 1.2×10^3/mm^3 (1.2×10^9/L) in neonates. Both neoplastic and nonneoplastic disorders are associated with absolute monocytosis (**Tables 19-1** and **19-2**). The most common cause of reactive monocytosis is a chronic infection secondary to many agents, including tuberculosis, *Listeria*, syphilis, subacute bacterial endocarditis, and certain protozoal and rickettsial infections. In general, a chronic infection is more likely than an acute infection to exhibit monocytosis. In rare cases, either chronic Epstein-Barr or cytomegalovirus infection in children results in sustained monocytosis and neutrophilia. Other causes of reactive monocytosis include nonhematopoietic neoplasms such as Hodgkin's disease and occasional non-Hodgkin's lymphomas. Often recovery from agranulocytosis is preceded by monocytosis; this is common in patients with cyclic neutropenia. A

Table 19-1   Causes of Reactive Monocytosis

Chronic infections, many agents
Hodgkin's disease
Recovery of agranulocytosis
Collagen vascular diseases
Gastrointestinal disorders (immune-mediated)
Non-Hodgkin's lymphomas
Sarcoidosis
Multiple myeloma
Hemolytic anemia
Chronic neutropenia
Rare carcinomas
Splenectomy
Immune thrombocytopenic purpura

Table 19-2   Disorders With Circulating Neoplastic Monocytes

Myelodysplasia, especially chronic myelomonocytic leukemia
Acute myelomonocytic leukemia
Acute monocytic leukemia
Chronic myelogenous leukemia
Other chronic myeloproliferative disorders
Malignant histiocytosis
Various pediatric myeloproliferative/myelodysplastic disorders that are linked
  to constitutional or acquired monosomy 7

variety of immune-mediated disorders also are associated with mature reactive monocytosis, including collagen vascular diseases and gastrointestinal disorders such as ulcerative colitis and regional enteritis. Other less common causes of reactive monocytosis include hemolytic anemia, chronic neutropenia, and postsplenectomy states.

Likewise, patients with primary hematopoietic neoplasms can exhibit a peripheral blood monocytosis, but in these disorders the monocytes are part of the neoplastic clone (*see Table 19-2*). For example, monocytosis is a defining feature of myelodysplastic disorders such as chronic myelomonocytic leukemia. In addition, both acute myelomonocytic and acute monocytic leukemias demonstrate a dominant monocytic component. However, in these acute leukemias the monocytes demonstrate marked immaturity, whereas more mature circulating monocytes are evident in chronic myelomonocytic leukemia and chronic myelogenous leukemia. Other chronic myeloproliferative/myelodysplastic disorders can sometimes demonstrate an increase in peripheral blood monocytes, and circulating neoplastic monocytic/histiocytic cells occasionally may be identified in the peripheral blood of patients with malignant histiocytosis. In particular, monocytosis with immaturity can be striking in very young children with constitutional or acquired myeloproliferative/myelodysplastic disorders frequently associated with monosomy 7 (see Chapter 26).

19.1 Pathophysiology

Monocytes are derived from bone marrow myeloid progenitor cells, and regulatory factors linked to monocyte production include granulocyte-monocyte colony-stimulating factor (GM-CSF) and monocyte colony-stimulating factor (M-CSF). The proposed stages of monocyte differentiation within the bone marrow include monoblasts, promonocytes, and mature monocytes, although neither monoblasts nor promonocytes are typically identified in normal bone marrow specimens.

Monocytes circulate briefly in the peripheral blood and migrate to tissues where they mature into a variety of cells composing the monocyte/histiocyte/immune accessory cell system. Members of this diverse cell family exhibit a variety of functions in both cellular and humoral immunity, in phagocytic and antimicrobial activities, and in tissue homeostasis and repair. Monocytes and other cells within this lineage secrete hundreds of proteins that modulate immune function, regulate hematopoiesis, stimulate inflammatory reactions, provide host defense against tumors, and remove either senescent blood cells or infectious organisms by phagocytosis. A partial list of proteins produced by cells within this complex lineage includes complement components, interferons, interleukins, prostaglandins, tumor necrosis factors, and colony-stimulating factors. Like neutrophils, monocytes contain granules within their cytoplasm that play a major role in the cell's function. These granules contain numerous enzymes, including lysozyme, acid phosphatase, collagenase, and elastase.

19.2 Clinical Findings

The predicted clinical features in patients exhibiting reactive monocytosis are diverse, because of the large variety of disorders linked to this relatively nonspecific peripheral blood finding. The most common cause of reactive monocytosis is chronic infection, and these patients are likely to be febrile with other symptomatology related to the specific type of chronic infection.

In patients in whom the monocytosis is a component of a hematopoietic neoplasm, additional blood abnormalities are expected. The clinical features in patients with primary hematopoietic neoplasms often include fatigue, fever, malaise, and signs of organ infiltration. Differentiation between reactive and neoplastic monocytosis is particularly challenging in young children because of the overlap between clinical and morphologic findings. Children with either chronic viral infections or juvenile rheumatoid arthritis can have splenomegaly and prominent monocytosis with some immature forms. Likewise, young children may develop clonal myeloproliferative/myelodysplastic disorders characterized by hepatosplenomegaly, variable lymphadenopathy, and marked leukocytosis with monocytosis and neutrophilia (see Chapter 26).

19.3 Diagnostic Approach

Because blood monocytosis occurs frequently in certain hematologic neoplasms, it is imperative that a distinction between reactive and neoplastic monocytosis be made. In patients with primary hematologic neoplasms such as chronic myelomonocytic leukemia, acute myelomonocytic and monocytic leukemias, and chronic myelogenous leukemia, the monocytes are an integral part of the neoplastic clone. The determination of the reactive or neoplastic nature of a blood monocytosis often requires the integration of a variety of hematologic, morphologic, and other laboratory and clinical parameters. A general approach to monocytosis includes:

1. A complete blood count with differential.
2. An evaluation of monocytes for evidence of nuclear immaturity or other atypical features.
3. An evaluation of other peripheral blood cells for evidence of atypia, dysplasia, or immaturity.

4. Correlation of clinical and hematologic findings.
5. Appropriate cultures to assess for possible chronic infection.
6. A bone marrow examination for culture or assessment with monocyte-specific stains for hematopoietic neoplasm.
7. A cytogenetic/molecular evaluation for possible hematopoietic neoplasm.

19.4 Hematologic Findings

19.4.1 Blood Cell Measurements

In healthy children and adults, the absolute monocyte count is characteristically less than $1.0 \times 10^3/mm^3$ ($1.0 \times 10^9/L$). Depending on the cause of the monocytosis, many other peripheral blood abnormalities may be evident. For example, reactive monocytosis secondary to infection may be accompanied by a neutrophilia (**Image 19-1**). In affected patients, the platelet count is highly variable, although a mild to moderate anemia (most likely anemia of chronic disease) also may be evident. The WBC count also is highly variable in patients with a neoplastic monocytosis, but it is typically elevated, with increased numbers of monocytes and a variable proportion of immature myeloid and monocytic elements. In patients with hematopoietic neoplasms, the hemoglobin, hematocrit, and platelet count may be markedly reduced.

19.4.2 Peripheral Blood Smear Morphology

Evidence of monocyte immaturity, such as finely dispersed nuclear chromatin, nucleoli, and variable abnormal nuclear configurations, suggests that the monocytes are part of a neoplastic process (**Image 19-2**). Circulating monoblasts also suggest a neoplastic process. Reactive monocytes characteristically exhibit indented or folded nuclei, relatively mature nuclear chromatin, and cytoplasm that is frequently vacuolated (*see Image 19-1*). Cytoplasmic granulation also may be prominent. In addition to evaluating monocyte morphology, an evaluation of the morphology of other cell types in the peripheral blood can be helpful in distinguishing benign from neoplastic monocytosis. If there is either prominent dyspoiesis of any lineage or substantial left shift, the patient probably has a neoplastic hematologic disorder with involvement of many cell lines, including the monocyte lineage. This multilineage dyspoiesis with atypical monocytes is especially prominent in myelodysplastic disorders.

19.4.3 Bone Marrow Examination

Bone marrow examination may be warranted in selected patients with blood monocytosis. Indications for bone marrow examination in this patient population include culture or evaluation for a possible hematopoietic neoplasm.

19.5 Ancillary Tests

1. Blood or bone marrow culture.
2. Serologic studies for infectious agents.
3. Cytogenetic/molecular studies in patients with possible hematopoietic neoplasm.
4. Urine/serum lysozyme levels (highest in monocytic leukemias).
5. Special stains for monocytic differentiation on bone marrow aspirate smears if monocytic leukemia is suspected (ie, α-naphthol butyrate esterase).
6. Flow cytometric immunophenotyping for suspected acute leukemia.

19.6 Course and Treatment

The clinical course varies with the underlying disorder, as does the treatment of patients with monocytosis. In general, patients with a neoplastic monocytosis follow an aggressive disease course requiring antileukemic therapy.

19.7 References

Cline MJ. Laboratory evaluation of benign quantitative granulocyte and mono-cyte disorders. In: Bick RL, ed. *Hematology Clinical and Laboratory Practice, Vol 2.* St Louis, Mo: Mosby; 1993:1155–1160.

Dinauer MC. The phagocyte system and disorders of granulopoiesis and granu-locyte function. In: Nathan DG, Orkin SH, eds. *Nathan and Oski's Hematology of Infancy and Childhood, Vol 1.* 5th ed. Philadelphia, Pa: Saunders; 1998:889–967.

Foucar K. Constitutional and reactive myeloid disorders. In: Foucar K, ed. *Bone Marrow Pathology.* 2nd ed. Chicago, Ill: ASCP Press. In press.

Foucar K, Foucar E. The mononuclear phagocyte and immunoregulatory effec-tor (M-PIRE) system: evolving concepts. *Semin Diagn Pathol.* 1990;7:4–18.

Herrod HG, Dow LW, Sullivan JL. Persistent Epstein-Barr virus infection mim-icking juvenile chronic myelogenous leukemia: immunologic and hemato-logic studies. *Blood.* 1983;61:1098–1104.

Kirby MA, Weitzman S, Freedman MH. Juvenile chronic myelogenous leukemia: differentiation from infantile cytomegalovirus infection. *Am J Pediatr Hematol Oncol.* 1990;12:292–296.

Luna-Fineman S, Shannon KM, Atwater SK, et al. Myelodysplastic and mye-loproliferative disorders of childhood: a study of 167 patients. *Blood.* 1999;93:459–466.

Nathan CF. Secretory products of macrophages. *J Clin Invest.* 1987;79:319–326.

Papadimitriou JM, Ashman RB. Macrophages: current views on their differenti-ation, structure, and function. *Ultrastruct Pathol.* 1989;13:343–372.

Stockman JA III, Ezekowitz RAB. Hematologic manifestations of systemic diseases. In: Nathan DG, Orkin SH, eds. *Nathan and Oski's Hematology of Infancy and Childhood, Vol 2.* 5th ed. Philadelphia, Pa: Saunders; 1998:1841–1891.

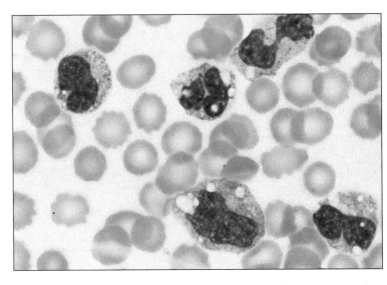

Image 19-1 Blood smear from a septic infant. Prominent cytoplasmic vacuolization of both neutrophils and monocytes is evident. (Wright's)

Image 19-2 Blood smear from a child with chronic myelomonocytic leukemia. A striking monocytosis with some nuclear immaturity and dyspoiesis is evident. (Wright's)

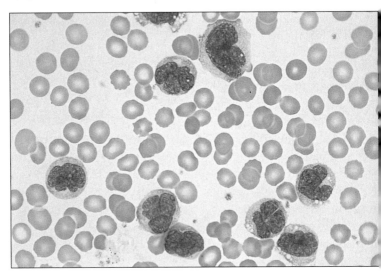

20   Neutropenia

In normal adults, the range for absolute neutrophil count is 1.5 to $7.0 \times 10^3/mm^3$ (1.5 to $7.0 \times 10^9/L$). Both patient age and race have an impact on the established lower limit of the normal range. For example, in neonates and infants, the lower limit is approximately $2.5 \times 10^3/mm^3$ ($2.5 \times 10^9/L$), whereas the lower limit of normal for children and adults is $1.5 \times 10^3/mm^3$ ($1.5 \times 10^9/L$). Approximately one fourth of healthy black children and adults demonstrate an absolute neutrophil count that ranges from 1.0 to $1.5 \times 10^3/mm^3$ (1.0 to $1.5 \times 10^9/L$). Because these patients demonstrate no evidence of clinically significant neutropenia, this value is presumed to represent a normal race variation.

Consequently, the definition of neutropenia varies by patient age and race. An absolute neutrophil count less than $2.5 \times 10^3/mm^3$ ($2.5 \times 10^9/L$) constitutes neutropenia in infants; an absolute neutrophil count less than $1.5 \times 10^3/mm^3$ ($1.5 \times 10^9/L$) is generally used to define neutropenia in all other patient age groups. Neutropenias are subclassified into mild, moderate, and severe based on the absolute neutrophil count. A mild neutropenia generally ranges from 1.0 to $1.5 \times 10^3/mm^3$ (1.0 to $1.5 \times 10^9/L$), while moderate neutropenias range from 0.5 to $1.0 \times 10^3/mm^3$ (0.5 to $1.0 \times 10^9/L$). Patients with severe neutropenia ($<0.5 \times 10^3/mm^3$ [<0.5

Table 20-1   Causes of Neutropenia

Infections
Idiosyncratic drug reactions
Autoimmune/other immune disorders
Neoplasms replacing bone marrow
Megaloblastic anemia
Constitutional neutropenic disorders
Hypersplenism
Acquired idiopathic neutropenia
Bone marrow ablative therapies

$\times 10^9$/L]) are at the greatest risk for serious bacterial infection, usually of endogenous origin.

Causes of neutropenia are listed in **Table 20-1**. Neutropenia can be the result of either a constitutional bone marrow defect or an acquired abnormality, and there are prominent age variations in the most common causes of neutropenia. In addition, an isolated neutropenia must be distinguished from multilineage cytopenias.

The primary causes of neutropenia, based on patient age, are listed in **Table 20-2**. Infection is by far the most common cause of neutropenia in neonates. However, neonates also may develop neutropenia from maternal factors such as hypertension, drug treatments given to the mother during late gestation, and maternal antibodies that cross the placenta and attack fetal granulocytes. Although only rarely encountered in clinical practice, a variety of distinct constitutional neutropenic disorders also may manifest during the neonatal period (**Table 20-3**). Of these rare hereditary disorders, the more prevalent are cyclic neutropenia, Kostmann's syndrome, and Chédiak-Higashi syndrome (see Chapter 22). Severe sustained neutropenia characterizes Kostmann's syndrome and Chédiak-Higashi syndrome, whereas patients with cyclic neutropenia exhibit episodic loss of neutrophils followed by a rebound recovery.

As with neonates, infection is a common cause of neutropenia in older children. Other causes of neutropenia in infants and children include autoimmune disorders, bone marrow neoplasms, myeloablative therapy, and idiosyncratic drug reactions. In adults, idiosyncratic drug reactions are the most common cause of neutropenia in ambulatory patients. Numerous drug treatments are linked to acquired neutropenia, and patients should always be

Table 20-2   Age-Related Causes of Neutropenia

Patient Age	Causes of Neutropenia
Neonate	Infections
	Maternal hypertension and/or drug treatment
	Maternal antibody production
	Constitutional disorders such as cyclic neutropenia, Kostmann syndrome, and Chédiak-Higashi syndrome
Infant/child	Infections
	Autoimmune neutropenia
	Neoplasms replacing bone marrow
	Idiosyncratic drug reactions
	Myeloablative therapies
	Constitutional neutropenic disorders (rare)
	Megaloblastic anemia (rare)
	Copper deficiency (rare)
Adult	Idiosyncratic drug reactions
	Infections
	Neoplasms replacing bone marrow
	Myeloablative therapies
	Autoimmune disorders including white cell aplasia
	Aplastic anemia
	Hypersplenism
	Megaloblastic anemia
	Large granular lymphocytosis

queried regarding medications. Other common causes of neutropenia in adults include infections; bone marrow replacement disorders; myeloablative therapy; megaloblastic anemia; and various autoimmune/immune disorders, including acquired white cell aplasia. Neutropenia secondary to splenic pooling of neutrophils can be present in patients with hypersplenism (*see Table 20-2*).

20.1 Pathophysiology

Normal numbers of circulating neutrophils are maintained by adequate bone marrow proliferation, unimpeded bone marrow maturation and release into blood, and normal survival time in blood. Defects both within and outside the bone marrow may be

Table 20-3 Constitutional Disorders Associated With Neutropenia

Disorder	Age of Onset	Type of Defect*
Cyclic neutropenia	Early infancy	Proliferation
Kostmann's syndrome	Birth/early infancy	Proliferation
Shwachman-Diamond syndrome	Birth/early infancy	Proliferation
Immunodeficiency disorders/ reticular dysgenesis	Early infancy	Proliferation
Chédiak-Higashi syndrome	Early infancy	Maturation
Myelokathexis	Early infancy	Maturation
Fanconi's anemia	Infancy/childhood/ adulthood (rare)	Proliferation
Dyskeratosis congenita	Infancy	Proliferation

*See Table 20-4 for mechanisms that cause neutropenic disorders.

responsible for neutropenia, and these mechanisms can be broadly classified as proliferation, maturation, survival, and distribution defects (**Table 20-4**). Often, more than one of these mechanisms is operational in the production of neutropenia. For example, a patient with an infection may develop neutropenia because of bone marrow suppression by the infectious agent, decreased neutrophil survival, and increased egress of neutrophils from the blood to infection sites. Likewise, the mechanisms that are operative in patients who develop neutropenia secondary to idiosyncratic drug reactions also are overlapping and variable. In some of these patients, the drug causes abrupt loss of the granulocyte lineage (ie, proliferation defect), while drug-induced immune-mediated neutrophil destruction is operative in other patients (ie, a survival defect).

20.2 Clinical Findings

Because of the variety of underlying causes, patients with neutropenia have diverse clinical manifestations. However, all neutro-

Table 20-4 Mechanisms Causing Neutropenia

Mechanism	Comments
Proliferation defect	Failure of granulocytic lineage
	Often only scattered myeloblasts and promyelocytes present
	Occurs in many constitutional neutropenias, many idiosyncratic drug reactions, bone marrow replacement disorders, aplastic anemia, and following myeloablative therapy
Maturation defect	Granulocytic lineage abundant but maturation does not proceed normally, and many cells die within the bone marrow
	Occurs in neutropenias associated with megaloblastic anemia and rare constitutional disorders such as myelokathexis
Survival defect	Bone marrow production and release of neutrophils is increased, but cells are rapidly removed from blood
	Occurs in many infections and immune disorders characterized by antineutrophil antibody production
Distribution abnormality	Total body granulocyte pool is normal, but number of circulating neutrophils is reduced
	Occurs in patients with hypersplenism and patients with defective release of bone marrow neutrophils (rare)
	Seldom the primary mechanism responsible for neutropenia

penic patients must be assessed for possible underlying infections that may be either the cause or the consequence of the neutropenia. Secondary infections in neutropenic patients are often derived from endogenous organisms, and commonly involved sites include skin, oral pharynx, gingiva, gastrointestinal tract, and the anal region. The detection of infection may be challenging in neutropenic patients, because many of the clinical "clues" to a specific site of infection are the consequence of the migration of huge numbers of neutrophils to that site. Consequently, in severely neutropenic patients, findings such as swelling, induration, erythema, and even infiltrates on chest radiograph are less conspicuous.

20.3 Diagnostic Approach

The evaluation of a patient with neutropenia requires the integration of multiple clinical and laboratory parameters. Although the appropriate workup varies with patient age, in general, the evaluation of a neutropenia should include the following steps:

1. A detailed history for evidence of recurrent infections, findings suggestive of a constitutional disorder, symptoms of a current infection, and symptoms of an underlying immunologic disorder or occult neoplasm.
2. An investigation for drug therapy, toxin, or alcohol exposure.
3. A physical examination for possible splenomegaly, evidence of occult infection, or evidence of neoplasm.
4. A complete blood count with differential. Serial complete blood counts may be necessary to document either a cyclic pattern or neutrophil recovery in patients with transient neutropenia.
5. A morphologic review of blood smear for evidence of hematopoietic neoplasms, infection-related changes, megaloblastic features, and features of constitutional disorders such as Chédiak-Higashi syndrome.
6. An evaluation of other hematopoietic lineages for morphologic or numeric abnormalities.
7. A laboratory workup for possible infection, if clinically suspected.
8. In selected patients, a laboratory assessment of immune status, tests for collagen vascular disorders, or serologic studies for viral infections.
9. Various radiographic studies in selected patients, including those with suspected constitutional neutropenic disorders, to assess for constitutional bony defects, evidence of neoplasm, or evidence of infection.
10. A bone marrow examination. This is generally required in adult patients with new-onset neutropenia. Likewise, bone marrow evaluation is necessary in children with suspected neoplasms, aplasia, and selected infections. However, many children develop transient neutropenia following presumed viral infections. In these children, who are otherwise healthy and have only isolated neutropenia, a "watch and wait" approach is often taken. A bone marrow examination is unlikely to be considered in these children unless spontaneous neutrophil recovery is not evident within 1 to 2 months.

20.4 Hematologic Findings

20.4.1 Blood Cell Measurements

The neutrophil count is less than $1.5 \times 10^3/mm^3$ ($1.5 \times 10^9/L$). Depending on the cause of the neutropenia, the other hemogram parameters are highly variable.

20.4.2 Peripheral Blood Smear Morphology

Although the total number is decreased, the morphology of granulocytes is generally normal, except in rare constitutional disorders such as Chédiak-Higashi syndrome. Toxic changes and left shift may be evident in infected patients. Monocytosis may be present and is partly compensatory.

20.4.3 Bone Marrow Examination

Bone marrow findings vary with the mechanism responsible for the neutropenia (**Tables 20-4** and **20-5**). In patients with proliferation defects, the granulocytic lineage is largely absent. This may be the consequence of some hematopoietic regulatory defect or the bone marrow may be effaced by a neoplasm or fibrosis. In patients with constitutional neutropenias such as Kostmann's syndrome, the myeloid lineage is virtually absent except for rare myeloblasts and promyelocytes, which often are enlarged and binucleate (**Image 20-1**). In patients with maturation defects, the granulocytic lineage is hyperplastic, and morphologic abnormalities are generally prominent. The defective myeloid elements generally die within the medullary cavity, often by apoptosis. In patients with survival defects, the granulocytic lineage also is hyperplastic. However, as a consequence of the rapid release of mature forms into the blood, the granulocyte maturation pyramid may exhibit left shift in patients with survival defects. If the survival defect is immune-mediated, bone marrow macrophages may contain ingested neutrophils (**Image 20-2**).

20.5 Ancillary Tests

Numerous ancillary tests may be warranted in selected neutropenic patients, including tests for folate and vitamin B_{12} levels, collagen

Table 20-5 Bone Marrow Findings in Nonneoplastic Neutropenic Disorders

Disorder	Comments
Aplastic anemia (proliferation defect)	All lineages absent or reduced
Radiation/chemotherapy (proliferation defect)	All lineages suppressed or absent
Myelophthisis (proliferation effect)	Bone marrow replaced by infiltrative disorder
Drug-induced neutropenia (proliferation or survival defect)	Variable; most cases exhibit almost complete granulocytic aplasia with occasional blasts and promyelocytes
	Other cases characterized by granulocytic hyperplasia with a decrease in mature forms (eg, drug-induced immune destruction)
Immune-mediated neutropenia (survival or proliferation defect)	Generally granulocytic hyperplasia with decreased mature neutrophils is found, although immune mechanisms also are responsible for suppressing granulocyte and other lineages
	Prominent ingestion of neutrophils by macrophages possible
	Immune aberrations may be primary or secondary to neoplastic or nonneoplastic disorders
Vitamin B_{12} or folate deficiency (maturation defect)	Markedly hypercellular bone marrow with pronounced megaloblastic changes; intramedullary cell death
Infection-associated neutropenia (proliferation or survival defect)	Variable bone marrow morphology; some infections (especially viral) suppress progenitor cells, inducing hypoplasia
	Other infections cause decreased neutrophil survival, and bone marrow shows granulocytic hyperplasia

vascular disease, immune status, granulocyte antibody studies, cytogenetics, serologic tests for infectious agents, neutrophil survival studies, and copper levels.

20.6 Course and Treatment

The management of a patient with neutropenia includes the following components:

1. Prompt antibiotic therapy for infected patients.
2. The determination and management of the underlying cause of neutropenia.
3. Possible recombinant human colony-stimulating factor therapy to stimulate neutrophil production.

The development of recombinant human colony-stimulating factor has been a major breakthrough in the treatment of neutropenias of diverse etiology, including both constitutional and acquired neutropenic disorders. The most consistent increases in absolute neutrophil count are achieved with granulocyte colony-stimulating factor therapy. In these patients, brisk neutrophilia with prominent toxic changes results from pharmacologic doses of granulocyte colony-stimulating factor (see Chapter 16).

20.7 References

Al-Mulla ZS, Christensen RD. Neutropenia in the neonate. *Clin Perinatol.* 1995;22:711–739.

Alter BP. Arms and the man or hands and the child: congenital anomalies and hematologic syndromes. *J Pediatr Hematol Oncol.* 1997;19:287–291.

Bux J, Behrens G, Jaeger G, et al. Diagnosis and clinical course of autoimmune neutropenia in infancy: analysis of 240 cases. *Blood.* 1998;91:181–186.

Claas FH. Immune mechanisms leading to drug-induced blood dyscrasias. *Eur J Haematol Suppl.* 1996;60:64–68.

Foucar K. Constitutional and reactive myeloid disorders. In: Foucar K, ed. *Bone Marrow Pathology.* 2nd ed. Chicago, Ill: ASCP Press. In press.

Foucar K, Duncan MH, Smith KJ. Practical approach to the investigation of neutropenia. *Clin Lab Med.* 1993;13:879–894.

Haurie C, Dale DC, Mackey MC. Cyclical neutropenia and other periodic hematological disorders: a review of mechanisms and mathematical models. *Blood.* 1998;92:2629–2640.

Peterson L, Foucar K. Granulocytosis and granulocytopenia. In: Bick RL, ed. *Hematology: Clinical and Laboratory Practice.* St Louis, Mo: Mosby; 1993:1137–1154.

Reed WW, Diehl LF. Leukopenia, neutropenia, and reduced hemoglobin levels in healthy American blacks. *Arch Intern Med.* 1991;151:501–505.

Shimizu H, Sawada K, Katano N, et al. Intramedullary neutrophil phagocytosis by histiocytes in autoimmune neutropenia of infancy. *Acta Haematol.* 1990;84:201–203.

Sievers EL, Dale DC. Non-malignant neutropenia. *Blood Rev.* 1996;10:95–100.

Uetrecht JP. Reactive metabolites and agranulocytosis. *Eur J Haematol Suppl.* 1996;60:83–88.

van der Klauw MM, Wilson JH, Stricker BH. Drug-associated agranulocytosis: 20 years of reporting in the Netherlands (1974–1994). *Am J Hematol.* 1998;57:206–211.

Welte K, Boxer LA. Severe chronic neutropenia: pathophysiology and therapy. *Semin Hematol.* 1997;34:267–278.

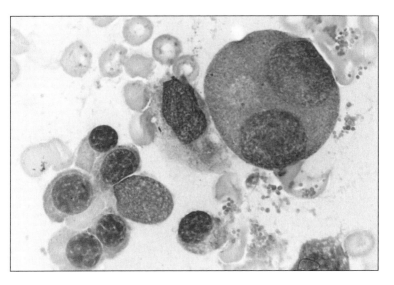

Image 20-1 Hypocellular bone marrow aspirate smear highlighting the rare myeloblasts and giant binucleate promyelocytes seen in patients with Kostmann's syndrome (constitutional neutropenia). (Wright's)

Image 20-2 Imprint smear of bone marrow from a child with autoimmune neutropenia. A macrophage contains numerous ingested neutrophils. (Wright's)

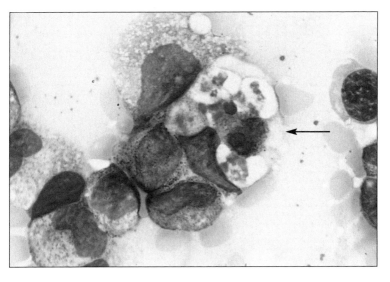

21 Functional Defects of Granulocytes

In this chapter disorders linked to impaired neutrophil function are reviewed. Adequate neutrophil function is essential for protection from invading bacteria and fungi. Patients with significant neutrophil function defects, especially from constitutional disorders, are susceptible to recurrent bacterial and fungal infections. All genetic disorders of neutrophil function are extremely rare and infrequently encountered in clinical practice. In contrast, acquired neutrophil function defects are much more common but generally are not severe. In fact, many acquired neutrophil function defects, although apparent by various in vitro tests using normal donor neutrophils as controls, may lack clinical significance.

21.1 Pathophysiology

Neutrophil function is a very complex and highly regulated process requiring normal levels and functional activity of various cytoplasmic components and membrane proteins, as well as an external environment that contains adequate chemotactic factors, complement levels, cytokines, and normal endothelial cell function. A series of interrelated activities are required to accomplish neutrophil destruction of invading bacteria and fungi. Neutrophils must be produced in adequate numbers by the bone marrow and appropriately released into the peripheral blood (see Chapters 16 and 20). Circulating neutrophils must be able to sense chemotactic factors released in the vicinity of bacterial or fungal invasion. Appropriate ligands on the surface of the neutrophil are necessary to bind these chemotactic factors, which include immunoglobulins, complement components, bacterial metabolites, and denatured neutrophil proteins. These neutrophils must then attach to endothelial cells, egress through the blood vessel wall, and migrate to the specific site of invasion. Adhesion of neutrophils to endothelial cells is accomplished by the binding of neutrophil adhesion molecules (integrins such as CD11b/CD18 and the selectin ligand CD15s) to the surface of the endothelial cells.

Neutrophil migration is a complex process that involves repetitive sequential series of receptor binding, signal transduction, and remodeling of the neutrophil cytoskeleton. Neutrophils must subsequently recognize, bind, surround tightly with cell membrane, phagocytose, and finally destroy these invading bacteria or fungi. This destruction is achieved by degranulation (fusion of a granule with phagolysosome) and activation of nicotinamide adenine dinucleotide phosphate (NADPH)–dependent oxidase. Neutrophil granules contain microbicidal enzymes, which are of high concentration when released into the small phagolysosomes.

Both chemotaxis and microbial phagocytosis/destruction require the integrated activity of cytoplasmic cytoskeletal proteins, cytoplasmic granules, and surface membrane constituents of neutrophils. In addition, many factors external to granulocytes are essential for normal function. For example, the complement system, various immunoglobulins, and several inflammatory cytokine mediators are all required for many of these neutrophil activities. Cytokines such as the colony-stimulating factors also enhance functional activities of mature neutrophils by binding to specific cell membrane receptors. Once microorganisms have been engulfed by neutrophils, an oxidative reaction called "respiratory burst" is often required for their destruction.

Any abnormality in this complex series of neutrophil functions can result in increased susceptibility to bacterial or fungal infections, including infections with low-virulence organisms. These neutrophil function abnormalities can be either constitutional (genetic) or acquired, and are generally classified as defects in adhesion, motility, granule formation, and phagocytic/killing activity (**Table 21-1**). In some disorders, especially in acquired conditions, more than one type of defect is evident. Because sophisticated methodologies to investigate neutrophil function are relatively new, multiple types of neutrophil function defects have been only recently categorized. In addition to intrinsic neutrophil abnormalities, disorders in the complement cascade and immunoglobulins also cause neutrophil dysfunction.

All constitutional neutrophil function defects are exceedingly rare; these hereditary disorders are typically manifested during infancy and early childhood. Hereditary neutrophil function disorders are often severe, and, consequently, patients develop numerous recurrent and progressive bacterial and fungal infections, often associated with poor wound healing.

Chédiak-Higashi syndrome was the first recognized constitutional neutrophil function disorder. This autosomal recessive, multisystem disease is the consequence of defects in granule structure and function that affect many cells throughout the body. Because of abnormalities in melanosome structure, affected patients often have oculocutaneous albinism; platelet granule defects are linked to bleeding disorders. Abnormal granules are apparent within all granulated hematopoietic cells and even within lymphocytes (see Chapter 22). Because of this defective cytoplasmic granulation, many cells die within the bone marrow, resulting in peripheral blood neutropenia and thrombocytopenia. Although neutrophil defects are primarily responsible for the increased susceptibility to infection in patients with Chédiak-Higashi syndrome, functional defects of eosinophils, basophils, and monocytes also are present. The abnormal cytoplasmic granulation in Chédiak-Higashi syndrome results in both impaired motility (ie, defective chemotaxis) and defective degranulation.

Chronic granulomatous disease is another type of constitutional neutrophil function disorder that is rarely encountered in clinical practice. Most cases of this disease are X-linked recessive disorders, although three autosomal recessive subtypes of chronic granulomatous disease also have been described. The onset of disease is characteristically within the first year of life, although milder forms may not manifest until adulthood. Patients with this disease frequently have lymphadenopathy, hepatosplenomegaly, and anemia of chronic disease. Dominant sites of recurrent infection include lung, skin, gastrointestinal tract, and lymph node; widespread multiorgan granuloma formation is a hallmark of this disease. Older patients often demonstrate restrictive lung disease;

Table 21-1 Classification of Constitutional and Acquired Functional Defects of Neutrophils

General Type of Defect	Constitutional Disorders	Acquired Disorders/ Conditions*
Adhesion defects	Leukocyte adhesion deficiency (Types 1 and 2)	Aging Alcohol-induced Drug effects (corticosteroids, epinephrine, aspirin) Diabetes Renal disorders Chronic infections Paraproteinemias Sickle cell anemia
Defects in granule structure/ function	Chédiak-Higashi syndrome Specific granule deficiency	Chronic myeloproliferative disorders, AML, myelodysplasia (hematologic neoplasms) Severe thermal injury Trauma surgery Pregnancy
Motility/ chemotaxis defects	Chédiak-Higashi syndrome Complement disorders Leukocyte adhesion deficiency Neutrophil actin deficiency Other actin and microtubular defects Specific granule deficiency Hyperimmunoglobulinemia E syndrome with associated chemotactic defects of neutrophils and monocytes Storage disease (eg, Gaucher's)	Autoimmune disorders (collagen vascular disorders) Diabetes Renal failure Numerous medications interfere with neutrophil migration (eg, colchicine, numerous anti-inflammatory agents) Chronic infections (including HIV-1) Malnutrition Hematologic neoplasms Thermal injury Bone marrow transplant Paroxysmal nocturnal hemoglobinuria Graft-versus-host disease Recombinant interleukin-2 therapy
Phagocytic/ killing defects	Chronic granulomatous disease (several types) Complement disorders Myeloperoxidase deficiency Specific granule deficiency Immunodeficiency disorders with decreased immunoglobulins Thalassemia major	Autoimmune disorders (collagen vascular disorders) Thermal injury Hematologic neoplasms Diabetes Trauma/surgery After bone marrow transplant Graft-versus-host disease Malnutrition Chronic infections (including HIV-1) Sickle cell anemia

Abbreviation: AML = acute myelogenous leukemia.
*Many acquired disorders/conditions are associated with multiple types of neutrophil function defects as determined by in vitro studies; clinical significance variable.

severe gastrointestinal disease is seen less frequently. Patients with chronic granulomatous disease demonstrate multiple types of defects related to the generation of NADPH oxidase that result in a failure to undergo oxidative reactions (respiratory burst). Consequently, ingested organisms are not killed.

Two types of leukocyte adhesion deficiency (LAD types 1 and 2) have been described. These rare genetic disorders of neutrophil adhesion/chemotaxis are characterized by severe, recurrent bacterial infections. In LAD type 1 the adhesion molecule CD11/CD18 is defective, whereas defects in selectin-dependent leukocyte rolling adherence characterize the more uncommon LAD type 2. Multiple mutations have been identified in the gene encoding the β2 subunit of CD18, which is a component of three major adhesion molecules (integrins). Reduced expression of these three integrins in patients with LAD type 1 results in two key functional defects: (1) neutrophils fail to adhere to and migrate through the endothelium and (2) neutrophils cannot bind CD3bi opsonized microorganisms.

In general, acquired neutrophil function disorders are much less severe than constitutional defects. Either in patients with a wide variety of diseases/conditions or in patients receiving numerous types of therapeutic agents, neutrophils may demonstrate many functional aberrations by in vitro techniques when compared with control neutrophils obtained from normal volunteers (**Table 21-1**). Whether these in vitro aberrations represent true functional defects or a physiologic response to the underlying disorder is unknown, especially in patients with nonneoplastic conditions. In contrast, in patients with hematologic neoplasms such as acute myelogenous leukemia (AML) or myelodysplasia (MDS), neutrophil function abnormalities are a reflection of a defective myeloid clone and are linked to increased susceptibility to bacterial infections. However, in both AML and MDS, the concurrent decrease in absolute neutrophil count is a key factor in the increased risk of bacterial infections. Neutrophil function defects also are readily identifiable in patients with chronic myeloproliferative disorders, especially chronic myelogenous leukemia, although generally these defects are not clinically significant.

In the nonneoplastic acquired disorders/conditions/drug treatments listed in **Table 21-1**, the significance of the detection of in vitro neutrophil defects is less clear-cut. Although some patients, such as those with either chronic renal failure or poorly controlled diabetes mellitus, are clearly at increased risk for bacterial infections, the cause of this increased susceptibility is complex, involving many environmental factors that interfere with neutrophil function. The significance of drug-mediated neutrophil function defects is similarly unclear, because drug interference with neutrophil function has typically been documented using in vitro techniques with very high drug concentrations. Consequently, these neutrophil function defects may not be clinically relevant, except in patients receiving exceptionally high doses of the specific medication.

Finally, there are physiologic age variations in neutrophil function. Neonates, especially those born prematurely, frequently demonstrate impaired functional activities of neutrophils and monocytes, including defects in bone marrow release, cellular activation, and chemotaxis. This, in part, explains the increased susceptibility of newborns to serious bacterial infections. Likewise, elderly patients may develop aberrations in neutrophil adhesion, resulting in mild functional impairment.

21.2 Clinical Findings

Most constitutional neutrophil function defects are manifested in infancy or early childhood, whereas acquired defects are substantially more prevalent in adults. The clinical findings vary, depending on the severity of the defect. However, patients with profound neutrophil function defects characteristically present with severe recurrent bacterial and (less often) fungal infections that involve skin, oral cavity, sinuses and lung, lymph nodes, and gastrointestinal tract. Progressive organ damage can result from these recurrent infections. Recurrent pneumonias may lead to bronchiectasis, and recurrent infections along the gastrointestinal tract may cause fistulas and abscesses.

In patients with either adhesion or motility defects, inadequate numbers of neutrophils reach infection sites. The lack of pus is a unique feature in such patients, and there may be few localizing clinical signs and symptoms of infection.

21.3 Diagnostic Approach

Although a neutrophil function defect should be considered in children and adults with severe recurrent bacterial and fungal infections, in actual practice most patients with recurrent infections do not exhibit a demonstrable neutrophil function defect. However, in the subgroup of patients with a likely defect, the approach should include both the distinction between a constitutional and acquired defect and an attempt to categorize the nature of the abnormality. In general, the evaluation of these patients should comprise the following elements:

1. A complete blood count with differential.
2. A quantitative and morphologic evaluation of neutrophils and other lineages.
3. A detailed history regarding the frequency, severity, sites, and types of recurrent infections; age of onset; and family history.
4. A physical examination to assess for scars, abscesses, and pulmonary infiltrates; a careful evaluation of skin, oral cavity, respiratory tract, and anal region.
5. An evaluation for other features of constitutional neutrophil function defects, such as oculocutaneous albinism in Chédiak-Higashi syndrome.
6. An evaluation for evidence of underlying disorders and drug treatments linked to acquired neutrophil function defects in adults.
7. An assessment of immune status, complement component levels, immunoglobulin levels, and CH_{50}.
8. Testing for HIV-1 in appropriate situations.

A variety of specialized tests of neutrophil function also should be considered; because these tests are ordered infrequently in clinical practice, most are performed only in specialized referral laboratories. The appropriateness and sequence of specialized neutrophil function testing should be determined on an individual basis. These specialized tests include

1. Nitroblue tetrazolium test (indirect measurement of respiratory burst activity).
2. Myeloperoxidase stain of neutrophils.
3. Flow cytometric evaluation of neutrophil surface membrane for expression of CD11/CD18 (adhesion molecules) or CD15s (selectin ligand).
4. Assessment of neutrophil motility, chemotaxis, and adhesion properties.
5. Superoxidase generation (other tests of oxidation, including flow cytometric tests).

6. Electron microscopy to evaluate neutrophil granules, especially in patients with possible specific (secondary) granule deficiency.

21.4 Hematologic Findings

21.4.1 Blood Cell Measurements

Depending on both the nature of the neutrophil function defect and whether the patient is actively infected, the blood cell measurements are variable. Patients with ongoing infection often demonstrate an absolute neutrophilia with toxic changes. Extremely high elevations of the absolute neutrophil count are characteristic of constitutional leukocyte adhesion disorders, because of the inability of these cells to bind to endothelium and consequently migrate to tissues. In affected patients, the absolute neutrophil count may exceed $100 \times 10^3/mm^3$ ($100 \times 10^9/L$). In contrast, neutropenia is a frequent finding in Chédiak-Higashi syndrome secondary to ineffective granulopoiesis from intramedullary cell death. Patients with recurrent infections also may develop anemia of chronic disease.

21.4.2 Peripheral Blood Smear Morphology

Except for the massively enlarged granules that characterize Chédiak-Higashi syndrome, morphologic findings in patients with neutrophil function defects generally are not distinctive, although both bilobed nuclei with abnormal nuclear membranes and absent secondary granules have been noted in cases of neutrophil-specific granule deficiency (*see Image 22-1*). Other morphologic aberrations, such as Pelger-Huët and May-Hegglin anomalies, are described in Chapter 22.

21.4.3 Bone Marrow Examination

Granulocytic hyperplasia is an anticipated finding in patients with neutrophil function defects who suffer from recurrent infections. In addition, granulomas may be evident, especially in patients with recurrent fungal infections. Indications for bone marrow examination in patients with neutrophil function abnormalities include assessment for infection, unexplained blood cytopenia, and evaluation for possible secondary hemophagocytic syndrome or secondary lymphoproliferative disorder (notably in patients with Chédiak-Higashi syndrome).

Other Laboratory Tests

Test 21.1 Nitroblue Tetrazolium Dye Test

The nitroblue tetrazolium (NBT) test is used to indirectly detect the production of superoxide by neutrophils, such as during a respiratory burst.

Principle. NBT is a soluble yellow dye that is converted to an insoluble blue-black compound when neutrophils are capable of undergoing oxidative metabolism. This insoluble material precipitates within neutrophil cytoplasm and can be seen by light microscopy. Neutrophils that fail to reduce NBT lack this oxidative capability.

Specimen. Heparinized blood can be used for activated NBT tests.

Procedure. Stimulated neutrophils are incubated with NBT. The dye is reduced by oxidative enzymes within granules in neutrophils and monocytes. Following incubation, blood smears are prepared and stained with Wright's stain. A differential cell count is performed by separating neutrophils into those containing or lacking the blue-black precipitate. Appropriate controls are used.

Interpretation. Indirect evidence of production of superoxide is present when neutrophils contain the blue-black precipitate. Neutrophils that fail to reduce NBT are evident in chronic granulomatous disease, as well as in other neutrophil enzyme deficiency disorders, some complement deficiency conditions, and agammaglobulinemias. Abnormal test results also can be useful in identifying female carriers. Normal ranges should be determined within individual laboratories.

Notes and Precautions. The NBT test cannot be performed on ethylenediaminetetraacetic acid (EDTA)–anticoagulated specimens. Likewise, heparin forms complexes with NBT that are ingested by neutrophils, making heparin an undesirable anticoagulant for examining spontaneous NBT-reducing activity. However, the incubated NBT-reducing activity using stimulated neutrophils is not affected by heparin anticoagulation. Although the NBT test is still used frequently to assess superoxide production, it probably will be replaced eventually by flow cytometric methods that employ fluorescence detection methods to measure oxidant production.

Test 21.2 **Myeloperoxidase Stain**

Purpose. This cytochemical stain is used to evaluate the presence of myeloperoxidase within neutrophil granules.

Principle. The myeloperoxidase enzyme of granulocyte primary granules reduces substrate dyes in a colorimetric reaction, producing an insoluble compound that precipitates within the cytoplasm of neutrophils.

Specimen. Freshly prepared air-dried blood smears are used for this test.

Procedure. A colorless substrate (usually benzidine dihydrochloride) and hydrogen peroxide are layered on the peripheral blood smear. During the incubation, the myeloperoxidase present within neutrophil primary granules converts hydrogen peroxide into water and oxygen, which oxidizes the substrate and produces a blue-black precipitate. After counterstaining, cells are viewed under a light microscope, and the proportion of positive neutrophils is determined.

Interpretation. Normal neutrophils demonstrate strong positive granular reactivity throughout the cytoplasm. In patients with myeloperoxidase deficiency, no staining or weak staining may be identified; Sudan black B staining is typically negative in these patients.

Notes and Precautions. Optimal pH is essential for this enzymatic reaction. Myeloperoxidase is degraded by exposure to light, and the test should generally be performed within a few hours of obtaining the specimen.

21.5 Ancillary Tests

Many tests have been developed to assess different types of neutrophil function activities (see "Diagnostic Approach" above). The decision to perform these sophisticated tests should be determined on a case-by-case basis. Likewise, the sequence of testing strategies in patients with a presumed neutrophil function abnormality should be determined individually. Additional specialized tests of neutrophil function include

1. Adherence of neutrophils to nylon wool fiber or to plastic tissue culture plates.
2. Measurements of various granule constituents, such as lactoferrin, as well as degranulation.
3. Assessment of bacterial killing ability, in addition to respiratory burst.
4. Flow cytometric methods to assess neutrophil oxidant production.

21.6 Course and Treatment

In patients with severe neutrophil function defects (typically constitutional defects), significant morbidity and mortality is associated with recurrent bacterial or fungal infections; prompt antibiotic therapy for established or suspected infections is essential. In addition, antibiotic prophylaxis is commonly prescribed. Despite aggressive management, affected patients may develop severe organ failure, most commonly pulmonary failure, as a result of tissue destruction from repeated infections. Response to immune-modulating agents such as recombinant human interferon-γ has been achieved in patients with chronic granulomatous disease, presumably through stimulation of the macrophage oxidative pathway, although this mechanism was not documented in a recent clinical trial. Bone marrow transplantation has been attempted, with suboptimal results, in small numbers of patients with constitutional neutrophil function defects. Because the specific gene mutations in many of the constitutional disorders of granulocyte function are known, the potential for gene therapy to correct these genetic abnormalities is being actively investigated. Genetic tests also can be used for prenatal diagnosis using chorionic villus biopsy samples.

21.7 Acknowledgment

The author is grateful to Richard S. Larson, MD, for reviewing this chapter.

21.8 References

Azuma H, Oomi H, Sasaki K, et al. A new mutation in exon 12 of the gp91-phox gene leading to cytochrome b-positive X-linked chronic granulomatous disease. *Blood.* 1995;85:3274–3277.

Babior BM. NADPH oxidase: an update. *Blood.* 1999;93:1464–1476.

Bogomolski-Yahalom V, Matzner Y. Disorders of neutrophil function. *Blood Rev.* 1995;9:183–190.

Dinauer MC. The phagocyte system and disorders of granulopoiesis and granulocyte function. In: Nathan DG, Orkin SH, eds. *Nathan and Oski's Hematology of Infancy and Childhood, Vol 1.* 5th ed. Philadelphia, Pa: Saunders; 1998:889–967.

Fletcher J, Haynes AP, Crouch SM. Acquired abnormalities of polymorphonuclear neutrophil function. *Blood Rev.* 1990;4:103–110.

Gorlin JB. Identification of (CA/GT)n polymorphisms within the X-linked chronic granulomatous disease (X-CGD) gene: utility for prenatal diagnosis. *J Pediatr Hematol Oncol.* 1998;20:112–119.

Hampton MB, Kettle AJ, Winterbourn CC. Inside the neutrophil phagosome: oxidants, myeloperoxidase, and bacterial killing. *Blood.* 1998;92:3007–3017.

Larson RS. Immunodeficiency disorders. In: Collins RD, Swerdlow S, eds. *Pediatric Hematopathology.* New York, NY: Churchill-Livingstone; 1999.

Malech HL, Bauer TR Jr, Hickstein DD. Prospects for gene therapy of neutrophil defects. *Semin Hematol.* 1997;34:355–361.

Matzner Y. Acquired neutrophil dysfunction and diseases with an inflammatory component. *Semin Hematol.* 1997;34:291–302.

Pedersen TL, Yong K, Pedersen JO, et al. Impaired migration in vitro of neutrophils from patients with paroxysmal nocturnal haemoglobinuria. *Br J Haematol.* 1996;95:45–51.

Romano M, Dri P, Dadalt L, et al. Biochemical and molecular characterization of hereditary myeloperoxidase deficiency. *Blood.* 1997;90:4126–4134.

Roos D, de Boer M, Kuribayashi F, et al. Mutations in the X-linked and autosomal recessive forms of chronic granulomatous disease. *Blood.* 1996;87:1663–1681.

Wolach B, Sonnenschein D, Gavrieli R, et al. Neonatal neutrophil inflammatory responses: parallel studies of light scattering, cell polarization, chemotaxis, superoxide release, and bactericidal activity. *Am J Hematol.* 1998;58:8–15.

22 Granulocytic Disorders With Abnormal Morphology

Both hereditary and acquired disorders are associated with morphologic abnormalities of neutrophils. These abnormalities include both nuclear and cytoplasmic aberrations. Nuclear defects include hyposegmentation and hypersegmentation; cytoplasmic abnormalities include various types of inclusions, hypergranular cytoplasm, and hypogranular cytoplasm.

Although all hereditary disorders with abnormal neutrophils are rare, the more prevalent of these genetic disorders include Pelger-Huët anomaly, May-Hegglin anomaly, Chédiak-Higashi syndrome, and Alder-Reilly anomaly (**Table 22-1**). Pelger-Huët anomaly is characterized by either bilobed or nonsegmented neutrophil nuclei. The nuclear chromatin of these cells tends to be uniformly dense, their cytoplasm is unremarkable, and they demonstrate no significant functional abnormalities. The neutrophils in May-Hegglin anomaly contain large blue cytoplasmic inclusions that resemble Döhle bodies. Similar inclusions also are evident in other granulated cells. Additional hematologic abnormalities include thrombocytopenia, enlarged platelets, and variable neutropenia. Many of these patients are asymptomatic. In contrast, patients with Chédiak-Higashi syndrome suffer from recurrent severe pyogenic infections and often die in childhood. Chédiak-Higashi syndrome is characterized by giant cytoplasmic granules

Table 22-1 Hereditary Granulocytic Disorders of Abnormal Morphology

Disorder	Granulocyte Feature	Other Blood, Bone Marrow Abnormalities	Inheritance	Other Findings
Pelger-Huët anomaly	Bilobed or nonsegmented neutrophil nuclei; cytoplasm normal	No other lineage abnormalities No functional abnormalities	Autosomal dominant	No associated findings
May-Hegglin anomaly	Large blue cytoplasmic inclusions resembling giant Döhle bodies	Thrombocytopenia Enlarged platelets Variable neutropenia Inclusions also in eosinophils, basophils, and monocytes	Autosomal dominant	Many patients are asymptomatic
Chédiak-Higashi syndrome	Giant cytoplasmic granules	Neutropenia, thrombocytopenia All granulated cells and even lymphocytes/ natural killer cells affected Represent fused lysosomes Functional defects of neutrophils Some patients develop infection, usually Epstein-Barr virus–associated hemophagocytic syndrome (accelerated phase) or Epstein-Barr virus–induced lymphoproliferative disorders	Autosomal recessive	Partial oculocutaneous albinism Frequent pyogenic infections Both neutrophil function defects and immunodeficiency from decreased natural killer cell function Mild bleeding tendency Progressive peripheral neuropathy
Alder-Reilly anomaly	Intense azurophilic granulation of neutrophil cytoplasm	Eosinophils and basophils contain large basophilic granules Vacuolated/abnormally granulated lymphocytes in some sera	Autosomal recessive	Associated with several different types of genetic mucopolysaccharide disorders

Specific granule deficiency	Absence of secondary granules in cytoplasm imparts a pale appearance; nuclear hyposegmentation also present	Abnormal granules (subset) in platelets and eosinophils	Autosomal recessive	Recurrent infections
Myelokathexis	Shape abnormalities, pyknotic nuclei; hypersegmentation	Striking bone marrow abnormalities affecting all stages of granulopoiesis Neutropenia; intramedullary death of granulocytes Functional defects of neutrophils and monocytes	Not well characterized	Growth retardation Skeletal abnormalities
Hereditary hypersegmentation of neutrophils	Increased mean nuclear lobe index	No other abnormalities	Autosomal dominant	No associated findings
Hereditary giant neutrophils	Enlarged overall neutrophil size with hypersegmentation	Only a subset of neutrophils affected Other lineages unremarkable	Autosomal dominant	No associated findings

that are present within all granulated cells and even in natural killer cells/lymphocytes within the blood, bone marrow, and solid tissues. These giant granules represent fused lysosomes and are linked to many functional defects. Other abnormalities include neutropenia and thrombocytopenia, which are likely secondary to ineffective hematopoiesis. As a consequence of immunosuppression from decreased natural killer cell function, patients with Chédiak-Higashi syndrome may develop secondary viral infections (especially Epstein-Barr virus) that induce either florid hemophagocytic syndromes or lymphoproliferative disorders.

Intense azurophilic granulation of neutrophil cytoplasm characterizes the Alder-Reilly anomaly, which is associated with several types of genetic mucopolysaccharide disorders. Abnormalities of eosinophils, basophils, and lymphocytes also are evident in patients with these disorders.

Acquired morphologic neutrophilic abnormalities are substantially more common than their hereditary counterparts and are associated with both neoplastic and nonneoplastic hematologic disorders, as well as with other conditions (**Table 22-2**). Morphologic abnormalities of both neutrophil nuclei and cytoplasm are common in patients with hematologic neoplasms such as myelodysplasia, acute myeloid leukemias, and chronic myeloid leukemias, especially in transformation, reflecting the clonal nature of even mature blood elements in these neoplasms. For example, patients with these hematologic malignancies may demonstrate neutrophil pseudo–Pelger-Huët nuclei in conjunction with hypogranular cytoplasm. Less commonly, nuclear hypersegmentation may be evident in neutrophils from affected patients with clonal hematopoietic neoplasms. These morphologic aberrations are associated with functional defects.

Other causes of acquired neutrophil hypersegmentation include vitamin B_{12} or folate deficiency, occasional drug treatments, iron deficiency, and renal insufficiency (*see Table 22-2*). Acquired Pelger-Huët change also is associated with certain drug exposures, notably colchicine and sulfonamide therapy. This nuclear segmentation defect can be found in patients with mycoplasma infection, HIV-1 infection, and (rarely) in bone marrow transplant recipients. Several morphologic abnormalities of neutrophils, including pseudo–Pelger-Huët nuclear hyposegmentation, giant neutrophils, and neutrophils with Howell-Jolly–like cytoplasmic inclusions, have been described in patients with AIDS. Finally, intense cytoplasmic granulation is an acquired abnormality in

Table 22-2 Acquired Neutrophil Disorders With Abnormal Morphology

Morphologic Abnormality	Other Hematologic Findings	Comments/Causes
Pseudo–Pelger-Huët change	Dependent on underlying cause	Found in patients with hematologic neoplasms (myelodysplasia, AML, CML) Small neutrophils with pseudo–Pelger-Huët nuclei and vacuolated cytoplasm described in myelodysplasia and AML associated with del(17p) Result of drug exposure (colchicine, sulfonamides) Linked to mycoplasma and HIV-1 infections Rare finding after bone marrow transplantation
Hypersegmentation of neutrophils	Varies depending on cause Pancytopenia and macrocytosis in patients with folate or vitamin B_{12} deficiency Cytoplasmic hypogranulation and other lineage dyspoiesis common in myelodysplasia or myeloid leukemias	Vitamin B_{12} or folate deficiency Myelodysplasia, acute myeloid leukemia, other myeloid neoplasms Corticosteroid therapy and certain chemotherapeutic agents Also noted in patients with iron deficiency anemia or renal insufficiency
Hypogranular cytoplasm	Often found in association with nuclear segmentation abnormalities Dyspoiesis of other lineages common	Myelodysplasia Acute myeloid leukemias Chronic myeloid neoplasms, often in transformation
Intense cytoplasmic granulation	Marked neutrophilia with left shift	Pharmacologic doses of recombinant human CSF Neoplasms producing CSF
Giant neutrophils	Other hematologic abnormalities common in AIDS patients, especially cytopenias	Advanced HIV-1 infection Pharmacologic G-CSF therapy
Pseudo–Howell-Jolly bodies in neutrophils	Other blood abnormalities common in AIDS patients especially cytopenias	Seen occasionally in AIDS patients

Abbreviations: AML = acute myeloid leukemia; CML = chronic myelogenous leukemia; CSF = colony-stimulating factor.

patients receiving pharmacologic doses of recombinant human colony-stimulating factor.

22.1 Pathophysiology

The pathophysiology of hereditary granulocytic disorders is linked to the underlying genetic defect. The cause of acquired neutrophil abnormalities is not always clear-cut. In patients with vitamin B_{12} or folate deficiency, the basic defect is an inability to undergo cell division (see Chapter 5), whereas the various nuclear and cytoplasmic abnormalities identified in patients with hematologic neoplasms are the consequence of acquired clonal genetic defects. The cause of medication- or infection-associated morphologic abnormalities of neutrophils is generally unknown, but these changes should regress following successful treatment of the infection or cessation of the drug treatment.

22.2 Clinical Findings

Associated clinical findings in patients with hereditary neutrophil disorders are listed in **Table 22-1**. The clinical findings in patients with acquired neutrophil disorders are variable, linked to the specific underlying disorder. Patients with hematologic neoplasms often experience fatigue, malaise, and fever if secondary infection has occurred. Likewise, splenomegaly and hepatomegaly may be evident in some of these patients.

22.3 Diagnostic Approach

When a morphologic neutrophilic abnormality is encountered, it is essential to determine whether it is a hereditary or an acquired defect. The cause of acquired defects, either neoplastic or nonneoplastic, also must be determined. The integration of clinical findings, other hematologic parameters, the history, and the physical examination generally allow for these distinctions. The evaluation of a patient with neutrophil morphologic abnormalities generally includes the following steps:

1. A complete blood count (CBC) with differential.
2. A morphologic review of neutrophils and other lineages.
3. A family history and possible evaluation of other family members.
4. An evaluation for evidence of underlying infection.
5. An evaluation for evidence of bleeding.
6. An evaluation for evidence of a hematologic neoplasm.
7. An assessment for drug treatments and other conditions linked to specific morphologic abnormalities of neutrophils.
8. An evaluation for phenotypic abnormalities that occur in constitutional neutrophil disorders.
9. An evaluation for possible secondary lymphoproliferative disorders or infection-associated hemophagocytic syndrome in selected patients with genetic disorders, especially Chédiak-Higashi syndrome.

22.4 Hematologic Findings

22.4.1 Blood Cell Measurements

Several of the hereditary and acquired granulocytic disorders with abnormal morphology are associated with cytopenias, most notably neutropenia and/or thrombocytopenia. Anemia also may be evident in patients with recurrent chronic infections and in patients with underlying hematologic malignancies.

22.4.2 Peripheral Blood Smear Morphology

The various morphologic abnormalities of neutrophil nuclei and cytoplasm in patients with either hereditary or acquired granulocytic disorders are delineated in **Tables 22-1** and **22-2** (**Image 22-1**). In addition, enlarged platelets characterize May-Hegglin anomaly; cytoplasmic abnormalities of other granulated cells or lymphocytes/natural killer cells may be encountered in patients with May-Hegglin anomaly, Chédiak-Higashi syndrome, and

Alder-Reilly anomaly (*see Table 22-1*). In patients with acquired neutrophil abnormalities, other blood findings suggestive of myeloid neoplasms may be evident; multilineage abnormalities also are evident in megaloblastic anemia (**Image 22-2**).

22.4.3 Bone Marrow Examination

Bone marrow examination generally is not required in patients with hereditary granulocytic disorders, unless warranted for cultures, assessment for a secondary neoplasm, or a possible infection-associated hemophagocytic or lymphoproliferative disorder. In contrast, bone marrow examination may be necessary to determine whether an acquired neutrophil disorder is the consequence of a hematologic neoplasm.

22.5 Ancillary Tests

Various tests of neutrophil function may be warranted in selected patients with morphologic neutrophil abnormalities. In addition, assessment of vitamin B_{12} or folate levels is appropriate in selected patients demonstrating nuclear hypersegmentation. Cytogenetic studies are warranted for patients with likely hematologic neoplasms.

22.6 Course and Treatment

The clinical course is highly variable in patients with hereditary and acquired morphologic neutrophil disorders. For example, patients with Pelger-Huët anomaly, hereditary hypersegmentation of neutrophils, and hereditary giant neutrophils and most patients with May-Hegglin anomaly are asymptomatic. In contrast, those with Chédiak-Higashi syndrome experience severe recurrent infections, infection-associated hemophagocytic syndrome, and secondary neoplasms. Allogeneic bone marrow transplantation has been successful in some patients with this syndrome. Likewise, patients with hematologic neoplasms demonstrate a variable disease course, typically requiring aggressive multiagent chemotherapy or possible bone marrow transplantation (see Chapters 26, 27, and 32).

22.7 References

Bassan R, Viero P, Minetti B, et al. Myelokathexis: a rare form of chronic benign granulocytopenia. *Br J Haematol*. 1984;58:115–117.

Bogomolski-Yahalom V, Matzner Y. Disorders of neutrophil function. *Blood Rev*. 1995;9:183–190.

Brunning RD. Morphologic alterations in nucleated blood and marrow cells in genetic disorders. *Hum Pathol*. 1970;1:99–124.

Carmel R, Green R, Jacobsen DW, et al. Neutrophil nuclear segmentation in mild cobalamin deficiency: relation to metabolic tests of cobalamin status and observations on ethnic differences in neutrophil segmentation. *Am J Clin Pathol*. 1996;106:57–63.

Davey FR, Erber WN, Gatter KC, et al. Abnormal neutrophils in acute myeloid leukemia and myelodysplastic syndrome. *Hum Pathol*. 1988;19:454–459.

Dinauer MC. The phagocyte system and disorders of granulopoiesis and granulocyte function. In: Nathan DG, Orkin SH, eds. *Nathan and Oski's Hematology of Infancy and Childhood, Vol 1*. 5th ed. Philadelphia, Pa: Saunders; 1998:889–967.

d'Onofrio G, Mancini S, Tamburrini E, et al. Giant neutrophils with increased peroxidase activity: another evidence of dysgranulopoiesis in AIDS. *Am J Clin Pathol*. 1987;87:584–591.

Haddad E, Le Deist F, Blanche S, et al. Treatment of Chédiak-Higashi syndrome by allogenic bone marrow transplantation: report of 10 cases. *Blood*. 1995;85:3328–3333.

Lai J-L, Preudhomme C, Zandecki M, et al. Myelodysplastic syndromes and acute myeloid leukemia with 17p deletion: an entity characterized by specific dysgranulopoiesis and a high incidence of P53 mutations. *Leukemia*. 1995;9:370–381.

Malech HL, Nauseef WM. Primary inherited defects in neutrophil function: etiology and treatment. *Semin Hematol*. 1997;34:279–290.

Masat T, Feliu E, Tassies D, et al. Pseudo–Pelger-Huët anomaly after bone marrow transplantation. *Hematol Pathol*. 1991;5:89–91. Letter.

Slagel DD, Lager DJ, Dick FR. Howell-Jolly body–like inclusions in the neutrophils of patients with acquired immunodeficiency syndrome. *Am J Clin Pathol*. 1994;101:429–431.

Stockman JA III, Ezekowitz RAB. Hematologic manifestations of systemic diseases. In: Nathan DG, Orkin SH, eds. *Nathan and Oski's Hematology of Infancy and Childhood, Vol 2.* 5th ed. Philadelphia, Pa: Saunders; 1998:1841–1891.

van Hook L, Spivack C, Duncanson FP. Acquired Pelger-Huët anomaly associated with *Mycoplasma pneumoniae* pneumonia. *Am J Clin Pathol.* 1985;84:248–251.

Zittoun J, Zittoun R. Modern clinical testing strategies in cobalamin and folate deficiency. *Semin Hematol.* 1999;36:35–46.

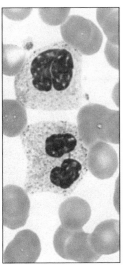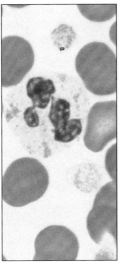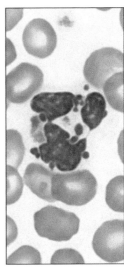

Image 22-1 Blood smears illustrating morphologic abnormalities in Pelger-Huët anomaly (left), May-Hegglin anomaly (center), and Chédiak-Higashi syndrome (right). (Right photo, courtesy of Dr P. Ward.) (Wright's)

Image 22-2 Composite of neutrophils in peripheral blood. Acquired nuclear hypersegmentation in a patient with alcohol-associated folate deficiency (left). An acquired mononuclear pseudo–Pelger-Huët anomaly in a hypogranular neutrophil from a patient with acute myelogenous leukemia (right). (Courtesy of Dr Lee Gates.) (Wright's)

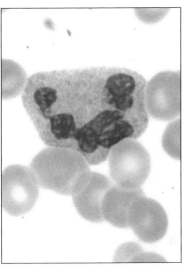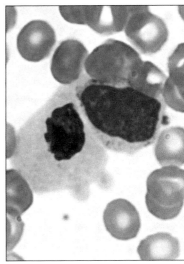

PART
IV

Reactive Disorders
of Lymphocytes

23 Infectious Mononucleosis and Other Reactive Disorders of Lymphocytes

The hallmark of reactive lymphocytosis is a transient increase in the number of lymphocytes in the blood. The lymphocytosis usually represents a specific response to an underlying disorder or condition (**Table 23-1**). The most common cause of a reactive lymphocytosis is infectious mononucleosis (IM) caused by Epstein-Barr virus (EBV). Infections with several other agents, primarily viruses, also can elicit a reactive lymphocytosis. In some of these disorders, such as cytomegalovirus (CMV) infection, the clinical and peripheral blood picture is similar to that of EBV-IM, and these disorders are referred to as "IM-like syndromes". Other less frequent causes of reactive lymphocytosis include viral hepatitis, childhood viral infections, and drug reactions. Some benign lymphocytoses are characterized by lymphocytes with nonreactive morphology; these disorders include whooping cough, infectious lymphocytosis, transient stress lymphocytosis, and persistent polyclonal B-cell lymphocytosis associated with cigarette smoking. This chapter focuses on IM but also addresses other causes of benign lymphocytosis.

23.1 Pathophysiology

IM is caused by an acute primary infection with EBV. The route of transmission of EBV seems to be intimate contact with saliva from

Table 23-1   Causes of Benign Lymphocytosis

Reactive morphology
    Infectious mononucleosis (EBV)
    Infectious mononucleosis–like syndromes
        Cytomegalovirus
        Toxoplasmosis
        Adenovirus
        Acute HIV infection
        Human herpesvirus-6
    Other viral infections
        Viral hepatitis
        Rubella
        Roseola
        Mumps
        Chickenpox
    Drug reactions
Nonreactive morphology
    Whooping cough
    Infectious lymphocytosis
    Transient stress lymphocytosis
    Persistent polyclonal B-cell lymphocytosis

Abbreviations: EBV = Epstein-Barr virus; HIV = human immunodeficiency virus.

a previously infected person. EBV infects B lymphocytes in the oropharynx, which then disseminate the virus throughout the reticuloendothelial system, provoking an intense immunologic response. The immune response is responsible for the immunopathology and the symptoms of EBV-IM. The majority of the reactive lymphocytes in the blood during the acute infection are T lymphocytes with cytotoxic-suppressor (CD8) phenotype. The cellular response is complex and is responsible for control of the acute infection. A humoral response also is elicited during acute IM and is characterized by non–EBV-specific responses, such as the production of heterophil antibody and EBV-specific antibodies, including those directed against viral capsid antigen (VCA), early antigen (EA), and Epstein-Barr nuclear antigen (EBNA). The humoral response seems to be important for preventing recurrent infections.

23.2 Clinical Findings

IM typically occurs in persons between the ages of 10 and 25 years. Characteristic symptoms include sore throat, fever, headache, malaise, nausea, and anorexia. Lymphadenopathy, usually cervical, is almost always present. More than 50% of patients have splenomegaly, and mild hepatitis may be present. Acute EBV infections are also common in early childhood but often are asymptomatic or characterized by clinical symptoms not recognized as IM. IM is rare in persons older than 40 years, since most patients are immune to the virus by that time. When it does occur, the presenting features may be atypical, including prolonged fever, often without pharyngitis and lymphadenopathy.

23.3 Approach to Diagnosis

In a patient suspected of having IM, the initial laboratory workup should include the following:

1. CBC count with leukocyte differential.
2. Morphologic examination of the peripheral blood smear.
3. Testing for IM heterophil antibody.

The appearance of increased numbers of reactive lymphocytes in the blood is one of the earliest laboratory signs of IM and is essential for the diagnosis. The diagnosis of IM is confirmed by detection of the heterophil antibody.

23.4 Hematologic Findings

23.4.1 Blood Cell Measurements
Hemoglobin and hematocrit measurements usually are normal in IM. Mild hemolysis occasionally is present in persons with IM, but clinically significant anemia is uncommon, occurring only in about 1% to 3% of patients. When anemia is present, it is usually an autoimmune hemolytic anemia caused by RBC autoantibodies. RBC autoantibodies with anti-i, anti-N, and anti-I specificities have

been described in IM. An absolute lymphocytosis greater than 4.0 $\times$ $10^3/mm^3$ (4.0 $\times$ $10^9/L$) usually is present. The total leukocyte count is increased and ranges from 10 to 30 $\times$ $10^3/mm^3$ (10.0-30.0 $\times$ $10^9/L$); counts exceeding this range are rare. The leukocytosis begins about 1 week after the onset of symptoms, peaks during the second or third week, and persists for 2 to 8 weeks. A mild to moderate neutropenia often is present and is most prominent during the third or fourth week of the illness. Rarely, agranulocytosis may complicate IM. Mild thrombocytopenia (100-150 $\times$ $10^3/mm^3$ [100-150 $\times$ $10^9/L$]) is present in about one third of patients with IM; severe thrombocytopenia is rare. The neutropenia and thrombocytopenia apparently are secondary to an immune mechanism.

23.4.2 Peripheral Blood Smear Morphologic Findings

The most striking morphologic finding in the peripheral blood smear from a patient with IM is the presence of an increased number of reactive lymphocytes. Reactive lymphocytes are benign activated cells with a characteristic morphologic appearance. Various terms are used to describe these cells, including "atypical", "variant", "transformed", and "Downey cells".

Reactive lymphocytes in the blood of patients with IM have a heterogeneous appearance. However, they usually are large with abundant cytoplasm. The most commonly encountered cells are large lymphocytes with abundant pale blue cytoplasm and coarse but dispersed chromatin. Nucleoli are absent or indistinct. Peripheral or radiating basophilia of the cytoplasm often is present, and scattered azurophilic granules may be noted (**Image 23-1**). Immunoblasts also are observed frequently in IM. They are typically seen early in the disease, but are few, usually comprising only 1% or 2% of the total lymphocyte population. Immunoblasts are medium to large lymphocytes with moderate amounts of basophilic cytoplasm, round to oval nuclei with a coarsely reticular chromatin pattern, and visible nucleoli (**Image 23-2**). In some cases, reactive lymphocytes are small with minimal basophilic cytoplasm, condensed chromatin, and indented or lobulated nuclei (**Image 23-3**). This type of cell is uncommon in IM but may be prominent in some patients, especially young children. Large granular lymphocytes also are increased frequently in IM and contribute to the morphologic heterogeneity of the lymphocytes in this disorder. In addition, circulating plasma cells often are present in small numbers in IM.

Table 23-2   Minimal Morphologic Criteria for Diagnosis of Infectious Mononucleosis

50% Mononuclear cells (lymphocytes and monocytes) in blood smear
At least 10 reactive lymphocytes per 100 leukocytes
Marked lymphocyte heterogeneity

The minimal morphologic criteria (**Table 23-2**) for the diagnosis of IM include the following: (1) at least 50% mononuclear cells in the blood smear, (2) at least 10 reactive lymphocytes per 100 leukocytes, and (3) marked lymphocyte heterogeneity.

The erythrocytes in blood smears from patients with IM usually are normochromic and normocytic, but spherocytes and increased polychromasia may be apparent if an autoimmune hemolytic anemia is present. The platelets have normal morphologic features, but the number may be slightly decreased.

23.4.3 Bone Marrow Examination

A bone marrow biopsy is not indicated to diagnose IM.

Other Laboratory Tests

Test 23.1 Tests for Detection of Heterophil Antibody

Purpose. Heterophil antibodies are produced in EBV-IM; they appear within the first 2 weeks of illness and usually are undetectable 3 to 6 months after the acute illness. The diagnosis of IM is confirmed by the detection of heterophil antibodies.

Principle. The IM heterophil antibody is of the IgM class and reacts with beef, sheep, and horse erythrocytes; it does not react with guinea pig kidney tissue. This characteristic separates the IM heterophil antibody from cross-reacting Forssman-type antibodies.

Specimen. Serum or plasma.

Procedure. Most clinical laboratories use one of the several commercially available rapid tests or "monospot tests" to detect heterophil antibodies.

Interpretation. The presence of heterophil antibodies in conjunction with the characteristic appearance of the peripheral blood smear is highly specific for the diagnosis of IM. When serial studies are done, heterophil antibody test results are positive in more than 96% of the teenagers and young adults with IM. False-positive results occur but are uncommon. Heterophil antibodies are not present in other conditions associated with a reactive lymphocytosis, such as the CMV mononucleosislike syndrome.

A small percentage of teenagers and young adults with EBV-IM do not produce heterophil antibodies. These cases represent heterophil-negative IM. The incidence of heterophil negativity is much higher in infants and young children. About 75% of children with IM from ages 2 to 4 years and fewer than 25% of children with IM younger than 2 years produce heterophil antibodies. When the heterophil antibody cannot be detected, EBV-specific serologic tests can be used to confirm the diagnosis of EBV-IM. These tests are based on the detection of antibodies produced against specific antigens encoded by the EBV, such as VCA, EA, and EBNA (see Test 23.2).

Test 23.2 **EBV-Specific Serologic Tests**

Purpose. EBV-specific serologic tests can be used to establish the diagnosis of EBV-IM. These tests are especially useful in patients with suspected heterophil-negative EBV-IM.

Principle. EBV-specific serologic tests are based on the detection of antibodies produced against specific antigens encoded by the virus. During the EBV infection, there is sequential appearance and disappearance of different antibodies (**Table 23-3**). Almost all patients develop antibodies of the IgG and IgM types to VCA early in the course of the disease. The IgM anti-VCA titers diminish rapidly during convalescence and usually are undetectable at 12 weeks, while the IgG anti-VCA titers persist for life. Antibody to EA (anti-EA) appears during the acute phase of the disease and then declines. Antibodies to EBNA do not appear until symptoms have resolved and then persist indefinitely.

Table 23-3 Serologic Profile in Infectious Mononucleosis (EBV)

Antibody	Acute (0-3 mo)	Recent (3-12 mo)	Past (>12 mo)
Heterophil	Pos*	Neg†	Neg
EBV-specific			
VCA-IgM	Pos	Neg	Neg
VCA-IgG	Pos	Pos	Pos
EA	Pos or neg	Pos or neg	Neg
EBNA	Neg	Pos	Pos

Abbreviations: EBV, Epstein-Barr virus; Pos, detectable antibody; Neg, no detectable antibody; VCA, viral capsid antigen; EA, early antigen; EBNA, Epstein-Barr nuclear antigen.
* Occasionally negative in teenagers and young adults; frequently negative in children younger than 4 years.
† Heterophil antibody may persist for about 3 to 12 months in some persons.

Procedure. Assays for EBV-specific antibodies are usually done with indirect immunofluorescence microscopy. Enzyme-linked immunosorbent assays, Western blot analysis, and other immunoassays are also available.

Interpretation. An acute primary infection is indicated by the following: (1) the presence of IgM anti-VCA, (2) high titers of IgG anti-VCA, (3) detection of anti-EA, and (4) the absence of anti-EBNA. The presence of IgG anti-VCA and anti-EBNA with absence of IgM anti-VCA indicates a remote infection.

23.5 Practical Approach to the Diagnosis of IM

A practical diagnostic approach for IM that is useful in most clinical settings is shown in **Table 23-4**. This approach uses the blood smear morphologic findings and a commercially available rapid test for heterophil antibody as the initial diagnostic workup in patients suspected of having EBV-IM. Four diagnostic possibilities exist:

1. If the peripheral blood smear does not exhibit the morphologic features of IM and the results of the rapid test are negative for heterophil antibody, the diagnosis of IM usually is excluded.

Table 23-4 Workup of Patients With Clinically Suspected Infectious Mononucleosis (IM)*

Reactive Lymphocytosis[†]	Rapid Test for Heterophil Antibody	Diagnosis of IM	Further Diagnostic Tests
Absent	Negative	Not confirmed	Not indicated
Present	Positive	Confirmed	Not indicated
Absent	Positive	Inconclusive	EBV serologic tests
Present	Negative	Suspicious for IM or IM-like illness	Repeat rapid heterophil test in 1-2 weeks; EBV serologic tests, tests for CMV, etc (see text)

Abbreviations: EBV = Epstein-Barr virus; CMV = cytomegalovirus.
*Modified from Horwitz CA. Practical approach to diagnosis of infectious mononucleosis. *Postgrad Med*. 1979;65:179–184.
†Blood smear meets minimal morphologic criteria for IM (see Table 23-2).

No further testing for IM is indicated. Other causes for the patient's symptoms should be considered.

2. If the morphologic features of IM are present in the blood smear and the results of the rapid test for heterophil antibody are positive, the diagnosis of IM is confirmed. No further testing is required. Determination of the heterophil titer is unnecessary since it does not correlate with clinical course.

3. When the results of the rapid test are positive for the heterophil antibody but the blood smear lacks the morphologic characteristics of IM, the diagnosis of IM is not confirmed. Another blood smear could be evaluated in a few days, because occasionally the appearance of reactive lymphocytes lags behind positive serologic findings. Since heterophil antibodies in some persons may persist for more than a year after acute IM, it also may be useful to ask the patient about past symptoms of IM. Another approach in this situation is to perform EBV-specific serologic tests to determine whether the rapid slide test result was a false-positive or whether there is additional evidence for IM.

4. If the blood smear meets the minimal morphologic criteria for IM and the results of the rapid test for heterophil antibody are

negative, the diagnosis of IM still should be suspected. The serologic findings frequently lag behind the appearance of reactive lymphocytes, and retesting may yield a positive result in 1 to 2 weeks. If a negative rapid test result persists, the patient may still have IM but may not produce the heterophil antibody. In this instance, EBV-specific serologic tests may be necessary to establish the diagnosis. Other disorders that may result in an IM-like syndrome unrelated to EBV, such as acute CMV infection, also should be considered (see "Infectious Mononucleosis–Like Syndromes").

23.6 Course and Treatment

IM is a self-limited disease. In patients with normal immunity, the syndrome resolves within days or weeks; persistence of symptoms beyond several months is unusual. Only symptomatic therapy is available. Steroid therapy is controversial but occasionally is used for the treatment of severe complications related to IM, including severe pharyngitis with obstructing tonsils, autoimmune hemolytic anemia, and other severe cytopenias. Rare complications include splenic rupture, neurologic complications, myocarditis, and pericarditis.

23.7 Other Causes of Reactive Lymphocytosis

Although IM is the most common cause of reactive lymphocytosis, other benign conditions also are associated with an increase in circulating lymphocytes. Selected tests that are useful in the diagnosis of several of these conditions are listed in **Table 23.5**.

23.7.1 Infectious Mononucleosis–Like Syndromes

Infections with several other agents, primarily viruses, also are associated with lymphocytosis (**Table 23-1**). In some of these disorders, the clinical and peripheral blood picture is similar to that of EBV-IM, and these disorders are referred to as "IM-like syndromes". The most common of these is caused by acute CMV infection. CMV-induced IM-like syndromes usually occur in adults

Table 23-5 Selected Tests in the Differential Diagnosis of Benign Lymphocytosis

Disease	Test	Interpretation
EBV-IM	Heterophil test (see Test 23.1)	Positive results in association with characteristic blood smear morphologic features indicate EBV-IM
	EBV-specific serologic tests (see Test 23.2)	IgM and IgG antibodies to viral capsid antigens indicate acute infection
Cytomegalovirus	pp65 Antigenemia assay	Positive results indicate acute infection
	Serologic test for antibody using EIA or other method	Change from negative to positive result or fourfold or greater rise in titer in paired serum samples indicates acute infection
Toxoplasmosis	Serologic tests by EIA for *Toxoplasma gondii*-specific antibodies	Elevated *Toxoplasma gondii*-specific IgM and IgG antibody indicates acute infection
Adenovirus	Culture	Positive results in acute infection
Acute HIV infection	Test for HIV–specific antibody by EIA with confirmation (eg, Western blot) of positive results	Positive results indicate infection with HIV
Human herpesvirus 6	Virus isolation by culture or detection of viral DNA	Detection of virus or DNA indicates acute infection
Hepatitis A, B, C	Serologic tests by EIA	Hepatitis A–specific IgM is positive in acute infection. Presence of hepatitis B surface antigen in absence of antibody indicates acute infection. Antibody to hepatitis C virus present in acute infection
Rubella	Serologic test for antibody using EIA or other method	Rise in antibody titers in paired serum samples or presence of rubella virus–specific IgM indicates acute infection
Bordetella pertussis	Culture of nasal swab; direct flourescent-antibody staining procedure for clinical specimens or cultures	Identification of bacteria indicates acute infection

Abbreviations: EBV = Epstein-Barr virus; IM = infectious mononucleosis; EIA = enzyme immunoassay.

between the ages of 20 and 30 years. The clinical syndrome may be indistinguishable from EBV-IM, but pharyngitis and lymphadenopathy typically are less severe than in EBV-IM. The peripheral blood morphologic features are indistinguishable from those of EBV-IM. The pathogenesis of CMV infection is less well understood than that of EBV-IM, but the peripheral lymphocytosis, like that of EBV-IM, is a T-cell response consisting primarily of T-cytotoxic-suppressor cells.

Patients undergoing seroconversion to HIV also occasionally have an IM-like syndrome. Predominant symptoms include fatigue, malaise, and fever. Generalized lymphadenopathy may occur near the end of the acute illness. The symptoms of the acute viral syndrome usually subside within a few weeks.

Other rare causes of an IM-like syndrome include infection with human herpesvirus 6 (also the causative agent of roseola), adenovirus, and *Toxoplasma gondii*, a nonviral agent.

23.7.2 Other Viral Infections

Occasionally, patients with viral hepatitis have a reactive lymphocytosis. Patients with rubella, roseola, mumps, and chickenpox also may have a reactive lymphocytosis. The morphologic features of the lymphocytes in these disorders are similar to those of IM, but the lymphocytosis often is less intense and not as long lasting. In addition, circulating plasma cells frequently are prominent.

23.7.3 Drug Reactions

Lymphocytosis also may be observed in patients with drug reactions, especially to phenytoin therapy. The leukocyte count is variable in these patients, and eosinophilia and neutrophilia may accompany the lymphocytosis. These patients also frequently exhibit circulating plasma cells.

23.7.4 Whooping Cough

Acute bacterial infections rarely cause lymphocytosis. An exception is whooping cough, in which a striking lymphocytosis may be seen. Whooping cough (pertussis) usually occurs in infants and young children who have not been immunized and is characterized clinically by severe paroxysmal coughing and prominent lymphocytosis. The causative organism, *Bordetella pertussis*, produces a soluble factor that seems to have a role in the accumulation of lymphocytes in the blood by preventing them from homing normally back to lymphoid tissue. In whooping cough, the peak lymphocyte counts average about $10.0 \times 10^3/mm^3$ ($10.0 \times 10^9/L$); counts higher than $30.0 \times 10^3/mm^3$ ($30.0 \times 10^9/L$) are not unusual. Neutrophilia also may be present. Unlike the previous disorders, the lymphocytes in whooping cough appear mature with condensed chromatin patterns and scant cytoplasm; they frequently exhibit cleaved or convoluted nuclei (**Image 23-4**). Surface marker studies show that these cells are predominantly of the T-helper (CD4+) phenotype. Adults with pertussis do not have peripheral lymphocytosis.

23.7.5 Infectious Lymphocytosis

Infectious lymphocytosis is a benign illness of young children that is presumably of viral origin. The patients often are asymptomatic, but fever, abdominal pain, or diarrhea may be present. Organomegaly does not occur. The symptoms resolve within a few days. Leukocyte counts in infectious lymphocytosis range from 35.0 to $100.0 \times 10^3/mm^3$ (35.0-$100.0 \times 10^9/L$). The predominant lymphocyte has been reported to be a T cell or natural killer cell, but increased numbers of B lymphocytes also have been observed. The lymphocytes appear morphologically mature, and eosinophilia may be present in the later stages of the disease. The lymphocytosis may persist for several weeks.

23.7.6 Transient Stress Lymphocytosis

Transient stress lymphocytosis occasionally is observed in patients with trauma, myocardial infarction, status epilepticus, and other acute medical conditions. In transient stress lymphocytosis, the lymphocytosis is mild to moderate, averaging about 6.0 to 8.0 $\times 10^3/mm^3$ (6.0-$8.0 \times 10^9/L$). The lymphocytes in transient stress lymphocytosis consist of mature or mildly reactive-appearing lymphocytes. Large granular lymphocytes occasionally are prominent in these patients. The lymphocytosis resolves quickly, often within a few hours, followed by a neutrophilia. The lymphocytosis in this situation represents an expansion of the normal lymphocyte population and is thought to be secondary to epinephrine release.

23.7.7 Persistent polyclonal B-cell Lymphocytosis

Persistent polyclonal B-cell lymphocytosis is a stable, presumably benign lymphocytosis diagnosed almost exclusively in women. The cause of the lymphocytosis is unknown, but there is a strong association with cigarette smoking. The patients usually are asymptomatic. The lymphocytosis has been documented over decades in some patients. The absolute lymphocyte counts in this disorder are typically mildly elevated but may exceed 10.0 × 10^3/mm^3 (10.0 × 10^9/L) with total leukocyte counts greater than 15.0 × 10^3/mm^3 (15.0 × 10^9/L). Flow cytometry shows a B-cell population (CD19+) with a normal κ/λ ratio. The hemoglobin level, platelet count, and neutrophil count are normal. A polyclonal increase in IgM often is present, and an association with HLA-DR7 has been reported. Morphologically, the lymphocytes appear mature; binucleate forms or bilobed nuclei are present in a variable proportion of the cells. Recently, a high frequency of isochromosome (3q+) has been reported in the nonbinucleate cells. In addition, multiple bcl-2/Ig gene rearrangements have been identified in several of these patients.

23.8 Differential Diagnosis

The differential diagnosis of a patient with a benign lymphocytosis occasionally includes a malignant lymphoproliferative disorder, most notably acute lymphoblastic leukemia (ALL) and chronic lymphocytic leukemia (CLL). Confusion of a reactive lymphocytosis with ALL is most likely to occur when the leukocyte count is unusually high (ie, >30 × 10^3/mm^3 [>30 × 10^9/L]). This problem is compounded when the serologic test results are negative. Familiarity with the morphologic appearance of reactive lymphocytes, however, will aid in this differential diagnostic dilemma. In addition, anemia and thrombocytopenia are almost always present in acute leukemia but usually absent or mild in benign reactive conditions such as IM. Moreover, the diagnosis of ALL should not be confirmed without a bone marrow aspirate and biopsy and other ancillary studies, including immunophenotypic analysis (see Chapter 28).

Benign reactive lymphocytosis occasionally can be difficult to distinguish from chronic lymphoproliferative disorders such as CLL. This is more of a problem in patients older than 40 years because of the relative frequency of CLL in comparison with reactive disorders such as IM in this age group. In addition, when IM occurs in an older patient, the clinical findings may be atypical for IM. The morphologic characteristics of the lymphocytes in CLL (*see Image 33-1*) may be helpful in this differential diagnosis since, in general, they appear mature and more monotonous than the lymphocytes in a reactive process. However, immunophenotypic studies and a bone marrow biopsy are required to confirm a diagnosis of CLL or other chronic lymphoproliferative disorder (see Chapter 33).

23.9 **References**

Cohen JI, Corey RC. Cytomegalovirus infection in the normal host. *Medicine.* 1985;64:100–114.

Foucar KM. Reactive lymphoid proliferations in blood and bone marrow. In Foucar K. *Bone Marrow Pathology.* 2nd ed. Chicago, Ill: ASCP Press. In press.

Groom DA, Kunkel LA, Brynes RK, et al. Transient stress lymphocytosis during crisis of sickle cell anemia and emergency trauma and medical conditions. *Arch Pathol Lab Med.* 1990;114:570–576.

Hickey SM, Strasburger VC. What every pediatrician should know about infectious mononucleosis in adolescents. *Pediatr Clin North Am.* 1997;44:1541–1556.

Horwitz CA. Practical approach to diagnosis of infectious mononucleosis. *Postgrad Med.* 1979;65:179–184.

Horwitz CA, Henle W, Henle G, et al. Clinical and laboratory evaluation of infants and children with Epstein-Barr virus–induced infectious mononucleosis: report of 32 patients (aged 10–48 months). *Blood.* 1981;57:933–938.

Horwitz CA, Henle W, Henle G, et al. Heterophil-negative infectious mononucleosis and mononucleosis-like illnesses: laboratory confirmation of 43 cases. *Am J Med.* 1977;63:947–957.

Horwitz CA, Henle W, Henle G, et al. Infectious mononucleosis in patients aged 40 to 72 years: report of 27 cases, including 3 without heterophil-antibody responses. *Medicine.* 1983;62:256–262.

Kubic VL, Kubic PT, Brunning RD. The morphologic and immunophenotypic assessment of the lymphocytosis accompanying *Bordetella pertussis* infection. *Am J Clin Pathol.* 1990;95:809–815.

Mazzulli T, Drew LW, Yen-Lieberman B, et al. Multicenter comparison of the digene hybrid capture CMV DNA assay (version 2.0), the pp65 antigenemia assay, and cell culture for detection of cytomegalovirus viremia. *J Clin Microbiol.* 1999;37;958–963.

Mossafa H, Malaure M, Maynadie M, et al. Persistent polyclonal lymphocytosis with binucleated lymphocytes: a study of 25 cases. *Br J Haematol.* 1999;104:486–493.

Peterson L, Hrisinko MA. Benign lymphocytosis and reactive neutrophilia: laboratory features provide diagnostic clues. *Clin Lab Med.* 1993;13:863–877.

Steeper TA, Horwitz CA, Ablashi DV. The spectrum of clinical and laboratory findings resulting from human herpesvirus-6 (HHV-6) in patients with mononucleosis-like illnesses not resulting from Epstein-Barr virus or cytomegalovirus. *Am J Clin Pathol.* 1990;93:776–783.

Steeper TA, Horwitz CA, Hanson M, et al. Heterophil-negative mononucleosis-like illnesses with atypical lymphocytosis in patients undergoing seroconversions to the human immunodeficiency virus. *Am J Clin Pathol.* 1988;89:169–174.

Teggatz JR, Parkin J, Peterson L. Transient atypical lymphocytosis in patients with emergency medical conditions. *Arch Pathol Lab Med.* 1987;111:712–714.

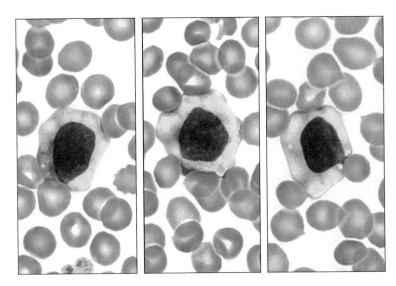

Image 23-1 Reactive lymphocytes from a patient with infectious mononucleosis. These cells exhibit abundant cytoplasm with radiating basophilia and correspond to Downey type II lymphocytes.

Image 23-2 Reactive lymphocytes from a patient with infectious mononucleosis. The cell on the right has an increased amount of pale blue cytoplasm, a common change in reactive lymphocytes. The cell on the left is large with a moderate amount of basophilic cytoplasm, coarse reticular chromatin, and a visible nucleolus. These are morphologic features of an immunoblast or a Downey type III lymphocyte.

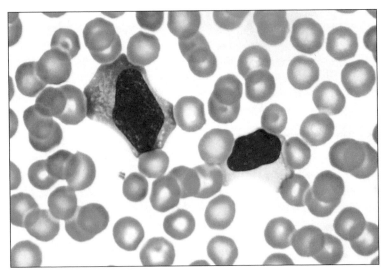

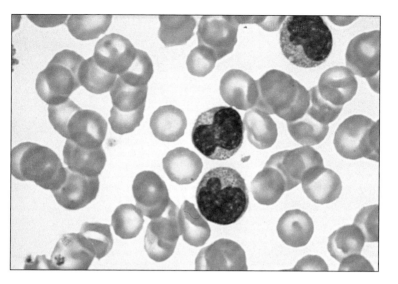

Image 23-3 Reactive lymphocytes from a patient with infectious mononucleosis. This morphologic type of reactive lymphocyte, referred to as a "Downey type I lymphocyte", is rare in infectious mononucleosis but may be prominent in young children. These cells are small with minimal cytoplasm, indented nuclei, and condensed chromatin.

Image 23-4 Blood smear from a child with whooping cough shows lymphocytes with scant cytoplasm, condensed chromatin, and cleaved nuclei.

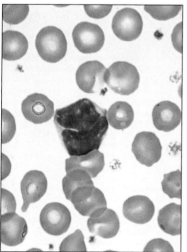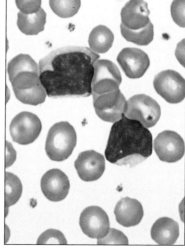

24 Lymphocytopenia

Lymphocytopenia in adults usually is defined as a total lymphocyte count in the blood of less than $1.0 \times 10^3/mm^3$ ($1.0 \times 10^9/L$). In children younger than 16 years, absolute lymphocyte counts are higher; the lower reference value is about $2.0 \times 10^3/mm^3$ ($2.0 \times 10^9/L$). Since approximately 80% of circulating lymphocytes in the blood are CD3+ T lymphocytes and about two thirds of the T lymphocytes are CD4+ (helper) T lymphocytes, most patients with lymphocytopenia have a decrease in the absolute number of T lymphocytes and CD4+ T lymphocytes in particular.

24.1 Pathophysiology

Table 24-1 lists the major conditions associated with lymphocytopenia. The pathogenesis of the lymphocytopenia in many of these disorders has not been established. However, the mechanisms that are known or postulated are discussed within each major diagnostic category.

Table 24-1 Major Conditions Associated With Lymphocytopenia*

Congenital immunodeficiency disorders
  Severe combined immunodeficiency disease
  Congenital thymic aplasia (DiGeorge syndrome)
  Wiskott-Aldrich syndrome
Nutritional deficiencies
  Protein-calorie malnutrition
  Zinc deficiency
Infectious diseases
  Viral infections (eg, HIV-1, influenza, hepatitis)
  Tuberculosis
  Typhoid fever
  Pneumonia
  Sepsis
  Other
Autoimmune disorders
  Rheumatoid arthritis
  Systemic lupus erythematosus
  Myasthenia gravis
Systemic diseases
  Burns
  Protein-losing enteropathy
  Sarcoidosis
  Renal insufficiency
  Hodgkin disease
Iatrogenic
  Radiation therapy
  Neoplastic chemotherapy
  Antilymphocyte globulin
  Glucocorticoid therapy
  Anesthesia and surgery
  Thoracic duct drainage or rupture
Idiopathic
  Idiopathic CD4+ T-lymphocytopenia

* Modified from Kipps TJ. Lymphocytosis and lymphocytopenia. In: Beutler E, Lichtman MA, Coller BS, et al, eds. *Williams Hematology*. 5th ed. New York, NY: McGraw-Hill; 1995:963–968.

24.1.1 Congenital Immunodeficiency Disorders

Patients with congenital immunodeficiency disorders may exhibit an associated lymphocytopenia. In many of these disorders, the lymphocytopenia is secondary to decreased lymphocyte production. For example, severe combined immunodeficiency disease (SCID), a syndrome characterized by profound defects in cellular and humoral immunity, almost always is associated with prominent lymphocytopenia. SCID is caused by a heterogeneous group of genetic abnormalities. The most common form is X-linked. The genetic defect in X-linked SCID has been identified as a mutation of the gamma chain of the interleukin-2 receptor. The early lymphoid progenitor cells lack intact interleukin receptors and fail to be stimulated by the growth factors essential to the normal development and differentiation of T cells and the late phase of B-cell development. The remainder of the cases of SCID result from autosomal recessive inheritance. The most common causes of the autosomal recessive cases are inherited deficiencies of the purine-degradation enzymes adenine deaminase and nucleoside phosphorylase.

Infants with congenital thymic aplasia (DiGeorge syndrome) usually exhibit profound lymphocytopenia. Aplasia of the thymus and the parathyroid gland probably results from a defect in embryogenesis of the third and fourth pharyngeal pouches. The T-cell areas of all tissues, including lymph nodes and spleen, are depleted.

Wiskott-Aldrich syndrome, an X-linked recessive disease characterized by eczematoid dermatitis, thrombocytopenia, and recurrent opportunistic infections, also is associated with lymphocytopenia. The lymphocytopenia in this disorder is caused by premature destruction of the lymphocytes secondary to a cytoskeletal membrane defect.

24.1.2 Nutritional Deficiencies

Nutritional deficiencies are associated with lymphocytopenia. Protein-calorie malnutrition is a common cause of lymphocytopenia worldwide and probably is due to decreased production of lymphocytes. Deficiency of zinc, an element required in protein synthesis, is also associated with lymphocytopenia and is characterized by decreased numbers of circulating CD4+ T cells and increased CD8+ T cells.

24.1.3 Infectious Diseases

Lymphocytopenia is prominent in AIDS and is due to selective loss of the CD4+ T lymphocytes. The lymphocytopenia in AIDS is, in part, secondary to a direct cytopathic effect of the HIV. It also could reflect impaired lymphocyte production due to defective expression of immunostimulatory cytokines or to increased expression of inhibitors of T-lymphocyte production. The host immune response also may contribute to the progressive loss of T lymphocytes in HIV-positive patients.

Some patients with other viral or bacterial infections also exhibit lymphocytopenia (*see Table 24-1*). The pathogenesis of the decrease in circulating lymphocytes for most infectious diseases is unclear. In viral infections, the lymphocytes may be destroyed by the virus, travel to the respiratory tract, or be trapped in spleen and lymph nodes.

24.1.4 **Autoimmune Disorders**

The lymphocytopenia seen in autoimmune disorders such as systemic lupus erythematosus is likely mediated by autoantibodies.

24.1.5 **Systemic Diseases**

Lymphocytopenia is associated with severe burns and is possibly related to redistribution of the T lymphocytes to the tissues. Lymphocytes are lost through the intestinal lymphatics in association with protein-losing enteropathies, severe congestive heart failure, or other primary diseases of the gut or intestinal lymphatics. The lymphocytopenia of renal insufficiency and sarcoidosis may be secondary to defective T-lymphocyte proliferative responses.

24.1.6 **Iatrogenic**

Radiotherapy induces lymphocytopenia through death of lymphocytes by direct exposure. T-helper lymphocytes are more sensitive than are T-suppressor cells; the helper/suppressor ratio can be decreased for months after exposure to radiation. Chemotherapeutic agents, such as alkylating agents, can cause profound lymphocytopenia that may persist for years. The administration of anti-lymphocyte globulin leads to lymphocytopenia by destruction of lymphocytes. The mechanism by which glucocorticoids cause lymphocytopenia is not completely clear but may be due to redistribution of lymphocytes away from the peripheral blood component and to cell destruction. Lymphocytopenia often is associated with anesthesia and surgical stress and is secondary to redistribution, perhaps related to endogenous steroid release. In thoracic duct drainage, lymphocytes are lost from the body.

A syndrome of isolated CD4+ T-cell depletion in the absence of evidence for a retroviral infection has been identified. The cause of this condition is unknown.

24.2 Clinical Findings

The signs and symptoms of patients with lymphocytopenia are those characteristic of the underlying disease process associated with the lymphocytopenia. Whether the patient exhibits clinical signs of immunodeficiency depends on the pathophysiology of the disease, the duration of the disorder, the lymphocyte subsets affected, and the degree of functional disturbance of cellular or humoral immunity. In general, patients with cellular immunodeficiency disorders have recurrent infections with low-grade or opportunistic infectious agents. In congenital disorders, growth retardation, wasting, and a short life span often are observed. A high incidence of malignant neoplasms, especially lymphomas, also is observed in some patient groups.

SCID is the most severe congenital immune deficiency state involving both cellular and humoral immunity. Affected patients suffer from recurrent bacterial, fungal, viral, or protozoan infections starting as early as 3 months of age. Transfusion with nonirradiated blood products may lead to severe graft-vs-host reactions. Persistent pulmonary infection, diarrhea, and wasting dominate the clinical picture. Infants with congenital thymic aplasia have severely impaired cellular immunity. They also have hypocalcemia and other congenital anomalies, including cardiac defects. Those who survive the neonatal period are susceptible to overwhelming viral, fungal, and bacterial infections. Wiskott-Aldrich syndrome also appears in early childhood with a triad of eczematoid dermatitis, thrombocytopenia with bleeding, and recurrent opportunistic infections. Patients are at high risk for developing malignant neoplasms, most commonly lymphomas and leukemias.

Patients with AIDS have repeated life-threatening infections. Opportunistic infections are prominent and include *Pneumocystis carinii* pneumonia, *Mycobacterium avium-intracellulare* complex pneumonia or disseminated disease, cryptosporidiosis diarrhea, oral candidiasis, hepatitis B, and cytomegalovirus and herpesvirus infections. Malignant neoplasms (Kaposi sarcoma, lymphoma), autoimmune diseases (thrombocytopenia), and neurologic disorders also occur in patients with AIDS.

24.3 Approach to Diagnosis

A clinical history—including the age and sex of the patient, family history, history of medication use, social and medical history, and physical examination—is needed to determine the subsequent workup. Unless the cause of the lymphocytopenia is clinically apparent or the lymphocytopenia is transient, the approach to the diagnosis should involve a comprehensive assessment of the integrity of the immune system. A thorough workup of patients with immunodeficiency diseases such as the congenital disorders can be complex and should be performed at referral medical centers that have expertise and experience in the diagnosis and treatment of these disorders.

In many cases, the workup of patients with lymphocytopenia includes the following:

1. CBC count with differential and platelet count. A bone marrow aspirate and biopsy may be indicated if the reason for the lymphocytopenia is unclear or to confirm a suspected diagnosis.
2. Quantitative immunoglobulin determination.
3. Immunophenotypic analysis of peripheral blood lymphocytes by flow cytometry.
4. Ancillary tests such as skin tests to evaluate cellular immunity.
5. Other tests dependent on the clinical setting to determine the underlying cause. These include tests for HIV, antinuclear antibodies (systemic lupus erythematosus), and lymph node biopsy (sarcoidosis).
6. Cultures for patients suspected of having infection.

24.4 Hematologic Findings

24.4.1 Blood Cell Measurements

In adults, the lymphocyte count is less than $1.0 \times 10^3/\text{mm}^3$ ($1.0 \times 10^9/\text{L}$) in lymphocytopenia. In children, it is less than $2.0 \times$

$10^3/mm^3$ (2.0×10^9/L). Granulocytopenia also may be present. The presence or absence of thrombocytopenia depends on the underlying condition. Thrombocytopenia with small platelets is characteristic of the Wiskott-Aldrich syndrome. Normochromic normocytic anemia is present in many of the diseases associated with lymphocytopenia.

24.4.2 Bone Marrow Examination

Findings depend on the underlying disorder and recent therapeutic approaches. In some congenital immunodeficiency states, lymphocytes are decreased.

The bone marrow in patients with HIV is usually hypercellular, even in the setting of peripheral cytopenias. Dysplasia may be present in all cell lines. Plasma cells frequently are increased, especially late in the course of the diseases. Lymphohistiocytic aggregates are frequent in bone marrow core biopsy specimens and may be large and atypical. These must be distinguished from lymphomas, since the occurrence of lymphomas is increased in AIDS and may involve the bone marrow. Disseminated infections, especially *M avium-intracellulare* complex and histoplasmosis, often involve the bone marrow. The marrow granulomas in association with these agents may be loosely formed or absent.

Other Laboratory Tests

Test 24.1 Quantitation of Immunoglobulins

Purpose. Immunodeficiency states associated with lymphocytopenia often are combined with deficient production of immunoglobulins. Quantitation of serum immunoglobulins aids in evaluating the presence and severity of any immunoglobulin abnormality.

Immunoglobulin production is altered when there is a defect in the B-cell population alone or when a combined defect involving B and T lymphocytes exists. Defects in antibody production also can result from severe defects in T-lymphocyte function, since in humans, all antigens seem to be T-lympho-cyte dependent.

Principle, Specimen, Procedure. See Test 37.4.

Interpretation. The level of serum immunoglobulins depends on the cause of the lymphocytopenia. In SCID and congenital thymic aplasia, serum immunoglobulin concentrations are normal. In Wiskott-Aldrich syndrome, serum IgG concentrations are low, but the concentrations of IgA and IgE are elevated. In AIDS, polyclonal hypergammaglobulinemia is often present.

Test 24.2 Immunophenotypic Analysis of Peripheral Blood Lymphocytes

Purpose. Lymphocyte markers are used to identify and enumerate lymphocyte subsets, which aids in diagnosing and classifying disorders associated with lymphocytopenia.

Principle. Labeled monoclonal antibodies bind to determinants on T cells, B cells, their subsets, and other hematopoietic cells. Labeled cells can then be enumerated with flow cytometry (see Chapter 48).

Specimen. Fresh peripheral blood sample anticoagulated with heparin.

Procedure. Flow cytometry involves a fluid system that delivers the cell sample past an excitation light beam in a single-file stream. The scattered light and any fluorescence emitted from this interaction (from dyes used to stain specific cell mole-cules) are collected and converted to electrical signals. They then can be analyzed to give quantitative information about specific cell characteristics (see Chapter 48).

Interpretation. About 60% to 80% of circulating lymphocytes are T cells, 10% to 20% B cells, and 5% to 10% natural killer cells. The T-cell population consists of T-helper (CD4+) and T-suppressor (CD8+) cells; the T-helper cells outnumber the T-suppressor cells 2 to 1.

In X-linked SCID, T lymphocytes are absent. The number of B lymphocytes is normal or elevated, but they fail to mature and function normally. Natural killer cell levels are normal or high. In autosomal recessive SCID, the number of T and B lymphocytes is markedly decreased. Congenital thymic aplasia is associated with a markedly decreased number of T lympho-cytes. In Wiskott-Aldrich syndrome, the number of T cells may be normal at first but decrease progressively, whereas the number of B cells expands progressively.

In AIDS, CD4+ cells are depleted and an inverted CD4/CD8 ratio is found. In patients with HIV, there is a strong association between CD4+ lymphocyte levels and development of opportunistic infections, progression to AIDS, and eventual death. Measurement of the CD4 subset is useful not only for assessing prognosis but also for making management decisions and for evaluating response to therapy.

24.5 Course and Treatment

The clinical course and treatment of lymphocytopenia depends on the underlying cause. The prognosis for patients with SCID is dismal without therapy. This disorder can be rapidly fatal if affected infants are not rendered immunocompetent by bone marrow transplantation. Transplants of fetal thymic tissue reverse the T-cell defects in children with congenital thymic aplasia. In the past, patients with Wiskott-Aldrich syndrome usually died within the first year of life, but improved management with splenectomy, intravenous immune globulin therapy, and other measures, including bone marrow transplantation, has improved their life expectancy.

Patients with HIV are being treated with antiretroviral agents. Most patients with AIDS eventually die of infection and/or malignant neoplasms associated with AIDS, although survival continues to increase with advances in treatment.

24.6 References

Bagby GC. Leukopenia and leukocytosis. In: Goldman L, Bennett JC, eds. *Cecil Textbook of Medicine.* 21st ed. Philadelphia, Pa: W.B. Saunders; 2000:919–933.

Bonilla FA, Rosen FS, Geha RS. Primary immunodeficiency diseases. In: Nathan DG, Orkin SH, eds. *Nathan and Oski's Hematology of Infancy and Childhood.* Philadelphia, Pa: Saunders; 1998:1023–1050.

Castelino DJ, McNair P, Kay TWH. Lymphocytopenia in a hospital population–what does it signify? *Aust N Z J Med.* 1997;27:170–174.

Hoxie JA. Hematologic manifestations of HIV infection. In: Hoffman R, Benz, Jr EJ, Shattel SJ, et al, eds. *Hematology: Basic Principles and Practice. 3rd ed.* New York, NY: Churchill-Livingstone; 2000:2430–2457.

Kim N, Rosenbaum GS, Cunha BA. Relative bradycardia and lymphopenia in patients with babesiosis. *Clin Infect Dis.* 1998;26:1218–1219.

Kipps TJ. Lymphocytosis and lymphocytopenia. In: Beutler E, Lichtman MA, Coller BS, et al, eds: *Williams Hematology.* 5th ed. New York, NY: McGraw-Hill; 1995:963–968.

Laurence J. T-cell subsets in health, infectious disease, and idiopathic CD4+ T lymphocytopenia. *Ann Intern Med.* 1993;119:55–62.

Rosen FS, Cooper MD, Wedgwood RJP. The primary immunodeficiencies. *N Engl J Med.* 1995;333:431–440.

Schoentag RA, Cangiarella J. The nuances of lymphocytopenia. *Clin Lab Med.* 1993;13:923–936.

Toft P, Svendsen P, Tonnesen E, et al. Redistribution of lymphocytes after major surgical stress. *Acta Anaesthesiol Scand.* 1993;37:245–249.

PART
V

**Reactive Disorders
of Lymph Nodes**

25 Reactive Disorders of Lymph Nodes

The immediate and most important problem for the clinician or surgeon when a patient presents with lymphadenopathy is to determine whether the patient has (1) a benign, reactive hyperplasia caused by infectious or noninfectious agents or (2) a malignant disease. The term "lymphadenopathy" refers to an enlarged lymph node or group of nodes. It is a common physical finding that requires an explanation as to its cause. Lymphadenopathy is often a transient response to localized infection and, in infected patients, the pathologic condition should be sought in the area drained by the node. In other patients, the lymphadenopathy may be due to metastatic malignancy or the response to a systemic disease. Lymphadenopathies caused by a neoplastic proliferation of lymphoid cells are known as "malignant lymphomas" and are discussed in Chapters 34 and 35.

25.1 Pathophysiology

Enlargement of the lymph nodes is caused by a proliferation of lymphoid cells and the associated cells of the mononuclear phagocytic system. In addition, there is frequently a variable degree of vascular proliferation. The intensity and pattern of reaction depends on the nature and duration of the antigenic stimulus and on the age and immune status of the patient.

As noted in **Table 25-1**, a wide variety of disorders are associated with lymphadenopathy. These disorders may be divided into five categories: infections, autoimmune, iatrogenic, malignant, and others. In approximately 40% to 60% of patients who undergo lymph node biopsy, no specific diagnosis can be reached. Of the specific benign lymphadenopathies, the most common causes encountered are infectious mononucleosis, toxoplasmosis, tuberculosis, and HIV.

25.2 Clinical Findings

The cause of the lymphadenopathy frequently is not apparent from microscopic changes observed in a lymph node biopsy specimen alone. The patient's clinical history, physical examination, and the results of other tests are usually essential for an accurate diagnosis. Certain benign lymphadenopathies, such as Kikuchi-Fujimoto lymphadenitis, are much more common in women than in men (4:1), whereas malignant lymphadenopathies are more common in men. Infectious mononucleosis is rarely seen in patients older than 35 years. Sexual behavior, drugs, previous surgery/biopsy, vaccination, occupation, exposure to pets, and duration of lymphadenopathy are important aspects of the clinical history (**Table 25-2**).

Lymphadenopathy with a duration of several months and an increase in the size of the lymph node strongly suggests a malignant condition. Fever and weight loss are common symptoms in many benign and malignant lymphoproliferative disorders. A sore throat is frequently present in infectious mononucleosis. The presence of toothache, earache, or lesions in the region drained by the enlarged lymph nodes may explain the cause of lymphadenopathy in some patients.

Once a significant lymph node enlargement has been detected, a careful physical examination must be done to seek other sites of lymphadenopathy, and the presence or absence of splenomegaly should be noted. The location of the enlarged lymph node is important because certain lymph nodes are more frequently affected than others by certain disease processes (**Table 25-3**). In inflammatory disorders, the lymph nodes are frequently tender, whereas in malignant lymphomas they are usually firm, rubbery, and painless.

Table 25-1   Causes of Lymphadenopathy

Infections
  Viral
    Infectious mononucleosis*
    Cytomegalovirus*
    HIV†
    Postvaccinal lymphadenitis‡
  Bacterial
    *Staphylococcus**
    *Streptococcus**
    *Mycobacterium tuberculosis**
    Cat-scratch disease‡
    Syphilis*
    Chancroid‡
  Protozoal
    Toxoplasmosis*
  Fungal
    *Cryptococcus**
    Histoplasmosis*
    Coccidioidomycosis*
    Chlamydial*
    Lymphogranuloma venereum‡

Autoimmune
  Sjögren's syndrome‡
  Rheumatoid arthritis*

Iatrogenic
  Drug hypersensitivity (phenytoin, phenylbutazone, methyldopa,
    meprobamate, hydralazine)*
  Serum sickness*
  Silicone‡

Malignant
  Hodgkin's lymphoma*
  Non-Hodgkin's lymphoma*
  Acute and chronic leukemias*
  Metastatic cancer*

Other disorders
  Castleman's disease*
  Kikuchi-Fujimoto lymphadenitis‡
  Sarcoidosis*
  Dermatopathic lymphadenopathy‡
  Histiocytosis X*
  Sinus histiocytosis with massive lymphadenopathy*
  Abnormal immune response*

*Localized or generalized lymphadenopathy.
†Generalized lymphadenopathy.
‡Localized lymphadenopathy.

Table 25-2 Useful Clinical Information in the Evaluation of Lymphadenopathy

Clinical Parameter	Description
History	Sex, age, duration of lymphadenopathy, symptoms, sexual behavior, drug history, pets, occupation
Physical examination	Location of lymphadenopathy; size, tenderness, and texture of lymph node; presence or absence of splenomegaly; ear-nose-throat examination or genital-pelvic examination (depending on site of lymphadenopathy)

Table 25-3 Correlations Between Lymph Node Locations and Disease Origin

Lymph Node Groups	Associated Causes
Occipital	Scalp infections, insect bites, ringworm infection
Posterior auricular	Rubella
Anterior auricular	Eye or conjunctival infections
Posterior cervical	Toxoplasmosis, scalp infections, cat-scratch disease
Submental/ submandibular	Dental infections, metastatic disease (oral cavity)
Anterior cervical	Infections of pharynx and oral cavity, tuberculosis, Epstein-Barr virus, nasopharyngeal carcinoma
Supraclavicular	Malignant lymphomas, metastatic disease (lung, gastrointestinal tract)
Mediastinal	Sarcoidosis, histoplasmosis, coccidioidomycosis, tuberculosis, lymphoma, metastatic disease
Axillary	Cat-scratch disease, pyogenic infections of upper arms, brucellosis, dermatopathic lymphadenopathy, lymphoma, metastatic disease (breast)
Epitrochlear	Viral diseases, sarcoidosis, tularemia, infections of hands, lymphoma
Abdominal/ retroperitoneal	Tuberculosis, lymphoma, metastatic disease
Inguinal	Herpes, lymphogranuloma venereum, syphilis, gonococcal infection, AIDS, lymphoma, metastatic disease

A rocklike lymph node usually indicates metastatic tumor. The lymph node size is of little help in establishing the diagnosis. With inguinal lymphadenopathy, a genital and perineal examination is imperative. A careful ear, nose, oral, and throat examination is indicated in patients with cervical lymphadenopathy to identify a possible source of infection or a primary tumor.

Lymphadenopathy in the supraclavicular area is always of pathologic significance, usually due to lymphoma or metastatic malignancy, especially in the lung or gastrointestinal tract.

25.3 Diagnostic Approach

Following a clinical history and physical examination, the workup for a patient with lymphadenopathy should include the following elements:

1. Complete blood cell count, including evaluation of the peripheral blood smear.
2. Erythrocyte sedimentation rate (ESR).
3. Throat culture and culture for gonorrhea (if clinically indicated).
4. Chest radiograph and computed tomography (CT) when needed.
5. Serologic tests for infectious disorders and autoimmune disorders.
6. Blood chemistry tests, including transaminase levels, serum calcium, and angiotensin-converting enzyme levels (test for sarcoidosis).
7. Tuberculin skin test.
8. Lymph node fine-needle aspiration (FNA).
9. Lymph node biopsy for histologic examination and culture.
10. Bone marrow aspirate (culture when indicated) and biopsy examination.

25.4 Hematologic Findings

The hematologic findings in reactive lymphadenopathies vary greatly depending on the cause of the disease. Examination of the peripheral blood smear may be particularly helpful.

25.4.1 Blood Cell Measurements

When anemia is present, it is usually mild, normochromic, and normocytic. The leukocyte count is usually elevated. The platelet count may be normal, decreased, or increased, depending on the cause of the lymphadenopathy.

25.4.2 Peripheral Blood Smear Morphology

The RBCs are usually normochromic and normocytic, or they may sometimes be macrocytic, as often seen in patients with AIDS. Neutrophilic leukocytosis is often present in pyogenic infections or in the early stages of viral infections such as infectious mononucleosis. The presence of many reactive (atypical) or transformed lymphocytes, together with the characteristic clinical setting, suggests infectious mononucleosis. Such lymphocytosis is also frequently found in CMV infection and toxoplasmosis.

25.4.3 Bone Marrow Examination

Examination of the bone marrow aspirate is rarely helpful in diagnosing benign lymphadenopathies. The bone marrow biopsy specimen may show granulomas in patients with tuberculosis, sarcoidosis, or disseminated fungal disease. Special stains for organisms and cultures may occasionally be helpful in the diagnosis.

Other Laboratory Tests

Test 25.1 Serologic Tests for Infectious Agents

Purpose. A variety of infectious diseases and autoimmune disorders associated with lymphadenopathy may be detected with immunoassays.

Principle. Specific and nonspecific antibodies and antigens produced by infection with various organisms are detected by methods such as complement fixation and enzyme-linked immunosorbent assay (ELISA) methods.

Specimen. Serum is used as a specimen. (Urine and cerebrospinal fluid are rarely used.) Specimens from the acute and convalescent phases are needed to detect rises in titer in complement fixation tests.

Procedure. A variety of methods can be used. The indirect immunofluorescent technique is performed by incubating serum dilutions with organisms fixed to glass slides. Specific antibody adheres to the organism. In complement fixation tests, specific antibody attaches to antigen (organism) with complement binding.

ELISA methods are extremely sensitive and are used for detecting antibodies to a variety of bacteria, viruses, and parasites. In this technique, an enzyme such as alkaline phosphatase is conjugated to an antispecies immunoglobulin such as antihuman IgG or IgM. An antigen specific to the infectious agent is used to coat a polystyrene well. Dilutions of the patient's serum are added and allowed to react. Excess serum is removed by washing. To detect the antibody specific to the infectious agent, the enzyme-linked antihuman immunoglobulin is then added and allowed to bind. Unbound immunoglobulin is removed by washing. The appropriate substrate for the enzyme is added to measure the enzyme activity, correlating to the amount of bound antihuman immunoglobulin.

Other tests include Western blot (for HIV infection) and polymerase chain reaction (PCR) technology. The PCR assays for infectious diseases associated with lymphadenopathy include HIV, cytomegalovirus (CMV), Epstein-Barr virus (EBV), tuberculosis, and cat-scratch disease.

Interpretation. Serologic tests are available for infectious mononucleosis; CMV lymphadenitis; HIV lymphadenitis; toxoplasmosis; histoplasmosis; lymphogranuloma venereum; cat-scratch disease; syphilis; and autoimmune disorders such as rheumatoid arthritis, systemic lupus erythematosus (SLE), and Sjögren's syndrome. A variety of techniques are used, including immunofluorescence, complement fixation, latex fixation, and ELISA. Even when the same basic procedure is used, the results from different laboratories may vary; reference values change frequently owing to modifications in techniques and reagents. It is therefore important to be familiar with the particular method used and the reference values given by the laboratory.

In children and young adults with lymphadenopathy, the detection of heterophil antibodies (monospot test) may be very helpful in the diagnosis of infectious mononucleosis. However, this test may be negative in approximately 50% of patients in the first 2 weeks of illness. Tests for EBV and/or CMV also may be useful. Other serologic tests that may be helpful include ELISA for HIV, toxoplasmosis, and cat-scratch disease.

Test 25.2 **Fine-Needle Aspiration**

Purpose. FNA is done either to render a diagnosis or to decide whether a (surgical) lymph node biopsy should be performed.

Principle. This simple technique is less risky, associated with less patient discomfort, and less costly than a surgical biopsy. It is particularly useful in the diagnosis of metastatic malignancy.

Specimen. Cells are aspirated from the lymph node and can be submitted for cytologic analysis, flow cytometry, microbial culture, or molecular diagnostics.

Procedure. A 23- or 25-gauge needle attached to a disposable syringe is inserted into the lymph node and tissue is aspirated. Small amounts of the aspirated material are smeared across glass slides and stained with Diff-Quik®, May-Grünwald, Giemsa, and/or Papanicolaou methods. Accuracy of the FNA may be improved by performing flow cytometry on the same specimen. A portion of the aspirated material is submitted to the flow cytometry laboratory in heparin (green-top tube) or citrate (yellow-top tube) anticoagulant. When indicated, a sterile specimen also may be submitted for culture.

Interpretation. FNA can provide a rapid diagnosis in metastatic malignancy, reactive hyperplasia, and some lymphomas when interpreted by an experienced cytopathologist. In select cases, immunohistochemistry and/or flow cytometry done on the aspirated material can provide additional information such as the demonstration of light chain restriction and/or aberrant phenotypic expression.

Notes and Precautions. FNA does not replace a lymph node biopsy but is a complementary diagnostic technique. The main purpose of FNA is to decide whether a lymph node biopsy is indicated. A diagnosis of metastatic malignancy often obviates the need for a surgical biopsy. Cytologic suspicion of lymphoma is an indication for lymph node biopsy.

Test 25.3 **Lymph Node Biopsy**

Purpose. Lymph node biopsy is the final step in the workup for a patient with lymphadenopathy. It provides a histopathologic diagnosis and, if indicated, sterile tissue should be submitted for culture. Frequently, a specific diagnosis cannot be made. It is then the responsibility of the pathologist to provide the physician with a differential diagnosis.

Principle. Biopsy should be performed when a significantly enlarged lymph node persists and/or increases in size and other tests have failed to provide a diagnosis. A lymph node biopsy should not be performed if a viral infection such as infectious mononucleosis is suspected, because histopathologic features often resemble malignant lymphoma.

Specimen. If several enlarged lymph nodes are present, an attempt should be made to remove the largest node. The lymph node should be submitted to the laboratory, intact and unfixed, as soon as possible.

Procedure. Histologic interpretation of lymph node biopsy specimens is often difficult, and special care is required in specimen handling. The major reason for difficulty in interpretation is technical and results from improper handling of the biopsy specimen. It is extremely important that the complete lymph node be submitted intact and fresh to the pathology laboratory, where a portion of fresh tissue should be frozen for possible immunologic or molecular studies and another portion submitted for flow cytometry, when indicated. If clinically indicated, sterile culture should be performed. A portion of the tissue should then be fixed in formalin and another portion should be fixed in B5 or a similar fixative. (For a more detailed discussion of the handling of lymph node specimens, see Chapter 34.)

Interpretation. Optimal interpretation of a lymph node biopsy specimen often requires the collaboration of an experienced surgeon, a hematopathologist, and a hematologist/oncologist. Reactive lymphoproliferative disorders may be difficult to differentiate from malignant disorders, in both lymph nodes and extranodal sites. Detailed clinical information, excellent histologic sections, and sometimes special marker studies are important to attain a correct diagnosis.

The most helpful approach to the histologic diagnosis is the pattern approach, or the low-magnification appearance of the lymph node. **Table 25-4** lists the most common patterns of

Table 25-4   Patterns Observed in Reactive Lymphadenopathies

Follicular pattern
  Nonspecific hyperplasia (most common)
  Rheumatoid arthritis
  AIDS
  Castleman's disease
  Toxoplasmosis
  Syphilis
Macronodular pattern
  Progressive transformation of germinal centers
Interfollicular pattern
  Viral lymphadenitis (infectious mononucleosis, cytomegalovirus)
  Dermatopathic lymphadenitis
  Postvaccinal lymphadenitis
Mixed pattern (follicular and interfollicular)
  Viral lymphadenitis (infectious mononucleosis, cytomegalovirus)
  Toxoplasmosis
  Kimura's disease
  Lymphogranuloma venereum
Sinusoidal pattern
  Nonspecific histiocytosis
  Sinus histiocytosis with massive lymphadenopathy
  Langerhans cell histiocytosis (histiocytosis X)
  Whipple's disease
  Monocytoid B-cell hyperplasia
  Early metastatic disease
  Lymphangiogram effect
Diffuse pattern
  Infectious mononucleosis
  Abnormal immune response
  Drug reactions
  Metastatic disease
Necrotizing pattern
  Cat-scratch disease
  Kikuchi-Fujimoto lymphadenitis
  Infarction
  Toxoplasmosis
Granulomatous pattern
  Sarcoidosis
  Tuberculosis
  Fungal disease
  Leprosy
  Drug exposure

Table 25-5   General Features Differentiating Benign Hyperplasia From Malignant Lymphoma in Lymph Node

Feature	Benign Hyperplasia	Malignant Lymphoma
Architecture	Distorted	Often effaced
Sinuses	Open or focally compressed	Often obliterated
Normal cell components	Hyperplastic	Often obliterated
Cell type	Mixture, often transformed cells	Atypical, often monomorphic cells
Immunophenotype	Polyclonal	Usually monoclonal

cellular infiltrate and the disorders associated with each. Once the general pattern is determined at low power, a higher-power examination determines the cellular components present. **Table 25-5** outlines features that may be useful in differentiating benign hyperplasia from malignant lymphoma. For a detailed histopathologic description of the various disorders listed in **Table 25-4**, see textbooks on lymph node pathology. **Images 25-1 to 25-13** show the characteristic morphologic features observed in several benign lymph node disorders.

Notes and Precautions. As previously noted, a number of benign disorders may clinically and histopathologically resemble a malignant lymphoproliferative disorder. Therefore, a hematopathologist should be consulted if the primary pathologist reviewing the tissue does not have experience in examining lymph nodes. In addition, if adequate specimen is available, fresh tissue should be frozen for possible future phenotypic and genotypic studies. Immunoperoxidase studies, flow cytometry studies, in situ hybridization studies, and gene rearrangement studies can be extremely helpful in the final diagnosis in difficult cases. These studies are described in more detail in Chapter 34.

In 40% to 60% of patients only a diagnosis of reactive, nonspecific hyperplasia can be made. However, even a nonspecific diagnosis is helpful to the clinician and reassuring to the patient, because the main aim of the lymph node biopsy is to exclude a malignant disease or a treatable disorder.

The term "atypical hyperplasia" refers to a condition the pathologist cannot distinguish as a benign or malignant process. Patients with such conditions must have a careful follow-up and a repeat biopsy if there is persistent lymphadenopathy or if new lymphadenopathy develops. In 18% to 25% of affected patients (adults and children), a specific diagnosis is made on repeat biopsy. In adults (particularly in older patients), approximately 50% of patients whose lymph nodes are interpreted as atypical hyperplasia are subsequently diagnosed with malignant lymphoma.

25.5 Ancillary Tests

25.5.1 Chest Radiograph

A chest radiograph, although normal in most cases, is often indicated. It may show enlarged mediastinal lymph nodes, which may indicate malignant lymphoma, tuberculosis, sarcoidosis, histoplasmosis, or metastatic malignancy. In addition, primary lung parenchymal lesions may be detected.

25.5.2 Serum Chemistry

Elevated serum calcium levels and angiotensin-converting enzyme may suggest sarcoidosis. Elevated transaminase levels are frequently seen in infectious mononucleosis.

25.5.3 Tuberculin Skin Test

A positive tuberculin skin test may be helpful in differentiating tuberculosis from sarcoidosis.

25.6 Course and Treatment

As expected, the clinical course and treatment of lymphadenopathy depend on the cause of the disease.

25.7 References

Ferry JA, Harris NL. *Atlas of Lymphoid Hyperplasia and Lymphoma*. Philadelphia, Pa: Saunders; 1997.

Fessas PH, Pangalis GA. Reactive, non-specific and reactive specific lymphadenopathies. In: Pangalis GA, Pollack A, eds. *Benign and Malignant Adenopathies: Clinical and Laboratory Diagnosis*. London, England: Hardword Academic Publishers; 1993:31–46.

Ioachim HL. *Lymph Node Biopsy*. 2nd ed. Philadelphia, Pa: Lippincott; 1994.

Jaffe ES. *Surgical Pathology of Lymph Nodes and Related Organs*. Philadelphia, Pa: Saunders; 1995.

Kjeldsberg CR. Childhood lymphoproliferative disorders: a selective review. *Semin Diagn Pathol*. 1995;12:283–346.

Pangalis GA, Boussiotis VA, Fessas PH, et al. Clinical approach to patients with lymphadenopathy. In: Pangalis GA, Pollack A, eds. *Benign and Malignant Lymphadenopathies: Clinical and Laboratory Diagnosis*. London, England: Hardword Academic Publishers; 1993:19–30.

Peterson BA, Frizzera G. Benign lymphoproliferative disorders. *Semin Oncol*. 1993;20:553–657.

Said JW. AIDS-related lymphadenopathies. *Semin Diagn Pathol*. 1988;5:365–378.

Swerdlow SH, Sukpanichnant S, Glick AD, et al. Reactive states in lymph nodes resembling lymphomas or progressing to lymphomas: a selective review. *Mod Pathol*. 1993;6:378–391.

Van der Valk P, Meijer CJLM. The histology of reactive lymph nodes. *Am J Surg Pathol*. 1987;11:866–878.

Weiss LM. *Pathology of Lymph Nodes*. New York, NY: Churchill-Livingstone; 1996.

Williamson HA. Lymphadenopathy in a family practice. *J Fam Pract*. 1985;20:449–452.

Zardarvi IM, Jain S, Bennet S. Flow cytometric algorithm on fine needle aspiration for the clinical workup of patients with lymphadenopathy. *Diagn Cytopathol*. 1998;19:274–278.

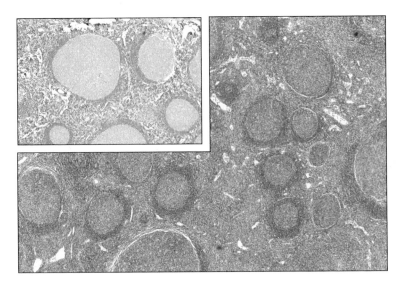

Image 25-1 Follicular hyperplasia. Multiple reactive follicles are visible. Immunoperoxidase demonstrates expression of Bcl-2 protein within the mantle zone but not within the follicle center (inset). For a comparison with follicular lymphoma see Image 34-8.

Image 25-2 Fine-needle aspirate of reactive lymph node shows a characteristic mixed cell population that includes a tingible body macrophage, large transformed lymphocytes, and many small lymphocytes.

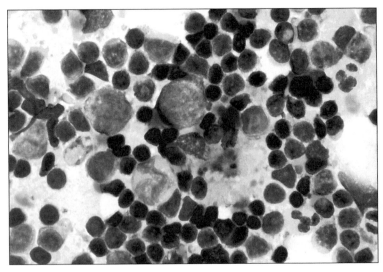

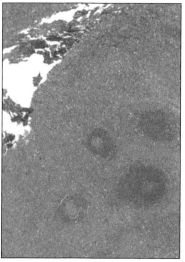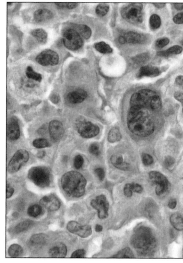

Image 25-3 Infectious mononucleosis. A prominent interfollicular infiltrate of large transformed lymphocytes and plasma cells is shown (left). Lymphoid cells are seen at various stages of transformation (right), including cells that resemble those seen in Hodgkin's lymphoma and anaplastic large cell lymphoma cell.

Image 25-4 Infectious mononucleosis. A "starry sky" pattern and sheets of large transformed cells are shown (left). Many large transformed lymphocytes, plasmacytoid lymphocytes, and plasma cells are visible (right). These cells could be mistaken for those seen in non-Hodgkin's large cell lymphoma.

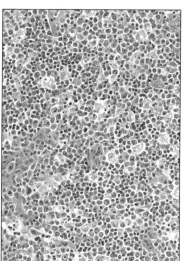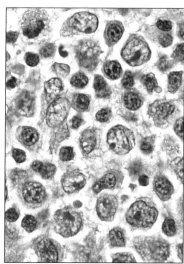

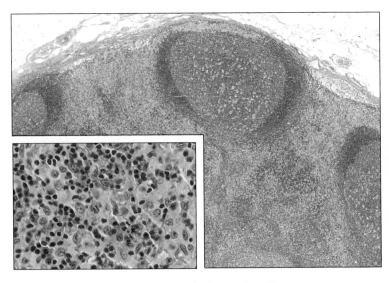

Image 25-5 Dermatopathic lymphadenopathy. The paracortex is expanded by numerous histiocytes. The paracortex contains various types of histiocytes, including Langerhans' cells and interdigitating dendritic cells (inset). The brown pigment represents melanin or lipid.

Image 25-6 Toxoplasmosis. A large germinal center contains epithelioid histiocytes (left). Monocytoid B cells with abundant pale cytoplasm are seen within sinusoids (right).

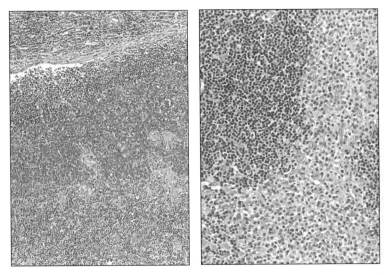

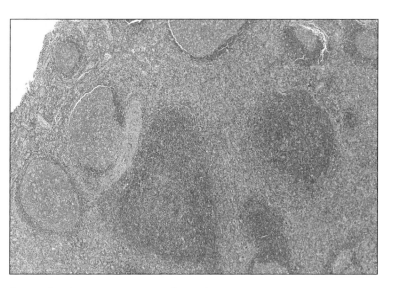

Image 25-7 Progressive transformation of germinal centers. This section demonstrates follicular hyperplasia and shows two large nodules containing predominantly small lymphocytes.

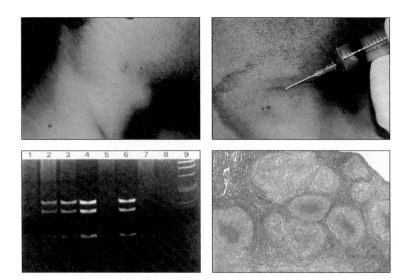

Image 25-8 Cat-scratch disease. A hard, immobile, tender mass in the neck is shown (top left). Pus is aspirated from the mass (top right). Polymerase chain reaction assay was done on the pus with primers specific for the *Bartonella henselae* citrate synthase gene. The DNA band pattern is shown (bottom left). Lanes 2 and 3 show pus specimen from the patient; lanes 1, 5, 7, and 8 show pus specimens from patients without cat-scratch disease. Lane 4 shows *B henselae* DNA; lane 6 shows pus specimen from another patient with cat-scratch disease; lane 9 shows the molecular size marker. Histopathologic features typical of lymph node biopsy specimens from patients with cat-scratch disease are shown (bottom right) (courtesy of Michael Giladi, MD; with permission from *N Engl J Med.* 1999;34:108).

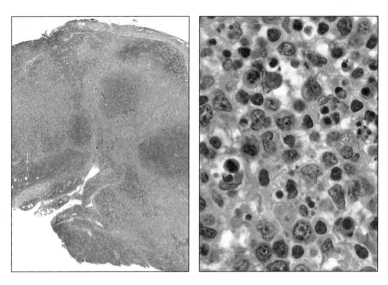

Image 25-9 Kikuchi's lymphadenitis. There is a localized eosinophilic zone of necrosis (left). Other areas in the node show a diffuse infiltrate of large cells. At higher power, transformed lymphocytes, histiocytes (some with crescent-shaped nuclei), plasmacytoid monocytes, and apoptotic debris can be seen (right).

Image 25-10 Castleman's disease, hyaline vascular variant. There is proliferation of lymphoid follicles of varying size and shape containing several germinal centers (left). Mantle zone cells are arranged in concentric rings ("onion skin" pattern) around atrophic hyalinized germinal centers (right). A follicle is penetrated by a blood vessel ("lollipop follicle").

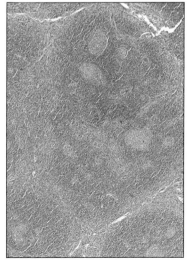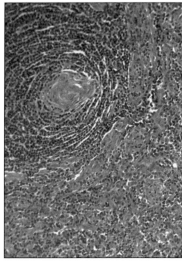

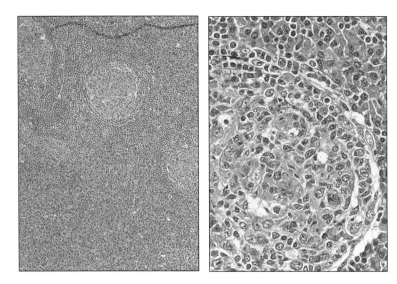

Image 25-11 Castleman's disease, plasma cell variant. Follicular hyperplasia is represented, and an interfollicular expansion of plasma cells is shown (left). Higher-power view of the same section shows sheets of plasma cells surrounding a germinal center (right).

Image 25-12 Sinus histiocytosis with massive lymphadenopathy (Rosai-Dorfman disease). Multiple histiocytes are seen within distended sinuses. Histiocytes contain intact-appearing lymphocytes (emperipolesis) (inset).

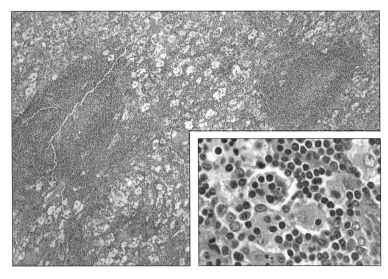

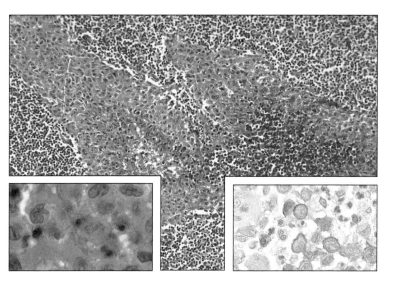

Image 25-13 Langerhans' cell histiocytosis. Sheets of Langerhans' cells within distended lymph node sinuses are shown. The cells' characteristic nuclear grooves are also shown (left inset). An immunoperoxidase study demonstrates expression of CD1a (right inset).

PART
VI

Acute Leukemias

26 Myelodysplastic Syndromes

Myelodysplastic syndromes (MDSs) are clonal disorders involving bone marrow stem cells and lead to ineffective and disorderly hematopoiesis. They manifest as irreversible quantitative and qualitative defects of hematopoietic cells caused by the abnormal division, maturation, and production of erythrocytes, granulocytes, and platelets. The clinical and morphologic features may be similar to those of acute myeloid leukemia (AML); some MDSs evolve into AML.

26.1 Pathophysiology

The mechanisms that contribute to the development of an MDS are poorly understood. It is possible that some are caused by exposure to agents that have adverse effects on hematopoietic stem cells, which leads to the disruption of normal hematopoiesis. The cytotoxic effects of radiotherapy, alkylating agents, and some other chemotherapeutic drugs play an important role in the etiology of therapy-related MDSs.

Regulatory abnormalities in the production of hematopoietic growth factors may contribute to the etiology of the stem cell defect in an MDS. In MDSs and AML, the absence of growth-inducing bone marrow proteins can uncouple the orderly pattern of growth and differentiation of myeloid hematopoietic cells. Because some growth factors such as interleukin-6 (IL-6) and colony-stimulating factor–1 (CSF-1) are produced by bone marrow fibroblasts, defects or alterations in the supportive marrow stromal elements may contribute to the pathogenesis of MDS.

Point mutations of *ras* oncogenes occur in 10% to 15% of patients with an MDS and less frequently (≈5%) point mutations of *fms* (receptor of colony-stimulating factor) are identified. Alterations of the *p53* (5%–10%) and *Rb* (5%–10%) genes also occur. The role these mutations play in the development of MDSs is unclear, but they may be useful as clonal markers of malignancy. Mouse double minute (MDM-2 [≈70%]), *bcl*-2 (≈30%), and multiple drug resistant–1 (MDR-1 [≈30%]) proteins commonly are overexpressed in patients with MDSs.

Numerous complex cytogenetic abnormalities have been identified in patients with MDSs. It is uncertain whether the cytogenetic changes cause or result from an MDS. The cytogenetic changes that have been described are not specific for MDSs and are similar to those observed in patients with AML.

26.2 Clinical Findings

MDSs are most commonly diagnosed in patients between 60 and 75 years of age. Relatively few patients are younger than 50; however, an MDS may develop at any age, even in young children. Men are afflicted slightly more often than women. Signs and symptoms are generally related to blood cytopenias. Fatigue, weakness, and malaise are common due to anemia. Less frequently, patients present with infections due to neutropenia or thrombocytopenia-related hemorrhage. A small percentage of patients have splenomegaly; hepatomegaly is rare.

26.3 Diagnostic Approach

A diagnosis of MDS should be considered for any adult patient with unexplained blood cytopenias or monocytosis. A complete blood count (CBC) and careful examination of a blood smear, bone marrow aspirate smears, and trephine biopsy sections are essential for diagnosis and classification. The type and severity of morphologic changes vary for different categories of MDS. Some patients present with profound dysplastic changes and increased myeloblasts. Others present with only subtle changes, and the diagnosis may be delayed for several months or until other possible causes of cytopenias have been eliminated.

After a clinical history and physical examination, laboratory diagnosis of MDS should proceed according to the following steps:

1. A complete blood count.
2. A blood smear examination for dysplastic changes.
3. Studies to assess vitamin B_{12}, folate, and other potential deficiencies.
4. Bone marrow aspiration and trephine biopsy morphologic examination.
5. Bone marrow cytogenetic studies.
6. Other studies, as clinically indicated, for serum biochemical parameters and to evaluate for possible toxic exposure (eg, arsenic poisoning and infectious disease).

Flow cytometry, molecular studies, and in vitro bone marrow culture studies may be performed when clinically indicated.

26.4 Hematologic Findings

The hematologic findings in MDSs are highly variable. In some patients, the diagnosis is obvious on examination of the blood smear. Other patients require a thorough evaluation to rule out secondary causes of cytopenias and myelodysplasia. The features generally used to define an MDS include various combinations of blood cytopenias, ineffective hematopoiesis, dyserythropoiesis, dysgranulopoiesis, dysmegakaryopoiesis, and increased myeloblasts. Ineffective hematopoiesis, characterized by blood cytopenias, and a normocellular or hypercellular bone marrow with normal or increased numbers of hematopoietic precursors are found in the majority of patients. The most common example is ineffective erythropoiesis, typified by anemia with reticulocytopenia and erythroid hyperplasia in the bone marrow.

26.4.1 Blood Cell Measurements

The CBC generally reveals a normocytic or macrocytic anemia with a low or normal reticulocyte count. The red cell distribution width (RDW) is often elevated as a result of RBC anisocytosis. Leukocyte counts vary from normal to markedly reduced. The leukocyte count is elevated in a minority of patients. The platelet count may be reduced or normal; patients rarely present with thrombocytosis, except in a special type of refractory anemia, the 5q– syndrome, discussed later in this chapter.

For the more indolent and prognostically favorable categories of MDS, anemia may be the only significant cytopenia. Patients with more aggressive types of MDS almost always present with pancytopenia or bicytopenia. The cytopenias typically progress with time, but the rate of progression is variable.

26.4.2 Blood Smear Morphology

The spectrum of morphologic changes on blood smears is listed in **Table 26-1**. The description of the various MDS categories in the classification section provides more morphologic details (**Images 26-1 to 26-3**).

26.4.3 Bone Marrow Examination

In most patients with an MDS, the bone marrow is hypercellular or normocellular; however, in about 10% the marrow is hypocellular. Iron stores are often increased. Myelofibrosis is occasionally observed, particularly in patients with a therapy-related MDS. The most important findings in the bone marrow are the dysplastic changes and, in some cases, increased myeloblasts (*see Table 26-1*).

Dyserythropoiesis

Dyserythropoiesis is the most common morphologic change. Many cases of refractory anemia and refractory anemia with ringed sideroblasts (RARS) involve only mild dyserythropoiesis. In the more severe categories of MDS, profound dyserythropoiesis with bizarre erythroid precursors is often observed (**Image 26-4**). Ringed sideroblasts may be found in any category of MDS but are most striking in RARS (**Image 26-5**).

Table 26-1   Hematologic Findings in Myelodysplastic Syndromes

Blood	Bone Marrow
Dyserythropoiesis	
Anemia	Erythroid hyperplasia (occasionally
Anisopoikilocytosis	hypoplasia)
Oval macrocytes	Nuclear-cytoplasmic asynchrony
Hypochromic cells	Megaloblastic(oid) chromatin
Dimorphic populations	Karyorrhexis
Decreased polychromatophilic cells	Multinuclearity
Basophilic stippling	Internuclear bridging
Nucleated RBCs	Nuclear fragments
Vacuolated RBCs	Ringed sideroblasts
Howell-Jolly bodies	PAS-positive erythroblasts
Dysgranulopoiesis	
Neutropenia	Increased myeloblasts and immature
Rarely neutrophilia	granulocytes
Immature granulocytes	Abnormally localized immature
Hypogranularity	precursors
Nuclear hyposegmentation	Maturation defects
(pseudo–Pelger-Huët change)	Hypogranularity
Nuclear "sticks"	Abnormal granules
Occasionally hypersegmentation	Abnormal nuclei
Hypercondensed chromatin	Myeloperoxidase-deficient neutrophils
Circulating myeloblasts (<5%)	Increased monocytes
	Increased basophils
Dysmegakaryopoiesis	
Thrombocytopenia	Increased or decreased megakaryocytes
Large platelets	Clusters of megakaryocytes
Hypogranular platelets	Micromegakaryocytes
Vacuolated platelets	Monolobation or hypolobation
Abnormal platelet granules	Odd-numbered nuclei
Micromegakaryocytes	Multiple widely separated nuclei
	Hypogranulation

Dysgranulopoiesis

Dysgranulopoiesis may be absent to severe (**Image 26-6**). Abnormal localization of immature precursors (ALIP) refers to the distribution of developing granulocytes on bone marrow trephine biopsy sections in some types of MDS. The most immature granulocyte precursors are normally located in groups along the bone trabecula or adjacent to blood vessels. As the granulocytes mature, they extend toward more central areas between bone trabeculae. In an MDS, the most immature granulocyte precursors may be found in clusters remote from the usual paratrabecular location. Some investigators have associated ALIP with a poor prognosis and a greater likelihood of transformation to AML.

Dysmegakaryopoiesis

Dysmegakaryopoiesis is found in many of the MDSs. In some cases, dysmegakaryopoiesis may be the primary manifestation (**Image 26-7**).

Increased Myeloblasts

Increased myeloblasts are found in patients with more aggressive types of MDS. The percentage of bone marrow myeloblasts is a defining feature of the classification of an MDS. Myeloblasts do not exceed 19% in the blood or bone marrow. Patients with symptoms of an MDS but 20% or greater myeloblasts have AML.

26.5 Classification of Myelodysplastic Syndromes

The classification of MDSs has evolved over the past 25 years as more has been learned about their pathology. The classification most commonly used since it was published in 1982 is the French-American-British (FAB) Cooperative Group Classification. The categories of the FAB classification are listed in **Table 26-2**. Recently, a new proposal for the classification of MDSs has been sponsored by the World Health Organization (WHO) and developed in a combined effort by the Society for Hematopathology in the United States and the European Association for Hematopathology. This new classification incorporates most of the FAB categories but refines some of them and adds new groups. In addition, some of the criteria for diagnosing MDSs have been modified. **Table 26-3** lists the proposed WHO categories of MDS. The major modifications from the FAB classification include

1. Reduction of the percentage of blasts for a diagnosis of AML from 30% to 20%.
2. Elimination of the category of refractory anemia with excess blasts in transformation.

Table 26-2   French-American-British (FAB) Classification of Myelodysplastic Syndromes

Refractory anemia
Refractory anemia with ringed sideroblasts
Refractory anemia with excess blasts
Refractory anemia with excess blasts in transformation
Chronic myelomonocytic leukemia

Table 26-3   Proposed World Health Organization Classification of Myelodysplastic Syndromes

Refractory anemia (RA)
Refractory anemia with ringed sideroblasts (RARS)
Refractory cytopenia with multilineage dysplasia (RCMD)
Refractory anemia with excess blasts (RAEB)
  Type 1 = 5 to 9% blasts in blood or marrow
  Type 2 = 10 to 19% blasts in blood or marrow
5q- syndrome
Therapy-related myelodysplastic syndrome
Myelodysplastic syndrome, unclassified

3. Recognition of two new categories of MDS—refractory cytopenia with multilineage dysplasia (RCMD) and the 5q-syndrome.
4. Shifting of the chronic myelomonocytic leukemia category from the MDSs to a newly defined group of disorders that exhibit overlapping features of an MDS and chronic myeloproliferative syndrome (MPS). These "bridging" disorders have been designated "myelodysplastic/myeloproliferative syndromes" (MDS/MPS) and are classified separately (**Table 26-4**).

The rest of this section describes each of the categories of MDS and MDS/MPS included in the proposed WHO classification.

26.5.1 **Refractory Anemia**

The major manifestation of refractory anemia (RA) is ineffective erythropoiesis characterized by anemia, reticulocytopenia, and erythroid hyperplasia in the bone marrow. The anemia may be normocytic or macrocytic with anisopoikilocytosis; oval macrocytes

Table 26-4   Proposed World Health Organization Classification of Myelodysplastic/Myeloproliferative Syndromes

Chronic myelomonocytic leukemia (CMML)
Atypical chronic myeloid leukemia (aCML)
Juvenile myelomonocytic leukemia (JMML)
Juvenile monosomy 7 syndrome

are common. A mild degree of neutropenia or thrombocytopenia may be present. However, there is no evidence of dysplastic changes in the neutrophils or platelets. Myeloblasts are not identified in the blood smear and monocytes are less than $1.0 \times 10^3/mm^3$ $(1.0 \times 10^9/L)$.

The bone marrow is usually hypercellular or normocellular with erythroid hyperplasia; occasionally the marrow is hypoplastic. Dyserythropoiesis may be noted but is not usually severe. Ringed sideroblasts are occasionally observed but make up less than 15% of the erythroblasts. Dysgranulopoiesis and dysmegakaryopoiesis are absent. Myeloblasts are less than 5% in the marrow. A thorough evaluation for other causes of anemia must always be performed before a diagnosis of RA is made. In some cases, the diagnosis is possible only after monitoring the patient for several months and eliminating all other possible causes. Most patients with RA follow a chronic course but may require RBC transfusion support. A small number evolve to a more aggressive MDS and bone marrow failure or AML.

26.5.2 Refractory Anemia With Ringed Sideroblasts

The clinical and morphologic features of RARS are similar to those of RA. However, in RARS 15% or more of the bone marrow erythroblasts are ringed sideroblasts (*see Image 26-5*). There is commonly a dimorphic anemia with normal erythrocytes and microcytic and/or hypochromic poikilocytes. Coarse basophilic stippling (including Pappenheimer bodies) is observed in some of the erythrocytes. Neutropenia and thrombocytopenia are absent or minimal, and there are no dysplastic changes in either lineage. There are no myeloblasts in the blood, and monocytes are less than $1.0 \times 10^3/mm^3$ $(1.0 \times 10^9/L)$.

The bone marrow is hypercellular or normocellular with erythroid hyperplasia and markedly increased iron stores. The numerous ringed sideroblasts are the most prominent feature of this condition. Mild to moderate dyserythropoiesis may be observed, but there are no dysplastic changes in granulocytes or megakaryocytes. Myeloblasts are rarely increased and never exceed 4%.

Ringed sideroblasts may be observed in any of the other categories of MDS, occasionally exceeding 15% of the erythroblasts. In some cases of RCMD (discussed later in this section), ringed sideroblasts number 15% or greater. This group is distinguished from RARS by the presence of bicytopenia or pancytopenia and dysplastic changes in more than one lineage. It is important to distinguish RCMD from RARS because of its more aggressive clinical course.

26.5.3 Refractory Cytopenia With Multilineage Dysplasia

In this category of MDS, there are one or more blood cytopenias and dysplastic changes in two or more of the major hematopoietic lineages. Bone marrow and blood myeloblasts are less than 5%. RCMD is distinguished from RA by the significant changes in the granulocyte and platelet/megakaryocytic lineages, as well as in the erythrocytes, and differs from refractory anemia with excess blasts (RAEB) by having less than 5% myeloblasts. In some instances, dysgranulopoiesis or dysmegakaryopoiesis are the major abnormalities (*see Image 26-6*). RCMD usually has a more aggressive course than RA and a greater propensity for evolution to AML. The clinical course is often similar to that of RAEB. In some respects, this category bridges RA and RAEB.

26.5.4 Refractory Anemia With Excess Blasts

Pancytopenia or bicytopenia are characteristic of RAEB. Dysplastic changes are commonly observed in erythrocytes, granulocytes, and platelets (*see Images 26-1 and 26-3*). Nucleated RBCs and immature granulocytes, including myeloblasts and (occasionally) micromegakaryocytes, may be found in the blood smears. Myeloblasts may constitute up to 19% of the leukocytes in the blood.

The bone marrow is normocellular or hypercellular, and granulocytic and/or erythroid hyperplasia are present. Myeloblasts are increased to at least 5% but less than 20%. Auer bodies may be present. Dyserythropoiesis is more severe in this condition than in RA or RARS. Dysgranulopoiesis is often prominent. Megakaryocytic hyperplasia with dysmegakaryopoiesis and megakaryocytic clusters may be observed on biopsy sections. The features that distinguish RAEB from RA and RARS include the severity of the pancytopenia or bicytopenia, dysplastic changes in more than one cell lineage, and the presence of 5% or greater myeloblasts in the blood or bone marrow. RAEB is distinguished from RCMD by the myeloblast percentage.

In the proposed WHO classification, RAEB is separated into two types by the following criteria:

1. Type 1 RAEB is characterized by 5% to 9% blasts in the blood or bone marrow.
2. Type 2 RAEB has 10% to 19% blasts in the blood or bone marrow.

The basis of this separation stems from the finding that patients with RAEB with greater than 10% myeloblasts often have a more aggressive course and a greater propensity for transformation to AML.

The FAB category of RAEB in transformation has been eliminated in the proposed WHO classification by the reduction of the required percentage of blasts from 30% to 20% for a diagnosis of AML. The presence of Auer rods no longer defines a distinctive category of transformation but is noted in RAEB or RCMD.

26.5.5 5q– Syndrome

A type of RA referred to as the "5q– syndrome" is generally associated with a particularly good prognosis. This syndrome is characterized by macrocytic anemia—often with thrombocytosis (≈50% of patients), erythroblastopenia, megakaryocyte hyperplasia with nuclear hypolobation, and an isolated interstitial deletion of chromosome 5. The 5q– syndrome is found predominantly in elderly women. Most patients have a stable clinical course but are often transfusion dependent.

26.5.6 Therapy-Related Myelodysplastic Syndromes and Acute Myeloid Leukemia

Therapy-related MDSs occur in patients previously treated with chemotherapy and/or radiotherapy. Alkylating drugs and the

Table 26-5 Features That May Cause Difficulty in Classifying Myelodysplastic Syndromes

Presence of Auer rods with <5% blasts
Isolated neutropenia or thrombocytosis
Leukocytosis or thrombocytosis
Hypocellular bone marrow
Significant leukocytosis or thrombocytosis
Myelofibrosis

type II topoisomerase inhibitors (epipodophyllotoxins) are the agents most commonly implicated. The median onset of therapy-related MDSs is approximately 5 years after initiation of alkylating agents and 2.5 to 3 years after first use of type II topoisomerase inhibitors. In many patients, there is evolution to frank AML in a short time. In a therapy-related MDS secondary to alkylating agents, patients present with unexplained cytopenias. In most cases, there is an obvious panmyelopathy. The dysplastic changes in the blood and bone marrow cells are often severe; however, the bone marrow myeloblast percentage is frequently less than 5%. Myelofibrosis, hypocellularity, and ringed sideroblasts are encountered more frequently than in de novo MDSs. The therapy-related MDSs associated with alkylating agents commonly have cytogenetic abnormalities affecting chromosomes 5 and/or 7. The type II topoisomerase inhibitor drugs more often are associated with monocytic or myelomonocytic leukemias and abnormalities of chromosome 11q23; occasionally they present as an MDS.

26.5.7 Myelodysplastic Syndrome, Unclassified

The proposed WHO criteria for diagnosis and classification of an MDS apply to most patients. However, occasional syndromes are difficult to place in defined categories because of one or more atypical or unusual features (**Table 26-5**). Some of the most common examples of conditions designated *MDS, unclassified* are discussed here.

In rare cases, patients with less than 5% blasts will present with Auer rods; they usually have the features of RCMD. The recommendation is to categorize these conditions as *MDS, unclassified*; the significance of the Auer bodies in the propensity for evolution to AML in this group is presently unclear.

Occasionally, patients with an MDS present with isolated neutropenia or thrombocytopenia without anemia and with dysplastic changes confined to the single lineage. The terms "refractory neutropenia" and "refractory thrombocytopenia" have sometimes been used to describe these conditions. A diagnosis of MDS in patients with neutropenia or thrombocytopenia without anemia should be made with caution, only when there is convincing evidence of dysplasia, and only after other causes have been ruled out.

Patients with features of RA or RAEB occasionally present with leukocytosis or thrombocytosis instead of the usual cytopenias. They may be diagnosed with MDS, unclassified, or they may be placed in the most appropriate category with notation of the unusual finding. Some of these conditions are more appropriately categorized as *atypical myeloproliferative disorders*.

Other Problems in Classifying Myelodysplastic Syndromes

Hypocellular Myelodysplastic Syndromes. In most MDSs, the bone marrow is hypercellular or normocellular. In about 10% of patients with de novo MDSs, however, there is a moderately to markedly hypocellular bone marrow; the incidence is higher in therapy-related MDSs. In a hypocellular MDS, the cellularity of the bone marrow is less than 30% in younger individuals and less than 20% in patients over 60 years of age. Except for hypocellularity, these conditions have the features of RA, RCMD, or RAEB. It seems appropriate to identify them with a designation of *hypocellular* following the appropriate classification. In some instances, it is difficult to distinguish a hypocellular MDS from aplastic anemia or hypocellular AML. Bone marrow cytogenetic studies are often helpful in distinguishing a hypocellular MDS from aplastic anemia. Distinction from hypocellular AML depends on careful enumeration of the blast percentage.

Myelofibrosis in Myelodysplastic Syndromes. Myelofibrosis is relatively common in patients with therapy-related MDSs and is present in about 10% to 15% of primary MDSs. Characterization of the MDS may be problematic because of the difficulty in obtaining a bone marrow aspirate adequate for morphologic assessment and accurate determination of the myeloblast percentage. With careful assessment of the blood smear and biopsy imprint preparations, along with the biopsy sections, some myelofibrotic MDSs can be subclassified into the appropriate category. In many instances, the designations *MDS with myelofibrosis* or *MDS, unclassified*, are more appropriate. These patients generally have pancytopenia with trilineage dysplasia. They may share features with the entity *acute panmyelosis with myelofibrosis* included in the classification of AML (see Chapter 27). Although the latter is theoretically distinguished by having 20% or more blasts, the degree of fibrosis may preclude obtaining an accurate assessment of blasts. Immunostains for CD34 on trephine biopsy sections may be useful in assessing the blast percentage.

Some patients with acute megakaryoblastic leukemia present with profound myelofibrosis, which must be differentiated from an MDS with fibrosis. MDSs with myelofibrosis are distinguished from the chronic myeloproliferative syndrome, chronic idiopathic myelofibrosis (CIMF), by the presence of blood cytopenias, trilineage dysplasia with increased and dysplastic megakaryocytes in the bone marrow sections, and the absence of splenomegaly. Occasionally, there is significant overlap of features between MDS with myelofibrosis and CIMF, precluding a definitive classification. The presence of myelofibrosis in MDS is an adverse prognostic finding.

26.6 Myelodysplastic/Myeloproliferative Syndromes

Some examples of myeloproliferative disorders bridge the MDSs and MPSs in their morphologic and clinical features. They do not clearly fit into the categories of either group of disorders. The WHO recognizes three myeloproliferative disorders that may have overlapping features of MDS and MPS (**Table 26-4**).

26.6.1 Chronic Myelomonocytic Leukemia

The designation *chronic myelomonocytic leukemia* (CMML) encompasses both myelodysplastic and chronic myeloproliferative syndromes. It is associated with a broad spectrum of clinical and hematologic presentations. Some patients present with the typical clinical and morphologic features of an MDS, including blood cytopenias, dysplastic hematopoiesis, and increased blasts. The morphologic features of CMML in these patients may be similar to those of RA, RCMD, or RAEB, with the addition of monocytosis of greater than $1.0 \times 10^3/mm^3$ ($1.0 \times 10^9/L$). In blood smears, the monocytes may exhibit dysplastic features in the form of hyperlobulated nuclei, increased basophilia of the cytoplasm, and abnormal granulation (**Image 26-8**). Blasts and promonocytes compose less than 20% of the leukocytes in the blood and bone marrow.

Other patients present with marked leukocytosis with monocytosis, organomegaly, and minimal or no dysplasia or increase in blasts; RBC and platelet counts may be normal. Cases of this type often were previously designated *Philadelphia chromosome–negative chronic myeloid leukemia* (CML).

Overall splenomegaly is present in one third to one half of patients with CMML; hepatomegaly is present in approximately one fifth. Some investigators have suggested separating CMML into MDS and MPS types based on presenting leukocyte counts, dysplastic features, and splenomegaly. A problem with this approach is that there is often a mixture of features in a given patient. Furthermore, regardless of the presenting features in CMML, it is not always predictable whether the disease will evolve clinically like an MDS or MPS.

26.6.2 Atypical Chronic Myeloid Leukemia

Atypical CML (aCML) is characterized by an increased leukocyte count composed predominantly of cells in the neutrophil lineage. Mature neutrophils predominate, but immature granulocytes usually account for more than 10% of the blood leukocytes. Monocytosis may occur but is fewer than 10% of the leukocytes. The bone marrow is hypercellular, and there is granulocytic hyperplasia with dysplastic changes. Some patients have dyserythropoiesis and dysmegakaryopoiesis. Several features of aCML are similar to those of CML, but unlike CML, basophilia is minimal or lacking, dysplasia is a prominent feature in the neutrophils, and anemia and/or thrombocytopenia are common. The Philadelphia chromosome and rearrangement of the *BCR* gene are absent. The prognosis for aCML is similar to that of aggressive MDSs, with reported median survival times of less than 2 years. Patients may manifest terminal bone marrow failure or AML. See Chapter 32.

26.6.3 Juvenile Myelomonocytic Leukemia

Juvenile myelomonocytic leukemia (JMML) was formerly referred to as *juvenile chronic myeloid leukemia*. The designation *JMML* is more appropriate because its morphologic and clinical features more closely mimic CMML than CML. Approximately 60% of cases are diagnosed in patients younger than 2 years of age.

However, cases have been diagnosed in children from less than 1 month of age to early adolescence. JMML arises from a stem cell defect that leads to deranged hematopoiesis. The disorder is characterized by leukocytosis in the range of 20 to 30×10^3/mm^3 (20 to 30 $\times 10^9$/L) composed of granulocytes and monocytes (**Image 26-9**). Immature and dysplastic forms can be identified, but dysplasia is usually not prominent. Blasts and promonocytes are less than 20% of the blood and bone marrow cells. The bone marrow is hypercellular with granulocytic hyperplasia. The degree of monocyte involvement is variable, from 5% to greater than 30% of the bone marrow cells. In vitro cell culture studies show spontaneous formation of high numbers of abnormal colony-forming units. Hypersensitivity of the neoplastic cells to granulocyte-monocyte colony-stimulating factor (GM-CSF) has been demonstrated repeatedly.

Other features of JMML are thrombocytopenia, hepatosplenomegaly, lymphadenopathy, skin rash, and an elevated hemoglobin F level. The latter can be a helpful diagnostic clue in the early stages of the disease. Results from cytogenetic studies are often normal; the most common reported abnormality is a monosomy 7. Mutated *ras* genes have been found in 30% of cases, and in about 10% of patients there is deletion of the *NF1* tumor suppressor gene. The deletion may lead to *ras* deregulation, which is important in leukemogenesis in these patients. These cases are associated with type I neurofibromatosis.

Unfavorable risk factors in JMML include age greater than 1 year, low platelet counts, elevated hemoglobin F levels, and abnormal cytogenetics. The disease course may wax and wane in some patients but most ultimately succumb to the disease. The only potentially curable treatment modality is allogeneic bone marrow transplant.

Juvenile Monosomy 7 Syndrome

Isolated juvenile monosomy 7 syndrome often presents with features of an MDS. Recurrent infections and hepatosplenomegaly are common findings, and neurofibromatosis has been observed. Patients usually have anemia and leukocytosis; thrombocytopenia is present in about half of affected patients. Monocytosis, leukoerythroblastosis, and defective neutrophil function are common. Dysplastic changes are generally observed, but myeloblasts are uncommon in the blood and only slightly elevated in the bone marrow. The bone marrow is hypercellular, and slight reticulin fibrosis may be present. Juvenile monosomy 7 syndrome may have features of RAEB but often is similar to JMML, and the two may be difficult to distinguish. Both share many of the same clinical features, such as the young age of the patient at diagnosis, a predominance in boys, hepatosplenomegaly, predominant myelomonocytic proliferation, increased frequency of neurofibromatosis, and a poor prognosis. However, patients with monosomy 7 syndrome more often transform to AML and suffer more infections.

Other Myelodysplastic Syndromes in Children

MDSs are primarily diagnosed in older adults and are uncommonly encountered in pediatric patients. JMML and isolated juvenile monosomy 7 syndrome have already been discussed. Other MDSs occur rarely in children. MDSs in children often evolve from genetically predisposing conditions such as Down's syndrome or Fanconi's anemia. The majority of cases are diagnosed before 5 years of age. The features and course of disease in children are similar to those in adults. About one third to one half of cases evolve to AML. In reports on childhood MDSs classified by FAB criteria, the categories of RAEB and RAEB-T are most common. The cytogenetic abnormalities seen most frequently are monosomy 7 and 7q–, alone or in combination with other changes. The next most common are trisomy 8 and various abnormalities of chromosome 3. Between 15% and 30% of cases of MDS in children show mutations of the *RAS* proto-oncogene.

The prognosis of children with an MDS is poor; about 30% to 50% of cases evolve to AML. The overall median survival time is 1 to 1.5 years. Infants younger than 1 year have a better prognosis than older children. Indications of poor prognosis are a fetal hemoglobin level of more than 10%, a platelet count of less than $40 \times 10^3/mm^3$ ($40 \times 10^9/L$), and complex chromosome abnormalities. The only realistic chance for cure is allogeneic bone marrow transplant.

26.7 Ancillary Tests

26.7.1 Cytogenetics

Bone marrow cytogenetic studies should be performed in every case of suspected MDS. The findings may provide important prognostic information, and in some instances the presence of a clonal chromosome abnormality is key in distinguishing an MDS from a secondary potentially reversible cause of myelodysplasia, such as alcohol, medication, a deficiency state, or chronic infection. Chromosome abnormalities may be detected by standard karyotyping of banded chromosomes or by fluorescence in situ hybridization (FISH) techniques when specific cytogenetic anomalies are suspected. (See Chapter 48 for descriptions of these techniques.)

Bone marrow clonal chromosome abnormalities are found in 30% to 50% of patients with a de novo MDS. Patients with RAEB and RCMD have a higher incidence of chromosome abnormalities than patients with RA or RARS. In therapy-related MDSs, cytogenetic abnormalities are observed in greater than 80% of patients. There are no cytogenetic abnormalities specific to MDSs; all of the karyotypic changes observed in MDSs also can be found in AML or other myeloproliferative disorders. In some cases, AML with specific cytogenetic abnormalities, such as t(8;21), t(15;17), or inv(16) (see Chapter 27), may present with a low myeloblast count in the range of an MDS (<20%). Despite low initial blast percentages, patients with these karyotypes should always be considered as having AML rather than an MDS.

Multiple cytogenetic changes, including deletions, trisomies, monosomies, and complex structural anomalies, have been identified in MDSs. The majority of patients show a loss of chromosome material rather than the reciprocal translocations or inversions that are common in patients with AML. Some of the most common recurring chromosome defects associated with MDSs are listed in **Table 26-6**. The single most common defect in a de novo MDS is 5q–. It is present in about 20% of patients—as an isolated finding in about 50% and in combination with other chromosome abnormalities in the other 50%. It has been found in association with all classes of MDS. 5q– as a single abnormality is associated with RA, characteristic megakaryocytic abnormalities, thrombocytosis, and a stable clinical course (5q– syndrome), as described earlier.

Monosomy 7 is the second most common cytogenetic abnormality in adults with an MDS and the most common in children. It is present in approximately 10% to 15% of cases of de novo MDSs and in 50% of cases of therapy-related MDSs. Abnormalities of chromosomes 5 and/or 7, alone or in combination with other rearrangements, are found in a high percentage of cases of therapy-related MDSs.

Table 26-6 Cytogenetic Abnormalities in Myelodysplastic Syndromes

Deletion 5q
Monosomy 7
Trisomy 8
Loss of Y chromosome
Deletion 20q
3q rearrangements
Various abnormalities of chromosome 11
Various abnormalities of chromosome 17p
Other complex chromosome defects

Source: Fenaux P, Morel P, Lai JL. Cytogenetics of myelodysplastic syndromes. *Semin Hematol.* 1996;33:127–138.

26.7.2 In Vitro Bone Marrow Cell Culture Studies

The colony-forming capacity of hematopoietic cells is diminished or absent in the majority of patients with an MDS. A leukemic-type in vitro growth pattern is often observed and is most commonly encountered in the more severe categories of MDS. In vitro culture of hematopoietic precursors sometimes may be valuable in assessing disease progression and prognosis.

26.7.3 Other Ancillary Laboratory Findings

Abnormalities in neutrophil function are reported in about half of patients with an MDS, in particular in juvenile monosomy 7 syndrome. Aberrant myeloid antigen expression may be identified. Occasionally, neutrophil myeloperoxidase staining is decreased or absent, and alkaline phosphatase levels may be increased or decreased. RBC metabolic abnormalities, changes in RBC membrane antigens, elevated levels of hemoglobin F, a positive acid hemolysis (Ham's) test, and various platelet function abnormalities have all been reported.

26.8 Differential Diagnosis of Myelodysplastic Syndromes

MDSs must be distinguished from other myeloproliferative disorders and from a variety of causes of secondary myelodysplasia, including nutritional deficiency states, infectious processes, drug effects, and toxic exposures. These conditions are often associated with one or more blood cytopenias and dysplastic changes that may be identical to those observed in MDSs. A thorough historical assessment and laboratory evaluation for secondary potentially reversible causes of myelodysplasia must always be performed before a diagnosis is made. **Table 26-7** lists conditions that may be considered in the differential diagnosis of MDSs.

In the MDSs that result primarily in anemia and dyserythropoiesis (RA and RARS), patients should always be evaluated for vitamin B_{12} and folate deficiency, exposure to drugs or toxins, arsenic poisoning, congenital dyserythropoietic anemia, and other causes of macrocytic anemia. When significant numbers of ringed sideroblasts are found, hereditary sideroblastic anemia, exposure to antituberculous drugs or chloramphenicol, alcohol toxicity, and chronic lead poisoning must be considered.

The cytopenias and myelodysplasia associated with AIDS may mimic a primary MDS (**Image 26-10**). Dysplastic changes in all hematopoietic cell lineages have been reported in patients with AIDS, and in the appropriate clinical setting it must be considered in the differential diagnosis. Other chronic infections and noninfectious causes of leukemoid reactions, particularly those associated with blood monocytosis, may be considered in the differential diagnosis.

MDSs with increased myeloblasts and generalized myelodysplasia must be distinguished from AML. The classes of AML that are most often considered are M2 (myeloid leukemia with maturation), M4 (myelomonocytic), and M6 (erythroleukemia). The distinction is based on the myeloblast percentage in the bone marrow and blood; 20% or greater is required for a diagnosis of leukemia. Diseases with t(8;21) or inv(16) with low blast counts are always considered AML, even when the presenting blast count is less than 20%. MDSs are problematic in the differential diagnosis of AML, mainly because of questions regarding the appropriateness of chemotherapy. Decisions to begin chemotherapy must be based on the patient's overall clinical status, not on blast counts alone.

26.9 Course and Treatment

Many therapeutic regimens have been used to treat patients with MDSs. Most have been relatively ineffective in changing the

Table 26-7 Considerations in the Differential Diagnosis of Myelodysplastic Syndromes

Megaloblastosis due to vitamin B_{12} or folate deficiency
Heavy metal intoxication: arsenic, lead, etc
Acute alcohol intoxication
Drug effects: primarily antineoplastic
Viral infection: parvovirus B19
Congenital dyserythropoietic anemia
Chronic infectious disease
AIDS
Acute myeloid leukemia (M2, M4, M6)
Any other condition with unexplained cytopenias or myelodysplasia

course of the disease, but several may result in limited clinical improvement. Protocols involving chemotherapeutic agents are generally reserved for patients with increased myeloblasts and/or severe pancytopenia. Conventional antileukemic chemotherapy is generally ineffective. However, some investigators report success in patients under 50 years of age. These younger patients may be candidates for allogeneic bone marrow transplantation, which is the only therapeutic modality with a reasonable chance of achieving a cure.

Growth factors (colony-stimulating factor) that regulate hematopoiesis by promoting proliferation and differentiation of progenitor cells have been used in treating MDSs. Granulocyte-monocyte colony-stimulating factor and granulocyte colony-stimulating factor (G-CSF), which enhance the function of mature granulocytes and monocytes and stimulate proliferation of the hematopoietic progenitor colonies, have been shown to increase neutrophil counts in patients with an MDS. However, their effect appears to be temporary. Other growth factors, including interleukin-3, erythropoietin, and combinations of growth factors, have been used with variable results.

26.9.1 **Prognosis and Prognostic Indicators in Myelodysplastic Syndromes**

In the majority of MDSs, the course of disease is chronic with gradually worsening blood cytopenias. Survival varies from several years to only a few weeks or months. Death results from evolution

Table 26-8   Survival and Evolution to Acute Myeloid Leukemia in Patients With MDS by FAB Classification*

FAB Type (% of Patients)	Leukemic Evolution (%)	Median Survival (Months)	Survival Range (Months)
RA (28)	12	50	18–64
RARS (24)	8	51	14–76+
RAEB (23)	44	11	7–16
RAEB-T (9)[†]	60	5	2.5–11
CMML (16)[‡]	14	11	9–60+

Abbreviations: MDS = myelodysplastic syndromes; FAB = French-American-British.
*From Third MIC Cooperative Study Group. Recommendations for a morphologic, immunologic, and cytogenetic (MIC) working classification of the primary and therapy related myelodysplastic disorders. *Cancer Genet Cytogenet.* 1988;32:1–9.
[†]RAEB-T is considered AML in the WHO proposed classification of MDS.
[†]CMML is included in the MDS-MPS bridging categories in the WHO classification.

to AML in approximately 30% of patients or from complications of blood cytopenias due to progressive bone marrow failure. The different categories of MDS have differing propensities for evolution to AML. Those associated with increased blasts and generalized myelodysplasia have the highest incidence and most rapid evolution to AML. **Table 26-8** compares the incidence of evolution to AML and length of survival for the FAB categories of MDS. Refractory anemia and RARS typically have the lowest incidence of leukemic evolution (<15%) and RAEB the highest (≈30%–40%). Therapy-related MDSs have a similar incidence of evolution to AML as RAEB.

Features with prognostic significance in MDSs are shown in **Table 26-9**. A predominance of good prognostic indicators are found in patients with RA and RARS. Mostly poor indicators are found in patients with the other de novo MDSs and therapy-related MDSs.

The International Prognostic Scoring System (IPSS) has been devised to predict prognosis in MDSs and is summarized in **Table 26-10**. The factors most useful for predicting the likelihood of evolution to AML include cytogenetic abnormalities, percentage of bone marrow myeloblasts, and number of cytopenias. For survival, these same variables, plus age and gender, are most important. Three prognostic cytogenetic groups are identified. Good outcomes are associated with normal cytogenetics, –Y alone, del(5q)

Table 26-9   Indicators of Good and Poor Prognoses in Myelodysplastic Syndromes

Good

Younger age

Normal or moderately reduced neutrophil and platelet counts

Low blast counts in the bone marrow and no blasts in the blood

No Auer rods

Ringed sideroblasts present

Normal karyotypes or mixed karyotypes without complex chromosome abnormalities

In vitro bone marrow culture reveals nonleukemic growth pattern

Poor

Advanced age

Severe neutropenia ($<0.5 \times 10^3$/mm^3[0.5×10^9/L]) or thrombocytopenia ($<50 \times 10^3$/mm^3 [50×10^9/L])

High blast count in the bone marrow or blasts in the blood

Auer rods

Absence of ringed sideroblasts

Abnormal localization of immature granulocyte precursors on bone marrow sections

All or mostly abnormal karyotypes or complex marrow chromosome abnormalities

In vitro bone marrow culture reveals leukemic growth pattern

Table 26-10   International Prognostic Scoring System for Survival and Evolution to Acute Myeloid Leukemia

Prognostic Variable	Score Value*				
	0	0.5	1.0	1.5	2.0
Bone marrow blast, %	<5	5-10	–	11–20	21–30†
Karyotype‡	Good	Intermediate	Poor	–	–
Cytopenias	0 or 1	2 or 3	–	–	–

*Scores for risk groups are 0 = low risk; 0.5–1.0 = intermediate-1; 1.5–2.0 = intermediate-2; 2.5 = high risk.

†The IPSS included the FAB category RAEB in transformation for this feature. The WHO classification considers patients with 20% to 30% blasts to have AML.

‡See description in text: good = normal, −Y, 5q–, 20q–; poor = chromosome 7 abns, or complex (3 or more) anomalies; intermediate = other abnormalities.

Abbreviations: IPSS = International Prognostic Scoring System; FAB = French-American-British; RAEB = refractory anemia with excess blasts; WHO = World Health Organization; AML = acute myeloid leukemia.

Source: Greenberg P, Cox C, LeBeau MM, et al. International scoring system for evaluating prognosis in myelodysplastic syndromes. *Blood.* 1997;89:2079–2088.

alone, and del(20q) alone. Poor outcomes are associated with abnormalities of chromosome 7 or complex chromosome abnormalities (three or more). Other cytogenetic anomalies are associated with intermediate outcomes.

26.10 **References**

Arico M, Biondi A, Pui CH. Juvenile myelomonocytic leukemia. *Blood*. 1997;90:479–488.

Bennett JM, Catovsky D, Daniel HT, et al. Proposals for the classification of the myelodysplastic syndromes. *Br J Haematol*. 1982;51:189–199.

Boultwood J, Lewis S, Wainscoat JS. The 5q– syndrome. *Blood*. 1994;84:3253–3260.

Brunning RD, McKenna RW. Tumors of the bone marrow: myelodysplastic syndromes. *Atlas of Tumor Pathology*. 3rd Series. Washington, DC: Armed Forces Institute of Pathology; 1994:143–194.

Fenaux P, Morel P, Lai JL. Cytogenetics of myelodysplastic syndromes. *Semin Hematol*. 1996;33:127–138.

Foucar K, Langdon RM, Armitage JO, et al. Myelodysplastic syndromes: a clinical and pathologic analysis of 109 cases. *Cancer*. 1985;56:553–561.

Gadner H. Pediatric experiences in myelodysplastic syndromes. In: Schmalzl F, Mufti GJ, eds. *Myelodysplastic Syndromes*. New York, NY: Springer-Verlag; 1992:31–37.

Greenberg P, Cox C, LeBeau MM, et al. International scoring system for evaluating prognosis in myelodysplastic syndromes. *Blood*. 1997;89:2079–2088.

Guyotat D, Campos L, Thomas X, et al. Myelodysplastic syndromes: a study of surface markers and in vitro growth patterns. *Am J Hematol*. 1990;34:26–31.

Haas OA, Gadner H. Pathogenesis, biology, and management of myelodysplastic syndromes in children. *Semin Hematol*. 1996;33:225–235.

Harris NL, Jaffe ES, Diebold J, et al. The World Health Organization Classification of Hematological Malignancies Report of the Clinical Advisory Committee Meeting, Airlie House, Virginia, November 1997. *Mod Pathol*. 2000;13(2):193–207.

Hofmann WK, Ottmann OG, Ganser A, et al. Myelodysplastic syndromes: clinical features. *Semin Hematol*. 1996;33:177–185.

Janssen JWB, Buschle M, Layton M, et al. Clonal analysis of myelodysplastic syndromes: evidence of multipotent stem cell origin. *Blood*. 1989;73:248–254.

Koeffler HP. Introduction: myelodysplastic syndromes. *Semin Hematol*. 1996;33:87–94.

Krsnik I, Srivastava PC, Galton DAG. Chronic myelomonocytic leukemia and atypical chronic myeloid leukemia. In: Schmalzl F, Mufti GJ, eds. *Myelodysplastic Syndromes*. New York, NY: Springer-Verlag; 1992:131–139.

Lambertenghi-Deliliers G, Orazi A, Luksch R, et al. Myelodysplastic syndrome with increased marrow fibrosis: a distinct clinico-pathological entity. *Br J Haematol*. 1991;78:161–166.

Luna-Fineman S, Shannon KM, Lange BJ. Childhood monosomy 7: epidemiology, biology, and mechanistic implications. *Blood*. 1995;85:1985–1999.

Mathew P, Tefferi A, Dewald GW, et al. The 5q– syndrome: a single-institution study of 43 consecutive patients. *Blood*. 1993;81:1040–1045.

Michels SD, McKenna RW, Arthur DC, et al. Therapy-related acute myeloid leukemia and myelodysplastic syndrome: a clinical and morphologic study of 65 cases. *Blood*. 1985;65:1364–1372.

Nand S, Godwin JE. Hypoplastic myelodysplastic syndrome. *Cancer*. 1988;62:958–964.

Park DJ, Koeffler HP. Therapy-related myelodysplastic syndromes. *Semin Hematol*. 1996;33:256–273.

Rosati S, Anastasi J, Vardiman J. Recurring diagnostic problems in the pathology of the myelodysplastic syndromes. *Semin Hematol*. 1996;33:111–126.

Third MIC Cooperative Study Group. Recommendations for a morphologic, immunologic, and cytogenetic (MIC) working classification of the primary and therapy related myelodysplastic disorders. *Cancer Genet Cytogenet*. 1988;32:1–9.

Tricot G, Vlietinck R, Boogaerts MA, et al. Prognostic factors in the myelodysplastic syndromes: importance of initial data on peripheral blood counts, bone marrow cytology, trephine biopsy and chromosomal analysis. *Br J Haematol*. 1985;60:19–32.

Tuzuner N, Cox C, Rowe JB, et al. Hypocellular myelodysplastic syndromes (MDS): new proposals. *Br J Haematol*. 1995;91:612–617.

Vardiman JW, Head D. Society for hematopathology: the myelodysplastic syndromes (MDS) and related disorders. *Mod Pathol*. 1999;12:101–106.

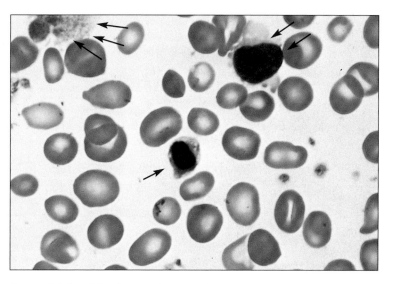

Image 26-1 Blood smear from a patient with a myelodysplastic syndrome. There is RBC anisopoikilocytosis with oval macrocytes. A nucleated RBC appears in the center of the field (one arrow), a micromegakaryocyte is seen at upper right (two arrows), and atypical platelets are evident at the upper left (three arrows).

Image 26-2 Blood smear from a patient with a myelodysplastic syndrome showing a hypogranular pseudo–Pelger-Huët neutrophil (arrow) and a lymphocyte.

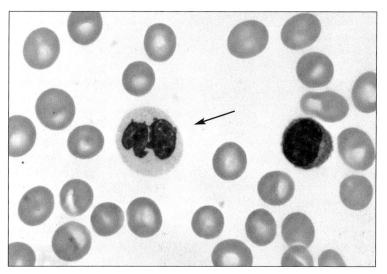

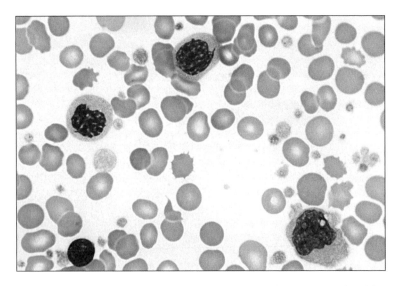

Image 26-3   Blood smear from a patient with refractory anemia with excess blasts. There are two dysplastic neutrophils with unsegmented nuclei and coarsely clumped nuclear chromatin.

Image 26-4   Bone marrow smear from a patient with a myelo-dysplastic syndrome. There is dyserythropoiesis with a multinucleated megaloblastoid erythroid precursor (arrow).

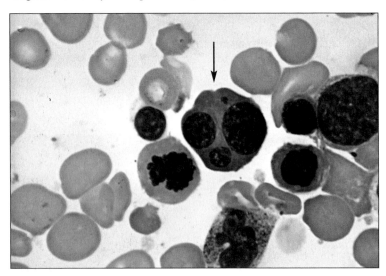

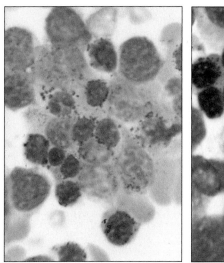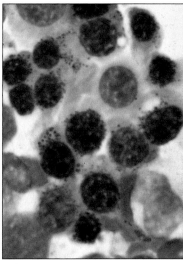

Image 26-5 Iron stains on a bone marrow smear from a patient with refractory anemia with ringed sideroblasts. Numerous ringed sideroblasts are visible. The smear on the right has a Wright's counterstain.

Image 26-6 Bone marrow aspirate smear from a patient with refractory cytopenia with multilineage dysplasia showing numerous neutrophil precursors. There is a shift toward immaturity, but the blast count is only 3%. There are obvious dysplastic changes in many of the cells.

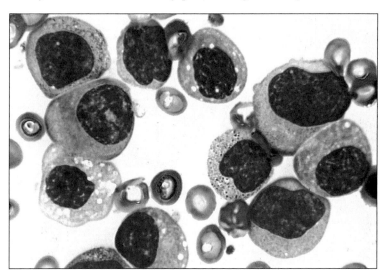

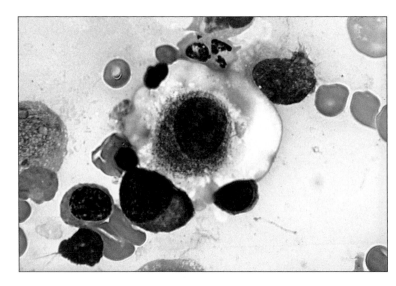

Image 26-7   A bone marrow aspirate smear from a patient with refractory anemia with excess blasts showing a dysplastic megakaryocyte and dyserythropoiesis. The megakaryocyte is uninucleated and small, and exhibits zoning of the cytoplasm.

Image 26-8   Blood smear from a patient with chronic myelomonocytic leukemia. Three atypical monocytes, two small lymphocytes, and a neutrophil are visible.

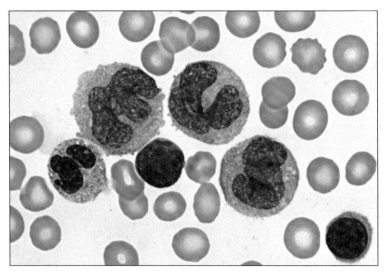

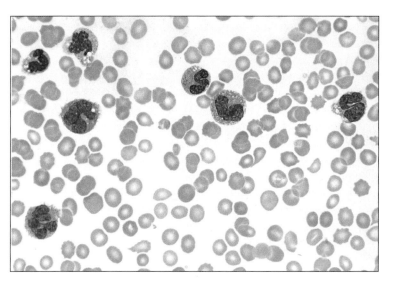

Image 26-9 Blood smear from a 2-year-old boy with juvenile myelomonocytic leukemia. The blood leukocyte count is $21 \times 10^3/mm^3$ ($21 \times 10^9/L$) with 30% monocytes. The remainder of the cells are mostly neutrophils, some exhibiting mild dysplastic changes. There is a moderate to marked thrombocytopenia and mild anemia.

Image 26-10 Bone marrow aspirate smear from a patient with AIDS showing myelodysplasia.

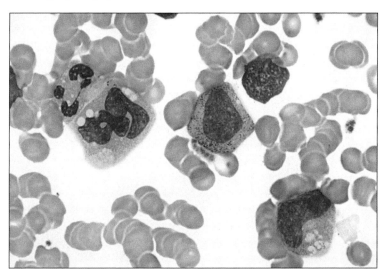

27   Acute Myeloid Leukemia

Acute myeloid leukemias (AMLs) are neoplastic proliferations arising in hematopoietic precursor cells. They result in overgrowth of myeloblasts and other immature cells of myeloid lineage. The malignant cells replace the bone marrow; circulate in the blood; and may accumulate in other tissues, including the lymph nodes, liver, and spleen. The overall incidence of AML in the United States is about 2.1 per 100,000 population per year. The age-specific incidence rate increases with age through the eighth decade. Eighty to ninety percent of acute leukemias in adults are AML.

27.1 Pathophysiology

The cause of AML is unknown, but studies suggest that genetic, environmental, and occupational factors may contribute to the etiology in some patients. Persons with Down syndrome, Bloom syndrome, Fanconi's anemia, neurofibromatosis, and several other genetic diseases are at higher risk of developing AML. Exposure to benzene and radiation, as well as treatment with alkylating agents and type II topoisomerase inhibitor drugs, increases the risk of AML.

AML originates in deranged clones of hematopoietic stem cells. Cell kinetic studies have shown that the rate of maturation of normal marrow cells is markedly reduced, leading to overgrowth of the malignant clone. The neoplastic cells replace the normal bone marrow cells, resulting in anemia, neutropenia, thrombocytopenia, and an outpouring of the neoplastic blasts into the peripheral blood. Death results from bone marrow failure, which leads to profound blood cytopenias, severe infections, and bleeding. The variants of AML are thought to represent maturation blocks that affect different stages of stem cell maturation.

27.2 Clinical Findings

The onset of symptoms may be insidious or abrupt; fatigue, malaise, pallor, weakness, and fever are the most common. An infection secondary to neutropenia is the initial manifestation in some patients. Hemorrhage in the form of petechiae, ecchymosis, or epistaxis is seen in less than 50% of patients. Bleeding is a particular problem in patients with acute promyelocytic leukemia, which is associated with disseminated intravascular coagulation (DIC).

Physical examination may reveal splenomegaly and lymphadenopathy, but both are usually less remarkable than in acute lymphoblastic leukemia (ALL). Sternal tenderness is common, and gingival hyperplasia may be a presenting sign in monocytic leukemias. Occasionally, an accumulation of blasts results in the formation of an extramedullary tumor mass or myeloid sarcoma. These tumors may form in any part of the body and occasionally precede other manifestations of leukemia. The clinical features of AML and their relationship to pathophysiology are summarized in **Table 27-1**.

27.3 Diagnostic Approach

The clinical manifestations already detailed are indications of a possible acute leukemia and dictate the series of laboratory tests that should be performed. After a complete history and physical examination, the laboratory evaluation for AML should proceed as follows:

Table 27-1 Clinical Features of Acute Leukemia Related to Pathophysiology

Pathophysiology	Clinical Features
Anemia	Weakness and pallor
Thrombocytopenia (occasionally DIC)	Bleeding or bruising
Granulocytopenia (immunosuppression)	Fever, infections
Leukemic infiltrates	Bone or joint pain, lymphadenopathy, hepatosplenomegaly
Leukemic cells in CSF (leptomeningeal leukemia infiltrates)	Neurologic symptoms (headache, vomiting, visual disturbance, etc)

Abbreviations: DIC = disseminated intravascular coagulation; CSF = cerebrospinal fluid.

1. A complete blood count.
2. Examination of a blood smear.
3. Bone marrow aspiration and trephine biopsy morphologic examination.
4. Cytochemical studies of blood and bone marrow.
5. Immunophenotyping of leukemic blasts by flow cytometry or immunocytochemistry.
6. Bone marrow cytogenetic studies.
7. Molecular analysis (in some cases).
8. Electron microscopy (in special cases).
9. Radiographic studies for assessment of extramedullary mass disease as clinically indicated.
10. Other laboratory tests, including coagulation studies, serum biochemistry studies, and febrile evaluation, as clinically indicated.

27.4 Hematologic Findings

The hematologic findings for AML vary. In many patients, the diagnosis is obvious from the blood smear examination. In others, the changes are subtle, and careful examination of blood smears and bone marrow by experienced individuals is required to make a

Table 27-2 Cytologic Features of Blasts in Acute Myeloid and Acute Lymphoblastic Leukemias

Feature	Acute Myeloid Leukemia	Acute Lymphoblastic Leukemia
Blast size	Large, often uniform	Variable, small to medium size
Nuclear chromatin	Usually finely dispersed	Coarse to fine
Nucleoli	1 to 4, often prominent	Absent or 1 or 2, often indistinct
Cytoplasm	Moderately abundant, granules often present	Usually scant, coarse granules sometimes present (~7%)
Auer rods	Present in 60%-70% of cases	Not present
Other cell types	Often dysplastic changes in maturing myeloid cells	Myeloid cells not dysplastic

diagnosis. Of first importance in the diagnosis is distinguishing AML from a reactive or other nonneoplastic condition. Secondly, AML must be distinguished from ALL because therapy differs significantly. Lastly, the subclassification of AML may provide prognostic or therapeutic insights.

The distinguishing features of AML and ALL are listed in **Table 27-2**. Evidence of these features, combined with results of the cytochemical, immunophenotypic, and cytogenetic studies, facilitates correct diagnosis and classification.

27.4.1 Blood Cell Measurements

Blood counts are abnormal in almost every case. In most patients, there is a reduction of at least two of the major normal cell lineages; often all three are reduced—ie, the patient has anemia, neutropenia, and thrombocytopenia. The anemia is usually normocytic and normochromic. The leukocyte count is elevated in more than 50% of patients due to the circulating blasts and other immature myeloid cells. Only about 20% of patients have leukocyte counts that exceed $100 \times 10^3/\text{mm}^3$ ($100 \times 10^9/\text{L}$).

27.4.2 Blood Smear Morphology

The decrease in the number of normal blood cells is apparent from examination of the peripheral blood smear. RBCs exhibit variable anisocytosis and poikilocytosis, and nucleated RBCs are often present. Neutropenia and thrombocytopenia are present in most cases. Dysplastic changes in the form of hypogranular and hyposegmented neutrophils and large atypical platelets may be observed. The number of leukemic blasts varies from numerous—with leukocyte counts greater than $100 \times 10^3/mm^3$ ($100 \times 10^9/L$)—to rare or absent. When blasts are sparse on the blood smear, the diagnosis of acute leukemia may be possible only with a bone marrow examination.

27.4.3 Bone Marrow Examination

A bone marrow examination should always be performed when a diagnosis of acute leukemia is considered. Complete clinical information is essential to the individual interpreting the bone marrow slides. Most errors in the diagnosis and classification of acute leukemia result from incomplete or erroneous clinical information, inadequate specimens, and technically poor blood and bone marrow preparations. The optimal morphologic evaluation for leukemia includes examination of well-prepared blood and bone marrow smears and trephine biopsy sections.

Bone marrow smears are usually hypercellular and consist predominantly of blasts and other immature and abnormal cells. Normal hematopoietic precursors are markedly reduced. There is retarded maturation of myeloid cells and variable dysplastic changes in granulocytic, erythroid, and megakaryocytic precursors. The number of blasts varies, but 20% or greater is required for a diagnosis of AML. Auer rods may be found in myeloblasts in 60% to 70% of patients.

The morphologic description of the blasts in the various categories of AML is provided in the section on classification. All morphologic criteria listed in **Table 27-2** should be considered when making an interpretation. Although there are usually distinctive features in AML and ALL, only the presence of unequivocal Auer rods always distinguishes them. When the morphologic findings are not distinctive for one of these major categories of acute leukemia, the appropriate diagnosis is usually determined by cytochemistry or immunophenotyping.

Trephine biopsy sections are usually markedly hypercellular, but occasionally a normocellular or even hypocellular marrow is encountered. Normal hematopoietic cells are replaced by a diffuse proliferation of leukemic cells. Scattered individual or clusters of megakaryocytes and other normal bone marrow elements may be observed.

27.5 The French-American-British Cooperative Group Classification

The French-American-British (FAB) classification of AML has been used widely since it was published in 1976. The classification is a lineage-based system that defines the categories primarily on morphology and cytochemistry, but immunophenotyping and other studies have been added in updated versions. The FAB classification has provided common terminology for hematologists and hematopathologists and a uniform base of comparison for studies published in the literature. The FAB classification of AML is shown in **Table 27-3**, and the case distribution of the categories is given in **Table 27-4**.

The blast percentage is the major feature that distinguishes AML from a myelodysplastic syndrome (MDS). The FAB classification requires a blast count of 30% or greater in the bone marrow for a diagnosis of AML. A World Health Organization (WHO) classification was proposed recently and incorporates the FAB classification while adding several distinctive cytogenetic categories of AML. In this proposed classification, the required percentage of blasts for a diagnosis of AML is 20% in the bone marrow or blood. This new criterion is based on compelling evidence that conditions with between 20% and 30% blasts behave clinically like AML and in most cases should be managed like acute leukemia. The WHO recommendation of 20% blasts for a diagnosis of AML is applied in the following discussion of FAB categories.

27.5.1 Myeloblastic Leukemia Minimally Differentiated (M0)
Criteria for the diagnosis of M0 are as follows:

1. Blasts are nongranular and may resemble lymphoblasts in some cases.
2. Less than 3% of blasts are myeloperoxidase positive by enzyme cytochemistry.
3. Blasts may express myeloperoxidase by immunohistochemical methods or by electron microscopy.
4. Blasts express myeloid antigens and are negative for lymphocyte antigens (in some cases, aberrant expression of lymphocyte antigens is observed).

Table 27-3 French-American-British (FAB) Classification of Acute Myeloid Leukemia

Myeloblastic leukemia minimally differentiated	M0
Myeloblastic leukemia without maturation	M1
Myeloblastic leukemia with maturation	M2
Hypergranular promyelocytic leukemia	M3
Microgranular (hypogranular) M3 variant	
Myelomonocytic leukemia	M4
With marrow eosinophilia (M4e)	
Monocytic leukemia	M5
Poorly differentiated (M5a)	
Differentiated (M5b)	
Erythroleukemia	M6
Megakaryoblastic leukemia	M7

Table 27-4 The Distribution of FAB Categories of AML

FAB Category	Sultan et al (n = 250)	Stanley et al (n = 358)
M0[*]	?	?
M1	21%	10%
M2	32%	45%
M3	16%	10%
Hypergranular		(7%)
Microgranular		(3%)
M4	16%	19%
With eosinophilia		(6%)
M5	12%	10%
Poorly differentiated		(6%)
Differentiated		(4%)
M6	3%	6%
M7[*]	?	?

Abbreviation: AML = acute myeloid leukemia
[*]Not included in these studies. The incidence of M0 is approximately 3% of AMLs. The incidence of M7 is up to 10% of AML in children.

Minimally differentiated AML includes the small number of cases that have a demonstrable myeloid lineage by immunophenotypic or ultrastructural findings but lack definitive cytologic and cyto-chemical criteria (**Image 27-1**). Two to three percent of cases of

AML are M0. There should be no expression of lineage-specific lymphocyte antigens by the leukemic blasts; lineage-associated antigens such as terminal deoxynucleotidyl transferase (TdT) and CD2, CD4, or CD7 sometimes are aberrantly expressed. Expression of these markers in AML should not be considered evidence of mixed lineage leukemia.

27.5.2 Myeloblastic Leukemia Without Maturation (M1)

Criteria for the diagnosis of M1 are as follows:

1. The myeloblast count must be 90% or greater of the nonerythroid cells.
2. The remaining cells must be either maturing granulocytes from promyelocytes onward or monocytes.
3. At least 3% of blasts must be myeloperoxidase or Sudan black B (SBB) positive.

The morphologic spectrum of myeloblasts may vary considerably in cases of M1 (**Image 27-2**). The blast nucleus is generally round. The cytoplasm may contain azurophilic granules. Auer rods are found in varying numbers of myeloblasts in approximately 50% of patients. Evidence of maturation to promyelocytes is minimal or absent. In many cases, the myeloblasts appear undifferentiated, and the myeloid nature of the leukemia is identified only after the myeloperoxidase stains are examined. When only 3% to 10% of the blasts are myeloperoxidase reactive, immunophenotyping studies should be performed to confirm the diagnosis.

27.5.3 Myeloblastic Leukemia With Maturation (M2)

Criteria for the diagnosis of M2 are as follows:

1. The myeloblast count is 20% to 89% of the nonerythroid cells.
2. Granulocytes from promyelocytes to mature neutrophils constitute more than 10% of cells.
3. Monocytic precursors are less than 20%.

This category is characterized by evidence of maturation beyond the myeloblast stage of development (**Image 27-3**). The maturing neutrophils often show dysplastic changes. Erythroid and megakaryocyte precursors may be dysplastic, and panmyelopathy is observed in some patients. Auer rods are found in about 70% of cases. Because of the obvious maturation in M2, the myeloid lineage of the leukemia is rarely in question. The finding of myeloperoxidase reactivity in the myeloblasts merely confirms the morphologic diagnosis.

The t(8;21)(q22;q11) bone marrow chromosome rearrangement is found in 20% to 25% of patients with M2. This category of AML is detailed in the section on the proposed WHO classification.

27.5.4 Hypergranular Promyelocytic Leukemia (M3)

Criteria for the diagnosis of M3 are as follows:

1. The majority of cells are abnormal promyelocytes with a characteristic pattern of heavy cytoplasmic granulation (**Image 27-4**).
2. The nucleus of the leukemic promyelocytes is often reniform.
3. Cells containing multiple Auer bodies are usually present.
4. In the microgranular variant, cytoplastic granules are fewer and smaller (**Image 27-5**).

Promyelocytic leukemia is a distinctive clinical, morphologic, ultrastructural, and cytogenetic entity and is discussed in detail in the section on the proposed WHO classification.

27.5.5 Myelomonocytic Leukemia (M4)

Criteria for the diagnosis of M4 are as follows:

1. The total percentage of myeloblasts and monoblasts is 20% or greater.
2. The total percentage of myeloblasts and granulocytes is 20% to 80%.
3. Twenty to seventy-nine percent of the bone marrow cells are of monocyte lineage.
4. If less than 20% of the marrow cells are monocytes, the diagnosis is still M4 if the blood monocyte count exceeds $5 \times 10^3/mm^3$ ($5 \times 10^9/L$).

Both granulocytic and monocytic differentiation are observed in varying proportions in the bone marrow (**Image 27-6**). The major criterion distinguishing M4 from M2 is the proportion of monoblasts, promonocytes, and monocytes, which collectively must equal 20% or greater. Monoblasts and early promonocytes cannot always be distinguished from granulocyte precursors in routine bone marrow smears. For this reason the additional criterion of nonspecific esterase reactivity in 20% or more of the cells or an elevated serum lysozyme of more than three times normal is included. Auer rods are present in the myeloblast component in approximately 60% of patients. The blood leukocyte count is often markedly elevated. Organomegaly, lymphadenopathy, and other tissue infiltration are common.

A variant of M4 has an inv(16) cytogenetic abnormality and increased and dysplastic bone marrow eosinophils (**Image 27-7**). It is designated M4 with marrow eosinophilia (M4e) in the FAB classification and is described in the discussion of the proposed WHO classification.

27.5.6 Monocytic Leukemia (M5)

The criterion for the diagnosis of M5 is as follows:

Eighty percent or more of all nonerythroid cells in the bone marrow are monoblasts, promonocytes, or monocytes.

There are two subcategories of M5 based on the percentage of the least mature monocyte precursors (monoblasts):

Poorly differentiated (M5a): 80% or more of the monocytic cells are monoblasts.
Differentiated (M5b): less than 80% of the monocytic cells are monoblasts; the remainder are promonocytes and monocytes.

Poorly differentiated monocytic leukemia is characterized by a predominance of monoblasts that are large and have moderately abundant, variably basophilic cytoplasm, which frequently contains delicate peroxidase-negative azurophilic granules (**Image 27-8**). Auer bodies are not observed. The nucleus is round with reticular chromatin and one or more prominent nucleoli. Because the morphology of the blasts is poorly differentiated in routine blood smears, the diagnosis is often made only with the aid of cytochemical stains. Monoblasts are nonspecific esterase positive and myeloperoxidase negative.

The leukemic cells in M5b manifest more obvious cyto-logic evidence of monocytic features. The nuclei have delicate chromatin and a characteristic folded or cerebriform appearance (**Image 27-9**). The promonocyte cytoplasm is usually less basophilic than that of M5a monoblasts and contains a variable number of azurophilic granules. Auer rods are rarely observed. The promonocytes are usually nonspecific esterase positive; some exhibit weak myeloperoxidase activity. In most cases of M5b, monoblasts constitute less than 20% of the marrow cells. Promonocytes are considered comparable to monoblasts for pur-poses of distinguishing leukemia from an MDS. The combination of monoblasts and promonocytes totals 20% or more.

Monocytic leukemia is associated with a relatively high inci-dence of organomegaly, lymphadenopathy, and tissue infiltration. The first clinical manifestations of leukemia are often extra-medullary tissue infiltrates, particularly in children with M5a.

27.5.7 Erythroleukemia (M6)

Criteria for the diagnosis of M6 are as follows:

1. Fifty percent or more of all nucleated bone marrow cells are erythroblasts.
2. Twenty percent or more of the remaining cells (nonerythroid) are myeloblasts.
3. Dyserythropoiesis is prominent.

Most patients with M6 present with pancytopenia and nucleat-ed RBCs in the blood. Many cases evolve from an MDS or present as a secondary leukemia in patients with prior alkylating agent chemotherapy. The predominant leukemic cells in the bone mar-row are erythroblasts. There is striking erythroid hyperplasia and dyserythropoiesis characterized by abnormalities of nuclear devel-opment, including megaloblastoid changes and karyorrhexis. Gigantoblasts with multiple nuclei are commonly present (**Image 27-10**). The leukemic erythroblasts may contain cytoplasmic vac-uoles that are positive by a periodic acid–Schiff (PAS) stain. There is often evidence of dysplastic megakaryocytes and platelets. Auer rods are present in myeloblasts in about 50% of patients. In rare cases, nearly 100% of the bone marrow cells are leukemic eryth-roblasts; the designations pure erythroleukemia, M6b, or eryth-remic myelosis have been used for this rare form of AML.

27.5.8 Megakaryoblastic Leukemia (M7)

Criteria for the diagnosis of M7 are as follows:

1. Twenty percent or more blasts are present in the bone marrow.
2. Blasts are of megakaryocyte lineage by expression of megakaryocyte-specific antigens and/or a positive platelet peroxidase reaction on electron microscopy.

In blood and bone marrow smears megakaryoblasts are usually medium to large cells. Nuclear chromatin is dense and homogeneous. Nucleoli are variably prominent. There is scant to moderately abundant cytoplasm, which may be vacuolated. An irregular cytoplasmic border is often noted, and occasionally projections resembling budding platelets are present. Transition forms between poorly differentiated blasts and recognizable micromegakaryocytes are often observed (**Image 27-11**). In some cases the majority of the leukemic cells consist of small lymphoidlike blasts. A bone marrow aspirate may be difficult to obtain because of frequent myelofibrosis. Trephine biopsy sections often reveal morphologic evidence of megakaryocytic differentiation that is not appreciated in the bone marrow aspirate smears.

Although many instances of M7 consist predominantly of poorly differentiated blasts, clues to their identity are often present. These include the presence of circulating micromegakaryocytes, atypical platelets, pseudopod projections on the surface of the blasts or zoning of the cytoplasm, myelofibrosis, and clusters of small megakaryocytes in trephine sections. More precise identification is accomplished with immunophenotyping or electron microscopy and ultracytochemistry. The more differentiated blasts are recognized by the presence of demarcation membranes and "bull's-eye" alpha granules by electron microscopy. Ultrastructural peroxidase activity is found in the nuclear envelope and endoplasmic reticulum but is absent from the granules and Golgi complexes of leukemic megakaryoblasts. This pattern of localization of the ultrastructural peroxidase reaction distinguishes megakaryoblasts from myeloblasts and is the earliest recognizable distinctive characteristic of megakaryoblasts. Immunophenotyping using monoclonal antibodies (MoAb) to megakaryocyte-restricted antigens (CD41 and CD61) may be diagnostic. The results of these studies are generally available in less time and at less expense than those from electron microscopy and ultracytochemistry.

The bone marrow chromosome abnormality +21 has been identified in some patients with M7. In addition there are a striking number of children with M7 who have a constitutional trisomy 21 chromosome abnormality (Down syndrome). In the first three years of life, megakaryoblastic leukemia is the most common type of leukemia in patients with Down syndrome. Neonates with Down syndrome may present with a transient myeloproliferative disorder (TMD) that may be indistinguishable from acute megakaryoblastic leukemia. Blood counts are elevated as high as $100 \times 10^3/\text{mm}^3$ ($100 \times 10^9/\text{L}$) in some cases of TMD, with numerous blasts, nucleated RBCs, megakaryoblasts, and micromegakaryocytes. The TMD spontaneously resolves in 2 to 14 weeks. The relatively common process in newborns with Down syndrome should not be mistaken for acute leukemia. Some patients with a history of TMD, however, later develop acute megakaryoblastic leukemia.

A variant of M7 with a t(1;22)(p13;q13) cytogenetic rearrangement has been described in young children. This leukemia is associated with marked organomegaly and prominent myelofibrosis. The leukemia may have features of a panmyelosis. The pattern of bone marrow and other organ involvement often resembles that of a metastatic tumor.

27.6 The World Health Organization Proposed Classification

A new classification of AML, proposed by WHO, was developed by the Society for Hematopathology in the United States and the European Association for Hematopathology. The WHO classification is shown in **Table 27-5**.

The proposed classification incorporates cytogenetic and molecular findings in addition to morphologic, cytochemical, and immunophenotypic features. The addition of categories with specific cytogenetic changes provides for a more precise diagnosis and introduces important prognostic correlations. The WHO proposal retains the FAB categories for cases of AML without distinctive cytogenetic rearrangements associated with specific clinical and prognostic features. In addition, the categories of acute basophilic leukemia, myeloid sarcoma, and acute panmyelosis with myelofibrosis have been added. The WHO classification also recognizes therapy-related AML as a distinct category.

Table 27-5   World Health Organization Proposed Classification
of Acute Myeloid Leukemia

I.	AML with recurrent cytogenetic translocations
	AML with t(8;21)
	AML with inv(16) or t(16;16)
	Promyelocytic leukemia with t(15;17)
	Promyelocytic leukemia with t(V;17)
	AML with 11q23 abnormalities
II.	AML with multilineage dysplasia*
	De novo AML with multilineage dysplasia
	AML following an MDS
III.	AML, NOS
	M0-M7 (FAB groups)
	Acute basophilic leukemia
	Myeloid sarcoma
	Acute panmyelosis with myelofibrosis
IV.	Therapy-related AML

Abbreviations: AML = acute myeloid leukemia; FAB = French-American-British classification; MDS = myelodysplastic syndrome; NOS = not otherwise specified.
*Classify using subgroups of category III.

A major change introduced in the WHO proposal is the reduction in the percentage of blasts required for a diagnosis of AML from 30% to 20%. The change eliminates the MDS category of refractory anemia with excess blasts in transformation. This was done because conditions with 20% to 30% blasts most commonly behave clinically like AML and should generally be managed as AML. The categories of the WHO classification of AML are described as follows.

27.6.1 Acute Myeloid Leukemia With Specific Cytogenetic Defects

This category includes four types of leukemia with distinctive morphologic, clinical, and prognostic features, in addition to specific cytogenetic and molecular findings.

Acute Myeloid Leukemia With t(8;21)(q22;q22)
The translocation results in a fusion product involving the *AML1* gene on chromosome 21 band q22 and the *ETO* gene on

chromosome 8 band q22. This group is one of the most common examples of association between a nonrandom reciprocal translocation and a specific subtype of AML. The morphologic features are nearly always those of the FAB M2 category and include large blasts, frequent and often large Auer rods, and striking dysplasia in the neutrophil lineage (*see Image 27-3*). Immunophenotypically, there is usually aberrant expression of the surface antigen CD19 and often expression of CD56. This category of AML is associated with a relatively favorable prognosis in adult patients.

Acute Myeloid Leukemia With inv(16)(p13;q22)

AML with inv(16)(p13;q22) or t(16;16)(p13;q22) generally has the morphologic features of myelomonocytic leukemia (FAB M4) with the addition of increased and dysplastic eosinophils (primarily an abundance of large basophilic staining granules) in the bone marrow (*see Image 27-7*).

The inv(16)(p13;q22) is a pericentric inversion of chromosome 16. The genes at the breakpoint junction are the β subunit of core binding factor (CBF) (CBFβ) at 16q22 and a gene encoding smooth muscle myosin heavy chain (MYH11) at 16p13.

AML with inv(16) constitutes approximately 8% of cases of adult AML and 25% to 30% of cases of FAB M4. The incidence among children with AML is not as well defined but appears to be as common as in adults. The incidence of extramedullary disease is approximately 50%, higher than for most types of AML; lymphadenopathy and hepatomegaly are particularly common. Granulocytic sarcoma concurrent with or preceding bone marrow involvement appears to be more common than in other leukemias. Some investigators have reported a high incidence of central nervous system relapse with intracerebral myeloblastomas. Complete remission rates of 76% and 92% have been reported. This category has a longer median survival time than other types of AML.

Promyelocytic Leukemia With t(15;17)(q22;q12-21)

This category of AML is associated with distinctive morphologic, clinical, and prognostic features and responds to a unique therapy. Promyelocytic leukemia with t(15;17) corresponds to FAB M3. In typical hypergranular promyelocytic leukemia the blood leukocyte count is usually decreased at presentation. The leukemic cell population is composed of abnormal promyelocytes (*see Image 27-4*). These cells are usually characterized by numerous red to purple cytoplasmic granules. The granules are often larger and darker staining than normal and may be so numerous that they obscure the nuclear borders. In some cases, a high percentage of the leukemic cells have basophilic cytoplasm. Cells containing multiple Auer rods are found in approximately 90% of patients. The Auer rods may be numerous and intertwined. Large globular inclusions of Auerlike material are found in the cytoplasm of occasional cells. The nuclei of many cells are reniform or bilobed. Myeloblasts are a minor component in most cases and rarely reach 20%. The abnormal promyelocytes are considered comparable to blasts for the purpose of diagnosing acute promyelocytic leukemia. In the microgranular variant of promyelocytic leukemia the blood leukocyte count is elevated, sometimes markedly. The leukemic cells have sparse and/or fine granulation and markedly irregular nuclei (*see Image 27-5*). Their identity as abnormal promyelocytes may be obscured by these features. Cells containing multiple Auer rods are usually present but less abundant than in typical hypergranular promyelocytic leukemia.

Typical hypergranular promyelocytic leukemia and the microgranular variant have the same characteristic ultrastructural, cytogenetic, molecular, and clinical features. They differ only in the size and number of granules, the prominence of the abnormal nuclear shape, and the magnitude of the blood leukocyte count.

The distinctive ultrastructural characteristics of the leukemic promyelocytes include Auer rods with a specific tubular substructure, markedly dilated endoplasmic reticulum, and stellate complexes of rough endoplasmic reticulum. The immunophenotype of most cases of promyelocytic leukemia differs from other AMLs by the lack of expression of HLA-DR and CD34 (**Image 27-12**). The t(15;17)(q22;q12-21) bone marrow chromosome rearrangement is not found in any other type of leukemia. The breakpoint regions are at the promyelocytic leukemia (*PML*) gene on band q22 of chromosome 15 and on band q12 at the first intron of the retinoic acid receptor α (*RARα*) gene on chromosome 17 (**Image 27-13**).

Acute promyelocytic leukemia may occur at any age but is most common in young and middle-aged adults; the median age at diagnosis is 35 to 40 years. Organomegaly is uncommon. The most outstanding clinical feature is the high frequency of DIC. Most patients experience severe DIC and hemorrhage prior to or during standard induction chemotherapy; hemorrhage is sometimes the cause of early death. When DIC and hemorrhage are adequately controlled, patients have an excellent chance for complete remission and prolonged survival.

The t(15;17) and resulting *PML-RARα* fusion gene imparts unique features to this leukemia that have led to a specific treatment regimen using all-*trans*-retinoic acid (ATRA). This treatment induces the leukemic cells to mature. Although a remission can be achieved with ATRA in most instances, relapse invariably occurs. Therefore, standard induction chemotherapy is generally given with or following ATRA. In adult patients who achieve a complete remission, the prognosis is better than for any other category of AML.

Promyelocytic Leukemia With t(V;17)(V;q12-21)

Uncommonly, a case with many of the morphologic and clinical features of promyelocytic leukemia has a variant cytogenetic translocation involving the *RARα* gene on chromosome 17 but not the *PML* gene on chromosome 15 (**Images 27-14** and **27-15**). A t(11;17) is one of the more common variant translocations, but other chromosomes also may be involved. Morphologically, promyelocytic leukemia with t(V;17) may have features intermediate between hypergranular promyelocytic leukemia (M3) and myeloblastic leukemia with maturation (M2) AML. As with typical M3, patients often experience DIC. Although this disease variant has many of the features of typical promyelocytic leukemia, it does not respond to ATRA therapy and may have an aggressive clinical course.

27.6.2 Acute Myeloid Leukemia With Multilineage Dysplasia

AML with multilineage dysplasia may present as a de novo AML or may evolve from an existing MDS. The morphologic features are similar in either case. The blast count is variable, and there is evidence of dysplasia in developing cells of more than one lineage; there is often an obvious panmyelopathy. There are no specific cytogenetic findings in this AML category, but trisomy 8 and abnormalities of chromosome 5 and/or 7 and complex cytogenetic rearrangements are common. These leukemias increase in incidence with age and may be the most common category of AML among older individuals.

Cases of AML with multilineage dysplasia sometimes overlap various FAB classes. They most often have the features of FAB M2 or M4, although cases of M1 and M6 also may exhibit multilineage dysplasia.

Many of the uncommon examples of hypocellular AML have multilineage dysplasia and may evolve from a hypocellular MDS. Hypocellular AML and MDS are defined by a bone marrow cellularity of less than 30% in patients under 60 years of age and less than 20% in patients over 60.

27.6.3 Acute Myeloid Leukemia, Not Otherwise Specified

Cases of AML that do not specifically fit either of the major WHO categories already discussed fall in the category of acute myeloid leukemia, not otherwise specified (AML, NOS) and are classified according to FAB criteria. In addition to the FAB categories there are three newly defined types of AML in this group, which are described here.

Acute Basophilic Leukemia

Although rare cases of acute leukemia with primarily basophil differentiation have been generally recognized, basophilic leukemia is not an FAB category. Recently, reports of cytologically undifferentiated leukemias with ultrastructural evidence of basophil differentiation have appeared. These poorly differentiated acute basophilic leukemias would most likely be classified as M0 if electron mi-croscopy were not used to confirm basophil lineage. Some cases may be classified as ALLs in the absence of immunophenotyping.

In differentiated cases, basophil granules that stain metachromatically with toluidine blue are identified with light microscopy (**Image 27-16**). In poorly differentiated cases, no or minimal basophil granules can be identified by light microscopy; this category is diagnosed by electron microscopic identification of early basophil granules. Blasts are myeloperoxidase negative by light microscopy but positive by electron microscopy, and cells express myeloid antigens.

Myeloid Sarcoma

Myeloid sarcomas are tumor masses of neoplastic immature myeloid cells in an extramedullary site (**Images 27-17** and **27-18**). Patients usually have evidence of myeloid leukemia in the bone marrow and blood, but some myeloid sarcomas occur without obvious leukemia. The most common sites for myeloid sarcomas are the subperiosteal bone, skin, lymph nodes, orbit, spinal canal, and mediastinum. Several categories of AML may present with myeloid sarcomas, but myelomonocytic and monocytic leukemias appear to be most frequent. Myelomonocytic leukemias with the inv(16) cytogenetic abnormality commonly have extramedullary tumors. Poorly differentiated monocytic leukemias in children (FAB M5a) often present with extramedullary lesions.

Acute Panmyelosis With Myelofibrosis

Acute panmyelosis with myelofibrosis is an uncommon form of acute leukemia occurring primarily in adults and rarely in children. Patients present with pancytopenia and panmyeloid proliferation. There are usually prominent megakaryocytic abnormalities; some cases are considered acute megakaryoblastic leukemias with profound myelofibrosis (**Image 27-19**). The degree of fibrosis varies. In most cases, there is marked reticulin fibrosis; collagen fibrosis is less common. The spleen is generally normal or minimally increased in size.

The disease has an aggressive course. The differential diagnosis includes chronic idiopathic myelofibrosis with myeloid metaplasia and MDS with myelofibrosis. The lack of splenomegaly and prominent dysplasia in the developing cells distinguishes this disorder from the myeloproliferative syndrome chronic idiopathic myelofibrosis. The elevated blast percentage distinguishes acute panmyelosis with myelofibrosis from an MDS.

27.6.4 Therapy-Related Acute Myeloid Leukemia

Therapy-related AMLs and MDSs occur in patients who have received chemotherapy for a neoplastic or nonneoplastic disorder. The two major types of drugs associated with therapy-related AMLs are alkylating agents and type II topoisomerase inhibitor drugs. The features of AMLs and MDSs associated with these two classes of drugs are detailed in Chapter 26.

Other Laboratory Tests

Test 27.1 Cytochemistry

Purpose. Cytochemical stains on blood and bone marrow smears are helpful in distinguishing AML from ALL and in subclassifying AML (**Tables 27-6** and **27-7**).

Table 27-6 Cytochemistry for Acute Leukemia

Reaction	Primary Normal Cells Manifesting Reaction	Major Diagnostic Utility
Myeloperoxidase	Neutrophil series, eosinophils (cyanide resistant), monocytes ±	Myeloid leukemia without maturation (M1), myeloid leukemia with maturation (M2), microgranular promyelocytic leukemia (M3)
Sudan black B	Neutrophil series, monocytes ±	M1, M2, microgranular M3
Chloroacetate esterase	Neutrophil series	M1, M2, microgranular M3, granulocytic sarcomas
Nonspecific esterase (α-naphthyl acetate or α-naphthyl butyrate)	Monocytes (inhibited by sodium fluoride)	Myelomonocytic leukemia (M4); monocytic leukemia, poorly differentiated (M5a); monocytic leukemia, differentiated (M5b)
Periodic acid–Schiff (PAS)		Erythroleukemia (M6), acute lymphoblastic leukemias
Terminal deoxynucleotidyl transferase (TdT)	T and B lymphocyte precursors	Acute lymphoblastic leukemias

Table 27-7 Cytochemical Profiles of Acute Leukemias

	MPO	SBB	CAE	NSE	PAS	AP
Acute myeloid leukemia	+	+	+	+ diffuse (M4, M5)	+/– (M5, M6, M7)	+/–
Acute lymphoblastic leukemia	–	–	–	–/+ (focal)	+ (75%)	+ T-ALL focal paranuclear

Abbreviations: MPO = myeloperoxidase; SBB = Sudan black B; CAE = chloroacetate esterase; NSE = nonspecific esterase; PAS = periodic acid–Schiff; AP = acid phosphatase.

Principle. Enzymatic activity in the cytoplasm is demonstrated by means of specific substrates and appropriate couplers, which provide localized color in the area of enzyme activity. The color is produced when one of the products of the enzyme action unites with the coupler.

Specimen. Smears are made from blood and bone marrow. Capillary blood from a fingerstick or anticoagulated blood may be used. Special fixatives are recommended for some stains, but most can be performed on air-dried smears. Ideally, all cytochemical stains should be made on recently prepared slides. Because this is often impractical, however, unstained smears can be stored away from light in a desiccator or refrigerator for some reactions. For the myeloperoxidase stain, a fresh smear is preferred.

Procedure. A variety of cytochemical stains are available, and a cytochemical profile exists for each hematopoietic cell lineage (*see Table 27-6*). Myeloperoxidase, which is present in primary granules, SBB, and specific esterase stains (chloroacetate esterase) are reactive in cells in the neutrophil lineage, variable in other granulocytic cells, and nonreactive in lymphocytes. These stains are therefore useful in differentiating between AML and ALL. The myeloperoxidase stain appears to have the best sensitivity and specificity of the three (**Image 27-20**). Sudan black B stains a variety of lipids in granulocytes and is especially useful when fresh specimens are unavailable and in occasional cases when the leukemic myeloblasts have an acquired myeloperoxidase deficiency. The specific esterase stain is less sensitive than SBB and peroxidase but may be useful in distinguishing granulocytic from lymphocytic cell proliferations in paraffin-embedded tissue sections.

Nonspecific esterase (using α-naphthol acetate or α-naphthol butyrate as substrates) stains monocytes and histiocytes diffusely and is used to identify monocytic leukemias (M4 and M5) (**Image 27-21**). NSE stains with the substrates already listed do not react with myeloblasts or neutrophil precursors to any significant degree.

The PAS reaction is not useful in differentiating acute leukemias. The typical block staining of lymphoblasts in ALL may occasionally be seen in AML. Positive reactions with PAS stain are frequently observed in poorly differentiated monocytic leukemia (M5a), erythroleukemia (M6), and megakaryoblastic leukemia (M7).

TdT is a DNA polymerase present in both T- and B-lymphocyte progenitors but absent in normal myeloid cells. A TdT assay is useful in distinguishing ALL from AML, although the myeloblasts in a small percentage of patients with AML may express TdT activity. The TdT assay is performed by flow cytometry, immunofluorescence micriscopy or immunohistochemical methods.

Interpretation. Factors relating to the interpretation and diagnostic utility of the special stains described are listed in **Tables**

27-6 and **27-7**. The myeloperoxidase (MPO) reaction primarily stains normal and leukemic myeloblasts and developing neutrophils; the intensity of the reaction increases with maturation. The reaction is in a diffuse granular pattern in the cytoplasm. Monocytes stain variably positive with MPO.

When an α-naphthol butyrate substrate is used, the NSE stain produces a diffuse cytoplasmic reaction in normal monocytes and monocytic leukemias (M4 and M5). Most mature T lymphocytes react to NSE with a dot of dense, localized positivity in the cytoplasm; some cases of ALL may show a similar pattern. A diffuse cytoplasmic reaction may be observed in epithelial cell malignancies. Positive staining with NSE also may be found in erythroblasts in megaloblastic anemia. In megakaryoblastic leukemia (M7), the α-naphthol acetate NSE stain often stains the blasts in a focal pattern in the cytoplasm. This is less common with a butyrate substrate.

Coarse granular PAS staining is characteristic of the blasts in ALL but is also found in erythroblasts in approximately 60% of patients with erythroleukemia (M6) and commonly in the blasts in poorly differentiated monocytic (M5a) and megakaryoblastic (M7) leukemias.

TdT is found in 95% of patients with ALL and in 5% to 10% of patients with AML. TdT reactivity in ALL is usually present in 80% to 100% of the blasts, whereas in AML the activity is typically weaker and present in a smaller percentage of cells.

Notes and Precautions. Considerable technical expertise is required to perform many of the staining techniques well. Experience in interpreting cytochemical stains in acute leukemia is required, because leukemic cells may not stain the same way as their normal counterparts. For example, one may observe neutrophils from patients with an AML (and an MDS) that stain negatively for myeloperoxidase. Occasionally, the immature cells in AML are negative with peroxidase stains but positive with SBB. Rare cases of SBB-positive granules in ALL also have been reported.

Test 27.2 **Immunophenotyping**

Purpose. Immunophenotyping leukemic blasts is important in distinguishing AML from ALL and in classifying cases of poorly differentiated AML.

Principle, Specimen, and Procedure. See Test 28.2.

Interpretation. Immunophenotyping has less therapeutic and prognostic significance for AML than for ALL. It is primarily important in distinguishing cases of AML from ALL when the morphologic and cytochemical profile of the leukemic cells is not definitive. In classifying AMLs, immunophenotyping is necessary to identify myeloblastic leukemia minimally differentiated (M0) and, often, megakaryoblastic leukemias (M7). Cases of myeloblastic leukemia without maturation (M1) with less than 10% myeloperoxidase-positive cells and the rare examples of NSE–negative monocytic leukemias (M5) also should be confirmed by immunophenotyping. Immunohistochemical stains on bone marrow sections can be particularly helpful in patients with myelofibrosis from whom an aspirate cannot be obtained for flow cytometry. An anti-CD34 antibody can be used to assess the number of blasts in biopsy sections, and myeloperoxidase and CD68 antibodies can be used to assess myeloid and monocytic cells, respectively.

Immunophenotypic classification of AML can be achieved by using panels of monoclonal antibodies with specificity for various myeloid antigens associated with maturation and differentiation. HLA-DR (Ia) reactivity is seen in most cases of AML except for promyelocytic leukemias (M3), which are also CD34 negative. The myelomonocytic and monocytic leukemias (M4 and M5) can usually be detected by their expression of both CD64 and CD36, along with CD14 in some cases, or by immunohistochemical stains for CD68 on paraffin-embedded tissue sections. Monoclonal antibodies that recognize platelet glycoprotein determinants CD41 and CD61 are used to identify megakaryoblastic leukemias. **Table 27-8** lists antibodies commonly used in the immunophenotypic characterization of AML.

27.7 Ancillary Tests

27.7.1 Cytogenetics

Bone marrow cytogenetic studies are essential in evaluating patients with acute leukemia and should always be performed.

Table 27-8 Antigen Expression in Acute Myeloid Leukemias

Antigen	M0, M1, M2	M3	M4, M5	M6	M7
CD13	+	+	+	+	+/–
CD33	+	+	+	+	+/–
HLA-DR	+	–/+	+	–/+	+/–
CD64	–/+	+/–	+	–	–
CD14	–/+	–	+	–	–
CD36	–/+	–	+	+	+
CD71	+/–	+/–	+/–	+	+/–
Glycophorin A	–	–	–	+/–	–
CD41 and CD61	–	–	–	–	+

They supplement the morphologic, cytochemical, and immuno-phenotypic studies in the characterization of AML and may contribute to the distinction between AML and ALL in selected cases. Most importantly, cytogenetic studies provide the most reliable independent indicators of prognosis; cytogenetics are incorporated into the WHO classification to define specific categories of AML. Chromosome abnormalities are found in most patients with AML when sensitive banding techniques are used. Structural changes are common and may involve a single rearrangement or multiple complex abnormalities. Fluorescence in situ hybridization (FISH) techniques are highly effective for detecting both numeric and structural chromosome abnormalities. In some cases with apparently normal cytogenetic studies, molecular translocations are identified by FISH or polymerase chain reaction (PCR) techniques (see Chapter 48).

Several specific chromosome rearrangements have been incorporated into the WHO classification of AML (*see Table 27-5*). Survival study data indicate that AMLs may be separated into low-, intermediate-, and high-grade diseases based on bone marrow cytogenetic findings (**Table 27-9**).

27.7.2 Molecular Analysis

Molecular studies are valuable in bone marrow diagnosis for several reasons. They may establish clonality, detect specific chromosome translocations and other cryptic structural rearrangements, identify virus genomes associated with neoplasms, and detect minimal residual disease. Molecular studies have proven

Table 27-9 Prognostic Implications of Chromosome Findings in Acute Myeloid Leukemia

Prognostic Group	Chromosome Findings
Favorable	Inv(16) or t(16;16) t(8;21) Single miscellaneous defects
Intermediate	t(15;17) +8 t(6;9) t(9;11) (children) Normal
Unfavorable	-7 or 5, del 7q t(11q23) inv(3q) Complex abnormalities

utility in diagnosing various lymphoproliferative disorders and play an increasingly important role in the diagnosis and management of patients with acute leukemia. Information provided by gene rearrangement studies and probes for detection of molecular translocations contributes directly to the classification of leukemias and may provide valuable treatment and prognostic information. The number of DNA probes available to detect specific genes associated with subtypes of leukemia that are clinically relevant is expanding. Some of the major fusion genes and the corresponding chromosome translocations in AML are listed in **Table 27-10**.

FISH and PCR studies for specific gene segments are proving to be highly sensitive indicators of minimal residual leukemia and early relapse. Another potentially important clinical application of molecular biology is in the measurement of expression of multiple drug resistance genes. These studies may prove useful in treatment design and prediction of response to therapy. Molecular diagnosis will continue to play an increasingly important role in the future.

27.7.3 Electron Microscopy and Ultracytochemistry

Electron microscopy may be useful in the characterization of acute leukemia when the leukemic blasts fail to manifest differentiating features on morphologic or cytochemical examination. Ultracytochemical peroxidase techniques are useful in characterizing

Table 27-10   Major Molecular Genetic Abnormalities in Acute Myeloid Leukemia

Cytogenetic Translocation	Molecular Genetic Abnormality
t(8;21)(q22;q22)	*ETO-AML1* fusion
inv(16)(p13;q22)	*MYH11-CBF*β fusion
t(15;17)(q22;q21)	*PML-RAR*α fusion
t(6;9)(p23;q34)	*DEK-CAN* fusion
t(9;11)(p22;q23)	*MLL-AF9* fusion

minimally differentiated and megakaryoblastic AMLs. Poorly differentiated basophilic leukemia may be diagnosed only by recognition of early basophil granules on ultrastructural examination. Rare cases of NSE–negative monocytic leukemia may be recognized by electron microscopy findings or an ultracytochemical esterase reaction. With the present immunophenotyping methods, however, and the array of monoclonal and polyclonal antibodies available for this purpose, the role of electron microscopy in the diagnosis of acute leukemias has been greatly diminished.

27.7.4 Coagulation Studies

Bleeding in AML is usually caused by thrombocytopenia. In patients with severe bleeding, however, DIC should be considered. DIC is particularly associated with acute promyelocytic leukemia (M3).

27.7.5 Serum Biochemistry

Serum uric acid levels are frequently elevated, especially in patients with high WBC counts and those undergoing induction chemotherapy. Uric acid is the end product of nucleic acid degeneration. Elevated serum levels of calcium and magnesium also may be seen. Similarly, serum lactate dehydrogenase levels are usually elevated.

27.7.6 Febrile Evaluation

The incidence of infection in patients with AML increases with the degree of neutropenia. Any patient with fever should be thoroughly evaluated for infection.

27.8 Differential Diagnosis

Differential diagnosis problems are often encountered in diagnosing and classifying AML. Difficulty in distinguishing AML from ALL or an MDS is most common. Other hematopoietic malignancies and, occasionally, leukemoid reactions, agranulocytosis, megaloblastic anemia, and other causes of disrupted hematopoiesis may be considerations. Distinguishing AML from ALL is most difficult when the blasts are poorly differentiated morphologically. An MDS may be considered in patients with a relatively low bone marrow blast count. In such situations, a diagnosis of AML is reached by the bone marrow blast percentage, the cytologic features of the blasts, and their cytochemical profile. When a diagnosis of AML cannot be made using these techniques, immunophenotyping studies nearly always clarify the issue. Other supplementary studies (eg, cytogenetics) are sometimes required. The features that define AML and distinguish it from ALL have already been covered in detail. **Table 27-11** lists the major differential diagnosis considerations for the individual FAB classes of AML and the studies most helpful in making a diagnosis.

27.9 Course and Treatment

All categories of AML are presently treated with the same basic chemotherapy regimens, except for cases of promyelocytic leukemia, in which ATRA therapy also may be used. Most patients undergo three phases of chemotherapy: induction, consolidation, and maintenance. The most common induction regimens include a combination of cytosine arabinoside, an anthracycline (daunorubicin or doxorubicin), and (often) 6-thioguanine. This combination induces a complete remission in approximately 70% of patients. The duration of complete remission can be prolonged and cure rates increased by administering consolidation chemotherapy shortly after the patient achieves remission with the same agents used for induction. Maintenance chemotherapy is less important in AML than in ALL, and its use is somewhat controversial; some studies show an improved remission duration but no apparent effect on cure rate.

Table 27-11   Differential Diagnosis of Acute Myeloid
                 Leukemia

FAB Category of AML	Considerations in the Differential Diagnosis	Studies Helpful in the Differential Diagnosis
M0, minimally differentiated	ALL, particularly L2 AML-M1, M5a, M7	Immunophenotype Cytochemistry (MPO, NSE), immunophenotype
	Poorly differentiated, basophilic leukemia	Electron microscopy
M1, without maturation	ALL, particularly L2	Cytochemistry (MPO), immunophenotype
	AML-M0, M5a, M7	Cytochemistry (MPO, NSE), immunophenotype
	Basophilic leukemia	Electron microscopy
M2, with maturation	Leukemoid reaction	Clinical history; % blasts, Auer rods, dysplasia; immunophenotypic aberrancy; cytogenetics
	Myelodysplastic syndrome	% blasts
	AML-M1, M3, M4, M6	FAB cytologic and cytochemical criteria
M3, promyelocytic		
Hypergranular	Agranulocytosis	Clinical history, cytology, Auer rods; immunophenotypic aberrancy; cytogenetics
	AML-M2	Cytology, eg, multiple Auer rods; immunophenotype; cytogenetics
Microgranular	AML-M4, M5b	Cytochemistry (MPO, NSE)
M4, myelomonocytic	Leukemoid reaction	% blasts, dysplasia, Auer rods; immunophenotypic aberrancy; cytogenetics
	Myelodysplastic syndrome	% blasts
	M2, M5, microgranular M3	Cytochemistry (MPO, NSE)
M5, monocytic		
M5a	ALL-L2	Cytochemistry (NSE), immunophenotype
	AML-M0, M1, M7	Cytochemistry (MPO, NSE), immunophenotype
M5b	M4, myelodysplastic syndrome	% monoblasts and promonocytes

Table 27-11 *Continued*

FAB Category of AML	Considerations in the Differential Diagnosis	Studies Helpful in the Differential Diagnosis
M6, erythroleukemia	Megaloblastic anemia and other secondary dyserythropoiesis, eg, drug effects, arsenic	Clinical history, % blasts, type of dyserythropoiesis, B_{12} and folate, arsenic levels
	Myelodysplastic syndrome	% blasts
	AML-M2	% erythroblasts
M7, megakaryoblastic	ALL	Immunophenotype
	AML-M0, M1, M5a	Cytochemistry (MPO, NSE), immunophenotype (CD41, CD61)

The median length of cure rate with standard chemotherapy regimens that include postinduction consolidation is about 30 months. Cure rates with chemotherapy alone are between 10% and 30%. Allogeneic bone marrow transplantation in first remission has achieved long-term disease-free survival in 45% to 60% of patients. This is presently the preferred treatment in suitable patients with a matched donor.

The most important indicators of treatment response and survival are

1. Age
2. Leukocyte count
3. A preexisting MDS
4. The speed at which remission is obtained
5. Cytogenetic findings

Young patients, particularly children, have higher remission and disease-free survival rates than older individuals. Very young patients (under 2 years of age) and patients over 60 years of age have the poorest treatment responses and survival rates. Patients with marked leukocytosis at diagnosis have a much poorer response than those with normal or mildly elevated leukocyte counts. Patients with a history of an MDS have a lower complete remission rate and a shorter survival time.

The rapidity of cytoreduction with chemotherapy and repopulation of the bone marrow with normal hematopoietic cells is a good indicator of remission duration and survival; patients who experience a rapid complete remission generally fare better than slow responders. Bone marrow cytogenetic findings also are important indicators of prognosis. The chromosome findings that indicate favorable and unfavorable prognosis are shown in **Table 27-9**.

27.10 References

Barbui T, Finazzi G, Falanga A. The impact of all-*trans*-retinoic acid on the coagulopathy of acute promyelocytic leukemia. *Blood.* 1998;91:3093–3102.

Bendeaux DH, Glosser L, Serokmann R, et al. Hypoplastic acute leukemia: review of 70 cases with multivariate regression analysis. *Hematol Oncol.* 1986;4:291–305.

Bennett JM, Catovsky D, Daniel M-T, et al. Proposals for the classification of the acute leukaemias. *Br J Haematol.* 1976;33:451–458.

Bennett JM, Catovsky D, Daniel M-T, et al. Criteria for the diagnosis of acute leukemia of megakaryocyte lineage (M7). *Ann Intern Med.* 1985;103:460–462.

Bennett JM, Catovsky D, Daniel M-T, et al. Proposed revised criteria for the classification of acute myeloid leukaemia. *Ann Intern Med.* 1985;103:620–625.

Bennett JM, Catovsky D, Daniel M-T, et al. Proposal for the recognition of minimally differentiated acute myeloid leukaemia (AML-M0). *Br J Haematol.* 1991;78:325–329.

Berger R, Bernheim A, Daniel M-T, et al. Cytologic characterization and significance of normal karyotypes in t(8;21) AML. *Blood.* 1982;59:171–178.

Bitter MA, LeBeau MM, Rowley JD, et al. Associations between morphology, karyotype, and clinical features in myeloid leukemias. *Hum Pathol.* 1987;18:211–225.

Brunning RD, McKenna RW. Tumors of the bone marrow: acute leukemias. In: Brunning RD, McKenna RW, eds. *Atlas of Tumor Pathology.* 3rd Series, Fascicle 9. Washington, DC: Armed Forces Institute of Pathology; 1994:19–142.

Fischer K, Fröhling S, Scherer SW, et al. Molecular cytogenetic delineation of deletions and translocations involving chromosome band 7q22 in myeloid leukemias. *Blood.* 1997;89:2036–2041.

Haferlach T, Löffler H, Nickenig C, et al. Cell lineage specific involvement in acute promyelocytic leukaemia (APL) using a combination of May-Grünwald-Giemsa staining and fluorescence in situ hybridization techniques for the detection of the translocation t(15;17)(q22;q12). *Br J Haematol.* 1998;103:93–99.

Harris NL, Jaffe ES, Diebold J, et al. The World Health Organization Classification of Hematological Malignancies Report of the Clinical Advisory Committee Meeting, Airlie House, Virginia, November 1997. *Mod Pathol.* 2000;13(2):193–207.

Hernández JA, Land KJ, McKenna RW. Leukemias, myeloma, and other lymphoreticular neoplasms. *Cancer.* 1995;75:381–394.

Holmes R, Keating M, Cork A, et al. A unique pattern of central nervous system leukemia in acute myelomonocytic leukemia associated with inv(16)(p13q22). *Blood.* 1985;65:1071–1078.

Kersey JH. Fifty years of studies of the biology and therapy of childhood leukemia. *Blood.* 1997;90:4243–4251.

Knuutila S. Lineage specificity in haematological neoplasms. *Br J Haematol.* 1997;96:2–11.

Licht JD, Chomienne C, Goy A, et al. Clinical and molecular characterization of a rare syndrome of acute promyelocytic leukemia associated with translocation (11;17). *Blood.* 1995;85:1083–1094.

Liu PP, Hajra A, Wijmenga C, et al. Molecular pathogenesis of the chromosome 16 inversion in the M4Eo subtype of acute myeloid leukemia. *Blood.* 1995;85:2289–2302.

Lu G, Altman AJ, Benn PA. Review of the cytogenetic changes in acute megakaryoblastic leukemia: one disease or several. *Cancer Genet Cytogenet.* 1993;67:81–89.

McKenna RW. A multifaceted approach to diagnosis and classification of acute leukemia. *Arch Pathol Lab Med.* 1991;115:328–330.

McKenna RW, Parkin J, Bloodfield C, et al. Acute promyelocytic leukaemia: study of 39 cases with identification of a hyperbasophilic microgranular APL variant. *Br J Haematol.* 1982;50:201–214.

Nucifora G, Rowley JD. AML1 and the 8;21 and 3;21 translocations in acute and chronic myeloid leukemia. *Blood.* 1995;86:1–14.

Peterson LC, Parkin JL, Arthur DC, et al. Acute basophilic leukemia: a clinical morphologic and cytogenetic study of eight cases. *Am J Clin Pathol.* 1991;96:160–170.

Soekarman D, von Lindern M, Daenen S, et al. The translocation (6;9)(p23;q34) shows consistent rearrangement of two genes and defines a myeloproliferative disorder with specific clinical features. *Blood.* 1992;79:2990–2997.

Stanley M, McKenna RW, Ellinger G, et al. Classification of 358 cases of acute myeloid leukemia by FAB criteria: analysis of clinical and morphologic features. In: Bloomfield CD, ed. *Chronic and Acute Leukemia in Adults.* Boston, Mass: Martinus Nijhoff; 1985:147–174.

Sultan C, Deregnaucourt J, Ko YW, et al. Distribution of 250 cases of acute myeloid leukaemia (AML) according to the FAB classification and response to therapy. *Br J Haematol.* 1981;47:545–551.

Tenen DG, Hromas R, Licht JD, et al. Transcription factors, normal myeloid development, and leukemia. *Blood.* 1997;90:489–519.

Vardiman JW, Head D. Society for Hematopathology: the myelodysplastic syndromes and related disorders. *Mod Pathol.* 1999;12:101–106.

Venditti A, Del Poeta G, Buccisano F, et al. Prognostic relevance of the expression of TdT and CD7 in 335 cases of acute myeloid leukemia. *Leukemia.* 1998;12:1056–1063.

Zeleznik-Le NJ, Nucifora G, Rowley JD. The molecular biology of myeloproliferative disorders as revealed by chromosomal abnormalities. *Semin Hematol.* 1995;32:201–219.

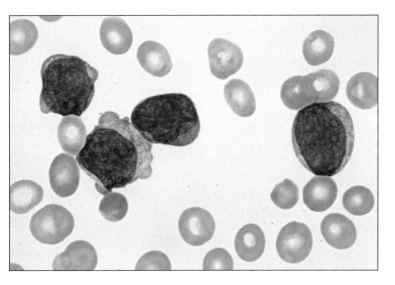

Image 27-1   Myeloblastic leukemia minimally differentiated (M0). The blasts are morphologically poorly differentiated. Myeloperoxidase and nonspecific esterase stains were negative. The myeloid lineage of the blasts was identified by flow cytometric immunophenotyping.

Image 27-2   Myeloblastic leukemia without maturation (FAB M1). More than 90% of the bone marrow cells are myeloblasts; approximately 10% are myeloperoxidase positive. One of the myeloblasts in this field contains a small Auer rod (arrow).

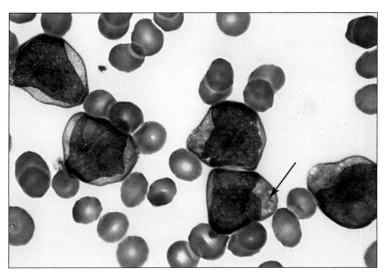

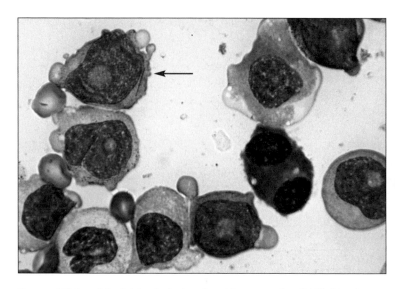

Image 27-3   Myeloblastic leukemia with maturation (M2). Myeloblasts number about 50% in the bone marrow. In addition to myeloblasts, dysplastic neutrophil precursors and a dysplastic erythroblast are depicted. One of the myeloblasts contains a large Auer rod (arrow). Bone marrow cytogenetics revealed a t(8;21)(q22;q22) rearrangement.

Image 27-4   Hypergranular promyelocytic leukemia (M3). Most of the cells are abnormal-appearing promyelocytes with heavy granulation and reniform nuclei. Multiple Auer rods are present in the cytoplasm of one of the cells (arrow). Cytogenetic studies revealed a t(15;17)(q22;q21) rearrangement.

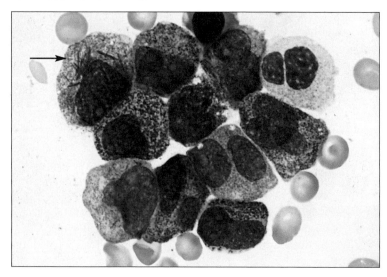

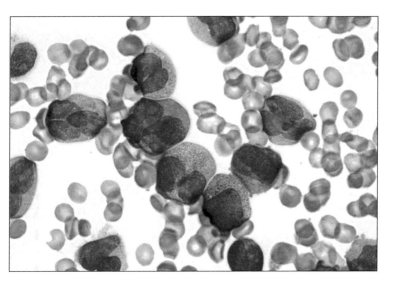

Image 27-5 Promyelocytic leukemia, microgranular (hypogranular) variant (M3v). The leukemic cells have smaller and fewer granules than the cells shown in Image 27-4. Most of the nuclei are folded or convoluted. A t(15;17) chromosome rearrangement was identified.

Image 27-6 Myelomonocytic leukemia (M4). Myeloblasts (one arrow) and promonocytes (two arrows) are depicted.

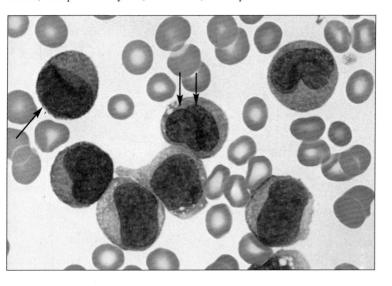

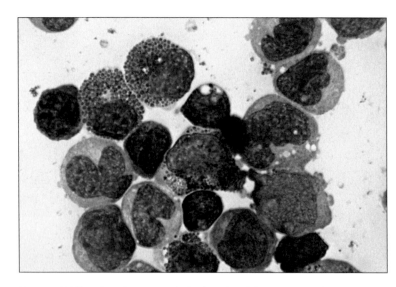

Image 27-7 Myelomonocytic leukemia with marrow eosinophilia (M4e). Increased bone marrow eosinophils with dysplastic granules characterize this leukemia. The eosinophil precursor in the center of the field contains large and irregular dark-staining granules in addition to the eosinophil granules. Cytogenetic studies revealed an inv(16)(p13;q22) rearrangement.

Image 27-8 Monocytic leukemia, poorly differentiated (M5a). The monoblasts have round nuclei and abundant cytoplasm. The lack of morphologic features typical of monocytes requires that a nonspecific esterase stain be performed to classify this type of monocytic leukemia.

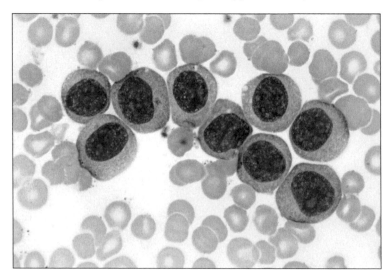

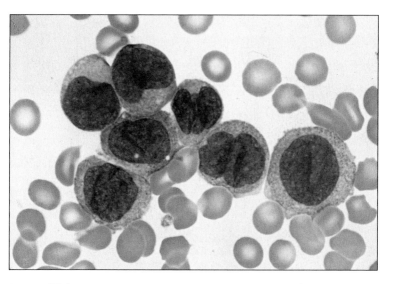

Image 27-9 Monocytic leukemia, differentiated (M5b). Promonocytes predominate.

Image 27-10 Erythroleukemia (M6). More than 50% of the bone marrow nucleated cells are erythroid. Myeloblasts constitute more than 20% of the nonerythroid cells. Markedly dysplastic changes are noted in the erythroblasts.

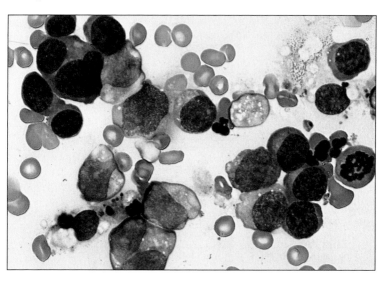

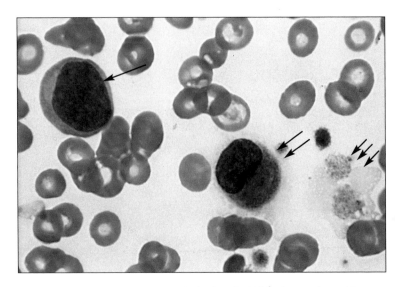

Image 27-11 Megakaryoblastic leukemia (M7). A megakaryoblast (one arrow), micromegakaryocyte (two arrows), and large atypical platelet (three arrows) are evident.

Image 27-12 Flow cytometric histograms of the neoplastic cells (red) from a patient with promyelocytic leukemia with t(15;17). The neoplastic cells exhibit significant orthogonal scatter, indicative of cytoplasmic granulation; express only dim, partial HLA-DR; and are negative for CD34, typical of promyelocytic leukemia.

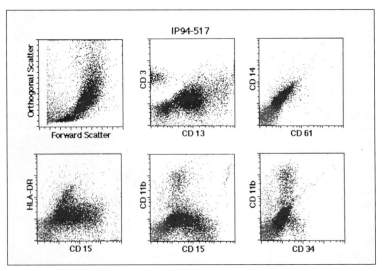

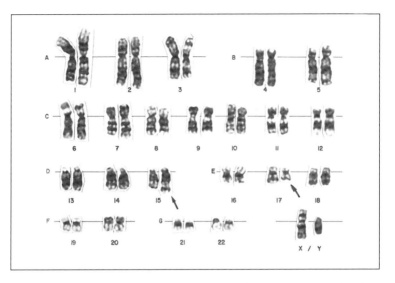

Image 27-13 Typical karyotype of neoplastic cells in promyelocytic leukemia. There is a t(15;17) rearrangement (arrows).

Image 27-14 Leukemic cells from the bone marrow of a 78-year-old woman with acute leukemia and mild DIC. The cells are heavily granulated, similar to those in promyelocytic leukemia.

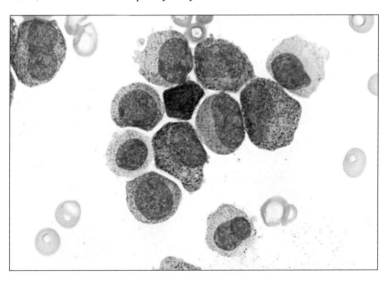

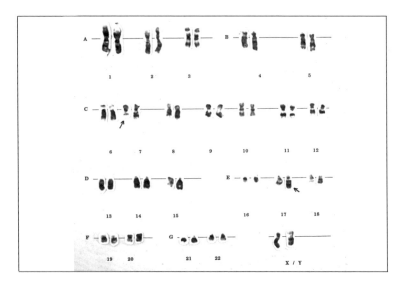

Image 27-15 Karyotype from the same patient as in Image 27-14. There is a t(V;17) [+ (7;17)] rearrangement. Fluorescence in situ hybridization (FISH) studies on the bone marrow failed to identify a *PML-RARα* fusion gene. The patient failed ATRA therapy.

Image 27-16 Acute basophilic leukemia. Blasts with coarse basophilic granules characterize this disease. The granules stained metachromatically with a toluidine blue stain. Basophil granules were identified by electron microscopy.

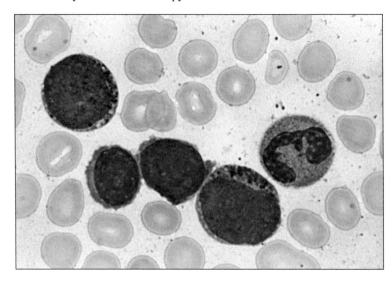

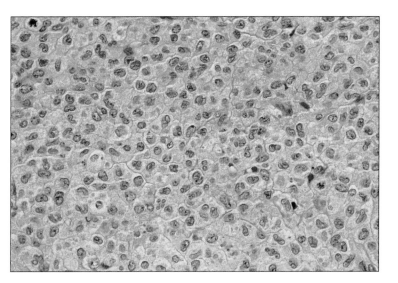

Image 27-17 A chest wall lesion from a 78-year-old man. The infiltrate consists of medium to large cells with abundant cytoplasm and irregular nuclei. A neoplastic monocytic infiltrate was suspected (myeloid sarcoma).

Image 27-18 CD68 immunoperoxidase stain on the same lesion as in Image 27-17. The cells are strongly positive for expression of CD68, supporting the diagnosis of a myeloid sarcoma. A bone marrow examination showed monocytic leukemia.

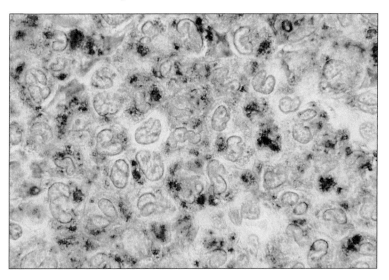

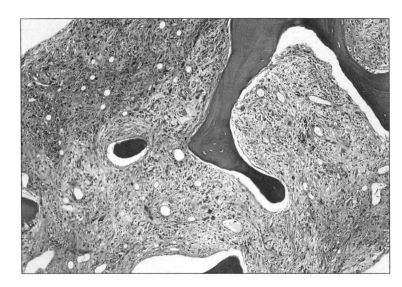

Image 27-19 Bone marrow section from a patient with acute panmyelosis with myelofibrosis. There is marked fibrosis with scattered and clustered abnormal hematopoietic cells. The patient presented with pancytopenia but no splenomegaly.

Image 27-20 Myeloperoxidase stain of a bone marrow smear in a patient with myeloblastic leukemia with maturation (M2). Most of the cells exhibit myeloperoxidase activity.

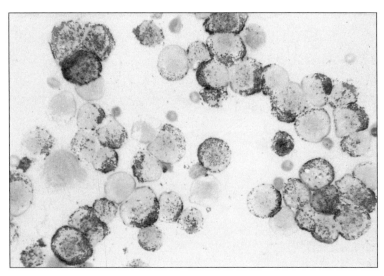

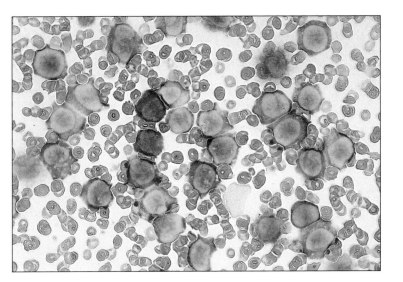

Image 27-21 Nonspecific esterase stain of a bone marrow smear in a patient with monocytic leukemia (M5). The monoblasts exhibit strong α-naphthol butyrate esterase reactivity.

28 Acute Lymphoblastic Leukemia

Acute lymphoblastic leukemia (ALL) is a systemic, neoplastic proliferation of lymphoblasts originating in lymphocyte progenitor cells of the bone marrow or thymus. About 70% of cases of ALL occur in patients under 17 years of age. It is the most common type of leukemia in this age group, accounting for approximately 80% to 85% of cases.

28.1 Pathophysiology

The incidence of ALL is higher in advanced than developing countries and higher among whites than among blacks. The etiology of ALL is unknown. Few data support a specific environmental factor. However, children exposed to radiation in utero or at a young age appear to have an increased incidence of ALL. Genetic factors presumably play a role in some cases. The monozygotic twin of a patient with ALL has a substantially increased risk of developing the disease. The incidence of ALL is significantly higher among individuals with certain genetic disorders such as Down syndrome and ataxia telangiectasia.

The leukemic blast cells in ALL express the immunopheno-type of committed precursors of B lymphocytes (~85%) or T lym-phocytes (~15%). The pattern of antigen expression varies from patient to patient. Although antigen expression in ALL is similar to stages of normal B-cell or T-cell maturation, asynchronous and/or aberrant antigen expression is commonly noted. In some cases, the blasts aberrantly express myeloid- as well as lymphoid-associated antigens.

28.2 Clinical Findings

Males are affected more frequently than females (1.4:1). ALL is most common between the ages of 2 and 10 years. The onset of clinical manifestations may be acute or insidious. The pre-senting signs and symptoms are similar to those of acute mye-loid leukemia (AML) and are usually related to blood cytopenias. Lethargy, malaise, fever, and infection are the most common. Pain in the joints and the extremities is a typical early complaint in children. Symptoms related to bleeding occur in approxi-mately 25% of patients. The most frequent physical findings are pallor, organomegaly, ecchymoses or petechiae, and lym-phadenopathy. In a minority of patients, the presenting clinical manifestations are caused by extramedullary leukemic infil-trates. Central nervous system (CNS), mediastinal, testicular, renal, and bone and joint involvement are most common, but any organ system can be affected. The CNS and the testicles are major sites of extramedullary relapse. The presenting clinical fea-tures in ALL related to pathophysiology are summarized in **Table 27-1**.

28.3 Diagnostic Approach

Patients generally present with one or more of the clinical mani-festations already discussed. These are indicators of a potential diagnosis of acute leukemia and dictate the types of laboratory tests that should be performed. A complete clinical history and physical examination should be supplemented by the following studies:

1. A complete blood count.
2. A peripheral blood smear examination.
3. Bone marrow aspiration and trephine biopsy morphologic examination.
4. Appropriate cytochemical studies on blood and bone marrow.
5. Immunophenotyping of leukemic blasts by flow cytometry or immunohistochemistry.
6. Bone marrow cytogenetic studies.
7. Molecular studies as indicated.
8. Cerebrospinal fluid examination.
9. Radiographic studies for assessment of extramedullary mass disease as indicated.
10. Other biochemical and microbiologic studies as indicated.

28.4 Hematologic Findings

The diagnosis of ALL is generally made or suspected from examination of a peripheral blood smear. There is nearly always evidence of cytopenia, and in most cases lymphoblasts can be identified. The number of recognizable blasts varies from none to several hundred thousand per cubic millimeter. The bone marrow is hypercellular and contains a high percentage of lymphoblasts. The three most important elements of the hematologic evaluation of ALL are

1. Differentiating ALL from other types of malignant lymphoproliferative disease or a nonneoplastic disorder.
2. Distinguishing ALL from AML.
3. Morphologic and immunologic classification of ALL.

The features that differentiate ALL from other disorders are discussed in the section on differential diagnosis. The cytologic features that distinguish ALL from AML are listed in **Table 27-2**. These cytologic features, together with cytochemical and immunophenotypic studies, facilitate correct diagnosis in nearly all patients. The classification of ALL is discussed in the sections on morphologic classification and immunophenotyping.

28.4.1 Blood Cell Measurements

Blood counts are abnormal in more than 90% of patients; there is usually bicytopenia or pancytopenia. Anemia is most common and may be mild to severe. The RBC indices are generally normochromic and normocytic, and the reticulocyte count is decreased. Approximately 75% of patients have platelet counts of less than $100 \times 10^3/mm^3$ ($100 \times 10^9/L$), and 15% of patients have platelet counts of less than $10 \times 10^3/mm^3$ ($10 \times 10^9/L$). Bleeding is generally found in patients with severely depressed platelet counts. Approximately 25% of patients present with leukopenia or leukocyte counts in the low normal range. Fifty percent of patients have leukocyte counts between 5 and $25 \times 10^3/mm^3$ (5 and $25 \times 10^9/L$), and 10% have leukocyte counts greater than $100 \times 10^3/mm^3$ ($100 \times 10^9/L$). Lymphoblasts are present in blood smears for the majority of patients, including most who present with leukopenia. The neutrophil count is usually reduced. The rate of infection parallels the severity of neutropenia.

28.4.2 Blood Smear Morphology

A decrease in normal blood cells is apparent from examination of blood smears. Anemia, usually normochromic-normocytic, is almost always noted, and a variable degree of neutropenia and thrombocytopenia is usually observed. There is frequently a leukoerythroblastic response with variably prominent granulocyte precursors and nucleated RBCs. Reactive lymphocytes are sometimes present; marked eosinophilia is rarely observed. Lymphoblasts are easily recognized in most patients. The number of lymphoblasts varies from a few scattered about the smear to a substantial number that cause a profound leukocytosis. Occasionally, no lymphoblasts are observed in blood smears, and the nature of the cytopenia is revealed only with a bone marrow examination.

28.4.3 Bone Marrow Examination

The bone marrow smears are hypercellular and consist mostly of lymphoblasts; normal hematopoietic cells are markedly reduced. The lymphoblasts are usually small, approximately twice the size of normal small lymphocytes, with sparse cytoplasm and a high nuclear/cytoplasmic ratio (**Image 28-1**). The nucleus is generally round or oval, but some cells have an indented or

Table 28-1 FAB Morphologic Classification of Acute Lymphoblastic Leukemias*

Cytologic Features	L1	L2	L3
Cell size	Small cells predominate	Large, heterogeneous in size	Medium to large and homogeneous
Amount of cytoplasm	Scant	Variable; often moderately abundant	Moderately abundant
Nucleoli	Not visible, or small and inconspicuous	One or more present, often large	One or more present, often prominent
Nuclear shape	Regular; occasional clefting or indentation	Irregular; clefting and indentation common	Regular; oval to round
Nuclear chromatin	Homogeneous in any one case	Variable; heterogeneous in any one case	Finely stippled and homogeneous
Basophilia of cytoplasm	Variable; usually moderate	Variable; occasionally intense	Intensely basophilic
Cytoplasmic vacuolation	Variable	Variable	Prominent

*Modified from Bennett JM, Catovsky D, Daniel M-T, et al. Proposals for the classification of the acute leukaemias. French-American-British (FAB) Co-operative Group. *Br J Haematol.* 1976;33:451–458.

convoluted nuclear outline. Nucleoli are either absent or small and indistinct. The cytoplasm is sparse and variably basophilic; a few vacuoles may be present. Cases of ALL with these morphologic features are designated L1 in the French-American-British (FAB) Cooperative Group classification of acute leukemias (**Table 28-1**).

In some patients, the majority of lymphoblasts are large, more than twice the size of a normal small lymphocyte. They have moderately abundant cytoplasm and a lower nuclear/cytoplasmic ratio (**Image 28-2**). The nuclear outline is frequently irregular; nucleoli vary from one to four in number and are often prominent. The cytoplasm is basophilic and may contain vacuoles. Cases with these features have been designated L2 in the FAB classification. A lower nuclear/cytoplasmic ratio and prominent nucleoli are the major features that distinguish L2 from L1 ALL.

In a minority of cases, the neoplastic cells are medium to large and morphologically homogeneous (**Image 28-3**). The nucleus is round to slightly oval. Two to four variably prominent nucleoli may be observed. The cytoplasm is moderately abundant and deeply basophilic, and it usually contains a large number of sharply defined, clear vacuoles. Cases with these features are designated *FAB L3*. The vacuoles are often the most striking cytologic feature of L3 ALL, which is cytologically identical to Burkitt's and Burkitt's-like lymphoma (small, noncleaved cell lymphoma).

The trephine biopsy sections in ALL are usually markedly hypercellular, although in rare cases the bone marrow is hypocellular. Normal hematopoietic cells are replaced by a uniform, diffuse proliferation of lymphoblasts. Scattered megakaryocytes and small collections of normoblasts or granulocytes may be present. In rare instances, part or all of the section is necrotic.

28.4.4 Classification of Acute Lymphoblastic Leukemia

The FAB Cooperative Group classification system has been the most widely used since it was published in 1976. This system separates ALL into the three morphologic categories already described: L1, L2, and L3. The categories are defined according to the cytologic features of the lymphoblasts (*see Table 28-1*). Cell size, the amount of cytoplasm, and the prominence of nucleoli are the most important characteristics in distinguishing L1 from L2. Nuclear features, cytoplasmic basophilia, and vacuolation are important defining characteristics of L3.

In pediatric patients, 80% to 88% of cases of ALL are classified as L1, 8% to 18% as L2, and 1% to 5% as L3. In adults, 35% to 40% of cases are L1, approximately 60% are L2, and 1% to 5% are L3. In the past, the FAB classification showed demonstrable prognostic significance in some studies because patients with L2 experienced earlier relapse and a shorter median survival time than patients with L1; patients with L3 had the shortest median survival time of all. With present-day protocols for treating higher risk ALL in children, the prognostic distinction between these morphologic groups is less clearly defined.

A new World Health Organization (WHO) proposal for the classification of ALL was recently developed through a joint effort of the Society for Hematopathology in the United States and the European Association for Hematopathology. This proposal emphasizes the immunophenotype and cytogenetic findings, which have

Table 28-2 World Health Organization Proposed Classification of Acute Lymphoblastic Leukemia

Acute lymphoblastic leukemia/lymphoma
  Synonyms: Former FAB L1/L2

  Precursor B acute lymphoblastic leukemia/lymphoma
    Cytogenetic subtypes:
      t(12;21)(p12;q22) TEL-AML1
      t(l;19)(q23;p13) PBX-E2A
      t(9;22)(q34;q11) ABL-BCR
      t(v;11)(v;q23) V-MLL

  Precursor T acute lymphoblastic leukemia/lymphoma

Burkitt's cell leukemia/lymphoma
  Synonyms: Former FAB L3

Biphenotypic acute leukemia

Abbreviation: FAB = French-American-British classification.

more clinical and prognostic relevance than morphology. The classification is shown in **Table 28-2** and is discussed in the sections on immunophenotyping and cytogenetics.

28.5 Variant Morphologic Features of Acute Lymphoblastic Leukemia

28.5.1 Acute Lymphoblastic Leukemia With Cytoplasmic Granules

Granules are observed in the cytoplasm of lymphoblasts in a small percentage of patients with ALL. They stain negative for myeloperoxidase but have been reported to be Sudan black B positive in rare cases. Several cases of ALL with cytoplasmic granules have been reported in children with Down syndrome or the Philadelphia (Ph[1]) chromosome t(9;22). The presence of cytoplasmic granules in lymphoblasts is important mainly because of the potential for confusion with myeloblasts.

28.5.2 Aplastic Presentation of Acute Lymphoblastic Leukemia

Rare patients with ALL present with pancytopenia and hypoplastic bone marrow. Leukemic blasts may not be identified initially. This hypocellular phase is typically followed by overt leukemia in a few weeks or months.

28.5.3 Acute Lymphoblastic Leukemia With Eosinophilia

Mild to marked eosinophilia is occasionally noted at diagnosis. In rare instances eosinophilia is profound and obscures a diagnosis of ALL. In some patients the primary clinical manifestations are related to hypereosinophilia. Eosinophilia generally resolves if a complete leukemic remission is achieved, but returns with relapse.

28.5.4 Relapse of Lymphoblastic Leukemia

In most cases, the morphology of the lymphoblasts at relapse is similar to the initial diagnostic bone marrow. In a minority of patients, there is an increase in lymphoblasts with L2-type features. Immunophenotypic and karyotypic changes also may be observed at relapse. A summary of the changes that may be observed in lymphoblasts at relapse is shown in **Table 28-3**.

28.5.5 Therapy-Related Acute Myeloid Leukemia

Therapy-related AML has been reported in approximately 2% of patients treated for ALL. The secondary leukemia results from the effect of chemotherapy on myeloid stem cells. There is a specific association with type II topoisomerase inhibitor drugs (primarily epipodophyllotoxins). The leukemia is frequently monocytic or has a monocytic component. An 11q23 chromosome rearrangement is usually found in AML secondary to type II topoisomerase inhibitors.

Other Laboratory Tests

Test 28.1 **Cytochemistry**

Purpose. Cytochemical stains are used primarily to help distinguish ALL from AML (*see Table 27-6*).

Table 28-3   Changes at Relapse of Acute Lymphoblastic Leukemia*

Morphology
    L1 → L2 (in a minority of cases)
TdT
    Positive → negative (~25%)
Immunologic
    Major phenotype change (rare)
    Gain or loss of an antigen (more common)
        eg, CD10+ → CD10–
        HLA-DR+ → HLA-DR–
Cytogenetic
    Clonal evolution common (~75%)
    One or more new structural abnormalities
Evolution to myeloid leukemia (lineage switch)
    Therapy-related in most cases
    Often associated with 11q23 chromosome abnormality

* Modified from Brunning RD, McKenna RW. Tumors of the bone marrow. Acute lymphoblastic leukemias. *Atlas of Tumor Pathology*. 3rd Series, Fascicle 9. Washington, DC: Armed Forces Institute of Pathology; 1994:100–142.

Principle, Specimen, and Procedure. See Test 27.1.

Interpretation. The cytochemical characteristics of lymphoblasts in ALL are listed in **Table 28-4**. Lymphoblasts are always myeloperoxidase negative but have been reported to be Sudan black B positive in rare instances. The periodic acid–Schiff (PAS) stain is positive in 70% to 75% of cases; the stain is distributed in coarse granules or clumps in the cytoplasm and generally corresponds to glycogen deposits (**Image 28-4**). The vacuoles in the blasts of L3 stain positively with the oil red O stain. The cytoplasm stains strongly with a methyl green–pyronine (MGP) stain but is PAS negative.

Terminal Deoxynucleotidyl Transferase. Terminal deoxynucleotidyl transferase (TdT) is a unique DNA polymerase found normally in the nuclei of cortical lymphocytes of human thymus and in a small number of bone marrow lymphoid cells. It is most commonly assayed by immunofluorescent or enzyme immunohistochemical microscopy techniques or by flow cytometry (**Image 28-5**). In more than 90% of cases of both precursor T-cell and precursor B-cell ALL, the lymphoblasts are TdT positive.

Table 28-4   Cytochemical Reactions in Acute Lymphoblastic Leukemia

	L1		L2	L3
Myeloperoxidase and Sudan black B	–		–	–
Nonspecific esterase	–/+	(focal)	–/+	–
Periodic acid–Schiff	+	(~75%)	+	–
Acid phosphatase	+	(T cell)	+	–
Oil red O	–		–	+
Methyl green–pyronine	+/–		+/–	+

Assessment of TdT is useful in distinguishing ALL from AML and from other lymphoproliferative disorders such as adult T-cell leukemia. A positive finding alone does not exclude AML, because myeloblasts are TdT positive in approximately 5% to 10% of cases of AML. However, the percentage of positive blasts and the reaction intensity are often less than in ALL.

Up to 10% of the normal lymphoid progenitor cells may be TdT positive in the bone marrow of patients without hematologic malignancies, particularly young children. They are commonly observed in the bone marrow recovery phase following chemotherapy for ALL. Therefore, the presence of a small number of TdT-positive cells in posttherapy bone marrow specimens should not be interpreted as residual disease or relapse of ALL without supporting morphologic or immunophenotypic evidence.

The TdT assay performed on spinal fluid may be useful in identifying or excluding CNS involvement in patients with ALL with relatively low spinal fluid cell counts and equivocal morphology.

Test 28.2 Immunophenotyping

Purpose. Immunophenotyping leukemic blasts is important in distinguishing ALL from AML and other lymphoproliferative disorders when the morphology and cytochemistry of the blasts are not definitive. In addition, the proposed WHO classification of ALL is based on immunophenotype (*see Table 28-2*) in recognition of its prognostic significance.

Principle. The abundance of lineage-restricted or lineage-associated monoclonal antibodies (MoAbs) and techniques available for immunophenotyping hematopoietic cells has added an important dimension to the diagnosis of acute leukemia.

In characterizing acute leukemias, it is important to use panels of MoAbs that include all of the major cell lineages to avoid misinterpretations and to recognize phenotypic aberrance and rare cases of biphenotypic leukemia. Flow cytometry is the preferred method of immunophenotyping acute leukemias. A discussion of flow cytometry in the characterization of hematologic disorders and a list of the common antigen cluster designations (CDs) of MoAbs used for this purpose are found in Chapter 48.

Specimen. Immunophenotyping can be performed by flow cytometry on cell suspensions from blood, bone marrow, body fluids, or other tissues such as fresh lymph node specimens. For immunophenotyping leukemias, blood or bone marrow are preferred. If blood is the source, there must be enough circulating leukemic cells to ensure valid results.

If flow cytometry cannot be performed, immunophenotyping can be performed using immunohistochemical methods on blood and bone marrow smears, touch preparations, body fluid cytospin preparations, frozen sections, and paraffin-embedded sections. Immunohistochemistry is particularly useful when live cell preparations are unavailable, making it impossible to perform flow cytometry.

Procedure. By using flow cytometry, a large number of cells can be immunophenotyped with MoAb panels in a relatively short time. An additional advantage of flow cytometry is that expression of two, three, or four antigens can be investigated simultaneously on the same cell (two-, three-, or four-color flow) (see Chapter 48). Many of the commercially available MoAbs also can be applied to immunohistochemical stains on smears and sections. The immunoalkaline-phosphatase techniques are preferable to immunoperoxidase methods for use on blood and bone marrow.

Interpretation. Table 28-5 shows the general immunophenotypic features of the major categories of the proposed WHO classification of ALL. Approximately 85% of cases of ALL type as precursor B cells, and the remainder are derived from precursor T cells.

Table 28-5 Immunophenotypic Categories of Acute Lymphoblastic Leukemia

	FAB Class	TdT	T-Cell Associated Antigens	B-Cell Associated Antigens	CIg	SIg
Precursor B cell	L1, L2	+	–	+	–/+*	–
Precursor T cell	L1, L2	+	+	–	–	–
B cell†	L3	–	–	+	–	+

Abbreviations: FAB = French-American-British classification; TdT = terminal deoxynucleotidyl transferase; CIg = cytoplasmic immunoglobulin; SIg = surface immunoglobulin.
*Approximately 20% of cases of precursor B cell ALL express cytoplasmic μ chains without light chains.
†B cell (SIg+) ALL is considered Burkitt's or Burkitt's-like lymphoma with secondary leukemic manifestations in the World Health Organization proposal.

Precursor B-Cell Acute Lymphoblastic Leukemia. Approximately 85% of cases of ALL are precursor B-cell type. They express various combinations of B-cell–associated antigens and are mostly TdT positive (**Figure 28-1**). The immunophenotype often parallels various stages of normal precursor B cell development, but there is frequent asynchronous and aberrant antigen expression. Cases of precursor B-cell ALL lack surface immunoglobulin (SIg), but about 20% contain cytoplasmic immunoglobulin (CIg) μ chains. These CIg+ cases are often referred to as pre-B ALL. All of the precursor B-cell ALLs express combinations of B-cell–associated antigens, including HLA-DR, CD10, CD19, CD20, and CD22. CD22 antigen is sometimes lacking on the cell surface but is almost always present in the cytoplasm. CD10 is expressed in approximately 80% of cases; lack of expression of CD10 is associated with a poorer prognosis. CD10-negative precursor B-cell ALL is most common in children under 2 years of age and in adults.

Precursor B-cell ALL may have morphologic features of either L1 or L2; in children, most cases are L1. Precursor B-cell ALL in children is generally associated with a favorable prognosis; however, some individual subsets have a less favorable outcome due to specific cytogenetic abnormalities or other factors that may negatively influence prognosis. Several cytogenetic groups of precursor B-cell ALL are included in the

Figure 28-1 Typical flow cytometric histograms of blood from a patient with precursor B-cell ALL. The cluster painted red represents the neoplastic lymphoblasts. They are CD45 and CD14 negative and express homogeneous and bright CD34, CD19, CD10, and CD38. They lack expression of both kappa and lambda light chains and express intracytoplasmic CD22 and nuclear TdT. (Photograph courtesy of Louis Picker, MD, Co-Director, Division of Hematopathology and Immunology, University of Texas Southwestern Medical Center, Dallas.)

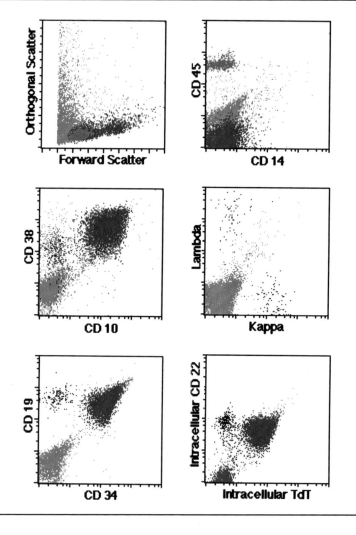

proposed WHO classification (*see Table 28-2*). These are discussed in the section on cytogenetics.

Precursor T-Cell Acute Lymphoblastic Leukemia. The lymphoblasts in precursor T-cell ALL are derived from cells in the thymocyte stages of development of T lymphocytes. They express various combinations of T-cell–associated antigens and are TdT positive in a vast majority of cases (**Figure 28-2**). CD2, CD5, and especially CD7 are expressed in a high percentage of cases. Cell surface expression of CD3, which is the most specific antigen for peripheral T cells, is lacking in approximately 70% of cases of precursor T-cell ALL. However, virtually all cases express cytoplasmic CD3. T-cell receptor gene rearrangements provide additional evidence of T-cell origin and clonality. Precursor T-cell ALL can be subclassified into early, intermediate, and mature stages of thymocyte development by using an appropriate MoAb panel, but these do not appear to have prognostic significance and, similar to precursor B-cell ALL, asynchronous antigen expression is quite common.

Precursor T-cell ALL may be either L1 or L2. In many cases, however, a distinct minor population of small blasts with little or no cytoplasm and markedly hyperchromatic nuclei, often with prominent nuclear convolution, may be identified in blood and bone marrow smears (**Image 28-6**). These contrast with a major population of larger leukemic blasts. Numerous mitotic figures are usually observed in trephine biopsy sections. These morphologic features are highly suggestive of a precursor T-cell ALL. The clinical and prognostic features of precursor T-cell ALL are summarized in **Table 28-6**.

B-Cell Acute Lymphoblastic Leukemia: Burkitt's Leukemia/ Lymphoma. The neoplastic cells in 2% to 5% of patients presenting with features of ALL express monoclonal surface immunoglobulin and pan B-cell antigens and usually lack expression of TdT. Leukemias with these characteristics have often been designated B-cell ALL because their immunophenotype (SIg+) is more mature than in precursor B-cell ALL. They have the morphologic features of Burkitt's lymphoma and are designated L3 in the FAB morphologic classification (*see Image 28-3*). Extramedullary mass disease is nearly always demonstrable and is often the most prominent feature. These cases are considered to be Burkitt's lymphomas with secondary leukemic manifestations in the proposed WHO classification.

Figure 28-2 Typical flow cytometric histograms of blood from a patient with precursor T-cell ALL. The cluster painted red represents the neoplastic lymphoblasts. They express bright CD7 and lack surface CD3. The blasts are weakly CD5 positive and CD1a and CD4 negative; they express CD8. They lack CD19 and CD34 and express cytoplasmic CD3 and TdT. Lack of expression of surface CD3 with positive cytoplasmic CD3 is found in approximately 70% of cases of precursor T-cell ALL. (Photograph courtesy of Louis Picker, MD, Co-Director, Division of Hematopathology and Immunology, University of Texas Southwestern Medical Center, Dallas.)

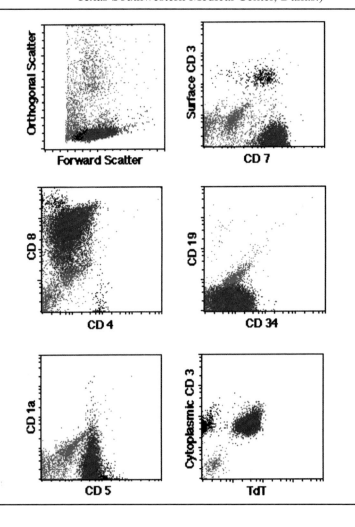

Table 28-6   Clinical Features of T-Cell Acute Lymphoblastic
Leukemia (ALL)

Older median age than for precursor B-cell ALL
Male predominance
Mediastinal mass in ~50% of cases
High blood leukocyte counts
Often chromosome rearrangements involving 14q11
Earlier relapse than precursor B-cell ALL
High incidence of central nervous system relapse
Shorter disease-free survival than for precursor B-cell ALL

Lymphoblastic Lymphoma/Leukemia. It is well recognized
that lymphoblastic neoplasms of both precursor T-cell and
precursor B-cell types may present primarily as extramedullary
tumors. This is particularly true of precursor T-cell neoplasms,
which are commonly associated with a mediastinal mass and
often with organomegaly and lymphadenopathy, with or without leukemic blood and bone marrow manifestations (**Image
28-7**). Morphologically and immunophenotypically, these neoplasms are identical to their ALL counterparts.

**Asynchronous and Aberrant Antigen Expression and Bipheno-
typic Acute Leukemia.** Many cases of precursor B-cell ALL
express combinations of early and late antigens not observed
in normal lymphocyte development. This type of asynchronous antigen expression is also found in T-cell ALL.

In some cases, the lymphoblasts aberrantly express one or
more myeloid-associated antigens in addition to lymphoid
antigens; less commonly, combinations of both B-cell– and T-
cell–associated antigens are present. In the past, these cases
were often referred to as *mixed lineage* or *biphenotypic
leukemias*. However, as more MoAbs have become available
to assess acute leukemias by flow cytometry, the finding of
aberrant antigen expression in ALL is recognized as a common
phenomenon.

Presently, most cases of ALL that express myeloid antigens are designated as *ALL with aberrant myeloid antigen
expression*. Most recent studies have shown no independent
prognostic significance associated with myeloid antigen
expression. The rare cases in which multiple and major antigens of both lymphoid and myeloid lineages are expressed

may still be referred to as *biphenotypic* or *mixed phenotype acute leukemias*. Such leukemias can be of two types: mixed lineage leukemia, in which the leukemic blasts coexpress multiple and major antigens of both lymphoid and myeloid lineage, or bilineal leukemia, in which individual leukemic cells express either lymphoid or myeloid antigens but not both (**Image 28-8**). In the latter, the two blast populations may have different morphologic, cytochemical, and ultrastructural features as well. There is an increased incidence of chromosome translocations involving 11q23, 14q32, or t(9;22) in mixed phenotype ALL. Translocations involving these chromosomes are associated with a poor prognosis.

Immunophenotypic Changes at Relapse. The consistency of major immunophenotype is generally maintained at relapse (*see Table 28-3*). Changes from a precursor T-cell to a precursor B-cell phenotype or vice versa have been reported only rarely. Losses or gains of individual antigens without a major evolution of immunophenotype are more common. Losses of TdT, HLA-DR, or CD10 expression are the most frequently reported alterations.

28.6 Ancillary Tests

28.6.1 Cytogenetics

Bone marrow cytogenetic studies supplement the morphologic and immunophenotypic studies. They have become such an important and routine part of the evaluation of patients with acute leukemia that in many treatment centers they are not considered ancillary tests. Their greatest value is in identifying prognostic groups; cytogenetic findings may be the single best predictor of remission duration and survival time. **Table 28-7** summarizes the relationship between bone marrow karyotype and prognostic group in ALL.

When studied with state-of-the-art cytogenetic techniques, 80% to 90% of patients with ALL have demonstrable karyotypic bone marrow chromosome abnormalities. Numeric abnormalities are most common, either alone or in combination with structural changes. The following discussion focuses on the most common

Table 28-7 Correlation of Prognosis With Bone Marrow Cytogenetic Findings in Acute Lymphoblastic Leukemia

Prognosis	Cytogenetic Findings
Favorable	Hyperdiploidy >50
	t(12;21)
Intermediate	Hyperdiploidy 47-50
	Normal (diploidy)
	del (6q)
	Rearrangements of 8q24
Unfavorable	Hypodiploidy (near haploidy)
	Near tetraploidy
	del 17p
	t(9;22)
	t(11q23), eg, t(4;11)

and clinically relevant changes. Those indicated with an asterisk are included in the proposed WHO classification of ALL.

Hyperdiploidy with more than 50 chromosomes (hyperdiploidy >50) is found in 25% to 30% of childhood ALLs (**Image 28-9**). It is associated with precursor B-cell immunophenotype and other favorable clinical features. Most patients are between 2 and 10 years of age and have low presenting blood leukocyte counts. The 5-year survival rate for children with hyperdiploidy >50 is approximately 80%.

Hypodiploidy is present in 3% to 9% of patients with ALL. Most of these patients have 45 chromosomes; chromosome 20 is commonly lost. Patients with hypodiploidy have an intermediate to unfavorable prognosis. A few have a near haploid karyotype. These individuals appear to have a particularly poor prognosis.

Pseudodiploidy (46 chromosomes with structural abnormalities) is found in approximately 40% of children with ALL and a higher percentage of adults. Pseudodiploidy is often associated with an unfavorable prognosis because of the frequency of specific chromosome translocations. Structural changes also may be found in the other numeric groups, except diploid. The most common and prognostically significant translocations are described here. Several of the important chromosome translocations and the resulting fusion gene products are listed in **Table 28-8**.

Table 28-8   Cytogenetic Translocations Associated With Specific Molecular Genetic Abnormalities in Acute Lymphoblastic Leukemia

Cytogenetic Translocation	Molecular Genetic Abnormality
t(9;22)(q34;q11)	*BCR-ABL* fusion (p185)
t(12;21)(p13;q22)	*TEL-AML1* fusion
t(1;19)(q23;p13)	*E2A-PBX* fusion
t(4;11)(q21;q23)	*MLL-AF4* fusion
t(8;14)(q24;q32)	*IGH-MYC* fusion
t(11;14)(p13;q11)	*TCRδ-RBTN2* fusion

Source: Kersey JH. Fifty years of studies of the biology and therapy of childhood leukemia. *Blood.* 1997;90:4243–4251.

A t(12;21)(p13;q22) "cryptic" chromosome rearrangement* is found in 22% to 27% of children with ALL. This translocation is not evident by routine cytogenetic studies but can be identified by polymerase chain reaction (PCR) or fluorescence in situ hybridization (FISH) techniques. It is associated with precursor B-cell ALL. It is not found with hyperdiploidy but may be associated with other cytogenetic abnormalities. The importance of identifying this cryptic rearrangement is its association with a favorable prognosis using treatment protocols for low-risk ALL. The molecular arrangement involves the *TEL* gene on chromosome 12 and the *AML1* gene on chromosome 21 forming a *TEL-AML1* fusion product.

Translocation (1;19)(q23;p13),* resulting in an *E2A-PBX* fusion gene, is found in about 25% of patients with CIg+ precursor B-cell ALL and 1% of Cig– precursor B-cell ALL. The overall incidence in children with ALL is 5% to 6%. Translocation (1;19) is particularly common in black children. It has been associated with a poor response to antimetabolite chemotherapy and an unfavorable prognosis in the past. Recent treatment protocols for higher risk ALL have significantly improved the long-term disease-free survival rate.

The Ph[1] chromosome* results from t(9;22)(q34;q11), which involves the breakpoint cluster region (BCR) on chromosome 22 and the Abelson proto-oncogene (ABL) on chromosome 9, producing a *BCR-ABL* fusion product. It is identified in approximately 3% of children and 20% to 25% of adults with ALL. The Ph[1]+ ALL is associated with an older age at onset, high presenting leukocyte count, L2 morphology, precursor B-cell immunophenotype, and CNS involvement. The prognosis is unfavorable in both children and adults. The karyotype of the chromosome rearrangement is indistinguishable from the t(9;22)(q34;q11) observed in chronic myeloid leukemia (CML). However, molecular analysis has shown that most cases of Ph[1]+ ALL differ from CML in the site of the breakpoint on the BCR. In CML, the molecular translocation results in a 210-kD *BCR-ABL* fusion product. In Ph[1]+ ALL, the most common *BCR-ABL* fusion gene is 185 kD.

Rearrangement of chromosome 11q23,* the site of the *MLL* gene, is found in less than 5% of childhood ALLs. t(4;11)(q21;q23) is the most common translocation involving 11q23. It is associated with markedly elevated leukocyte counts, splenomegaly, and a poor prognosis. The t(4;11) is often found in patients with congenital acute leukemia. An 11q23 abnormality in de novo acute leukemia is frequently associated with a mixed phenotype leukemia. It is also associated with therapy-related AMLs secondary to type II topoisomerase inhibitor drugs.

Reciprocal translocations involving chromosome 8q24, L3 morphology, and B-cell phenotype (SIg+) are found in approximately 3% of patients with ALL (*see Image 28-3*). These conditions are essentially all Burkitt's or Burkitt's-like lymphomas with leukemic manifestations. The most common translocation is t(8;14)(q24;q32); the *MYC* proto-oncogene on chromosome 8 assumes a position adjacent to the heavy chain gene. A large tumor cell burden, extramedullary disease, and CNS disease are common in these cases. Although associated with a poor prognosis in the past, new approaches to treatment in children have been highly effective in recent years.

Forty to fifty percent of cases of T-cell ALL involve translocations. In approximately 50% of them, breakpoints are in the locations of the T-cell receptor (TcR) genes; 14q11, the site of the *TCRδ* gene, appears to be the most commonly involved. The presence of these chromosome abnormalities correlates with an unfavorable prognosis.

Cytogenetic evolution from diagnosis to relapse is common in ALL (*see Table 28-3*). The karyotype changes at relapse are generally related to those at diagnosis, with the addition of new structural abnormalities.

28.6.2 Molecular Analysis

Leukemic lymphoblast genotype differs with the cytogenetic ALL groups. The genotype appears to define clinical and prognostic features of ALL. Leukemias often result from the fusion of genes critical for signal transduction or transcription. Molecular techniques can identify specific fusion genes.

A number of molecular techniques, such as Southern blot, PCR, and FISH, can be used to provide important information in some cases of ALL (see Chapter 48). These techniques are generally unnecessary for an initial diagnosis of ALL but may provide important prognostic information, particularly when cytogenetic studies are either unavailable or not sensitive enough to identify a significant translocation of genetic material. This is particularly important in the case of the cryptic t(12;21) discussed previously. Molecular techniques also are more sensitive than morphologic or cytogenetic examination for detecting minimal residual disease and early recurrence of ALL. Several of the important fusion gene products in ALL that may be identified by molecular studies are listed in **Table 28-8**.

28.6.3 **Cerebrospinal Fluid Analysis**

CNS involvement is the most significant extramedullary manifestation of ALL. It is most commonly encountered at diagnosis in precursor T-cell or B-cell (SIg+) ALL (Burkitts) but is found in precursor B-cell ALL as well (**Image 28-10**). The CNS is also a common site of relapse with or without bone marrow relapse. Due to the frequency of CNS relapse, CNS prophylactic therapy is included in ALL treatment protocols. Morphologic examination of cerebrospinal fluid (CSF) should be performed for all patients with ALL at diagnosis and periodically during the course of maintenance therapy. Cytocentrifuge preparations of CSF are preferred for morphologic examination. When the CSF is involved, the cell count varies from occasional to numerous lymphoblasts. When only a few are present, their identity may be difficult to establish. CD34, CD10, or TdT studies by immunocytochemical methods on cytocentrifuge CSF preparations may assist in characterizing the leukemic cells in equivocal cases.

28.7 **Differential Diagnosis**

A number of disorders may present with clinical or morphologic manifestations similar to those of ALL. Several are listed in **Table 28-9**. Most of these conditions can be distinguished

Table 28-9   Considerations in the Differential Diagnosis of Acute Lymphoblastic Leukemia

Acute myeloid leukemia
Increased normal bone marrow B-cell precursors (hematogones)
Metastatic small cell tumors
Reactive lymphocytosis
Hypoplastic anemia
Chronic lymphocytic leukemia
Adult T-cell leukemia
Prolymphocytic leukemia
Non-Hodgkin's lymphoma

from ALL by careful morphologic examination of blood and bone marrow. Cytochemistry, immunophenotyping, and electron microscopy or molecular studies may be required in some cases. Three of the most common and difficult considerations in the differential diagnosis are discussed in this section.

28.7.1 Acute Myeloid Leukemia

Categories of AML that are poorly differentiated morphologically are most likely to be confused with ALL. These categories—M0, M1, M5a, and M7—can be distinguished from ALL on the basis of the myeloperoxidase and nonspecific esterase stains and the profile of antigen expression by flow cytometry or immunohistochemical methods.

28.7.2 Increased Normal Bone Marrow Precursor B Cells

Bone marrow aspirate specimens from children and (occasionally) from adults may contain increased numbers of normal marrow precursor B cells. Many of these small lymphoid cells have morphologic features in common with ALL lymphoblasts (**Image 28-11**) and are frequently referred to as "hematogones". They are found in large numbers in normal infants and in a number of diverse disease processes in children past infancy, particularly in association with various types of blood cytopenias. When encountered in the bone marrow of children undergoing evaluation for cytopenias or organomegaly, a diagnosis of lymphoblastic leukemia or lymphoma may be considered. Regenerative bone marrow following chemotherapy for ALL also typically contains increased numbers of normal precursor B cells. In these patients, there is a potential for misinterpreting the cells as residual or recurrent leukemic lymphoblasts.

Normal precursor B cells may express an antigen profile similar to that of neoplastic lymphoblasts (eg, TdT, CD34, CD10, and various pan B-cell antigens). They do not express immunophenotypic aberrance, however, and they also differ from neoplastic lymphoblasts by displaying a maturational spectrum of antigen expression, in contrast to the incomplete maturational spectrum and antigen aberrance usually observed in ALL. DNA content is normal in hematogones, and there is no evidence of clonality by either cytogenetic or immunogenotypic analysis.

28.7.3 Metastatic Small Cell Tumors

Metastatic small cell tumors in children occasionally present with extensive bone marrow involvement in the absence of an identifiable primary tumor mass. Primary clinical manifestations may be related to blood cytopenias or a leukemoid reaction. The neoplastic cells in this group of tumors sometimes resemble lymphoblasts in bone marrow smears. Neuroblastoma is the most common of these; embryonal rhabdomyosarcoma, retinoblastoma, Ewing's sarcoma, and medulloblastoma also may mimic ALL. Clues to the correct diagnosis include the presence of neoplastic cells in clumps or clusters on bone marrow smears. Large numbers of bare nuclei and damaged cells also may be observed throughout the smears. The distinction between metastatic disease and ALL is usually apparent in trephine biopsy sections. In equivocal cases, immunophenotyping, electron microscopy, and enzyme immunocytochemistry using appropriate antibodies for the characterization of small cell tumors facilitate the correct diagnosis.

28.8 Course and Treatment

The prognosis for children with ALL has improved dramatically during the past three decades. In children with precursor B-cell ALLs that lack unfavorable prognostic features (**Table 28-10**), standard ALL induction chemotherapy produces a complete

Table 28-10 Prognostic Indicators in Acute Lymphoblastic Leukemia (ALL)*

	Favorable	Less Favorable
Clinical		
Age	2 to 10 y	<2 and >10 y
Sex	Female	Male
Race	White	Black
WBC count	$<10 \times 10^3/mm^3$ $(10 \times 10^9/L)$	$>50 \times 10^3/mm^3$ $(50 \times 10^9/L)$
Rapidity of cytoreduction	Bone marrow free of disease by day 14	Residual disease at day 14
Relapse	No relapse	Relapse
Morphologic	L1	?L2, ?L3
Immunophenotypic	CD10+ precursor B cell	CD10– precursor B-cell, precursor T-cell ALL, ?B-cell ALL (SIg)
Cytogenetic	Hyperdiploidy >50 chromosomes t(12;21)	Translocations [especially t(9;22) and t(4;11)] near haploidy, near tetraploidy, del 17p

Abbreviation: SIg = surface immunoglobulin.
*From Brunning RD, McKenna RW. Tumors of the bone marrow. Acute lymphoblastic leukemias. *Atlas of Tumor Pathology*. 3rd Series, Fascicle 9. Washington, DC: Armed Forces Institute of Pathology; 1994:100–142.

remission in more than 98% of patients; approximately 75% achieve long-term event-free survival and presumably are cured.

For high-risk types of ALL, treatment results are less favorable. More aggressive therapy, with higher doses of standard chemotherapy agents plus additional drugs, has improved long-term disease-free survival in children with T-cell ALL to 40% to 50% in some cancer treatment centers. Allogeneic bone marrow transplantation provides another potentially curative treatment for children with high-risk ALL and patients who relapse after standard chemotherapy. Adults with ALL fare worse than children. This is partly because of the higher frequency of bad prognostic features such as the t(9;22) chromosome rearrangement.

Several clinical, morphologic, immunophenotypic, and cytogenetic parameters have been identified as indicators of prognosis. **Table 28-10** lists some of the most commonly considered factors. The significance of these factors varies in different studies. Some former indicators of poor prognosis have less significance in predicting survival time because management of high-risk ALL has improved.

28.9 **References**

Behm FG. Morphologic and cytochemical characteristics of childhood lymphoblastic leukemia. *Hematol Oncol Clin North Am.* 1990;4:715–741.

Bennett JM, Catovsky D, Daniel M-T, et al. The morphological classification of acute lymphoblastic leukaemia: concordance among observers and clinical correlations. *Br J Haematol.* 1981;47:553–561.

Brunning RD, McKenna RW. Tumors of the bone marrow. Acute lymphoblastic leukemias. In: *Atlas of Tumor Pathology.* 3rd Series, Fascicle 9. Washington, DC: Armed Forces Institute of Pathology; 1994:100–142.

Cave H, Van Der Werff ten Bosch J, Suciu S, et al. Clinical significance of minimal residual disease in childhood acute lymphoblastic leukemia. *N Engl J Med.* 1998;339:591–598.

Chessells JM, Swansbury GJ, Reeves B, et al. Cytogenetics and prognosis in childhood lymphoblastic leukaemia: results of MRC UKALL X. *Br J Haematol.* 1997;99:93–100.

Copelan EA, McGuire EA. The biology and treatment of acute lymphoblastic leukemia in adults. *Blood.* 1995;85:1151–1168.

Faderl S, Kantarjian HM, Talpaz M, et al. Clinical significance of cytogenetic abnormalities in adult acute lymphoblastic leukemia. *Blood.* 1998;91:3995–4019.

Gassmann W, Loffler H, Thiel E, et al. Morphological and cytochemical findings in 150 cases of T-lineage acute lymphoblastic leukaemia in adults. *Br J Haematol.* 1997;97:372–382.

Harris NL, Jaffe ES, Diebold J, et al. The World Health Organization Classification of Hematological Malignancies Report of the Clinical Advisory Committee Meeting, Airlie House, Virginia, November 1997. *Mod Pathol.* 2000;13(2):193–207.

Homans AC, Barker BE, Forman EN, et al. Immunophenotypic characteristics of cerebral spinal fluid cells in children with acute lymphoblastic leukemia at diagnosis. *Blood.* 1990;76:1807–1811.

Hurwitz CA, Mirro J. Mixed lineage leukemia and asynchronous antigen expression. *Hematol Oncol Clin North Am.* 1990;4:767–794.

Kersey JH. Fifty years of studies of the biology and therapy of childhood leukemia. *Blood.* 1997;90:4243–4251.

Longacre TA, Foucar K, Crago S, et al. Hematogones: a multiparameter analysis of bone marrow precursor cells. *Blood*. 1989;73:543–552.

Pui CH. Childhood leukemias. *N Engl J Med*. 1995;332:1618–1630.

Pui CH, Behm FG, Crist WM. Clinical and biologic relevance of immunologic marker studies in childhood acute lymphoblastic leukemia. *Blood*. 1993;82:343–362.

Pui CH, Ribeiro PC, Hancock ML, et al. Acute myeloid leukemia in children treated with epipodophyllotoxins for acute lymphoblastic leukemia. *N Engl J Med*. 1991;325:1682–1687.

Shurtleff SA, Buijs A, Behm FG, et al. TEL/AML1 fusion resulting from a cryptic t(12;21) is the most common genetic lesion in pediatric ALL and defines a subgroup of patients with an excellent prognosis. *Leukemia*. 1995;9:1985–1989.

Uckun FM, Sather HN, Gaynon PS, et al. Clinical features and treatment outcome of children with myeloid antigen positive acute lymphoblastic leukemia: a report from the Children's Cancer Group. *Blood*. 1997;90:28–35.

Uckun FM, Sensel MG, Sun L, et al. Biology and treatment of childhood T-lineage acute lymphoblastic leukemia. *Blood*. 1998;91:735–746.

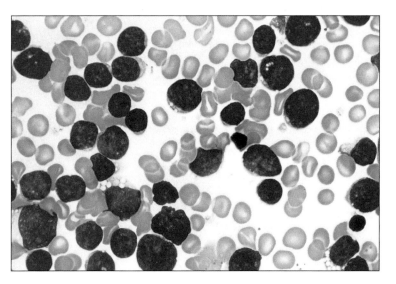

Image 28-1   Acute lymphoblastic leukemia (L1). The lymphoblasts are small with little cytoplasm and no nucleoli.

Image 28-2   Acute lymphoblastic leukemia (L2). The lymphoblasts are larger than those in L1, have more cytoplasm, and contain distinct nucleoli. (From Brunning RD, McKenna RW. Tumors of the bone marrow. In: *Atlas of Tumor Pathology*. 3rd Series, Fascicle 9. Washington, DC: Armed Forces Institute of Pathology; 1994:107.)

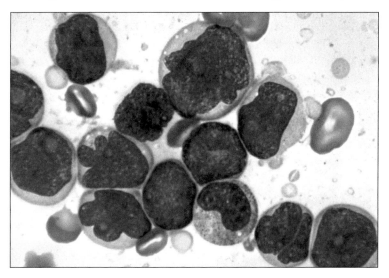

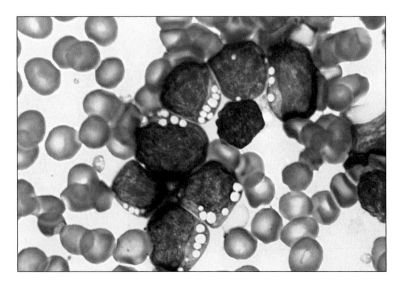

Image 28-3   Acute lymphoblastic leukemia (L3). The lymphoblasts are large and have a moderate amount of basophilic cytoplasm with sharply defined, clear vacuoles. The nuclei are round with relatively coarse chromatin.

Image 28-4   A periodic acid–Schiff (PAS) stain on a bone marrow smear from a child with acute lymphoblastic leukemia. The lymphoblasts exhibit coarse granular and block PAS positivity.

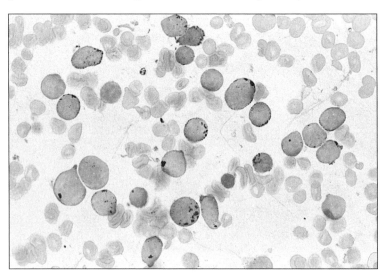

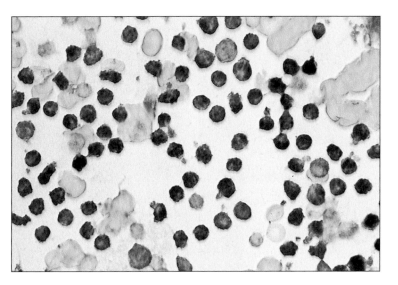

Image 28-5   Immunohistochemical (immunoperoxidase) reaction for terminal deoxynucleotidyl transferase (TdT) on a bone marrow smear from a child with acute lymphoblastic leukemia. The lymphoblasts show a nuclear distribution of reactivity for TdT.

Image 28-6   A blood smear from a young man with precursor T-cell acute lymphoblastic leukemia and a markedly elevated leukocyte count. The lymphoblasts are heteromorphous. The minor population consists of small lymphoblasts with hyperchromatic, convoluted nuclei.

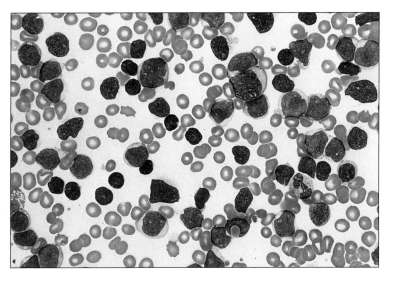

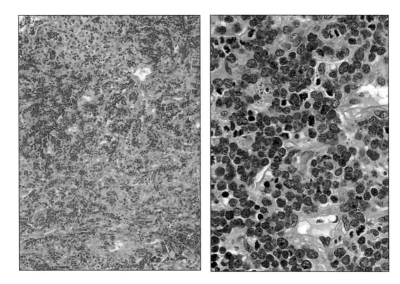

Image 28-7 Biopsy of a mediastinal mass from 10-year-old boy. Low magnification shows a lymphoid infiltrate (left). High magnification shows typical lymphoblast morphology and a high mitotic rate (right). The patient had a small number of precursor T lymphoblasts in the bone marrow aspirate.

Image 28-8 Bilineal leukemia. A blood smear from a neonate with congenital leukemia. The leukemic blast population expressed two separate morphologic, cytochemical, and immunophenotypic lineages: lymphoblasts (small) and monoblasts-promonocytes (large).

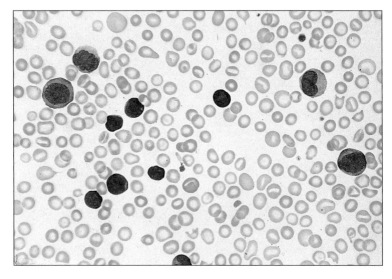

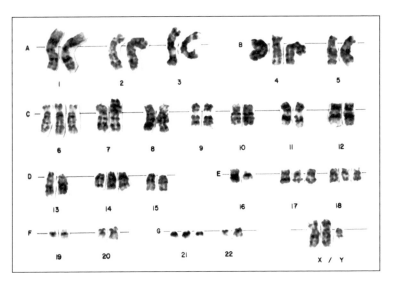

Image 28-9   A bone marrow karyotype from a 5-year-old girl with precursor B-cell acute lymphoblastic leukemia (ALL). There is hyperdiploidy with 53 chromosomes. Hyperdiploidy >50 is the most common cytogenetic abnormality in children with precursor B cell ALL and is associated with a favorable prognosis. (Photograph courtesy of Nancy Schneider, MD, Director, Division of Cytogenetics, University of Texas Southwestern Medical Center, Dallas. From Brunning RD, McKenna RW. Tumors of the bone marrow. In: *Atlas of Tumor Pathology*. 3rd Series, Fascicle 9. Washington, DC: Armed Forces Institute of Pathology; 1994:127.)

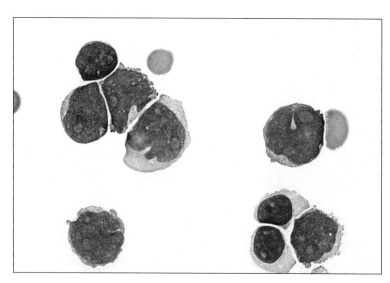

Image 28-10 Cerebrospinal fluid (CSF) relapse of acute lymphoblastic leukemia. The preparation is a cytocentrifuged CSF specimen. Several large lymphoblasts and two normal lymphocytes (lower right) are depicted.

Image 28-11 A bone marrow aspirate smear from a 2.5-year-old bone marrow transplant donor. There are several hematogones in the field. These normal precursor B cells may resemble leukemic lymphoblasts morphologically and immunophenotypically. (From McKenna RW. The bone marrow manifestations of Hodgkin's disease, the non-Hodgkin's lymphomas, and lymphoma-like disorders. In: Knowles DM, ed. *Neoplastic Hematopathology*. Baltimore, Md: Williams & Wilkins; 1992:1135–1180.)

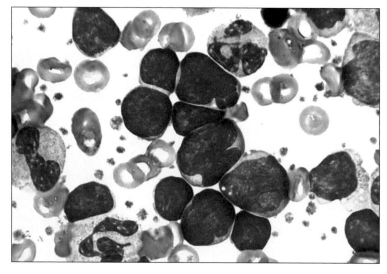

PART VII

Myeloproliferative Disorders

29   Myelofibrosis

The term "chronic myeloproliferative disorder" (MPD) was introduced 50 years ago to describe a group of closely related syndromes—chronic myelogenous leukemia (CML), polycythemia vera, myelofibrosis/myeloid metaplasia (MF/MM), and essential thrombocythemia (**Table 29-1**). These disorders have similar clinical and hematologic manifestations at some stage in their disease processes (**Table 29-2**) and must be distinguished from the newly recognized category of overlap myeloproliferative/myelodysplastic syndromes. (Polycythemia vera, essential thrombocythemia, and CML are described in Chapters 30, 31, and 32, respectively. Chronic myelomonocytic leukemia was discussed in Chapter 26. Juvenile and atypical CML are discussed briefly in Chapter 32.) This chapter is confined to a discussion of MF/MM, a clinical and pathologic state common to all of these disorders and to other hematologic and nonhematologic disorders.

29.1 Pathophysiology

A large number of synonyms have been used for MF/MM, including "idiopathic myelofibrosis", "chronic myelosclerosis", "agno-

Table 29-1 Classification of Chronic Myeloproliferative Disorders and Overlap Myelodysplastic/Myeloproliferative Syndromes

Chronic myeloproliferative
  Polycythemia vera (PV)
  Chronic myelogenous leukemia (CML)
  Essential thrombocythemia (ET)
  Myelofibrosis with myeloid metaplasia (MF/MM)

Myelodysplastic/myeloproliferative syndromes
  Chronic myelomonocytic leukemia (CMML)
  Juvenile myelomonocytic leukemia (JMML)
    Juvenile monosomy 7 syndrome
  Atypical chronic myeloid leukemia (aCML)

Table 29-2 Common Features of Myeloproliferative Disorders

Similar clinical manifestations
  Asymptomatic or fatigue, bleeding, and splenomegaly
Peripheral blood
  Anemia with variable red blood cell changes
  Variable degrees of leukocytosis with immature cells
  Variable degrees of eosinophilia and basophilia
  Qualitative and quantitative platelet abnormalities
Bone marrow
  Panmyelosis with variable degrees of myelofibrosis
Spleen
  Extramedullary hematopoiesis
Apparent "transitional" forms between various disorders
Accelerated phase or blastic crisis common in terminal stages

---

genic myeloid metaplasia", "aleukemic megakaryocytic myelosis", and "leukoerythroblastosis". These names usually indicate the feature of the disease most striking to the observer. The disorder is clonal in nature, arising from an abnormal multipotent hematopoietic stem cell. Unlike CML, no specific cytogenetic abnormality has been described for MF/MM. There are variable degrees of fibrosis in the bone marrow and a variable proliferation of the granulocytic, erythroid, and megakaryocytic series in the bone marrow, spleen, liver, and lymph nodes. The abnormal megakaryocyte precursors release growth factors such as platelet factor 4 and platelet-derived growth factor that stimulate fibroblastic proliferation, resulting in fibrosis in the marrow.

Figure 29-1 Conditions associated with myelofibrosis.

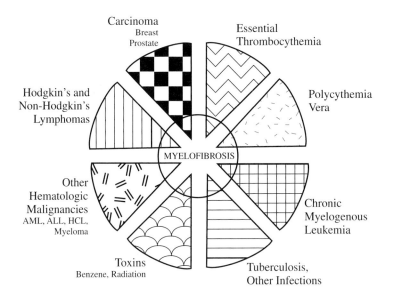

Abbreviations: AML = acute myeloid leukemia; ALL = acute lymphocytic leukemia; HCL = hairy cell leukemia.

Myelofibrosis also may be a secondary process consequent to a known cause, such as metastatic carcinoma (**Figure 29-1**). Patients suffering from MF characteristically have an enlarged spleen, possibly to a considerable degree. The cause of the spleno-megaly is a combination of vascular expansion, tremendous RBC pooling, hematopoietic hyperplasia, and fibrosis.

Studies have not demonstrated a correlation between the extent of marrow fibrosis and duration of disease, splenic weight, or degree of splenic myeloid metaplasia. Likewise, studies have been unable to document a progression of marrow fibrosis as a cause for the increase in splenomegaly.

Several theories have been postulated to explain extra-medullary hematopoiesis in MF. One states that circulating hema-topoietic precursors are filtered from the peripheral blood by the spleen and accumulate there. If they do not undergo phagocytosis, these cells proliferate and are released, resulting in the leuko-erythroblastosis characteristic of MF. Autonomous hematopoiesis may occur later in the course of the disease. The characteristic fea-tures of this disorder are listed in **Table 29-3**.

Table 29-3   Characteristics of Idiopathic Myelofibrosis

Insidious onset with weakness, weight loss, pallor
Splenomegaly
Normochromic anemia
Red blood cell morphology
    Prominent poikilocytosis (teardrop forms) and anisocytosis
Nucleated red blood cells common in peripheral blood
White blood cell count
    Elevated ($<30 \times 10^3/\text{mm}^3$ [$30 \times 10^9/\text{L}$]), normal, or rarely decreased
    Immature granulocytes, occasional myeloblasts; eosinophilia and
      basophilia
Platelet count
    Increased, normal, or decreased
    Giant platelets, micromegakaryocytes, and megakaryocytic fragments
Bone marrow
    Panmyelosis with increasing myelofibrosis
    Osteosclerosis may be present

29.2 Clinical Findings

MPDs usually have an insidious onset. The patient may present with a history of weakness or may be relatively asymptomatic. In MF/MM, patients exhibit a variety of symptoms, including malaise, weight loss, bleeding, diarrhea, and fever. Splenomegaly is the main physical finding and may be associated with abdominal discomfort, pain, dyspepsia, or dyspnea. Other features that may be present include hepatomegaly, petechiae and bleeding (usually secondary to thrombocytopenia, abnormal platelet function, or both), ascites, jaundice, portal hypertension, cirrhosis, and (rarely) lymphadenopathy.

29.3 Diagnostic Approach

Following a clinical history and physical examination with attention to the presence of splenomegaly, the laboratory diagnosis of MF/MM proceeds in the following sequence:

1. A complete blood count.

2. Examination of the peripheral blood smear.
3. Examination of the bone marrow aspirate and biopsy.
4. Cytogenetic and molecular studies, including *bcr* rearrangement.

Figure 30-1 presents an algorithm for the differential diagnosis of MF, the other chronic MPDs, and myelodysplastic syndromes (MDSs). **Table 29-1** also lists the most recently revised World Health Organization (WHO) classification of overlap syndromes, those disorders with features of both chronic MPDs and myelodysplasia.

29.4 Hematologic Findings

The hematologic findings in MF are variable and depend on the stage of the disease. As expected, there is considerable overlap among the different chronic MPDs. MDSs, whether de novo or therapy related, may be extremely difficult to differentiate from MF/MM. MDSs usually do not have significant splenomegaly, hepatomegaly, or the teardrop RBC morphology present in MF. In the differential diagnosis of MF/MM, other conditions associated with bone marrow fibrosis and leukoerythroblastosis must be considered (**Tables 29-1** and **29-4**; **Figure 29-1**).

29.4.1 Blood Cell Measurements
Initially in MF/MM, there is a slight anemia that becomes progressively more severe. The leukocyte count may be slightly increased, usually less than $30 \times 10^3/mm^3$ ($30 \times 10^9/L$), or decreased. The platelet count is initially normal or high. As the disease progresses, thrombocytopenia and leukopenia are common.

29.4.2 Peripheral Blood Smear Morphology
In MF, the whole spectrum of granulocytic precursors may be seen, and the blood smear resembles a granulocytic leukemoid reaction. The percentage of blasts varies from 0 to 10%, and the presence of blasts in the peripheral blood does not necessarily indicate an accelerated phase or blast crisis. Eosinophilia and basophilia may be present, but are usually less marked than in CML. In

Table 29-4   Conditions Associated With Myelofibrosis and/or Leukoerythroblastosis

Nonmalignant	Malignant
Tuberculosis	Chronic myeloproliferative disorders
Gaucher's disease	Acute and chronic leukemias
Radiation	Myelodysplastic syndromes
Renal osteodystrophy	Hodgkin's disease
Paget's disease of bone	Non-Hodgkin's lymphomas
Benzene	Metastatic carcinomas
Congenital syphilis	Plasma cell myeloma

addition to immature granulocytes, there are usually a small number of nucleated RBCs that, together with the immature granulocytes, constitute the "leukoerythroblastic picture" (**Image 29-1**). The RBC morphology usually includes a significant degree of anisocytosis, poikilocytosis, and polychromasia. Teardrop forms (dacryocytes) and ovalocytes are common in MF. Smaller microcytic cells may be present in patients who have developed iron deficiency secondary to bleeding. Platelets often exhibit abnormal morphology and may be extremely large. Fragments of megakaryocytes or micromegakaryocytes also may be seen.

29.4.3 Bone Marrow Examination

In MF, attempts to aspirate the bone marrow often yield a dry tap. A bone marrow biopsy must be performed in patients for whom a diagnosis of a chronic MPD is being considered. Early in the course of MF, the bone marrow may not show striking abnormalities except for hypercellularity with an increased number of all cell lines. All stages of cell differentiation are represented. This is the "cellular phase," or early stage of MF (**Image 29-2**). Usually, an increased proportion of neutrophilic precursors and megakaryocytes are seen. The megakaryocytes occur in clusters, are frequently abnormal in size and shape, and may be difficult to recognize as megakaryocytes. The marrow sinusoids are characteristically distended.

A reticulin stain is necessary to detect early fibrosis. The amount of fibrosis increases as the disease progresses (**Image**

29-3). The marrow gradually becomes less cellular, and the megakaryocytes persist until fibrosis is the predominant feature (**Image 29-4**). Formation of collagen in the marrow is associated with the appearance of extramedullary hematopoiesis of spleen, liver, and (sometimes) lymph nodes. However, the degree of marrow fibrosis need not correlate with the duration of the disease and splenic myeloid metaplasia. In addition to MF, increasing osteosclerosis may be seen.

Other Laboratory Tests

Test 29.1 Leukocyte Alkaline Phosphatase

Purpose. The leukocyte alkaline phosphatase (LAP) score may be useful in differentiating CML from polycythemia vera, essential thrombocytosis, and any of the MDSs.

Principle, Specimen, and Procedure. See Test 16.1.

Interpretation. In CML, the LAP score is characteristically zero or markedly decreased, but it is usually elevated in other chronic MPDs. In MF/MM, however, the LAP score may be high, normal, or low. Low scores are particularly common in patients with low granulocyte counts. Therefore, a low LAP score does not rule out MF/MM.

Test 29.2 Cytogenetic Studies

Purpose. Cytogenetic studies may be useful in distinguishing CML from other chronic MPDs, the overlap myeloproliferative/myelodysplastic syndromes, and primary myelodysplasias.

Principle, Specimen, and Procedure. See Test 32.2.

Interpretation. The Philadelphia (Ph[1]) chromosome, which is present in most patients with CML, is absent in those with MF. Several chromosome changes have been observed with the MPDs, but none is specific except for the Ph[1] chromosome.

29.5 Ancillary Tests

29.5.1 Platelet Aggregation Studies

Bleeding problems occur with all of the MPDs. The bleeding may be caused by thrombocytopenia or by a defect in platelet function. The latter manifests as impairment of in vitro platelet aggregation, most typically impaired responses to epinephrine and collagen. These studies are usually not helpful in differentiating among chronic MPDs and MDSs.

29.5.2 Blood Biochemistry

Serum uric acid level is frequently elevated. Complications include gouty arthritis, urate stones, and nephropathy, particularly in patients with a high leukocyte count. The serum alkaline phosphatase level may be elevated, possibly reflecting extramedullary hematopoiesis in the liver. Increased lactate dehydrogenase levels are seen as well.

29.5.3 Radiology

Osteosclerosis has been demonstrated in approximately 50% of patients with MF/MM. The bones most frequently affected are (in order of frequency) femur, pelvis, vertebrae, radius, tibia, and sternum. Foci of rarefaction also may be seen.

29.5.4 Biopsy of Tissue Other Than Bone Marrow

Extramedullary hematopoiesis may be associated with lymph node enlargement. Biopsy of a lymph node usually reveals intact architecture and a mixed proliferation of hematopoietic cells in the sinuses. Atypical megakaryocytes may predominate. This extramedullary hematopoiesis can exhibit such bizarre morphology that it may be mistaken for a malignant lymphoma or metastatic carcinoma. A chloroacetate esterase stain is helpful in confirming the presence of granulocytic precursors.

29.6 Course and Treatment

Patients with MF/MM usually show a progressive deterioration associated with increasing splenomegaly and fibrosis of the bone marrow. Anemia becomes progressively more severe, requiring blood transfusions. The median survival time is 4 to 5 years after diagnosis. In 10% to 12% of patients, there is an expansion of the malignant clone in the form of an accelerated phase or overt acute leukemic transformation (blast crisis). During the course of MF, many patients exhibit morphologic and cytogenetic evidence of dyspoiesis. Terminally, the clinical and laboratory picture may be indistinguishable from acute myeloid leukemia.

Therapy for MF/MM is mainly symptomatic. Androgen therapy has been used in patients who are markedly anemic and/or thrombocytopenic. In patients with painful splenomegaly, splenectomy or local radiation may be beneficial. Allopurinol may be indicated in patients with high serum uric acid levels.

29.7 Special Diagnostic Considerations

29.7.1 Acute Myelofibrosis (Acute Panmyelosis With Myelofibrosis)

According to the newly proposed WHO classification of acute myeloid leukemia (AML), acute MF is a rare AML characterized by pancytopenia, minimal poikilocytosis and anisocytosis (in contrast to MF/MM), bone marrow fibrosis, and panmyelosis. Most of the cells are immature, and megakaryocytes or megakaryoblasts are prominent. Also, in contrast to MF/MM, splenomegaly is minimal or absent. Acute MF is fulminant and usually fatal. It may be impossible to distinguish acute megakaryoblastic leukemia (M7 [see Chapter 27 for classification schema]) from acute MF.

29.7.2 Undifferentiated or Atypical Myeloproliferative Syndromes

Approximately one third of patients are diagnosed as having an "atypical" or "undifferentiated myeloproliferative syndrome." Their clinical and laboratory findings do not fit precisely into any specific disease category. Thus, some patients exhibit MM in the spleen and liver with a classic leukoerythroblastic blood smear, but the bone marrow shows only panmyelosis with minimal fibrosis. This may closely resemble CML; however, in contrast to CML, affected patients have normal or elevated LAP scores and lack the Ph[1] chromosome. To exclude polycythemia vera, the RBC mass

Table 29-5 Differential Characteristics of Chronic Myeloproliferative Syndromes

Variable	Myelofibrosis With Myeloid Metaplasia	Essential Thrombocythemia
Hemoglobin	Decreased	Normal or decreased
Leukocyte count	Usually <30 × 10³/mm³ (30 × 10⁹/L)	Usually <20 × 10³/mm³ (20 × 10⁹/L)
Differential count	Moderate number of immature granulocytes	Usually normal
Eosinophilia and/or basophilia	Usually present	May be present
RBC morphology	Anisocytosis and teardrop poikilocytosis	Normal or hypochromic, microcytic
Nucleated RBCs	Common	Rare
Platelet count	Normal, increased, or decreased	Increased
Bone marrow	Hypercellular with increasing fibrosis	Hypercellular with megakaryocytosis
LAP	Variable, usually increased	Usually normal
Ph¹	Absent	Absent
bcr-abl rearrangement	Absent	Absent
Splenomegaly	Marked	Absent or mild

Abbreviations: LAP = leukocyte alkaline phosphatase; Ph¹ = Philadelphia chromosome.

must be normal. Still other patients may have severe MF but only minimal MM. A summary of the differential characteristics of the various myeloproliferative syndromes is shown in **Table 29-5**.

29.8 References

Harris NL, Jaffe ES, Diebold J, et al. The World Health Organization Classification of Hematological Malignancies Report of the Clinical Advisory Committee Meeting, Airlie House, Virginia, November 1997. *Mod Pathol.* 2000;13(2):193–207.

Hasselbalch H. Idiopathic myelofibrosis: a clinical study of 80 patients. *Am J Hematol.* 1990;34:291–300.

Chronic Myelogenous Leukemia	Polycythemia Vera
Decreased	Normal or increased
Usually $<50 \times 10^3/mm^3$ $(50 \times 10^9/L)$	Usually $<20 \times 10^3/mm^3$ $(20 \times 10^9/L)$
Many immature granulocytes	Usually normal
Present	May be present
Usually normal	Normal or hypochromic, microcytic
Rare	Rare
Normal, increased, or decreased	Normal or increased
Marked myeloid hyperplasia	Hypercellular with decreased iron stores
Decreased	Usually increased
Present	Absent
Present	Absent
Moderate	Absent or mild

Jandl JH. Chronic myeloproliferative syndromes. In: Jandl JH. *Blood*. 2nd ed. Boston, Mass: Little, Brown; 1996:923–951.

Thiele J, Zankovich R, Steinberg T, et al. Agnogenic myeloid metaplasia (AMM)—correlation of bone marrow lesions with laboratory data: a longitudinal study of 114 patients. *Hematol Oncol*. 1989;7:327–343.

Vardiman J. The overlap between MDS and chronic myeloproliferative disorders, including CMML. *Mod Pathol*. 1999;12:104–106.

Visani G, Finelli C, Castelli U, et al. Myelofibrosis with myeloid metaplasia clinical and haematological parameters predicting survival in a series of 133 patients. *Br J Haematol*. 1990;75:4–9.

Wolf BC, Neiman RS. Hypothesis-splenic infiltration and the pathogenesis of extramedullary hematopoiesis in agnogenic myeloid metaplasia. *Hematol Pathol*. 1987;1:77–80.

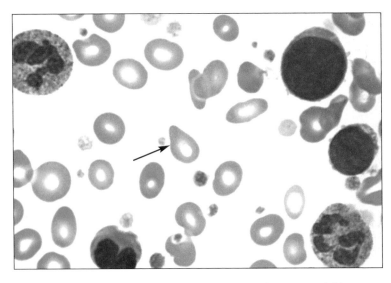

Image 29-1   Myelofibrosis. Peripheral smear shows a myeloblast (upper left corner), a dysplastic binucleated RBC, and a rare teardrop RBC (arrow).

Image 29-2   Myelofibrosis, early stage. Bone marrow biopsy section shows panhyperplasia.

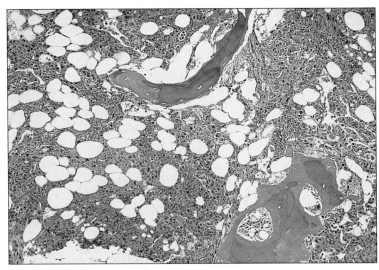

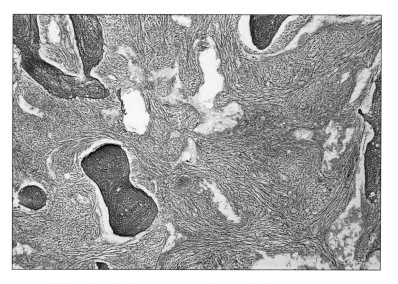

Image 29-3 Myelofibrosis, advanced stage. Reticulin stain of a bone marrow biopsy shows marked (4+) fibrosis. Compare this with the normal reticulin fiber content shown in Image 30-3.

Image 29-4 Myelofibrosis, end stage. Prominent fibrosis, osteosclerosis, and dilated sinuses are seen in this bone marrow biopsy section.

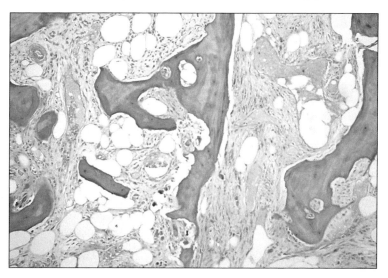

30   Polycythemia: Primary and Secondary

Polycythemia (erythrocytosis) is defined as an increase in the concentration of RBCs in the peripheral blood measured by the RBC count, the hemoglobin, or the hematocrit. It is caused by an increase in the total number of RBCs or a decrease in plasma volume. The terms "erythrocytosis" and "polycythemia" are often used synonymously, although the latter term implies an increase in multiple hematopoietic cell lines. For simplicity, however, the terms are used interchangeably in this chapter. Polycythemia can result from an intrinsic bone marrow defect, altered erythropoietin regulatory activity, or decreased plasma volume (**Table 30-1**).

30.1 Types of Polycythemia

30.1.1 Polycythemia Vera (Primary Erythrocytosis)

Primary vera (PV), or primary erythrocytosis, is a chronic myeloproliferative disorder that occurs when all hematopoietic cell lines undergo uncontrolled proliferation with intact maturation. By definition, the erythroid proliferation is dominant. The abnormal cells are derived from a single parent cell and, hence, are clonal.

Table 30-1 Differential Diagnosis of Polycythemia*

Nonneoplastic

    Increased erythropoietin production, appropriate response

        High altitude

        Chronic obstructive pulmonary disease

        Left-to-right cardiovascular shunt

        High-oxygen affinity hemoglobinopathy

        Congenital deficiency of red blood cell diphosphoglycerate

    Increased erythropoietin production, inappropriate response

        Tumor

            Uterine leiomyoma

            Adenocarcinoma of kidney

            Cerebellar hemangioblastoma

            Hepatocellular carcinoma

        Renal disease

    Increased plasma volume or relative (stress) polycythemia

Neoplastic: polycythemia vera

*Modified with permission from Berlin NI. Diagnosis and classification of the polycythemias. *Semin Hematol.* 1975;12:340.

The proliferation is erythropoietin-independent. The disease has an estimated annual incidence of 1 case per 100,000 population; there is a slight predominance in men; and most patients are older than 50 years. The diagnostic features of PV are separated into major and minor criteria:

Major criteria
1. Elevated RBC mass (men, >36 mL/kg; women, >32 mL/kg)
2. Normal arterial oxygen saturation (≥92%)
3. Splenomegaly

Minor criteria
1. Platelet count greater than $400 \times 10^3/\text{mm}^3$ ($400 \times 10^9/\text{L}$)
2. WBC count greater than $12 \times 10^3/\text{mm}^3$ ($12 \times 10^9/\text{L}$)
3. Elevated leukocyte alkaline phosphatase (LAP) level
4. Elevated vitamin B_{12} level or vitamin B_{12}–binding capacity

A diagnosis of PV can be made when all three major criteria are present or when the first two major criteria plus any two minor criteria are identified. These relatively stringent criteria may exclude patients in the earlier stages of the disease. More recent

Table 30-2 Disorders Associated With Physiologically Inappropriate Erythrocytosis

Organ	Disorder
Kidney	Cystic renal disease
	Hydronephrosis
	Adenocarcinoma
	Transplant rejection
Liver	Hepatocellular carcinoma
Uterus	Leiomyoma
Ovary	Ovarian carcinoma
Adrenal glands	Pheochromocytoma
	Adrenal cortical hyperplasia
Brain	Cerebellar hemangioblastoma

criteria also require that a bone marrow biopsy demonstrate characteristic histopathologic findings.

30.1.2 Secondary Polycythemia

Patients with secondary polycythemia have an erythropoietin-mediated, absolute increase in RBC mass that may be physiologically appropriate or inappropriate (**Table 30-2**). Physiologically appropriate polycythemia results from a hypoxic stimulus such as residing at a high altitude, chronic pulmonary or cardiac disease, high oxygen–affinity hemoglobinopathies, or increased carboxyhemoglobin levels. Patients with physiologically inappropriate secondary polycythemia do not exhibit tissue hypoxia but have excess production of either erythropoietin or anabolic steroids. Disorders associated with this type of secondary polycythemia include renal disorders such as cystic disease and hydronephrosis; various erythropoietin-producing tumors such as uterine, liver, and cerebellar tumors; and adrenal cortical hypersecretion.

30.1.3 Relative Polycythemia

In patients with relative or stress polycythemia, the primary disorder is one of decreased plasma volume rather than true or absolute polycythemia. Although the hematocrit is elevated, the RBC mass is normal or decreased. This is sometimes known as "stress erythrocytosis".

30.2 Pathophysiology

Bone marrow production of RBCs is largely regulated by erythropoietin, a glycoprotein cytokine that induces committed bone marrow stem cells to mature into RBCs and also prevents apoptosis of later-stage erythroid cells. The erythropoietin precursor substance is produced in the peritubular interstitial cells of the kidney in response to tissue hypoxia. Once oxygen delivery to the tissues is increased, erythropoietin production is suppressed.

In patients with PV, an acquired stem cell defect results in unregulated production of all hematopoietic elements. The production of RBCs in this disorder is independent of erythropoietin.

The excess RBC production in secondary polycythemia is erythropoietin-mediated. In patients with physiologically appropriate secondary polycythemia, the tissue hypoxia responsible for erythropoietin production can result from decreased oxygen in the atmosphere, impaired oxygen–carbon dioxide exchange in the lungs, or decreased delivery of oxygen to tissues (*see Table 30-1*). In all of the disorders associated with secondary polycythemia, the erythropoietin production decreases if the tissue hypoxia is alleviated.

Physiologically inappropriate polycythemia occurs when high levels of erythropoietin, erythropoietinlike substances, or anabolic steroids drive the bone marrow to produce excessive numbers of RBCs in the absence of tissue hypoxia. The disorders associated with this type of secondary polycythemia are listed in **Table 30-2** and include a variety of neoplasms from the kidney, liver, uterus, ovary, adrenal gland, and brain. The nonneoplastic disorders associated with physiologically inappropriate polycythemia are mainly renal diseases.

The relative or stress polycythemia present in patients with decreased plasma volume can be secondary to either dehydration or excess water loss (renal or gastrointestinal abnormalities). Decreased plasma volume is also is a contributing factor to the polycythemia frequently observed in heavy smokers.

30.3 Clinical Findings

Patients with PV are generally middle-aged and present with symptoms related to increased blood volume or thromboembolic or hemorrhagic phenomena (**Image 30-1**). These patients often experience headache, weakness, light-headedness, and sweating. More than 35% of patients experience pruritus, which is postulated to be secondary to excessive histamine release by basophils. The frequency of peptic ulcer disease in these patients is four times that of the general population.

The thromboembolic and hemorrhagic episodes seen both at presentation and during the disease course in patients with PV are secondary to thrombocytosis, platelet function defects, and hyperviscosity. The uric acid level is often increased and is associated with gout in approximately 10% of patients. Some patients present with erythromelalgia, a vaso-occlusive process localized to the distal extremities, although this finding is more common in essential or primary thrombocythemia (see Chapter 31).

On physical examination, patients with PV almost invariably exhibit splenomegaly. They may be plethoric, with conjunctival and retinal venous engorgement.

The clinical findings in patients with secondary polycythemia vary greatly, depending on the underlying cause. For instance, patients with physiologically appropriate secondary polycythemia may have manifestations of cardiopulmonary disease such as cyanosis, clubbing, and increased respiratory rate. However, many other patients with the same disease may have no specific clinical findings. Splenomegaly is not a clinical manifestation of secondary polycythemia, and thrombotic events are not expected.

In patients with relative polycythemia, the underlying cause of the decreased plasma volume is usually apparent and includes such disorders as diarrhea, vomiting, dehydration, and renal disease. Splenomegaly, the physical finding that is the hallmark of chronic myeloproliferative disorders, is not present in patients with relative polycythemia.

30.4 Diagnostic Approach

Patients should be evaluated for possible primary or secondary polycythemia when the hemoglobin level is elevated with no obvious clinical cause. An algorithm to encompass all possible diagnostic explanations for polycythemia is very complex and includes tests rarely performed in routine clinical or laboratory practice. A simplified approach to the diagnosis of polycythemia, however, allows classification of most patients' diseases. **Figure 30-1**

Figure 30-1 Algorithm for diagnosis of chronic myeloproliferative disorders.

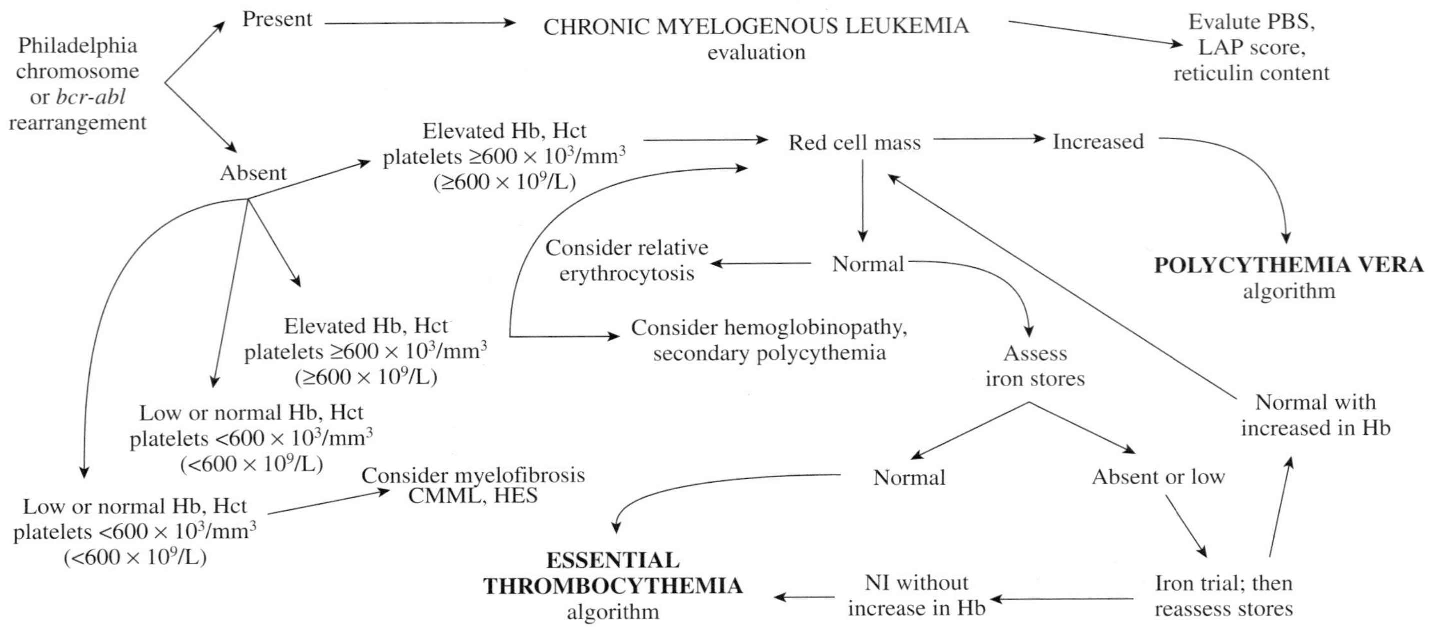

provides an algorithm for the diagnosis of chronic myeloproliferative disorders, including PV. The steps are as follows:

1. Eliminate cases of relative polycythemia by careful clinical evaluation for disorders associated with loss of plasma volume.
2. If the patient has an established diagnosis of renal disease or a neoplasm associated with polycythemia, it should be considered a possible cause of polycythemia.
3. Assess other hematologic features for abnormalities not explained by the clinical setting, notably leukocytosis and thrombocytosis.
4. Evaluate for diagnostic criteria of PV in patients in whom other unexplained hematologic abnormalities are identified. This includes measurement of arterial oxygen saturation and (if possible) RBC mass.
5. In patients with no other unexplained hematologic abnormalities, distinguish between physiologic and nonphysiologic secondary erythrocytosis. Most of the physiologically appropriate cases of polycythemia are secondary to pulmonary or cardiovascular disorders or to smoking. Causes such as high oxygen–affinity hemoglobinopathy, however, require more extensive laboratory investigation.
6. In the absence of PV or a physiologic cause for the polycythemia, a diverse group of disorders, including occult tumors and renal diseases, should be considered (*see Table 30-2*).

30.5 Hematologic Findings

The hematologic findings of PV differ from those of secondary and relative polycythemia. In PV, abnormalities are detected in all three cell lines in the blood, whereas secondary and relative polycythemia are generally associated only with RBC changes.

30.5.1 Blood Cell Measurements

In patients with PV, the hemoglobin level, hematocrit, WBC count, and platelet count are characteristically elevated. The RBC indices and red cell distribution width are generally normal but may be abnormal in patients with concurrent iron deficiency. Because more than 90% of patients with PV are iron deficient at diagnosis, the mean corpuscular volume may be particularly misleading. The percentage of reticulocytes is within normal limits.

Patients with secondary polycythemia have elevated hemoglobin and hematocrit levels with normal WBC and platelet counts. The RBC indices and red cell distribution width are generally normal. The absolute reticulocyte count is often elevated.

The elevated hematocrit value noted in patients with relative polycythemia is almost always less than 60% (0.60) and is not associated with an increased reticulocyte count.

30.5.2 Peripheral Blood Smear Morphology

In patients with PV, the erythrocytes are generally normocytic and normochromic, except when there is concurrent iron deficiency. Increased numbers of platelets and megakaryocyte fragments may be present. The WBC differential count occasionally shows basophilia and/or eosinophilia.

The peripheral blood smear morphology in secondary polycythemia is normal, except for the increase in normal-appearing RBCs. Polychromasia may be present.

No specific morphologic abnormalities are present in blood smears from patients with relative polycythemia.

30.5.3 Bone Marrow Examination

In patients with PV, both the bone marrow aspirate smear and biopsy are characteristically hypercellular with a panhyperplasia. In addition, the biopsy shows clusters of normal-appearing and atypical megakaryocytes (**Image 30-2**). Although an increase in reticulin fibers may be present at diagnosis (**Image 30-3**), there is generally a progressive increase in the amount of reticulin fibrosis throughout the course of the disease. As this fibrosis increases, there is an associated progressive decrease in the cellularity, which is sometimes referred to as the "spent phase" of PV. This occurs in 10% of patients with PV. Storage iron is often markedly decreased because of increased RBC production, bleeding, and the periodic phlebotomy that is sometimes used for treatment.

Bone marrow examination is generally not necessary to establish a diagnosis of secondary polycythemia. If a bone marrow specimen is obtained, erythroid hyperplasia is the major finding. In patients with relative polycythemia, bone marrow examination is not indicated.

Table 30-3 Laboratory Tests Used to Distinguish Types of Erythrocytosis

Laboratory Test	Polycythemia Vera	Secondary Erythrocytosis*	Relative Erythrocytosis
RBC mass†	Increased	Increased	Normal
Erythropoietin	Usually decreased	Normal to increased	Usually normal
PO_2	Usually normal	Decreased in some cases	Normal
Leukocyte alkaline phosphatase	Increased	Usually normal‡	Usually normal
Vitamin B_{12}	Increased	Normal	Normal
Vitamin B_{12}–binding proteins	Increased	Normal	Normal
Carboxyhemoglobin§	Usually normal	May be increased	May be increased
Uric acid	Increased	Normal	Normal
Serum iron	Decreased	Normal	Normal
Marrow iron stores	Decreased	Normal	Normal
Marrow biopsy histopathology	Panhyperplastic with megakaryo-cyte clustering	Erythoid hyperplasia	Normal
Hemoglobinopathy	Absent	Present in some cases	Absent
Platelet aggregation‖	Abnormal	Normal	Normal
Cytogenic abnormalities	May be present	Absent	Absent

*Includes both physiologically appropriate and inappropriate causes of erythrocytosis.
†Assay may be difficult to obtain in many clinical settings.
‡Can be elevated during pregnancy, with oral contraceptive drugs, and in inflammatory/infectious disorders.
§Increased in patients who smoke.
‖Study not warranted in most cases.

Other Laboratory Tests

Laboratory tests that can be used to distinguish PV from secondary polycythemia and relative polycythemia are shown in **Table 30-3**.

Test 30.1 **Arterial Oxygen Saturation**

Purpose. Arterial oxygen saturation is performed to determine whether there is hypoxemia.

Principle and Procedure. The standard nomogram and spectrophotometric techniques used to measure arterial oxygen saturation are detailed in clinical pathology texts.

Specimen. Arterial blood specimens for blood gas determinations are collected with a minimum amount of heparin, which is maintained under anaerobic conditions and analyzed promptly.

Interpretation. When the arterial oxygen saturation is less than the established normal range, hypoxia is present.

Notes and Precautions. Proper, prompt specimen handling is necessary to ensure the accuracy of the result. Normal range values are affected by altitude and need to be established for each laboratory.

Test 30.2 **RBC Mass**

Purpose. Measurement of the RBC mass can be used to distinguish true from relative polycythemia.

Principle. Erythrocyte mass is measured by a dilution technique using radiolabeled RBCs, with the degree of dilution directly proportional to RBC mass.

Specimen. Anticoagulated venous blood is used.

Procedure. A fixed number of the patient's erythrocytes are radiolabeled in vitro and intravenously injected back into the patient. After a 10- to 20-minute equilibrium period, a second sample of venous blood is drawn from the opposite arm. A scintillation counter is used to measure the radioactivity of the injected sample and the second venous sample. RBC mass is calculated using the following formula:

$$\text{RBC Mass} = \frac{\text{Injected Radioactivity}}{\text{Radioactivity of Erythrocytes After Mixing}}$$

Interpretation. An elevated erythrocyte mass is seen in primary and secondary polycythemia but not in relative polycythemia.

Notes and Precautions. Because RBC mass is related to lean body mass, spuriously low values can occur in patients with marked obesity. When chromium-51 is used to radiolabel the patient's erythrocytes, the patient should not have previously received antibiotics or ascorbic acid, which impair the labeling process, yielding spuriously low results. For many reasons, including concerns about radioisotopes, this assay may be difficult to obtain.

30.6 Ancillary Tests

Other laboratory tests that can be used on a selected basis to distinguish the three types of polycythemia are listed in **Table 30-3**. The characteristic test result for each type of polycythemia is included.

30.6.1 Platelet Aggregation Studies
Hemostatic problems, both thrombosis and hemorrhage, occur frequently in chronic myeloproliferative disorders. Only occasionally are platelet aggregation assays necessary for diagnostic purposes. The bleeding may be due to a defect in platelet function. The most common manifestation in vitro is a defect in aggregation in response to epinephrine and collagen. Some patients also display aggregation defects in response to adenosine diphosphate.

30.6.2 Cytokine Receptor Studies
Hematopoietic growth factors (cytokines) signal cells through interaction with cell surface receptors. Although only a research tool at the time of this printing, measurement of receptor site expression on RBCs and platelets may make greater diagnostic accuracy possible.

30.7 Course and Treatment

The increased blood viscosity associated with polycythemia causes a significant morbidity and even mortality in affected patients. Blood viscosity increases dramatically as the patient's hematocrit value rises from 50% to 60% (0.50 to 0.60). As viscosity increases, the oxygen-carrying ability of erythrocytes actually decreases. In patients with physiologically appropriate secondary polycythemia, this decrease in oxygen delivery leads to further erythropoietin release and a greater severity of polycythemia. In addition to impaired oxygen delivery, patients with increased blood viscosity are at risk for thrombosis, especially in slow flow rate venous channels.

30.7.1 Polycythemia Vera

PV typically follows an indolent, slowly progressive course with gradual evolution from a hypercellular bone marrow picture to bone marrow fibrosis, with an associated decline in peripheral blood counts (spent phase). Thrombosis and hemorrhage caused by increased blood viscosity, thrombocytosis, and platelet function abnormalities are causes of increased morbidity and mortality in patients with PV. With proper management, risks from these complications can be reduced substantially. Without treatment, patients with PV have a median survival time of about 18 months. With treatment, however, these patients can have survival times equal to those of age- and sex-matched control populations.

Treatment modalities that have been used successfully in patients with PV include periodic phlebotomy to reduce the viscosity and alkylating agent or radioactive phosphorus (^{32}P) therapy to reduce bone marrow production of all hematopoietic elements. Alkylating agent therapy has been associated with an increased incidence of both acute leukemia (**Image 30-4**) and non-Hodgkin's lymphoma. Therapy with ^{32}P also increases the risk of acute leukemia and so is generally reserved for patients older than 70 years.

Theoretically, less leukemogenic agents, including hydroxyurea and interferons, are used. Interferon-α is often used in younger patients, especially women of child-bearing age. Patients undergoing periodic phlebotomy should be monitored for the development of iron deficiency, because hypochromic erythrocytes have increased internal viscosity and decreased deformability, which enhances blood viscosity and further compromises tissue oxygen delivery.

Preventing the thrombotic complications that occur in more than 40% of patients during the course of their disease is the rationale for low-dose aspirin ($\leq$100 mg/d) prophylaxis. Higher doses cause gastrointestinal and other bleeding.

30.7.2 Secondary Polycythemia

The clinical course and proper management of patients with secondary polycythemia depends on the specific cause of the excessive RBC production. Although there is no curative treatment for some conditions, such as high oxygen-affinity hemoglobinopathies, others, such as certain cardiopulmonary disorders, can be alleviated with proper treatment. To reduce blood viscosity, periodic phlebotomy may be indicated for some patients with physiologically appropriate secondary polycythemia.

Management of the neoplasm is the primary treatment goal for patients with excessive erythropoietin production caused by a tumor. In a small number of patients with tumors of the kidney, adrenal gland, liver, or brain, erythropoietin production is the first sign that the patient has a neoplasm. Identification of these tumors before they are clinically obvious may be associated with improved survival. Management of nonneoplastic renal disease is necessary to reduce erythropoietin production in patients with physiologically inappropriate polycythemia.

30.7.3 Relative Polycythemia

In affected patients, the primary cause of the decreased plasma volume is often apparent and can usually be treated properly. Other factors that could aggravate the polycythemia, such as hypertension and smoking, should be addressed. The course of the disease and treatment vary with the underlying cause of the reduced plasma volume.

30.8 References

Berlin NI. Diagnosis and classification of the polycythemias. *Semin Hematol.* 1975;12:339–351.

Beutler E. Polycythemia vera. In: Beutler E, Lichtman MA, Coller BS, et al, eds. *Williams' Hematology.* 5th ed. New York, NY: McGraw-Hill; 1995:324–330.

Ellis JT, Peterson P, Geller SA, et al. Studies of the bone marrow in polycythemia vera and the evolution of myelofibrosis and second hematologic malignancies. *Semin Hematol.* 1986;23:144–155.

Fruchtman SM, Mack K, Kaplan ME, et al. From efficacy to safety: a PVSG report on hydroxyurea in patients with polycythemia vera. *Semin Hematol.* 1997;34:17–23.

Gruppo Ilaliano Studio Policitemia. Polycythemia vera: the natural history of 1213 patients followed for 20 years. *Ann Intern Med.* 1995;123:656–664.

Michiels JJ, Juvonen E. Proposal for revised diagnostic criteria of essential thrombocythemia and polycythemia vera by the Thrombocythemia Vera Study Group. *Semin Thromb Hemost.* 1997;23:339–347.

Peterson P, Ellis JT. The bone marrow in polycythemia vera. In: Berlin NI, Berk PD, Wasserman LR, eds. *Polycythemia and the Myeloproliferative Disorders.* Philadelphia, Pa: Saunders; 1994:31–53.

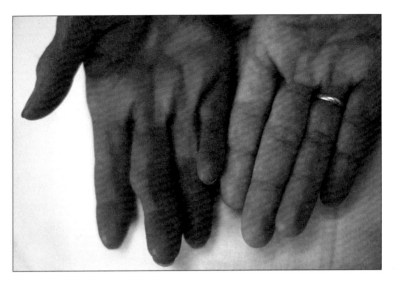

Image 30-1   Polycythemia vera. The hand on the left is that of a 62-year-old man with newly diagnosed and untreated PV. His ruddy color is readily explained by a hemoglobin level of 20.3 g/dL (203 g/L). In comparison, the hand of the 55-year-old man on the right shows a normal skin color. He has a normal hemoglobin level of 14.8 g/dL (148 g/L).

Image 30-2   Polycythemia vera. Bone marrow biopsy section from a patient with untreated PV shows hypercellularity, hyperplasia, and a near absence of fat. Erythroid and granulocytic precursors and megakaryocytes are increased. Note the clustering and atypical appearance of the megakaryocytes.

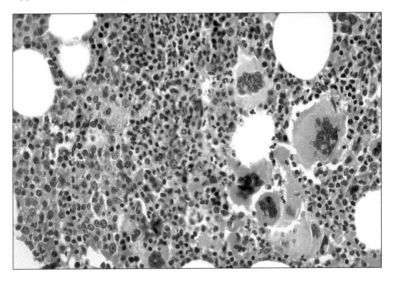

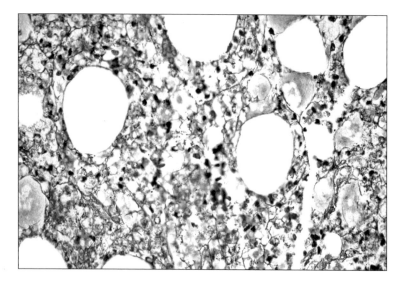

Image 30-3 Polycythemia vera. Reticulin stain of the same bone marrow biopsy shown in Image 30-2. The section shows normal reticulin fiber content with only thin, delicate reticulin fibrils. Compare this with Image 29-3.

Image 30-4 Acute leukemic transformation in polycythemia vera. Peripheral smear from a patient treated with myelosuppressive agents (chemotherapy) shows myeloblasts. Note the absence of platelets.

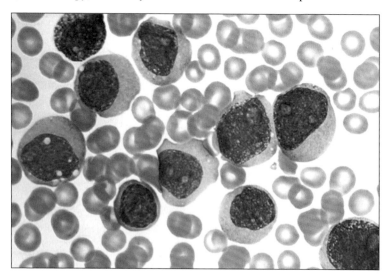

31 Thrombocytosis: Primary and Secondary

Thrombocytosis (thrombocythemia) is defined as an increase in the number of platelets in the peripheral blood and is usually due to an increase in the total number of megakaryocytes. The terms "thrombocytosis" and "thrombocythemia" are often used interchangeably, although the latter term implies a hematopoietic stem cell disorder. For simplicity, the terms are used interchangeably in this chapter. Thrombocytosis can be caused by an intrinsic stem cell defect or it may be a reaction to hemorrhage or other clinical states (**Table 31-1**).

31.1 Primary Thrombocytosis (Essential Thrombocythemia)

Primary thrombocytosis, or essential thrombocythemia (ET), is a chronic myeloproliferative disorder (MPD) that occurs when all hematopoietic cell lines undergo uncontrolled proliferation with intact maturation. By definition, megakaryocytic proliferation is dominant. The abnormal cells are derived from a single parent cell and hence are clonal. This disease may be the most common of the

Table 31-1 Classification of Thrombocytosis

Type	Examples
Primary	Essential thrombocythemia
	Polycythemia vera
	Chronic myelogenous leukemia
	Myelofibrosis with myeloid metaplasia
Secondary (reactive)	Hemorrhage
	Chronic iron deficiency
	Postsplenectomy (temporary)
	Chronic inflammatory/infectious states
	Collagen vascular disorders
	Ulcerative colitis
	Tuberculosis
	Malignancies
	Drugs: vincristine, high-dose erythropoietin

chronic MPDs, there is no sex predominance, and patients range from 20 to 70 years of age. The diagnostic features of ET are as follows:

1. Sustained platelet count greater than $600 \times 10^3/\text{mm}^3$ ($600 \times 10^9/\text{L}$).
2. Normal hemoglobin level (or normal RBC mass).
3. Stainable iron in the bone marrow or failure of hemoglobin to rise 1 g/dL (10 g/L) after 1 month of iron therapy.
4. Absence of the Philadelphia (Ph^1) chromosome or *bcr* rearrangement.
5. Collagen fibrosis of marrow either absent or less than one third of bone marrow area without both splenomegaly and leuko-erythroblastic reaction.
6. No known cause for reactive thrombocytosis.

These diagnostic criteria have been revised to allow a platelet count elevation of greater than $400 \times 10^3/\text{mm}^3$ ($400 \times 10^9/\text{L}$) in patients who experience a thrombosis, especially an arterial event. Similar to polycythemia vera (PV), the criteria require that a bone marrow biopsy demonstrate characteristic histopathologic findings.

An algorithm for the differential diagnosis of thrombocytosis is shown in **Figure 31-1**. *See Figure 30-1* for the differential diagnosis of ET and other chronic MPDs.

Figure 31-1 Algorithm for the evaluation of thrombocytosis.*

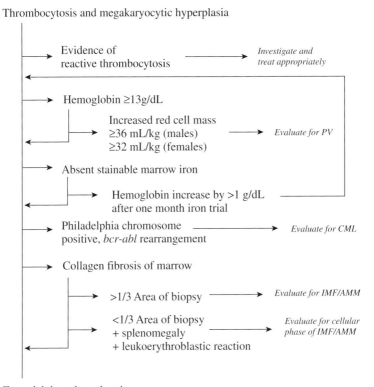

Thrombocytosis and megakaryocytic hyperplasia

Evidence of
reactive thrombocytosis → *Investigate and treat appropriately*

Hemoglobin ≥13g/dL

Increased red cell mass
≥36 mL/kg (males)
≥32 mL/kg (females) → *Evaluate for PV*

Absent stainable marrow iron

Hemoglobin increase by >1 g/dL
after one month iron trial

Philadelphia chromosome → *Evaluate for CML*
positive, *bcr-abl* rearrangement

Collagen fibrosis of marrow

>1/3 Area of biopsy → *Evaluate for IMF/AMM*

<1/3 Area of biopsy
+ splenomegaly → *Evaluate for cellular phase of IMF/AMM*
+ leukoerythroblastic reaction

Essential thrombocythemia

* Adapted with permission from Iland HJ, Laszlo J, Peterson P, et al. Essential thrombocythemia: clinical and laboratory characteristics at presentation. *Trans Assoc Am Physicians.* 1983;96:167. Abbreviations: PV = polycythemia vera; CML = chronic myelogenous leukemia; IMF/AMM = idiopathic myelofibrosis/agnogenic myeloid metaplasia.

31.1.1 Secondary Thrombocytosis

Patients with secondary thrombocytosis have an increased platelet number resulting from a hemorrhagic stimulus such as bleeding, chronic inflammatory or infectious states, a postsplenectomy state, certain medications, or a rebound phenomenon from a thrombocytopenic state (**see Table 31-1**).

31.1.2 Pathophysiology

The histopathologic hallmark of ET is megakaryocyte proliferation. Overproduction of platelets is the predominant physiologic feature. The recurrent thromboses and hemorrhages observed in patients suffering from this disorder are caused by the marked elevation in platelet count associated with distinctly abnormal platelet function. Although this entity has also been called "hemorrhagic thrombocythemia", thrombotic complications are generally a greater clinical hazard than is bleeding. Iron deficiency anemia may develop as a result of chronic gastrointestinal hemorrhage. Between hemorrhages, there may be a tendency toward polycythemia. As with other MPDs, ET is a clonal abnormality of the multipotential stem cell. The main features of this disorder are listed in **Table 31-2**.

Patients with ET may be asymptomatic and are often detected because of an elevated platelet count enumerated by an automated analyzer. More than 50% of symptomatic patients present with or because of a thrombotic event such as a myocardial infarct, a stroke, erythromelalgia, or other microcirculatory disturbances. Other complaints are weakness, headache, paresthesias, and dizziness. Bleeding may occur in the gastrointestinal tract and (less commonly) in the urinary tract or the skin. Splenomegaly is present in approximately 60% of patients but usually is not as prominent as in myelofibrosis with myeloid metaplasia. The liver may be slightly enlarged, but only rarely is there lymph node enlargement.

31.2 Hematologic Findings

The hemoglobin level is usually normal. Microcytic hypochromic anemia may develop if the patient has chronic bleeding. Almost one third of patients, however, exhibit an elevated hematocrit value, signifying a possible misdiagnosis of PV. The leukocyte count may be normal but is usually moderately increased. The striking feature in ET is the markedly elevated platelet count, by definition exceeding $600 \times 10^3/mm^3$ ($600 \times 10^9/L$) and very often greater than $1000 \times 10^3/mm^3$ ($1000 \times 10^9/L$).

31.2.1 Peripheral Blood Smear Morphology

Large clumps or swarms of platelets are usually seen (**Image 31-1**). In addition, the platelets show marked variation in size and shape, including giant platelets, microplatelets, and platelets with abnormal granularity. The leukocytes are slightly increased in number and may exhibit metamyelocytes, but promyelocytes are

Table 31-2 Characteristic Features of Essential Thrombocythemia

Insidious onset
Splenomegaly
Bleeding and thromboembolic (arterial and venous) phenomena
Sustained elevation of platelet count $>600 \times 10^3/\text{mm}^3$ ($600 \times 10^9/\text{L}$)
Normal hemoglobin level (unless iron-deficient from bleeding)
Slight neutrophilic leukocytosis
Marrow megakaryocytic hyperplasia and dysplasia

unusual. As with myelofibrosis, mild eosinophilia may be seen. The RBCs are usually normochromic and normocytic, but microcytic hypochromic RBCs can be found in patients with chronic blood loss.

31.2.2 Bone Marrow Examination

The bone marrow aspirate and biopsy show a preponderance of megakaryocytes. The aspirate also shows the resultant extensive platelet production. Megakaryocytes frequently occur in clusters and vary considerably in size and shape (**Image 31-2**). The biopsy specimen is normocellular to hypercellular without evidence of fibrosis. With one exception, the bone marrow findings in patients with untreated ET are difficult to separate from those of patients with PV. The exception is the demonstration of stainable iron in patients with ET, compared with its absence in patients with PV. As the disease progresses, a transition to acute myelogenous leukemia and/or myelofibrosis can occur, although the incidence of transformation appears to be less than in the other chronic MPDs.

Other Laboratory Tests

Test 31.1 Leukocyte Alkaline Phosphatase

Purpose. The leukocyte alkaline phosphatase (LAP) score may be useful in differentiating CML from ET and the other chronic MPDs.

Principle, Specimen, and Procedure. See Test 16.1.

Interpretation. In CML, the LAP score is characteristically zero or markedly decreased. In ET, the LAP score is usually normal or elevated.

Test 31.2 Cytogenetic Studies

Purpose. Cytogenetic studies may be useful in distinguishing CML from ET and the other chronic MPDs.

Principle, Specimen, and Procedure. See Test 32.2.

Interpretation. The Ph[1] chromosome, present in nearly all patients with CML, is absent in those with ET. Several chromosome changes have been observed in patients with ET, but none are specific.

Test 31.3 RBC Mass

Purpose. The RBC mass may be useful in differentiating PV from ET. The test should be performed only when the patient's iron stores are replete.

Principle, Specimen, and Procedure. See Test 30.2.

Interpretation. In ET, the RBC mass is normal; it is elevated in PV.

31.3 Ancillary Tests

31.3.1 Blood Biochemistry

Serum potassium levels may be artifactually elevated because of the release from platelets during clotting. Plasma potassium levels, however, are accurate. In addition, serum uric acid, alkaline phosphatase, and lactate dehydrogenase levels are elevated in more than 50% of untreated patients.

31.3.2 Platelet Aggregation Studies

See Chapter 30.

31.4 Course and Treatment

Patients with ET, especially younger patients, may not require therapy for years. Other patients may experience repeated hemorrhagic and thrombotic episodes. Blast crisis or myelofibrosis develops in a small percentage of patients.

When a patient of any age develops a thrombotic or bleeding episode, treatment is probably indicated. Current therapeutic options to reduce the platelet count include the antimetabolite hydroxyurea, interferon-α, and the oral imidazoquinazolin derivative anagrelide. The long-term consequences of these drugs with respect to controlling thrombotic events and the potential for leukemogenesis and teratogenesis are not fully known. Occasionally, vaso-occlusive events may require drugs that interfere with normal platelet function, such as low-dose aspirin (≤100 mg/d).

31.5 References

Blickstein D, Aviram A, Luboshitz J, et al. BCR-ABL transcripts in bone marrow aspirates of Philadelphia-negative essential thrombocythemia patients: clinical presentation. *Blood.* 1997;90:2768–2771.

Buss DH, O'Connor ML, Woodruff RD, et al. Bone marrow and peripheral blood findings in patients with extreme thrombocytosis. *Arch Pathol Lab Med.* 1991;115:475–480.

Iland HJ, Laszlo J, Case DC, et al. Differentiation between essential thrombocythemia and polycythemia vera with marked thrombocytosis. *Am J Hematol.* 1987;25:191–201.

Iland HJ, Laszlo J, Peterson P, et al. Essential thrombocythemia: clinical and laboratory characteristics at presentation. *Trans Assoc Am Physicians.* 1983;96:165–174.

Randi ML, Fabria F, Cella G, et al. Cerebral vascular accidents in young patients with essential thrombocythemia: relation to other known cardiovascular risk factors. *Angiology.* 1998;49:477–481.

Stoll DB, Peterson P, Exten R, et al. Clinical presentation and natural history of patients with essential thrombocythemia and the Philadelphia chromosome. *Am J Hematol.* 1988;27:77–83.

van Genderen PJJ, Mulder PGH, Waleboer M, et al. Prevention and treatment of thrombotic complications in essential thrombocythaemia: efficacy and safety of aspirin. *Br J Haematol.* 1997;97:179–184.

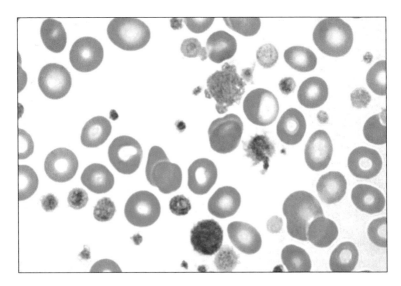

Image 31-1   Essential thrombocythemia. Peripheral smear from a patient with untreated ET shows an increased number of platelets, many of which are enlarged.

Image 31-2   Essential thrombocythemia. Bone marrow biopsy section from a patient with untreated ET shows megakaryocytic hyperplasia. Note the variation in both the size and shape of the abnormally clustered megakaryocytes.

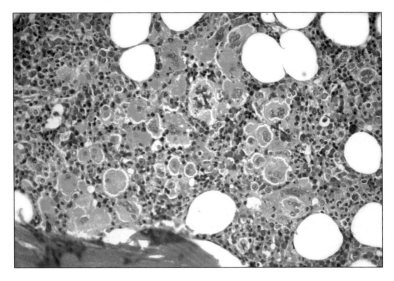

32 Chronic Myelogenous Leukemia

Chronic myelogenous leukemia (CML) is a chronic myeloproliferative disorder characterized by a clonal proliferation of myelogenous and B-lymphocytic cells that results in a large increase in total body granulocyte mass. In the majority of patients, there is a terminal blastic metamorphosis. CML composes approximately 20% of all adult leukemias and occurs most frequently in middle age. Variant or atypical forms are well known, and the disease also occurs in children.

32.1 Pathophysiology

CML is a clonal disorder originating from the multipotential hematopoietic stem cell. More than 95% of patients with CML have a translocation of one of the long arms of chromosome 22, usually to chromosome 9 [t(9;22)]. The presence of this abnormal chromosome, the Philadelphia (Ph[1]) chromosome, in a patient with leukocytosis and granulocytic hyperplasia in the bone marrow is diagnostic of CML. Variant chromosomal translocations also have been identified. Regardless of the specific translocation, the reciprocal chromosomal rearrangements are associated with translocation and activation of cellular oncogenes. The proto-oncogene c-*abl* on chromosome 9 is translocated to chromosome 22. The break point on chromosome 22 occurs within the *bcr* (breakpoint cluster region) gene. The result is the chimeric gene *bcr-abl*. This gene is expressed as the cytoplasmic fusion protein BCR-ABL, a tyrosine kinase. The length of the *bcr* sequence retained determines the size of the fusion protein. The patient with typical Ph[1]-positive CML expresses either a 210- or a 190-kd BCR-ABL protein.

CML is characterized by major regulatory defects that are probably due to activation of signal-transduction pathways critical to hematopoietic cell growth and function. Granulocytic hyperplasia, at all stages of maturation within the bone marrow, is explained by a combination of stem cell expansion, delays in cell cycle times, and delayed apoptosis. The average half-life of granulocytes in the blood in patients with CML is 5 to 10 times longer than normal. At the same time, the granulocyte turnover rate may be increased 10 times.

32.2 Clinical Findings

CML is seen most frequently in patients between 50 and 60 years of age and usually develops insidiously. The initial symptoms may include malaise, fatigue, weight loss, and upper abdominal fullness or discomfort. Physical examination usually reveals splenomegaly, but hepatomegaly is less common. Lymphadenopathy is very unusual; when present, it is often associated with the accelerated phase of the disease. As the disease progresses, the spleen may become markedly enlarged, and in general the extent of splenomegaly correlates with the size of the leukocyte count. **Table 32-1** provides a summary of the characteristic features of CML.

32.3 Diagnostic Approach

After a clinical history is obtained and a physical examination performed, the laboratory diagnosis of CML proceeds in the following sequence:

Table 32-1   Characteristics of Chronic Myelogenous Leukemia

Age	35-50 years; rarely in children
Physical examination	Splenomegaly
Leukocyte count	$50\text{-}200 \times 10^3/\text{mm}^3$ ($50\text{-}200 \times 10^9/\text{L}$)
Blood findings	Granulocytosis with entire spectrum of precursors from myeloblasts (<2%) to polymorphonuclear neutrophils; absolute basophilia; eosinophilia; normal or increased platelet count
Bone marrow findings	Granulocytic hyperplasia; basophilia and eosinophilia; megakaryocytic hyperplasia; variable degree of fibrosis
Leukocyte alkaline phosphatase score	Markedly decreased or zero
Chromosome analysis	Philadelphia chromosome (Ph^1)
Molecular studies	*bcr* rearrangement
Clinical course (untreated)	Chronic phase: 2-4 years
	Accelerated phase: weeks to months
	Blast phase: days to weeks

1. A complete blood count.
2. Examination of the peripheral blood smear.
3. A leukocyte alkaline phosphatase (LAP) score.
4. Examination of the bone marrow aspirate smear and biopsy.
5. Cytogenetic studies for the Ph^1 chromosome or molecular studies for the *bcr* rearrangement.

Table 32-2 compares the major findings in chronic and acute leukemias. (*See Figure 29-1* for an algorithm of the differential diagnosis of CML and other myeloproliferative disorders.)

32.4 Hematologic Findings

The hematologic findings in CML are characteristic but not diagnostic. Severe leukemoid reactions—due to infections, for example—can mimic CML. Other myeloproliferative disorders such as myelofibrosis may have similar blood and bone marrow findings.

Table 32-2 Comparison of Acute and Chronic Leukemia

Variable	Acute	Chronic
Age	All ages	Adults
Clinical onset	Sudden	Insidious
Lymphadenopathy	Slight	Moderate
Splenomegaly	Mild	Moderate to prominent
Anemia and thrombocytopenia	Marked	Mild
Leukemic cells	Immature	Mature
Course (untreated)	6 months or less	2-6 years

32.4.1 Blood Cell Measurements

The majority of patients have a slight anemia at the time of diagnosis. The anemia becomes more severe as the leukocyte count increases. The rise in leukocyte count is gradual, the majority of patients having counts ranging between 50 and $400 \times 10^3/\text{mm}^3$ (50 and $400 \times 10^9/\text{L}$) at the time of diagnosis. In contrast to acute myeloid leukemia (AML), the platelet count is normal or even elevated.

32.4.2 Peripheral Blood Smear Morphology

CML can be suspected from an examination of the peripheral blood. The striking feature is granulocytosis, with the presence of the entire spectrum of granulocytic precursors (**Image 32-1**). Mature granulocytes and metamyelocytes predominate. Promyelocytes and myeloblasts do not exceed 10% in the chronic phase. An absolute increase in basophils is characteristic of CML and may be useful in distinguishing CML from a leukemoid reaction. There are also increased numbers of eosinophils. Nucleated RBCs are infrequent. Thrombocytosis may result in megakaryocyte nuclei and giant platelets.

32.4.3 Bone Marrow Examination

The bone marrow is markedly hypercellular with a large increase in the myeloid/erythroid ratio—as much as 10:1 to 40:1. As in the peripheral blood, all stages of maturation of the granulocytic series are present, and there is usually an increased number of basophils and eosinophils. The number of erythroid precursors appears decreased. The megakaryocytes are usually increased in number and frequently show dyspoietic features. Megakaryocytic hyperplasia and platelet clumping can obscure the changes in the granulocytic line. Increased numbers of dyspoietic megakaryocytes are common to chronic myeloproliferative disorders (see Chapters 29 to 31). The marrow biopsy specimen may reveal reticulin fibrosis, which may become more severe as the disease progresses. Bone marrow fibrosis is associated with a higher incidence of splenomegaly and a poor prognosis. Marked fibrosis also is associated with the accelerated or blastic phase of the disease.

Bone marrow examination is of limited help in making a diagnosis of CML. It is indicated, however, to obtain material for cytogenetic and molecular studies (Ph[1] chromosome, *bcr* rearrangement) and to evaluate for the presence of marrow fibrosis.

Other Laboratory Tests

Test 32.1 Leukocyte Alkaline Phosphatase

Purpose. Together with cytogenetic studies, LAP is a useful confirmatory test in CML.

Principle, Specimen, and Procedure. See Test 16.1.

Interpretation. In patients with CML, the LAP score is 0 or markedly decreased. The diagnostic value of a low score is increased because LAP scores are usually elevated in the conditions with which CML is most commonly mistaken, such as leukemoid reactions, polycythemia vera, and myelofibrosis with myeloid metaplasia (**Table 32-3**). However, the LAP score in CML may be normal or elevated in the presence of infection, during pregnancy, after splenectomy, and during the accelerated or blastic phases of the disease.

Test 32.2 Cytogenetics

Purpose. The Ph[1] chromosome is present in 95% of patients with CML. In the presence of granulocytic hyperplasia and absolute

Table 32-3   Conditions Associated With Abnormal LAP

Decreased	Increased
Chronic myelogenous leukemia	Leukemoid reactions
PNH	Pregnancy; oral contraceptive use
Hypophosphatemia	Polycythemia vera
ITP	Myelofibrosis
Infectious mononucleosis	Hodgkin's disease
Pernicious anemia	Essential thrombocythemia
Myelodysplastic syndromes	G-CSF administration
Plasma cell myeloma	

Abbreviations: LAP = leukocyte alkaline phosphatase; PNH = paroxysmal nocturnal hemoglobinuria; ITP = idiopathic thrombocytopenic purpura; G-CSF = granulocyte colony-stimulating factor.

basophilia in the peripheral blood and bone marrow, it is diagnostic of CML.

Principle. The Ph[1] chromosome results from translocation of the greater part of the long arm of chromosome 22 to another chromosome, usually chromosome 9 (**Image 32-2**). This is an acquired somatic mutation of a common stem cell of granulocytic-monocytic, erythroid, megakaryocytic, and B-lymphocytic precursors. Persistence of the Ph[1] chromosome during the course of the disease is associated with an overall shorter survival time when compared with complete or partial cytogenetic remissions.

Specimen. Bone marrow is the tissue of choice. A buffy coat preparation of peripheral blood contains an adequate number of cells from the myelocytic stage or earlier. Bone marrow is aspirated directly into a syringe that has been rinsed with heparin. An aliquot of 0.5 to 1.0 mL of bone marrow is transferred immediately into either a sterile screw-top vial containing 2 mL of sterile tissue culture medium or a small (2- to 3-mL) sterile plain (red top) vacuum tube. This specimen should not be refrigerated. The sample can be transported to a reference laboratory with satisfactory results if it arrives within 24 hours. In special circumstances, lymph node biopsy specimen and splenic tissue also may be subjected to chromosome analysis.

Procedure. Chromosome charts are prepared by examining metaphase spreads of leukocytes from blood, bone marrow, or both. Chromosome analysis is performed following 24 to 48 hours of incubation at 37°C without phytohemagglutinin stimulation. Many techniques are available to study chromosomes. The simplest is a direct study, in which a cell suspension is made of leukocytes from blood or bone marrow and incubated with colchicine to arrest cell division at the metaphase stage. The cells are swollen by hypotonic saline treatment and fixed. The fixed cells are placed on a slide, flattened, and dried. The metaphase spreads are then stained, examined under the microscope, and photographed or digitally imaged.

Cell culture techniques are employed when the cells have a low mitotic index. Malignant leukocytes grow in vitro without stimulation, and peak cell division occurs 24 to 48 hours after the onset of cell culture. G- and Q-banding is used for detailed karyotypic analysis.

Interpretation. The Ph[1] chromosome is present in more than 95% of patients with CML, both in relapse and during apparent remission of the disease. During the accelerated phase or blast crisis, additional chromosome abnormalities are frequently found, often a duplication of the Ph[1] chromosome, isochromosome 17q, or loss of the Y chromosome. A small number of patients lack the Ph[1] chromosome. These patients may have a different disease from classic CML (discussed later in this chapter).

Although the Ph[1] chromosome translocation is the cytogenetic hallmark of CML, molecular detection of the rearrangement of genes involved in the translocation break point (the *bcr* locus on chromosome 22 and the *c-abl* proto-oncogene on chromosome 9) is a more sensitive marker for the disease. The *bcr-abl* rearrangement may be present in cytogenetically normal cases of CML. In combination with cytogenetic analysis, newer diagnostic modalities such as polymerase chain reaction (PCR) and fluorescent in situ hybridization (FISH) increase the ability to detect clonal abnormalities.

Test 32.3 **Southern Blot Hybridization**

Purpose. The *bcr-abl* rearrangement is present in most patients with CML. In the absence of the Ph[1] chromosome and in the appropriate clinical setting, it is diagnostic of CML.

Principle. The *bcr-abl* rearrangement results from a translocation in a very narrow region of the long arm of chromosome 22. Translocation of the c-*abl* oncogene into the *bcr* region alters a restriction enzyme site on the normal chromosome 22 and changes the normal germline configuration (banding pattern) of the *bcr* locus.

Specimen. Bone marrow is the tissue of choice.

Procedure. Cellular DNA is extracted and digested into varying length fragments by restriction endonucleases. These DNA fragments are separated according to length by agarose gel electrophoresis. A nitrocellulose film is then placed in contact with the gel surface, and the DNA in the gel is transferred ("blotted") onto the nitrocellulose film by either capillary action or vacuum force. The presence or absence of the *bcr-abl* rearrangement in the cellular DNA is then analyzed by DNA-DNA hybridization to a radioactive, usually phosphorus 32-labeled, nucleotide probe. The *Hin*dIII/*Bg*II DNA fragment corresponding to the *bcr-abl* junction is the most commonly used probe to detect this rearrangement in CML.

Interpretation. The *bcr-abl* rearrangement is present in 90% to 95% of patients with CML.

Test 32.4 **Fluorescent In Situ Hybridization**

Purpose and Principle. See Test 32.3.

Specimen. Bone marrow is the tissue of choice, but peripheral smears and touch imprints are acceptable in certain circumstances.

Procedure. Fluorescent in situ hybridization (FISH) is a highly sensitive technique using specific DNA probes to identify each chromosome. This technique labels the *bcr* and *abl* genes separately. After the probes are applied, the smear is counterstained with 4´,6-diaminodino-2-phenylindole (DAPI). Normal *bcr* and *abl* sequences stain different colors. If present, the *bcr-abl* fusion gene stains a third color. This third color is not a result of the mixing of light waves (electromagnetic radiation), but of gamma wavelengths in the atomic spectrum (**Images 32-3** and **32-4**).

Interpretation. The *bcr-abl* rearrangement is present in 90% to 95% of patients with CML.

32.5 Ancillary Test

Terminal deoxynucleotidyl transferase (TdT) is a marker for early lymphoid cells (see Chapter 28). In approximately one third of patients with CML in blast crisis, TdT is present. This test is performed because TdT-positive patients respond more frequently to vincristine and prednisone, drugs normally used for the treatment of acute lymphoblastic leukemia. Identification of TdT can be done on blasts in peripheral blood (if an adequate number of lymphoblasts are present), on bone marrow aspirate material, or on imprints from a biopsy specimen. With the use of an immunoperoxidase technique, TdT can also be demonstrated in histologic sections.

32.6 Special Diagnostic Considerations

32.6.1 Accelerated Phase and Blast Crisis in CML

There are three phases in the natural history of CML: the chronic phase, the accelerated phase, and the terminal blastic phase (blast crisis). The metamorphosis from the chronic phase to blast crisis can occur very rapidly or gradually over several months. The less fulminant transition is referred to as the "accelerated phase" or "acute transformation". The development of blast crisis occurs in the majority of patients from 2 to 6 years after diagnosis. The accelerated phase and blast crisis are associated with a maturation block similar to that in AML. Features associated with the accelerated phase include an increased number of basophils, additional chromosomal abnormalities, and myelofibrosis.

Blast crisis is usually myeloid (60% of patients), but lymphoid blast crisis (approximately 30% of patients) also occurs (**Image 32-5**). In some instances, myeloid-lymphoid hybrid blasts or granulocytic blast mixtures may be present. This mixture of blast crises is not surprising, because CML represents a lesion of the multipotential stem cell. Blast crisis is associated with a clonal expansion of any of several potential progeny. The type of blast crisis (myeloid vs lymphoid) influences the therapy undertaken because TdT-positive blasts dictate therapy normally used for acute lymphocytic leukemia. In addition to TdT positivity, lymphoid blasts usually have a lymphoblastic morphology and are CD10-positive.

Clinically, the accelerated phase and blast crisis are associated with marked malaise, fatigue, anorexia, bone pain, and weight loss. Lymphadenopathy may develop, and biopsy of affected lymph nodes reveals a predominance of blasts (granulocytic sarcoma or chloroma), which may be mistaken for large cell lymphoma. Increasing anemia and thrombocytopenia are other common features.

32.6.2 Atypical CML

In approximately 5% of patients who initially show a CML-like picture, the Ph^1 chromosome is absent on cytogenetic analysis. Some of these patients have the *bcr-abl* gene and can be reclassified as typical CML. Compared with patients with classic CML, Ph^1-negative, *bcr-abl*–negative patients are usually older and have a higher incidence of anemia, thrombocytopenia, and marrow blasts; they also have decreased megakaryocytes and a lower incidence of both basophilia and thrombocytosis. There is often multilineage dysplasia. Clinically, these patients experience a more aggressive disease course than that for typical CML. Atypical CML may be more closely allied with myelodysplastic syndrome and chronic myelomonocytic leukemia than with CML. Currently, it is recommended that this disease be classified within the myelodysplastic/myeloproliferative category (see Chapter 26).

32.7 Course and Treatment

CML has a constant, predictable course during the chronic phase, with a median survival time of 3.5 to 4 years. Approximately 20% of the patients survive 7 years or more after the initial diagnosis. The majority of patients die of complications associated with blast crisis, usually infection, hemorrhage, or both.

The principle of therapy for CML is to reduce the total granulocyte mass and relieve symptoms of hyperleukocytosis, thrombocytosis, and splenomegaly (hematologic remission). Ideally, therapy should also induce a cytogenetic remission (absence of detectable Ph^1 chromosome or *bcr-abl* rearrangement). Commonly used therapeutic agents for chronic phase disease are the antimetabolite hydroxyurea and interferon-α (IFN-α). The alkylating agent busulfan is not a first-line option because of its shorter median duration of chronic phase and shorter median survival. None of these agents induces a cytogenetic remission or delays the onset of blast crisis.

The only cure for CML is high-dose chemotherapy or a combination of chemotherapy and total body irradiation followed by allogeneic marrow transplantation, preferably early in the chronic phase.

32.8 **References**

Bennett JM, Catovsky D, Daniel MT, et al. The chronic myeloid leukaemias: guidelines for distinguishing chronic granulocytic, atypical chronic myeloid, and chronic myelomonocytic leukaemia. Proposals by the French-American-British Cooperative Leukaemia Group. *Br J Haematol.* 1994;87:746–754.

Dekmezian R, Kantarjian HP, Keating MJ, et al. The relevance of reticulin stain-measured fibrosis at diagnosis in chronic myelogenous leukemia. *Cancer.* 1987;59:1739–1743.

Faderl S, Talpaz M, Estrov Z, et al. The biology of chronic myeloid leukemia. *N Engl J Med.* 1999;341:164–172.

Harris NL, Jaffe ES, Diebold J, et al. The World Health Organization Classification of Hematological Malignancies Report of the Clinical Advisory Committee Meeting, Airlie House, Virginia, November 1997. *Mod Pathol.* 2000;13(2):193–207.

Hehlman R, Heimpel H, Hasford J, et al. Randomized comparison of interferon-α with busulfan and hydroxyurea in chronic myelogenous leukemia. *Blood.* 1994;84:4064–4077.

Radich JP, Gehly G, Gooley T, et al. Polymerase chain reaction detection of the BCR-ABL fusion transcript after allogeneic marrow transplantation for chronic myeloid leukemia: results and implications in 366 patients. *Blood.* 1995;85:2632–2638.

Rowley JD. The Philadelphia chromosome translocation: a paradigm for understanding leukemia. *Cancer.* 1990;65:2178–2184.

Sawyers CL. Chronic myeloid leukemia. *N Engl J Med.* 1999;340:1330–1340.

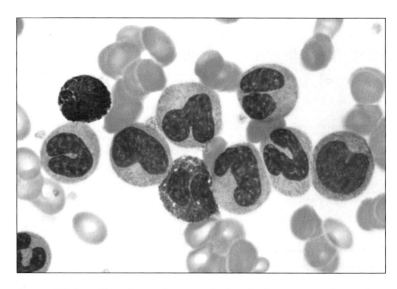

Image 32-1   Chronic myelogenous leukemia. A spectrum of granulocytes, from immature to mature, together with one basophil and one eosinophil, are seen in the peripheral blood smear.

Image 32-2   Chronic myelogenous leukemia karyotype 46, XY t(9;22). The classic Philadelphia chromosome is a translocation from the long arm of chromosome 22 to the long arm of chromosome 9.

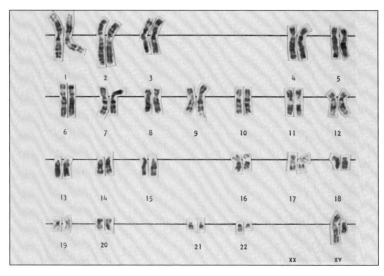

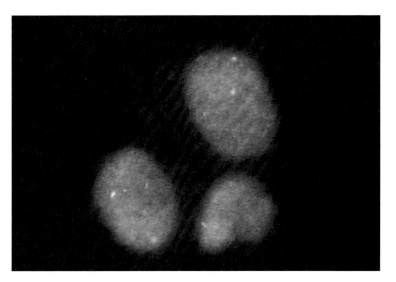

Image 32-3   Chronic phase chronic myelogenous leukemia. In situ hybridization studies performed on peripheral smear with *bcr* (red) and *abl* (green) probes. Counterstaining was done with DAPI. Green-red and yellow (product of green and red) hybridization signals are seen in two of the cells. Randomly distributed red and green signals correspond to *bcr* and *abl* on normal chromosomes 22 and 9. (Courtesy of R. K. Brynes, MD.)

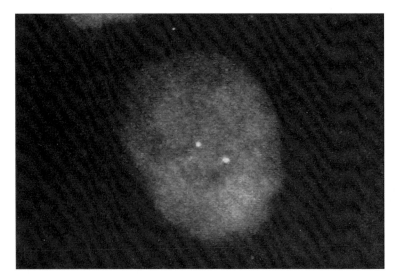

Image 32-4 Chronic phase chronic myelogenous leukemia. In situ hybridization studies performed on peripheral smear with *bcr* (red) and *abl* (green) probes. Counterstaining was done with DAPI. The yellow (product of green and red) hybridization signal corresponds to the *bcr-abl* fusion gene and is produced by overlapping red *bcr* and green *abl* probes. The remaining red and green signals were produced by *bcr* and *abl* on normal chromosomes 22 and 9. (Courtesy of R. K. Brynes, MD.)

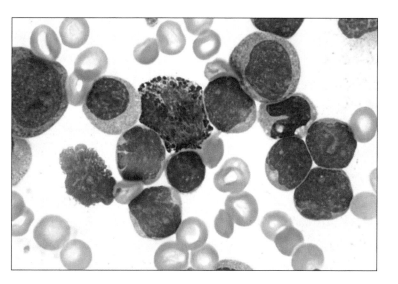

Image 32-5 Chronic myelogenous leukemia in blast crisis (transformation). Blasts and one basophil are present in this peripheral smear. (Courtesy of P. C. J. Ward, MD.)

PART
VIII

Chronic Lymphoid Leukemias

33 Chronic Lymphocytic Leukemia and Other Lymphoid Leukemias

The chronic lymphoid leukemias are a complex group of mature B- and T-cell lymphoproliferative disorders affecting primarily older adults. Chronic lymphocytic leukemia (CLL), a B-cell lineage neoplasm, is the most common and is the prototype of these disorders. The recently proposed World Health Organization (WHO) classification merges leukemias and lymphomas into a unified classification system that includes a variety of mature B- and T-cell neoplasms (see Chapter 34, Table 34-9). This chapter emphasizes the subset of mature B- and T-cell disorders than characteristically involve the blood and bone marrow (**Tables 33-1** and **33-2**). This discussion focuses on CLL and its variants and also includes the other chronic lymphoid leukemias.

33.1 Pathophysiology

The hallmark of CLL is absolute lymphocytosis in the peripheral blood and bone marrow; lymphadenopathy and splenomegaly also may be present. It typically occurs in middle-aged and elderly persons, and its incidence increases with advancing age.

CLL is a clonal disorder of B lymphocytes that express pan B-cell surface antigens, including CD19 and CD20. The cells display

Table 33-1 B-Cell Chronic Lymphoid Leukemias

Chronic lymphocytic leukemia, common
Chronic lymphocytic leukemia, mixed
B-cell prolymphocytic leukemia
Hairy cell leukemia
Leukemic phase of non-Hodgkin lymphoma
  Splenic marginal zone lymphoma
  Follicular lymphoma
  Mantle cell lymphoma
  Lymphoplasmacytic lymphoma

Table 33-2 T-Cell Chronic Lymphoid Leukemias

T-cell prolymphocytic leukemia
T-cell large granular lymphocyte leukemia
Adult T-cell leukemia/lymphoma
Sézary syndrome

---

surface immunoglobulin that is restricted to one or two classes of heavy chains, usually IgM or IgM and IgD. Since the lymphocytes are clonal, only a single light chain, κ or λ, is expressed. The CLL lymphocytes almost always react with antibodies against the CD5 antigen. This antigen initially was thought to be a specific pan T-cell antigen, but it is now known that a small subset of normal lymphocytes coexpresses B-cell antigens and CD5.

Abnormalities of T cells also have been identified in patients with CLL. Increased absolute numbers of T lymphocytes have been reported in untreated patients with CLL, although the level fluctuates during the course of the disease. Inversion of the normal T helper/suppressor ratio in the blood with decreased T-helper function usually is present. Natural killer (NK) function often is decreased or absent, even though the absolute number of NK cells in the blood may be increased in CLL.

Hypogammaglobulinemia eventually develops in almost all patients with CLL. The hypogammaglobulinemia probably results from impaired B-cell function, but abnormalities of T-cell regulation also may be important. Patients with CLL have impaired antibody and cell-mediated immunity to recall antigens, which is related to the hypogammaglobulinemia and T-cell abnormalities. Many patients develop autoantibodies; most are directed against mature hematopoietic cells. Autoimmune hemolytic anemia occurs during the course of disease in about 15% of patients, while immune thrombocytopenia and granulocytopenia are less common.

Clonal chromosome alterations are detected in about 50% to 60% of patients with CLL. The most common numeric abnormality is trisomy 12, present in 20% to 30% of the patients. The most common structural abnormality involves the long arm of chromosome 13 at chromosome band 13q14.

33.2 Clinical Findings

Most patients with CLL are older than 40 years; the disease is unusual before 30 years of age. There is a higher incidence of CLL among men; the ratio of affected men to women is approximately 2:1. Many patients are asymptomatic when the disease is diagnosed. Symptoms, when present, usually include weakness, easy fatigability, and weight loss. Fever, night sweats, or frequent viral and bacterial infections are more common as the disease progresses but may be present at diagnosis. The most common abnormality noted on physical examination is the presence of lymphadenopathy that varies from enlargement of only a single node or node group to enlargement of virtually all lymph nodes. Hepatomegaly or splenomegaly occurs at diagnosis but is less common.

The most widely used clinical staging system for CLL in the United States is the Rai system (**Table 33-3**). Patients with minimal evidence of disease, ie, lymphocytosis only, are considered to be in the earliest stage of disease, while those demonstrating compromise of bone marrow function, such as anemia and thrombocytopenia, are in advanced stages. The Rai system has been modified according to degree of risk: stage 0 indicates low risk; stages I and II, intermediate risk; and stages III and IV, high risk. The survival times correlate inversely with the clinical stage. Approximate survival times in these three categories are greater than 10, 6, and 2 years, respectively.

33.3 Approach to Diagnosis

A clinical history and physical examination are obtained. The laboratory diagnosis of CLL includes the following:

Table 33-3   Rai's Clinical Staging System for Chronic
Lymphocytic Leukemia

Stage 0:	Lymphocytosis in blood and bone marrow only
Stage I:	Lymphocytosis plus enlarged lymph nodes
Stage II:	Lymphocytosis plus enlarged liver and/or spleen; lymphadenopathy may be present
Stage III:	Lymphocytosis plus anemia (hemoglobin <11 g/dL [110 g/L]); lymph nodes, spleen, or liver may be enlarged
Stage IV:	Lymphocytosis and thrombocytopenia (platelet count <100 × 10³/mm³ [100 × 10⁹/L]); anemia and organomegaly may be present

1. A complete blood cell count.
2. Examination of the peripheral blood smear.
3. Examination of a bone marrow aspirate and biopsy specimen.
4. Immunophenotyping by flow cytometry.
5. Ancillary studies, such as serum immunoglobulin analysis and antiglobulin tests.

33.4 Hematologic Findings

CLL is characterized by a sustained peripheral blood lymphocytosis. Morphologically, the lymphocytes appear mature. Immunophenotypic analysis is useful for the diagnostic workup of CLL to confirm monoclonality of the lymphocytes and to aid in differentiating CLL from other lymphoproliferative disorders. A bone marrow aspirate and core biopsy often are performed to confirm the diagnosis and to provide prognostic information. Ancillary studies, such as immunoglobulin analysis and an antiglobulin test often are performed to evaluate the immune status of the patient and to evaluate for autoimmune disorders, such as autoimmune hemolytic anemia. Cytogenetic analysis is not done routinely but may be performed to aid in the diagnosis or to gain prognostic information.

Several benign diseases, such as infectious mononucleosis and acute cytomegalovirus infection, are also accompanied by peripheral lymphocytosis (see Chapter 23). These entities usually are distinguishable readily from CLL since they occur in younger patients, are characterized by fever and other acute symptoms, and exhibit lymphocytosis that differs morphologically and immunologically from that of CLL. Several malignant lymphoproliferative disorders, such as prolymphocytic leukemia, hairy cell leukemia, follicle center cell lymphoma, splenic marginal zone lymphoma, mantle cell lymphoma, and large granular lymphocyte leukemia, may closely resemble CLL and are discussed later in this chapter.

33.4.1 Blood Cell Measurements

Anemia (hemoglobin <11.0 g/dL [110 g/L]) is present in about 15% to 20% and thrombocytopenia (<100 × 10^3/mm^3 [100 × 10^9/L]) is present in about 10% of patients at diagnosis. The anemia typically is normochromic and normocytic. The reticulocyte count usually is normal unless the patient has an autoimmune hemolytic anemia, in which case it is elevated.

Usually, the absolute peripheral lymphocyte count is greater than 10 × 10^3/mm^3 (10 × 10^9/L), but the degree of lymphocytosis sometimes is milder (in the range of 5-10 × 10^3/mm^3 [5-10 × 10^9/L]). Extreme lymphocytosis higher than 500 × 10^3/mm^3 (500 × 10^9/L) may occur late in the disease.

33.4.2 Peripheral Blood Smear Morphologic Features

The RBCs usually are normochromic and normocytic. If autoimmune hemolytic anemia is present, spherocytes and increased numbers of polychromatophilic cells may be present in the blood smear. In most cases of CLL, the lymphocytes are small with condensed chromatin patterns and narrow rims of cytoplasm (**Image 33-1**). The lymphocytes tend to resemble one another and appear monotonous. Smudged or damaged lymphocytes often are prominent in the smear. Lymphocytes having the appearance of prolymphocytes frequently are present. Prolymphocytes are identified by their larger size, loosely condensed chromatin, single nucleoli, and small to moderate amounts of basophilic cytoplasm. In a typical case of CLL, prolymphocytes represent less than 10% of the total lymphocyte population.

33.4.3 Bone Marrow Examination

The bone marrow usually is hypercellular; greater than 20% to 30% of the nucleated cells are lymphocytes. The lymphocytes are similar morphologically to those in the blood. Histologic sections of trephine biopsy specimens show four possible morphologic patterns of bone marrow infiltration in CLL: (1) interstitial, with preservation of the marrow architecture and fat cells; (2) nodular (focal); (3) mixed interstitial and nodular (**Image 33-2**); and (4) diffuse, with replacement of the bone marrow space by CLL cells. The nodular infiltrates are located randomly throughout the biopsy and are not paratrabecular. The lymphocytes are small with condensed chromatin patterns. Proliferation centers may be present. Bone marrow histopathologic features in CLL have emerged as prognostic indicators independent of clinical stage. Patients with a diffuse pattern of involvement have a poorer prognosis than those with a nondiffuse pattern.

33.4.4 CLL, Mixed Cell Types

The term *CLL, mixed cell type,* is used for cases of CLL in which a heterogeneous population of lymphocytes is present. Two morphologic subtypes are included in this group: (1) CLL with mixed small and large cells and (2) CLL with increased prolymphocytes (CLL/PL). *CLL with mixed small and large cells* is characterized by a spectrum of morphologic features from small to large lymphocytes (**Image 33-3**). The large lymphocytes exhibit condensed chromatin and moderately abundant, lightly basophilic cytoplasm. In *CLL/PL*, the prolymphocytes make up 10% to 55% of the circulating lymphoid cells (**Image 33-4**). The distinction from CLL in prolymphocytoid transformation rests mainly on the absence of a history of typical CLL. The majority of patients with CLL/PL maintain a stable percentage of prolymphocytes, rather than the progressive accumulation seen in prolymphocytoid transformation of CLL.

Other Laboratory Tests

Test 33.1 Cell Surface Markers

Purpose. Immunophenotypic analysis is used to confirm a diagnosis of CLL in a patient with a peripheral blood lymphocytosis that is morphologically consistent with CLL. It documents that the disease is a B-cell disorder and confirms its clonality by identifying light chain restriction. Coexpression of B-cell antigens and CD5, positivity for CD23, and the low intensity of expression of CD20 and surface immunoglobulin are characteristic of CLL lymphocytes. These immunophenotypic findings help not only to confirm the diagnosis of CLL but also to differentiate it from other chronic lymphoproliferative disorders and lymphoma (**Tables 33-4** and **33-5**).

Principle. Labeled lineage-restricted or associated monoclonal antibodies combine with determinants on B lymphocytes, T lymphocytes, their subsets, and other hematopoietic cells (see Chapter 48). Labeled cells in suspension can then be characterized by flow cytometry.

Specimen. Fresh peripheral blood anticoagulated with heparin is the usual specimen for immunophenotypic analysis of the lymphocytes in CLL. Cell suspensions from bone marrow or other tissues, such as fresh lymph node, also can be used.

Procedure. See Chapter 48.

Interpretation. The lymphocytes in CLL are positive for the pan B-cell antigens CD19 and CD20. The cells express surface immunoglobulin that is restricted to a single light chain, κ or λ. In addition, IgM or IgM and IgD heavy chains usually are present on the surface of the lymphocytes; the presence of IgG or IgA is much less common. Concentration of the monoclonal surface immunoglobulin usually is low, with dim immunofluorescence intensity demonstrated by flow cytometry. The intensity of the positivity for the pan B-antigen CD20 also is dim. This contrasts with the strong intensity seen with other B-cell chronic lymphoproliferative disorders or non-Hodgkin lymphomas. The CLL cells almost always coexpress the CD5 antigen with the pan B-cell antigens. CLL lymphocytes are also positive for CD23. This finding aids in distinguishing CLL from mantle cell lymphoma, a CD5+ B-cell lymphoproliferative disorder that is negative for CD23. The lymphocytes of CLL almost always are negative for CD10.

33.5 Ancillary Tests

33.5.1 Direct Antiglobulin Test

Autoimmune hemolytic anemia develops in approximately 10% to 15% of patients with CLL at some time during the disease.

Table 33-4 Immunophenotype of B-Cell Chronic Lymphoproliferative Disorders

Antigen	CLL	B-Cell PLL	HCL	SMZL	FL	MCL
SIg	+(dim)	+	+	+	+	+
CD19	+	+	+	+	+	+
CD20	+(dim)	+	+	+	+	+
CD22	+/–	+	+	+	+	+
CD23	+	+/–	–	+/–	+/–	–
CD25	+/–	–	+	–	–	–
CD5	+	–	–	–	–	+
FMC7	–	+	+	+	+	+
CD11c	+/–	–	+	+/–	–	–
CD103	–	–	+	–	–	–
CD10	–	–	–	–	+	–
CD79b	–	+	+/–	+	+	+

Abbreviations: CLL = chronic lymphocytic leukemia; PLL = prolymphocytic leukemia; HCL = hairy cell leukemia; SMZL = splenic marginal zone lymphoma; FL = folliclular lymphoma; MCL = mantle cell lymphoma; SIg = surface immunoglobulin; + = most cases are positive for this antigen; – = most cases are negative; +/– = cases are variably positive.

The hemolysis is mediated by a warm-reacting IgG antibody, and the direct antiglobulin test (DAT) result usually is positive. The DAT result may be positive in approximately 25% of patients with CLL, but autoimmune hemolysis occurs only about half as frequently. Autoimmune thrombocytopenia and neutropenia also may occur in CLL, but laboratory demonstration of these antibodies is difficult.

33.5.2 Serum Immunoglobulin

Hypogammaglobulinemia occurs initially or during the course of the disease in most patients with CLL. All immunoglobulin classes—IgG, IgM, and IgA—usually are depressed. In about 5% of patients, a monoclonal protein, usually IgM, is present.

33.5.3 Cytogenetic Analysis

Clonal chromosome abnormalities can be detected in 50% to 60% of patients with CLL, and the karyotype of the malignant cells is useful for predicting the prognosis of patients with CLL. The most common numeric chromosome abnormality in CLL is

Table 33-5 Immunophenotype of T-Cell Chronic Lymphoproliferative Disorders

Antigen	T-Cell PLL	T-Cell LGLL	ATLL	SS
CD2	+	+	+	+
CD3	+	+	+	+
CD4	+	–	+	+
CD8	+/–	+	–	–
CD5	+	+/–	+	+
CD7	+	+/–	–	–
CD16	–	+/–	–	–
CD25	+/–	NA	+	+/–
CD57	NA	+/–	NA	NA

Abbreviations: PLL = prolymphocytic leukemia; LGLL= large granular lymphocyte leukemia; ATLL = adult T-cell leukemia/lymphoma; SS = Sézary syndrome; + = most cases are positive for this antigen; – = most cases are negative; +/– = cases are variably positive; NA = not available.

trisomy 12. This abnormality has been associated with CLL/PL. The most common structural abnormality involves the long arm of chromosome 13 at band 13q14. Other karyotypic abnormalities, including those of chromosomes 14q and 6q, also have been identified. Patients with trisomy 12 have a poorer prognosis than those with normal karyotypes, while patients with 13q abnormalities seem to have a prognosis similar to those those with normal karyotypes.

33.5.4 Lymph Node Biopsy

A lymph node biopsy is unnecessary for the diagnosis of CLL but may be performed to evaluate enlarged lymph nodes for evidence of transformation of the CLL to a more aggressive lymphoma such as Richter syndrome (see "Course and Treatment"). Lymph nodes involved with chronic phase CLL typically exhibit diffuse effacement by a monotonous infiltrate of small lymphocytes with round nuclear contours, inconspicuous nucleoli, and scant cytoplasm. Pseudonodules, also referred to as "proliferation" or "growth centers", frequently are present. These areas consist of larger cells with more prominent nucleoli and more readily apparent mitotic activity. Occasionally, the larger cells are mixed diffusely with the smaller lymphocytes but usually account for less than 30% of the total cells.

33.6 Course and Treatment

The clinical course of CLL is extremely variable. Many patients
have an indolent, almost benign course and live for more than 10
or 20 years without major complications from CLL. Others have a
more rapid downhill course and die within 1 to 2 years after diagnosis. Most patients with CLL, however, have a disease course
somewhere in between these two extremes, with a median survival
rate of 3 to 4 years. Since CLL tends to occur in elderly patients,
death often results from other unrelated illnesses in this age group.
Patients younger than 60 years of age almost always die as a result
of CLL or one of its complications, usually infections. Gram-positive organisms usually cause infections that occur early in the disease, but most deaths are due to infections by gram-negative bacteria or fungal infections. Infections by other organisms such as
viruses, *Pneumocystis carinii*, or *Mycobacterium tuberculosis* also
may contribute to death in CLL.

A minority of patients with CLL experience a morphologic
transformation to a more aggressive malignant neoplasm.
Prolymphocytoid transformation of CLL (**Image 33-5**) is the most
common form of transformation, occurring in about 15% of
patients. Prolymphocytoid transformation occurs after a chronic
phase of CLL and is associated with increasing numbers of circulating prolymphocytes, progressive anemia, thrombocytopenia,
lymphadenopathy, splenomegaly, and resistance to therapy. The
blood contains two distinct cell populations, typical CLL cells and
prolymphocytes. The prolymphocytes express the same
immunoglobulin isotype and the identical immunoglobulin gene
rearrangements as the original CLL cells, indicating that they
evolve from the original CLL clone.

Richter's syndrome occurs in about 5% to 10% of patients with
CLL and is characterized by the development of a rapidly progressive lymphoma. Classically, this manifests as a large cell lymphoma
(**Image 33-6**), but a spectrum of morphologic features, including
Hodgkin disease, has also been described. This transformation is
heralded by fever, weight loss, increasing organomegaly, and worsening cytopenias. Response to chemotherapy is generally poor.

Since patients with CLL are usually late in life and the disease
may be stable for many years, it is traditional to delay treatment of
early-stage CLL until the disease progresses. Signs of progressive
disease often include cytopenias, organ enlargement, and increased
susceptibility to infections. Treatment of CLL usually has involved

alkylating agents such as chlorambucil or cyclophosphamide, often combined with prednisone. Newer agents such as fludarabine are also active against CLL. Bone marrow transplantation is a therapeutic option, especially for younger patients with CLL.

33.7 Other Chronic Lymphoid Leukemias

33.7.1 Prolymphocytic Leukemia

Prolymphocytic leukemia (PLL) is a rare variant of CLL that occurs predominantly in older men and is characterized by leukocytosis, prominent splenomegaly, and minimal or absent lymphadenopathy. The leukocyte count frequently is elevated markedly, often greater than $100 \times 10^3/\text{mm}^3$ ($100 \times 10^9/\text{L}$). Prolymphocytes are the predominant cell in the blood, representing more than 55% of the lymphocytes. Prolymphocytes are characterized by large size, moderate rims of basophilic cytoplasm, moderately condensed chromatin patterns, and prominent nucleoli (**Image 33-7**). Anemia, thrombocytopenia, and neutropenia are common at diagnosis. The bone marrow usually is infiltrated extensively in a diffuse or mixed interstitial and nodular pattern. The spleen shows white and red pulp infiltration. Sections of lymph nodes show a diffuse pattern of infiltration with or without a pseudonodular pattern. Patients with PLL have an aggressive clinical course with shorter survival times than those with CLL.

About 80% of cases of PLL are of B-cell origin and express several pan B-cell antigens, including CD19 and CD20 (**Table 33-4**). Unlike CLL, prolymphocytes exhibit bright surface immunoglobulin, are positive for FMC7 and CD79b, and usually are negative for CD5. The most common cytogenetic abnormality in B-cell PLL seems to be a 14q+ chromosome with the break point at the heavy-chain immunoglobulin gene locus. About 20% of cases of PLL are T-cell in origin and express CD2, CD5, and CD7. Most have a CD4+, CD8– phenotype; a minority coexpress CD4 and CD8 or are CD4–, CD8+. Cytogenetic abnormalities of chromosome 14 with break points at q11 and q32 are common in T-PLL.

33.7.2 Hairy Cell Leukemia

Hairy cell leukemia (HCL) is a rare type of leukemia characterized by pancytopenia or other combinations of cytopenias, splenomegaly, minimal lymphadenopathy, and the presence of hairy cells in both the blood and bone marrow. The disease affects adults with a mean age of about 50 years and is more common in men than in women. Patients often have systemic symptoms such as weakness, weight loss, recurrent bacterial infections, or abdominal discomfort.

On peripheral blood films, hairy cells are one to two times the size of small lymphocytes and have round, oval, or kidney-shaped nuclei (**Image 33-8**). The chromatin patterns are stippled, and nucleoli usually are single, small, and inconspicuous. The cytoplasm is moderate to abundant and pale blue and has poorly defined borders or hairy projections. Although these cells are present in the blood of most patients with HCL, they may be rare and difficult to find.

The bone marrow in HCL often cannot be aspirated as a result of reticulin fibrosis. The trephine biopsy specimen is invaluable for establishing a diagnosis of HCL. The bone marrow sections show variable degrees of subtle patchy or diffuse interstitial infiltration by hairy cells. The hairy cells can be identified in sections by their abundant clear cytoplasm and well-spaced nuclei (**Image 33-8**). On high power, the hairy cell nuclei appear bland with round, oval, or indented nuclei. Extravasated RBCs commonly are present. Histologic sections of the spleen show red pulp infiltration by hairy cells with widening of the pulp cords and frequent blood-filled pseudosinuses lined by hairy cells.

A cytochemical stain detecting the presence of tartrate-resistant acid phosphatase is used widely to confirm the diagnosis of HCL. This stain is usually performed on blood smears and bone marrow aspirate smears or touch preparations of bone marrow.

Hairy cells are B cells and exhibit characteristic immunophenotypic features. They express strong monotypic surface immunoglobulin, CD19, CD20, CD22, and FMC7. They almost always are positive for CD25, CD11c, and CD103. They are negative for CD5 and CD10. Hairy cells in fixed sections react with several monoclonal antibodies directed against B cells, including CD20, CD79a, and DBA.44.

HCL is an indolent, slowly progressive disease with a median survival time of about 5 years. Until recently, the mainstay of therapy was splenectomy. During the past few years, however, effective medical therapies have become available that control the disease in most patients. These include the purine analogue 2-chlorodeoxyadenosine (2-CdA).

33.7.3 Leukemic Manifestations of Malignant Lymphoma

Splenic marginal zone B-cell lymphoma (SMZL) is recognized as an indolent non-Hodgkin lymphoma, but this disorder frequently exhibits leukemic manifestations. SMZL typically manifests in older men who have symptoms secondary to splenomegaly. Peripheral blood examination reveals anemia, thrombocytopenia, and a mildly to moderately elevated WBC count. The circulating malignant cells are small to medium-sized lymphocytes with condensed chromatin, inconspicuous nucleoli, and scant to moderate amounts of cytoplasm that may possess bipolar projections. On bone marrow biopsy sections, the infiltrate is interstitial, diffuse, or nodular and may be random or paratrabecular (**Image 33-9**). Intrasinusoidal infiltration also is frequent in SMZL and is highlighted by immunostaining for B-cell antigens. The cells are positive for CD19 and CD20 and may be positive for CD11c; they usually are negative for CD25 and CD103. They do not express CD5 or CD10.

Follicular lymphoma (FL) occasionally manifests with a peripheral lymphocytosis secondary to circulating lymphoma cells. Approximately 55% to 70% of patients with FL have bone marrow involvement; about 50% of the patients with bone marrow involvement have peripheral manifestations of the lymphoma. In most cases, the number of morphologically recognizable lymphoma cells is small and does not alter the differential count significantly. Occasionally, however, the involvement of the blood is characterized by a striking lymphocytosis that mimics CLL. The circulating cells in FL are small to medium-sized with smooth, evenly staining nuclei that frequently are cleaved or folded. Nucleoli are absent or inconspicuous. The cytoplasm is very sparse and pale blue. Bone marrow involvement in FL is characterized by a focal, paratrabecular, or diffuse pattern of infiltration (**Image 33-10**). Immunophenotypically, the cells in FL express the B-cell markers CD19 and CD20 and bright monotypic surface immunoglobulin. The cells are CD5– and usually CD10+.

Mantle cell lymphoma also may exhibit a de novo leukemic picture. Bone marrow biopsy specimens are involved by lymphoma in about 80% to 90% of cases; circulating lymphoma can be identified morphologically in about 80% of cases (**Image 33-11**). The pattern of infiltration in the bone marrow is focal random, focal paratrabecular, interstitial, or diffuse. Circulating mantle cell lymphoma cells are intermediate-sized with loosely condensed chromatin patterns, frequent nucleoli, and occasional cleaved or indented nuclei. As in CLL, they coexpress B-cell markers and CD5. Strong surface immunoglobulin, bright CD20 positivity, and negativity for CD23 in mantle cell lymphoma aid in differentiating this disorder from CLL. Mantle cell lymphoma, unlike CLL, is also positive for cyclin D1.

Lymphoplasmacytic lymphoma is discussed in Chapter 37.

33.7.4 Large Granular Lymphocyte Leukemia

Large granular lymphocyte leukemia (LGLL) is a rare chronic lymphoproliferative disorder characterized by mild to moderate blood lymphocytosis, neutropenia, polyclonal hypergammaglobulinemia, mild to moderate splenomegaly, and absence of lymphadenopathy. The disease occurs in adults with a median age of about 55 years; occasionally, patients are affected during their teenage years. Patients usually present with recurrent bacterial infections. Rheumatoid arthritis is present in about 25% to 30% of patients.

The lymphocyte in this disorder is a large granular lymphocyte, medium to large in size, with coarse chromatin, moderate pale cytoplasm, and prominent azurophilic granules (**Image 33-12**). The bone marrow in this disorder generally shows a mild to moderate increase in lymphocytes that are morphologically similar to those in the blood. Patients with LGLL usually have neutropenia, which often is severe. Anemia and/or mild thrombocytopenia is present in some cases. The involvement of the trephine biopsy sections usually is interstitial, with focal accentuation in some cases. The number of neutrophils generally is decreased only moderately with a normal maturation sequence.

In most cases of LGLL, the cells have a mature postthymic phenotype and are CD3+; most are CD8+ and CD4–. They usually express CD16 and CD57 and are CD56–, although variations in immunophenotype occur. Most cases fulfill criteria for a neoplastic disorder based on the demonstration of clonal T-cell receptor gene rearrangements. Despite clonality, the majority have a prolonged clinical course with little progression of symptoms. A subset of LGLL marks as NK cells. The usual phenotype of these cases is CD3–, CD4–, variable CD8, CD16+, CD56+, and CD57–. The NK LGLLs are more difficult to assess for clonality since they lack a clonal immunogenotypic marker.

33.7.5 Adult T-Cell Leukemia/Lymphoma

Adult T-cell leukemia/lymphoma (ATLL) first was described in persons from southwestern Japan but now has been identified in other areas, including the Caribbean and the United States. This disorder occurs in adults and is characterized by a proliferation of multilobated T lymphocytes in the blood, lymphadenopathy, splenomegaly, and skin lesions. Many patients have osteolytic lesions and hypercalcemia. ATLL is caused by a retrovirus, human T-cell lymphotropic virus I (HTLV-I). Most patients have a subacute or acute course that is refractory to therapy.

Leukocytosis is present and ranges from 25 to $500 \times 10^3/mm^3$ ($25\text{-}500 \times 10^9/L$). The malignant cells vary from small to large and have nuclei with a markedly irregular outline and deep nuclear indentations or lobulation (**Image 33-13**). The nucleoli usually are inconspicuous in the smaller cells but may be prominent in the larger cells, and the cytoplasm is scant. The bone marrow, lymph nodes, skin, liver, and spleen frequently are infiltrated by these cells.

The immunophenotype of the leukemic cells in ATLL is predominantly that of helper T cells that are CD2+, CD3+, and CD4+. They also express CD25.

33.7.6 Sézary Syndrome

Mycosis fungoides (MF) is a primary T-cell lymphoma of the skin. In a small percentage of patients with MF, Sézary syndrome (SS) develops, which is characterized by a generalized exfoliative erythroderma and a peripheral blood lymphocytosis. The lymphocytosis is caused by circulating abnormal lymphocytes called "Sézary cells". Sézary cells may be small or large with a small to moderate amount of cytoplasm; the nuclei have marked convolutions that give them a cerebriform appearance (**Image 33-14**). Nucleoli usually are absent or inconspicuous. Many of the Sézary cells show periodic acid–Schiff–positive cytoplasmic vacuoles around the nuclei.

The membrane immunophenotype of Sézary cells is that of a mature helper T lymphocyte, CD3+, CD4+, and CD8–. Patients with SS have a poorer prognosis than those with classic MF and frequently exhibit hepatosplenomegaly and lymphadenopathy. The bone marrow may be normal or show minimal infiltration but often is involved, especially when the WBC count is high.

33.8 References

Bennett JM, Catovsky D, Daniel M-T, et al. Proposals for the classification of chronic (mature) B and T lymphoid leukaemias. *J Clin Pathol.* 1989;42:567–584.

Brunning RD, McKenna RW. Small lymphocytic leukemia and related disorders. In: *Atlas of Tumor Pathology: Tumors of the Bone Marrow. Fascicle 9, Third Series.* Washington, DC: Armed Forces Institute of Pathology; 1994:255–322.

Catovsky D, Matutes E. Splenic lymphoma with circulating villous lymphocytes/splenic marginal-zone lymphoma. *Semin Hematol.* 1999;36:148–154.

Cohen PL, Kurtin PJ, Donovan KA, et al. Bone marrow and peripheral blood involvement in mantle cell lymphoma. *Br J Haematol.* 1998;101:302–310.

Diamandidou E, Cohen PR, Kurzrock R. Mycosis fungoides and Sézary syndrome. *Blood.* 1996;88:2385–2409.

Finn WG, Thangavelu M, Yelavarthi KK, et al. Karyotype correlates with peripheral blood morphology and immunophenotype in chronic lymphocytic leukemia. *Am J Clin Pathol.* 1996;105:458–467.

Franco V, Florena AM, Campesi G. Intrasinusoidal bone marrow infiltration: a possible hallmark of splenic lymphoma. *Histopathology.* 1996;29:571–575.

Harris NL, Jaffe ES, Diebold J, et al. World Health Organization classification of neoplastic diseases of the hematopoietic and lymphoid tissues: report of The Clinical Advisory Committee Meeting–Airlie House, Virginia, November 1997. *J Clin Oncol.* 1997;17:3835–3849.

Harris NL, Jaffe ES, Stein H, et al. A revised European-American classification of lymphoid neoplasms: a proposal from the International Lymphoma Study Group. *Blood.* 1994;84:1361–1392.

Huang JC, Finn WG, Goolsby CL, et al. CD5– small B-cell leukemias are rarely classifiable as chronic lymphocytic leukemia. *Am J Clin Pathol.* 1999;111:123–130.

Kroft SH, Finn WG, Peterson LC. The pathology of the chronic lymphoid leukaemias. *Blood Rev.* 1995;9:234–250

Loughran, Jr TP. Clonal diseases of large granular lymphocytes. *Blood.* 1993;82:1–14.

Matutes E, Brito-Babapulle V, Swanbury J, et al. Clinical and laboratory features of 78 cases of T-prolymphocytic leukemia. *Blood.* 1991;78:3269–3274.

Pangalis GA, Angelopoulou MK, Vassilakopouios TP, et al. B-chronic lymphocytic leukemia, small lymphocytic lymphoma, and lymphoplasmacytic lymphoma, including Waldenström's macroglobulinemia: a clinical, morphologic, and biologic spectrum of disorders. *Semin Hematol.* 1999;36:104–114.

Rozman C, Montserrat E. Chronic lymphocytic leukemia. *N Engl J Med.* 1995;333:1052–1057.

Tallman MS, Hakimian D, Peterson L. Hairy cell leukemia. In: Hoffman R, Benz EJ, Shattil SJ, et al, eds. *Hematology: Basic Principles and Practice.* 3rd ed. New York, NY: Churchill-Livingstone; 2000:1363–1372.

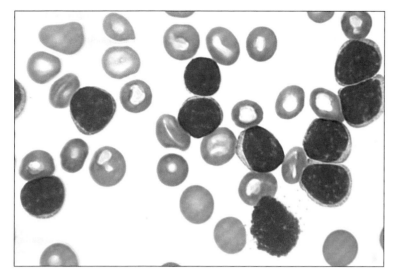

Image 33-1 Blood smear from a patient with chronic lymphocytic leukemia. The lymphocytes have scant cytoplasm and condensed chromatin patterns.

Image 33-2 Bone marrow trephine biopsy specimen from a patient with chronic lymphocytic leukemia shows a mixed interstitial and nodular pattern of infiltration.

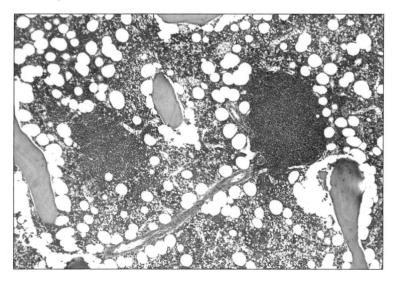

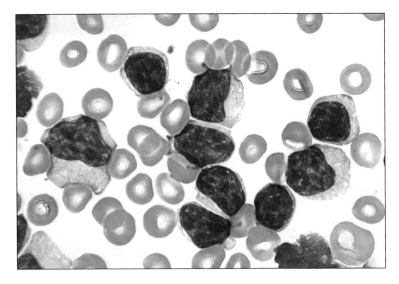

Image 33-3 Blood smear showing chronic lymphocytic leukemia, mixed cell type, with mixed small and large cells.

Image 33-4 Blood smear from a patient with chronic lymphocytic leukemia with increased prolymphocytes (CLL/PL) shows small lymphocytes with condensed chromatin and larger prolymphocytes with loosely condensed chromatin and nucleoli.

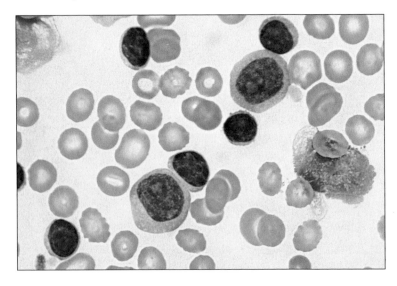

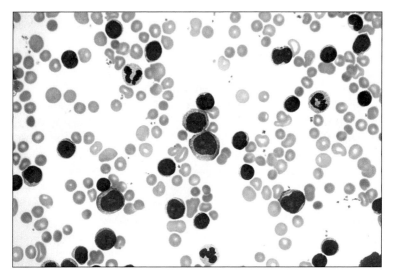

Image 33-5 Blood smear from a patient with prolymphocytoid transformation of chronic lymphocytic leukemia. The leukocyte count is markedly elevated, and prolymphocytes are increased compared with an earlier blood smear.

Image 33-6 Bone marrow core biopsy specimen showing Richter transformation. A large cell lymphoma occupies the majority of the specimen; a portion of the biopsy specimen shows the background "chronic phase" chronic lymphocytic leukemia.

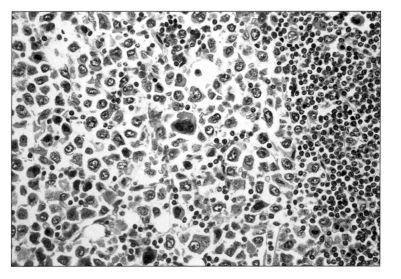

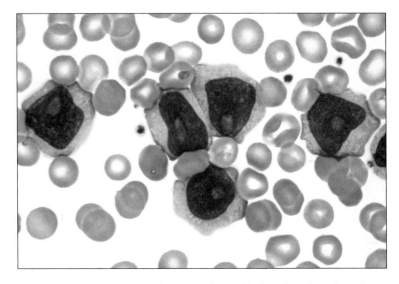

Image 33-7 Blood smear from a patient with B-cell prolymphocytic leukemia. The leukocyte count is elevated markedly, and the majority of the circulating cells are prolymphocytes.

Image 33-8 Bone marrow biopsy specimen showing diffuse infiltration by hairy cells with well-spaced nuclei. Inset shows a hairy cell with stippled chromatin pattern and an indistinct cytoplasmic border.

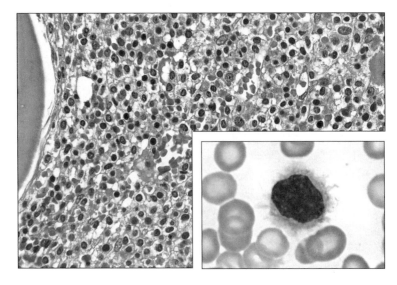

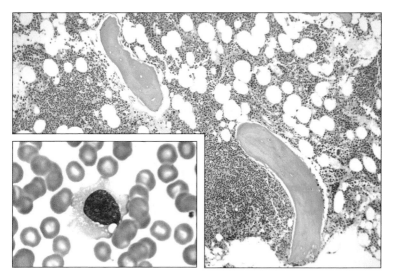

Image 33-9 Bone marrow core biopsy specimen showing involvement by a splenic marginal zone B-cell lymphoma. The lymphoid infiltrate in this case is focal and is both paratrabecular and nonparatrabecular. Inset shows a circulating lymphoma cell with abundant cytoplasm and a visible nucleolus.

Image 33-10 Bone marrow core biopsy specimen showing a paratrabecular pattern of involvement by follicle center cell lymphoma. Inset shows a circulating small cleaved cell lymphoma cell.

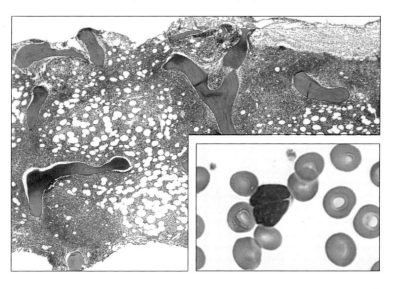

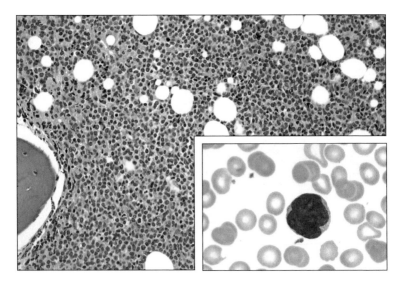

Image 33-11 Bone marrow core biopsy specimen showing diffuse involvement by mantle cell lymphoma. Inset shows a circulating lymphoma cell.

Image 33-12 Blood smear from a patient with large granular lymphocyte leukemia.

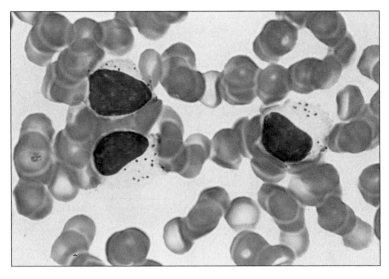

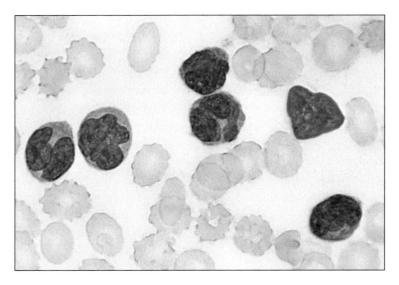

Image 33-13   Blood smear from a patient with adult T-cell leukemia/lymphoma shows multilobated lymphocytes.

Image 33-14   Blood smear shows Sézary cells with convoluted nuclei.

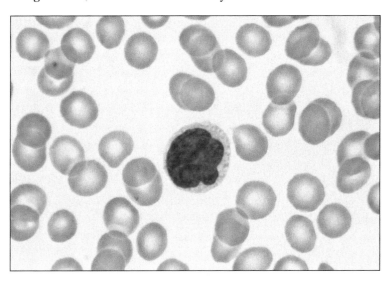

PART
IX

Lymphomas

34   Non-Hodgkin's Lymphoma

The term "malignant lymphoma" was first used by Billroth in his description of lymphoid neoplasia in 1871. Hodgkin's lymphoma (HL) and non-Hodgkin's lymphoma (NHL) are the two major categories of malignant lymphomas recognized. This chapter discusses the NHLs. These lymphomas are clonal lymphoproliferative disorders that are heterogeneous with respect to their clinical presentation, pathogenesis, and biologic behavior. In the United States, both the incidence and the mortality attributed to malignant lymphomas have steadily increased over the last four decades. Also, the overall incidence of NHL increased by about 75% between 1973 and 1991 and now accounts for approximately 50,000 new malignancies diagnosed annually. Increased frequencies have been observed in all age groups and may reflect demographic and socioeconomic factors. Although a substantial proportion of the increase is attributable to the HIV epidemic, it is important to note that significant increases in non–HIV-related cases also have been observed. Parallel with the increases in incidence, there have been corresponding increases in mortality.

The tremendous advances in the understanding of the molecular biology and immunology of the immune system and its effector cells has translated into several modifications in the classification of NHL. In this regard, the Revised European American Lymphoma (REAL) classification and the proposed World Health Organization (WHO) modification are favored over previous classification schemes that were based primarily on the morphologic features or clinical behavior of the tumors. The REAL/WHO scheme integrates the clinical, histopathologic, immunophenotypic, and molecular genetic characteristics of the lymphomas and defines distinct "real" biologic entities.

As stated earlier, the NHLs are a heterogeneous group of malignant neoplasms with diverse clinical manifestations, responses to therapy, and prognoses. Although the majority of lymphoid neoplasms arise in lymph nodes, an increasing number of NHLs of primary extranodal origin are recognized (especially in children and immunosuppressed patients). More so for the B-cell than the T-cell NHLs, the putative cell of origin for a substantial number of malignant lymphomas has been deduced from their morphologic and immunophenotypic characteristics, as well as their predilection for particular microanatomic areas of involvement.

Although NHLs may be conveniently grouped into indolent, aggressive, and highly aggressive neoplasms, it is important not to lose sight of the unique biologic characteristics of each individual lymphoma within the context of a particular patient's prognostic parameters. Indolent NHLs include such disorders as chronic lymphocytic leukemia/small lymphocytic lymphoma (CLL/SLL) and marginal zone B-cell lymphoma of mucosa-associated lymphoid tissue (MALT) type. Examples of aggressive lymphomas include mantle cell lymphoma (MCL) and diffuse large B-cell lymphoma (DLBCL). Burkitt's lymphoma (BL) and lymphoblastic lymphoma are considered highly aggressive NHLs.

There are considerable differences in the demographic and epidemiologic characteristics of the different lymphomas. For instance, follicular lymphomas are characteristically adult diseases and are more prevalent in Europe and North America than in Africa and Asia. By comparison, BL is more prevalent in equatorial Africa, with a peculiar predilection for presentation as a jaw tumor in children. Adult T-cell leukemia/lymphoma is most frequently seen in southwestern Japan and the Caribbean countries.

34.1 Pathophysiology

The NHLs are clonal proliferations of malignant lymphocytes. In many cases, the primary abnormality is a cytogenetic aberration that is consistently associated with a particular subtype of malignant lymphoma (**Table 34-1**). The cytogenetic abnormality is

Table 34-1 Common Cytogenetic Aberrations in Malignant Lymphoma

Subtype	Cytogenetic Abnormality	Implicated Genes	Frequency (%)
B cell			
FL	t(14;18)(q32;q21)	IgH/*bcl*-2	~90
	t(2;18)(p12;q21)	Igκ/*bcl*-2	<5
	t(3;14)(q27;q32)	*bcl*-6/IgH	~10
MCL	t(11;14)(q13;q32)	*bcl*-1/IgH	>90
MZBCL-MALT	Trisomy 3	Unknown	Variable
	t(11;18)(p21;q21)	*API2*/MLT	50
	t(1;14)(p22;q32)	*bcl*-10/IgH	*
LPL	t(9;14)(p13;q32)	*PAX-5*/IgH	*
Burkitt's	t(8;14)(q24;q32)	*c-myc*/IgH	75
	t(2;8)(p12;q24)	Igκ/*c-myc*	15
	t(8;22)(q24;q11)	*c-myc*/Igλ	10
DLBCL	t(3;14)(q27;q32)	*bcl*-6/IgH	~30
	t(14;18)(q32;q21)	IgH/*bcl*-2	30
PMLBCL	Amplification 9p	*REL*	*
B-CLL	del 13q14	Unknown	25–50
	Trisomy 12	Unknown	30
B-PLL	t(11;14)(q13;q32)	*bcl*-1/IgH	*
Precursor B-ALL	t(12;21)(p13;q22)	*ETV6-CBFA2 (TEL/AML1)*	22
	t(1;19)(q23;p13)	*PBX1/E2A*	~30
	t(9;22)(q34;q11)	*c-abl/bcr*	5–20
	t(4;11)(q21;q23)	*AF4/MLL*	10
ALL-FABL3	t(8;14)(q24;q32)	*c-myc*/IgH	6
T cell			
ALCL, T/NK	t(2;5)(p23;q35)	*ALK/NPM*	~40
T-PLL	inv 14(q11;q32) or complex translocations involving both chromosomes 14		75
Hepatosplenic γ/δ	Isochromosome 7q	Unknown	*
	Trisomy 8	Unknown	*
Precursor T-ALL	t(1:14)(p32;q11)	*SCL* (*tal*-1)/ TcR δ/α	15–30
	t(10;14)(q24;q11)	*HOX-11*/TcR δ/α	7
T-cell lympho-blastic with eosinophilia	t(8;13)(p11;q11-12)	*FGFR1/ZNF* 198	*

Abbreviations: FL = follicular lymphoma; MCL = mantle cell lymphoma; MZBCL = marginal zone B-cell lymphoma; MALT = mucosa-associated lymphoid tissue; LPL = lymphoplasmacytic lymphoma; DLBCL = diffuse large B-cell lymphoma; PMLBCL = primary mediastinal large B-cell lymphoma; B-CLL = B-chronic lymphocytic leukemia; PLL = prolymphocytic leukemia; ALL = acute lymphoblastic leukemia; ALCL = anaplastic large cell lymphoma; NK = natural killer.
*An insufficient number of patients were studied to permit accurate assessment of percentage of tumors with the cytogenetic aberration indicated.

frequently a nonrandom chromosomal translocation that leads to juxtaposition of a proto-oncogene (eg, c-*myc*) to one of the antigen receptor genes (immunoglobulin heavy chain or T-cell receptor). In addition to proto-oncogene activation, other mechanisms implicated in lymphoma genesis and progression include deregulation of anti-apoptosis genes (eg, *bcl-2*), and tumor suppressor gene inactivation (eg, *p53*). The role of microbiologic agents such as *Helicobacter pylori* organisms in the pathogenesis of gastric MALT lymphomas is also well established. Similarly, there is compelling evidence that certain oncogenic viruses play important roles in the development of such lymphoproliferative disorders as posttransplantation lympho-proliferative disease (Epstein-Barr virus [EBV]) and primary effu-sion lymphoma (human herpesvirus 8). These exciting discoveries notwithstanding, the precise causes of most NHLs are unknown. Nevertheless, it is believed that NHLs arise as a result of an interplay of multiple factors, including genetic aberrations, congenital or acquired immunosuppression, exposure to ionizing radiation, and chemical agents. A list of some of the conditions and factors associ-ated with the development of NHLs is provided in **Table 34-2**.

34.2 Clinical Findings

Clinical manifestations of NHL vary depending on histologic sub-type. More than two thirds of patients with NHL present with pain-less peripheral lymph node enlargement, most commonly in the cervical region. In up to 10% of patients, especially those with fol-licular lymphoma, the lymph nodes may fluctuate in size or even undergo apparent spontaneous remission lasting months and some-times years. Patients with follicular lymphoma usually have multi-ple sites of involvement, including extranodal disease within bone marrow, liver, or spleen. Although most patients are asymptomatic at presentation, about 20% of the patients have constitutional "B" symptoms, manifested by fevers, night sweats, weight loss, and pain. Such symptoms are more commonly seen in the aggressive types of lymphomas.

In addition to lymph nodes, NHLs can present in almost any organ system. Extranodal lymphomas may present diagnostic difficulties because of their unusual anatomic site of presenta-tion. The most common sites of extranodal lymphomas are the

Table 34-2 Predisposing Conditions and Factors in the Development of Non-Hodgkin's Lymphoma

Primary (congenital) immunodeficiency syndromes
Ataxia-telangiectasia
Wiskott-Aldrich
Common variable immunodeficiency
X-linked lymphoproliferative syndrome
Secondary/therapy-induced immunodeficiencies
Organ transplantation
Immunosuppressive therapy
Autoimmune disorders
Rheumatoid arthritis
Sjögren's syndrome
Hashimoto's thyroiditis
Microbiologic agents
Viruses
HIV
Epstein-Barr virus (PTLD)
Human T-cell lymphotropic virus 1 (ATL/L)
KSHV/HHV-8 (PEL)
Bacteria
Helicobacter pylori (gastric MALT-lymphoma)
Environmental factors
Pesticides
Benzene
Phenoxyherbicides
Chemotherapy
Ionizing radiation

Abbreviations: HIV = human immunodeficiency virus; PTLD = posttransplantation lymphoproliferative disorder; ATL/L = adult T-cell leukemia lymphoma; KSHV = Kaposi's sarcoma-associated herpesvirus; HHV-8 = human herpesvirus 8; PEL = primary effusion lymphoma; MALT = mucosa-associated lymphoid tissue.

gastrointestinal tract, lung, thyroid, salivary gland, orbit, gonads, central nervous system, bone, and skin. A comparison of the characteristic features in NHL and HL is presented in **Table 34-3**.

34.3 **Staging**

The purpose of staging a patient with lymphoma is to identify the extent of the disease and to choose the optimal therapy for each

Table 34-3   Comparison of Non-Hodgkin's and Hodgkin's Lymphomas

Feature	Non-Hodgkin's Lymphoma	Hodgkin's Lymphoma
B symptoms	20%	40%
Presentation	Often extranodal	Predominantly nodal
Involvement	Rarely localized	Usually localized
Peripheral blood	Affected in 10%–40%	Not affected
Bone marrow involvement	Frequent	Uncommon
Mediastinal involvement	Uncommon except for lymphoblastic and mediastinal large B-cell lymphoma	Common
Gastrointestinal involvement	Common	Extremely rare
Skin involvement	Common	Extremely rare
Central nervous system involvement	Occasionally	Extremely rare

Table 34-4   Stages of Lymphoma

Stage I: Disease limited to one anatomic region or two contiguous regions on the same side of the diaphragm

Stage II: Disease in more than two anatomic regions or in noncontiguous regions on the same side of the diaphragm

Stage III: Disease on both sides of the diaphragm, but limited to involvement of lymph nodes and spleen

Stage IV: Disease of any lymph node region with involvement of liver, lung, or bone marrow

patient (**Table 34-4**). Unfortunately, because NHLs represent a heterogeneous group of diseases with distinct natural histories and variable response to therapy, no general staging classification is helpful in dividing patients into specific therapy categories. The extent of staging studies depends on the tissue diagnosis, age of the patient, clinical symptoms, and physical examination. The Cotswald modification of the Ann Arbor staging classification for HL (*see Table 35-2*) also may be used in NHL, but it is less prognostically helpful than with HL. A National Cancer Institute modified staging system exists for intermediate- and high-grade lymphomas (**Table 34-5**). These staging classifications are often inappropriate

Table 34-5 National Cancer Institute Modified Staging for
Intermediate- and High-Grade Lymphomas

Stage	Characteristics
I	Localized nodal or extranodal disease (Ann Arbor stage I or IE)
II	Two or more nodal sites of disease or a localized extranodal site plus draining nodes with one of the following: performance status ≤70, B symptoms, any mass >10 cm in diameter (particularly gastrointestinal), serum lactate dehydrogenase >500, three or more extranodal sites of disease
III	Stage II plus any poor prognostic factor

for primary extranodal lymphomas, especially those in the gastrointestinal tract.

The most important part of the clinical history is to determine the presence or absence of systemic B symptoms and whether there are symptoms such as bone pain or gastrointestinal disorders related to extranodal involvement. It is also helpful to assess the duration of the disease to determine the growth rate of the tumor. The physical examination should include examination of all nodal areas, including Waldeyer's ring; periauricular, epitrochlear, and popliteal lymph nodes; and the presence or absence of hepatosplenomegaly. The skin, breasts, testicles, central nervous system, and lungs should be examined for possible extranodal involvement. Other staging studies usually include complete blood cell count, evaluation of renal and liver function, radiologic studies including chest radiograph, bilateral lower extremity lymphangiogram, abdominal pelvic computed tomography scan, and bilateral bone marrow needle biopsies and aspirate. Cerebrospinal fluid cytologic studies are indicated in intermediate- or high-grade lymphomas. The clinical staging procedures are summarized in **Table 34-6**.

34.4 Classification of Non-Hodgkin's Lymphoma

The diagnosis and classification of NHL are based primarily on the morphologic features of the tissue biopsy specimen and on immunologic characteristics, cytogenetic studies, and biologic behavior (**Table 34-7**). Many classification systems of NHL have been used over the years. In the 1990s, the Working Formulation in

Table 34-6 Staging Procedures for Non-Hodgkin's Lymphoma

1. Clinical history with special attention to duration and specific symptoms
2. Physical examination including all lymph node–bearing areas, liver, and spleen
3. Surgical biopsy with fine-needle aspiration
4. Complete blood cell count, including examination of peripheral blood smear
5. Bilateral bone marrow aspirates and biopsies
6. Liver and renal function tests
7. Serum lactate dehydrogenase and β_2-microglobulin levels
8. Serum protein electrophoresis
9. Radiologic studies including chest radiograph, bilateral lower extremity lymphangiogram, and abdominal-pelvic computed tomography
10. Cytologic examination of any effusions
11. Lumbar puncture for cerebrospinal fluid cytologic studies in intermediate and high-grade lymphomas

the United States and the Kiel classification in Europe were used successfully. The classification system used in this chapter is that proposed by the International Lymphoma Study Group (REAL classification) (**Table 34-8**) and recently modified in the WHO proposal (**Table 34-9**). This classification is based on the Kiel and Lukes-Collins classifications and includes the more recently described subtypes of NHL. Although several of the entities listed are considered provisional, recent studies have shown that the classification is clinically relevant. Undoubtedly, several modifications will take place when the system is tested in clinical trials. More studies are needed to define prognostic groups valuable to clinicians. Comparison of this classification with the Working Formulation and the Kiel classification is shown in **Tables 34-10** and **34-11**.

The REAL/WHO classification is based on current knowledge of histologic, immunologic, and genetic features; the clinical presentation and course of the disease; and the postulated normal cell counterparts. The classification is divided into B-cell and T-cell lymphomas; this distinction should be made whenever possible. In the REAL classification, the term "grade" refers to morphologic features such as cell size, density of chromatin, and proliferation rate. With regard to the clinical behavior of tumor, the terms "prognostic group" or "aggressiveness" are used. A number of the entities described in this classification have a range of morphologic grades and clinical aggressiveness.

Table 34-7 Principles of Classification of Non-Hodgkin's Lymphoma

Morphology

    Pattern

        Follicular

        Diffuse

        Interfollicular

        Sinusoidal

    Cytology

        Cell size

            Small (small lymphocytic lymphoma)

            Small to intermediate (mantle cell lymphoma, marginal zone B-cell lymphoma)

            Intermediate (follicular small cleaved cell, Burkitt's and lymphoblastic lymphoma)

            Large (large-cell lymphoma)

    Nuclear contour

        Round—small lymphocytes, noncleaved cells (Burkitt's lymphoma, centroblastic lymphoma)

        Irregular—mantle cell lymphoma

        Cleaved—follicular lymphoma

        Convoluted—mycosis fungoides, Sézary syndrome, lymphoblastic lymphoma (some)

        Multilobated—some large cell lymphomas

        Pleomorphic—anaplastic large cell lymphoma

        Monocytoid—marginal zone B-cell lymphoma

        Cerebriform—mycosis fungoides

    Chromatin pattern

        Clumped—small lymphocytic, centrocytic (small cleaved cell), mantle cell, marginal zone B cell

        Fine—lymphoblastic cells

        Vesicular—centroblasts

    Nucleoli

        Burkitt's lymphoma, immunoblastic large cell lymphoma

Immunologic characteristics

    Determination of B- and T-cell immunophenotype, and monoclonality using immunohistochemistry or flow cytometry and sometimes gene rearrangement studies

Cytogenetics and oncogenes

Biologic behavior

Table 34-8   List of Lymphoid Neoplasms Recognized by the International Lymphoma Study Group* (REAL) Classification)

B-Cell Neoplasms

I. Precursor B-cell neoplasm: B-precursor lymphoblastic leukemia/lymphoma

II. Peripheral B-cell neoplasms

   1. B-cell chronic lymphocytic leukemia/prolymphocytic leukemia/small lymphocytic lymphoma

   2. Lymphoplasmacytoid lymphoma/immunocytoma

   3. Mantle cell lymphoma

   4. Follicle center lymphoma, follicular
     Provisional cytologic grades: small cell, mixed small and large cell, large cell
     Provisional subtype: diffuse, predominantly small cell type

   5. Marginal zone B-cell lymphoma
     Extranodal (MALT type ± monocytoid B cells)
     Provisional category: nodal (± monocytoid B cells)
     Provisional category: splenic (± villous lymphocytes)

   6. Hairy cell leukemia

   7. Plasmacytoma/myeloma

   8. Diffuse large B-cell lymphoma[†]
     Subtype: primary mediastinal (thymic) B-cell lymphoma

   9. Burkitt's lymphoma

  10. Provisional category: high-grade B-cell lymphoma, Burkitt-like[†]

T-Cell and Putative NK-Cell Neoplasms

I. Precursor T-cell neoplasm: T-precursor lymphoblastic lymphoma/leukemia

II. Peripheral T-cell and NK-cell neoplasms

   1. T-cell chronic lymphocytic leukemia/prolymphocytic leukemia

   2. Large granular lymphocytic leukemia
     T-cell type
     NK-cell type

   3. Mycosis fungoides/Sézary syndrome

   4. Peripheral T-cell lymphoma[†]
     Provisional subtypes: medium-sized cell, mixed medium and large cell, large cell, lymphoepithelioid cell

   5. Angioimmunoblastic T-cell lymphoma

   6. Angiocentric lymphoma

   7. Intestinal T-cell lymphoma (± enteropathy-associated)

   8. Adult T-cell lymphoma/leukemia

   9. Anaplastic large cell lymphoma (ALCL), CD30+, T- and null-cell types

  10. Provisional subtype: anaplastic large cell lymphoma, Hodgkin's-like

Table 34-8   *Continued*

Hodgkin's Disease
  I. Lymphocyte predominance
  II. Nodular sclerosis
  III. Mixed cellularity
  IV. Lymphocyte depletion
  V. Provisional subtype: lymphocyte-rich classic Hodgkin's disease

Unclassifiable
  I. B-cell lymphoma, unclassifiable (low grade/high grade)
  II. T-cell lymphoma, unclassifiable (low grade/high grade)
  III. Hodgkin's disease, unclassifiable
  IV. Malignant lymphoma, unclassifiable

Abbreviations: MALT = mucosa-associated lymphoid tissue; NK = natural killer.
*From Harris NL, Jaffe ES, Stein H, et al. A revised European-American classification of lymphoid neoplasms: a proposal from the International Lymphoma Study Group. *Blood.* 1994;84:1361–1392.
†These categories are thought likely to include more than one disease entity.

34.5 B-Cell Neoplasms

34.5.1 Precursor B-Cell Lymphoblastic Leukemia/Lymphoma

Clinical Features

The majority of patients with precursor B-cell neoplasms are children, and the disease represents 80% of acute lymphoblastic leukemia (ALL) cases. B-cell lymphoblastic leukemia/lymphoma (B-LBL) probably represents less than 20% of lymphoblastic lymphomas, the majority being T-cell phenotype. A patient with greater than 25% lymphoblasts in the bone marrow is considered to have ALL. B-LBL often presents as cutaneous nodules. This tumor is highly aggressive but is often curable with chemotherapy.

Morphology

The morphologic features of B-LBL are essentially identical to those seen in precursor T-cell lymphoblastic leukemia/lymphoma (T-LBL). The cells are intermediate in size—between small and large cell lymphoma—with convoluted or round nuclei, delicate chromatin, indistinct nucleoli, and scant cytoplasm. Mitoses are frequently seen (especially in younger patients), and a "starry sky" pattern may be present.

Table 34-9 Proposed World Health Organization Classification for Neoplastic Diseases of Hematopoietic and Lymphoid Tissues (February 1998)

B-cell neoplasms
  Precursor B-cell lymphoblastic leukemia/lymphoma
  Peripheral B-cell neoplasms
    B-cell chronic lymphocytic leukemia/small lymphocytic lymphoma
      Variant: with monoclonal gammopathy/plasmacytoid differentiation
    B-cell prolymphocytic leukemia
    Lymphoplasmacytic lymphoma
    Mantle cell lymphoma
      Variant: blastic
    Follicular lymphoma
      Variants: grades 1, 2, and 3
               cutaneous follicle center lymphoma
    Marginal zone B-cell lymphoma (MALT type)
    Nodal marginal zone lymphoma +/- monocytoid B cells
    Splenic marginal zone B-cell lymphoma (+/- villous lymphocytes)
    Hairy cell leukemia
      Variant: hairy cell
    Diffuse large B-cell lymphoma
      Variants: centroblastic
               immunoblastic
               T cell- or histiocyte-rich
               anaplastic large B cell
    Diffuse large B-cell lymphoma
      Subtypes: mediastinal (thymic) large B-cell lymphoma
               intravascular large B-cell lymphoma
               primary effusion lymphoma
    Burkitt's lymphoma
      Variants: endemic
               sporadic
               atypical (pleomorphic)
               atypical with plasmacytoid differentiation (AIDS associated)
  Immunosecretory disorders (clinical or pathologic variants)
    Plasma cell myeloma (multiple myeloma)
      Indolent myeloma
      Smoldering myeloma
      Osteosclerotic myeloma (POEMS syndrome)
      Plasma cell leukemia
      Nonsecretory myeloma
    Plasmacytomas
      Solitary plasmacytoma of bone
      Extramedullary plasmacytoma
    Waldenström's macroglobulinemia (lymphoplasmacytic lymphoma, see above)

Table 34-9 *Continued*

Heavy chain disease (HCD)
  γ-HCD
  α-HCD
  μ-HCD
Immunoglobulin deposition diseases
  Systemic light chain disease
  Primary amyloidosis

T-cell neoplasms
  Precursor T-cell lymphoblastic leukemia/lymphoma
  Peripheral T-cell and NK-cell neoplasms
    T-cell prolymphocytic leukemia
      Variants: small cell
                   cerebriform cell
    T-cell large granular lymphocytic leukemia
    Aggressive NK-cell leukemia
    NK/T-cell lymphoma, nasal and nasal-type
    Sézary syndrome
    Mycosis fungoides
      Variants: pagetoid reticulosis
                   MF-associated follicular mucinosis
                   granulomatous slack skin disease
    Angioimmunoblastic T-cell lymphoma
    Peripheral T-cell lymphoma (unspecified)
      Variants: lymphoepithelioid (Lennert's)
                   T zone
    Adult T-cell leukemia/lymphoma (HTLV-I+)
      Variants: acute
                   lymphomatous
                   chronic
                   smoldering
                   Hodgkin's-like
    Anaplastic large cell lymphoma (T and null cell types)
      Variants: lymphohistiocytic
                   small cell
    Primary cutaneous CD30+ T-cell lymphoproliferative disorders
      Variants: lymphomatoid papulosis (types A and B)
                   primary cutaneous ALCL
                   borderline lesions
    Subcutaneous panniculitislike T-cell lymphoma
    Enteropathy-type intestinal T-cell lymphoma
    Hepatosplenic γ/δ T-cell lymphoma

Hodgkin's lymphoma (disease)
  Nodular lymphocyte predominance Hodgkin's lymphoma
  Classical Hodgkin's lymphoma
    Hodgkin's lymphoma, nodular sclerosis (grades I and II)
    Classic Hodgkin's lymphoma, lymphocyte-rich

Table 34-9 *Continued*

Hodgkin's lymphoma, mixed cellularity
Hodgkin's lymphoma, lymphocyte depletion

Immunodeficiency-related lymphoproliferative disorders*
  Congenital immunodeficiency-associated lymphoproliferative disorders†
    Atypical lymphoproliferative disorders
    Diffuse large B-cell lymphoma
  Posttransplantation and other iatrogenic lymphoproliferative disorders
    Polymorphic B-cell lymphoproliferative disorders
    Diffuse large B-cell lymphoma
    Plasmacytoma (+/- multiple myeloma)
    Peripheral T-cell lymphomas (cytotoxic, NK/T)
    Hodgkin's lymphoma
  AIDS-associated lymphoproliferative disorders
    Burkitt's and atypical Burkitt's lymphoma
    Diffuse large B-cell lymphoma
    Immunoblastic lymphoma (with plasmacytoid differentiation)
    Primary effusion lymphoma

Abbreviations: MALT = mucosa-associated lymphoid tissue; NK = natural killer; MF = mycosis fungoides; HTLV-I = human T-cell leukemia virus type I; ALCL = anaplastic large cell lymphoma.
*These disorders are seen with increasing frequency in immunodeficiency states. This list does imply an independent classification scheme for immunodeficiency-associated lymphoproliferative disorders. Those disorders occurring without known immunodeficiency are also listed with B-cell and T-cell neoplasms.
†The congenital immunodeficiencies most commonly associated with lymphoproliferative disorders include Wiskott-Aldrich syndrome, common variable immunodeficiency, ataxia-telangiectasis, severe combined immunodeficiency, X-linked lymphoproliferative disorder, and hyper-IgM syndrome. Each form of immunodeficiency disorder is associated with its own risk factors, which affect the pattern of lymphoproliferative disorder. Consequently, the lymphoproliferative disorders vary by type and frequency according to the form of underlying immune deficiency.
Source: Complete list of lymphoid neoplasms, including morphologic and clinical variants provided by personal communication from Elaine Jaffe, MD, as presented at the Clinical Advisory Committee meeting, November 3-5, 1997, Airlie, Virginia. (The proposed classifications for tumors of histiocytic and dendritic cell derivation are not included.)

The differential diagnosis based on morphologic features includes BL, granulocytic sarcoma, and the "lymphoblastoid" variant of MCL. In older individuals, B-LBL may resemble small lymphocytic lymphoma.

Immunophenotype

Immunophenotyping of this tumor shows the following features: terminal deoxynucleotidyl transferase (TdT) positive, CD79a+, CD19+, CD20–/+, CD22+, CD10+/–, SIg–, cytoplasmic μ–/+, CD34+/–. CD45 is often negative. The tumor may aberrantly coexpress myeloid markers CD13 and/or CD33. The major cytogenetic aberrations seen in B-LBL are summarized in **Table 34-1**.

Molecular and Cytogenetic Features
The cytogenetic changes are variable but frequently involve chromosomal translocations, which result in chimeric fusion products that are important for malignant transformation. In contrast to malignant lymphomas in adults, most pediatric leukemias arise from aberrant genetic recombinations that do not involve the antigen receptor genes. The oncogenic fusion proteins act through dysregulation of transduction pathways and frequently involve transcription factors.

34.6 Mature B-Cell Neoplasms

Tables 34-12 and **34-13** summarize the morphologic and immunophenotypic features of the seven small B-lymphocytic neoplasms discussed in this section.

34.6.1 B-Cell Chronic Lymphocytic Leukemia/Small Lymphocytic Lymphoma (B-CLL/B-SLL)
Clinical Features
This tumor occurs mainly in older individuals with a male:female ratio of 2:1. The majority of patients have bone marrow and peripheral blood involvement with or without lymphadenopathy or splenomegaly at time of diagnosis. A history of waxing and waning lymphadenopathy is not uncommon. Transformation to large B-cell lymphoma (Richter's syndrome) is seen in approximately 5% of patients. Follow-up biopsies occasionally show features of HL. EBV appears to be involved in such cases. B-cell CLL/SLL is an indolent disease that is usually incurable with currently available therapy.

Morphology
This tumor is principally composed of small lymphocytes that may be somewhat larger than normal lymphocytes (**Image 34-1**). A helpful diagnostic feature is the presence of proliferation centers consisting of larger lymphoid cells (prolymphocytes and paraimmunoblasts). Microscopically, they appear as vaguely delineated

Table 34-10 Comparison of the REAL Classification With the Working Formulation*

Revised European-American Lymphoma Classification	Working Formulation
Precursor B-lymphoblastic lymphoma/leukemia	Lymphoblastic
B-cell CLL/prolymphocytic leukemia/SLL	Small lymphocytic, consistent with CLL[†]; small lymphocytic, plasmacytoid
Lymphoplasmacytoid lymphoma	Small lymphocytic, plasmacytoid[†]; diffuse, mixed small and large cell
Mantle cell lymphoma	Small lymphocytic; diffuse, small cleaved cell[†]; follicular, small cleaved cell; diffuse, mixed small and large cell; diffuse, large cleaved cell
Follicle center lymphoma, follicular Grade I	Follicular, predominantly small cleaved cell[†]
Grade II	Follicular, mixed small and large cell[†]
Grade III	Follicular, predominantly large cell
Follicle center lymphoma, diffuse, small cell [provisional]	Diffuse, small cleaved cell[†]; diffuse, mixed small and large cell
Extranodal marginal zone B-cell lymphoma (low-grade B-cell lymphoma of MALT type)	Small lymphocytic[†]; diffuse, small cleaved cell; diffuse, mixed small and large cell
Nodal marginal zone B-cell lymphoma [provisional]	Small lymphocytic[†]; diffuse, small cleaved cell; diffuse, mixed small and large cell; unclassifiable
Splenic marginal zone B-cell lymphoma [provisional]	Small lymphocytic[†]; diffuse, small cleaved cell
Hairy cell leukemia	—
Plasmacytoma/myeloma	Extramedullary plasmacytoma
Diffuse large B-cell lymphoma	Diffuse, large cell[†]; large cell immunoblastic; diffuse, mixed small and large cell
Primary mediastinal large B-cell	Diffuse, large cell[†]; large cell immunoblastic
Burkitt's lymphoma	Small noncleaved cell, Burkitt's
High-grade B-cell lymphoma, Burkitt-like [provisional]	Small noncleaved cell, non-Burkitt's[†]; diffuse, large cell; large cell immunoblastic
Precursor T-lymphoblastic lymphoma/leukemia	Lymphoblastic
T-cell CLL/prolymphocytic leukemia	Small lymphocytic[†]; diffuse, small cleaved cell
Large granular lymphocytic leukemia (T-cell type, NK-cell type)	Small lymphocytic[†]; diffuse, small cleaved cell
Mycosis fungoides/Sézary syndrome	Mycosis fungoides

Table 34-10 *Continued*

Revised European-American Lymphoma Classification	Working Formulation
Peripheral T-cell lymphomas, unspecified [including provisional subtype: subcutaneous panniculitic T-cell lymphoma]	Diffuse, small cleaved cell; diffuse, mixed small and large cell[†]; diffuse, large cell; large cell immunoblastic[†]€
Hepatosplenic γ/δ T-cell lymphoma [provisional]	—
Angioimmunoblastic T-cell lymphoma	Diffuse, mixed small and large cell[†]; diffuse, large cell; large cell immunoblasts[†]
Angiocentric lymphoma	Diffuse, small cleaved cell; diffuse mixed small and large cell[†]; diffuse, large cell; large cell immunoblastic[†]
Intestinal T-cell lymphoma	Diffuse, small cleaved cell; diffuse, mixed small and large cell[†]; diffuse, large cell; large cell immunoblastic[†]
Adult T-cell lymphoma/leukemia	Diffuse, small cleaved cell; diffuse, mixed small and large cell[†]; diffuse, large cell; large cell immunoblastic[†]
Anaplastic large cell lymphoma, T- and null-cell types	Large cell immunoblastic

Abbreviations: CLL = chronic lymphocytic leukemia; MALT = mucosa-associated lymphoid tissue; NK = natural killer.

*From Harris NL, Jaffe ES, Stein H, et al. A revised European-American classification of lymphoid neoplasms: a proposal from the International Lymphoma Study Group. *Blood.* 1994;84:1361–1392.

[†]When more than one Working Formulation category is listed, these compose the majority of the cases.

pale areas, imparting a nodular pattern to the lymph node. The morphologic features of B-CLL and B-SLL are identical.

The differential diagnosis based on morphologic features would include MCL, follicular lymphoma (in cases with prominent proliferation centers), and rarely lymphoblastic lymphoma. Tumors that have plasmacytoid differentiation are considered a variant of B-CLL/SLL and are not considered a separate diagnostic category.

Immunophenotype

Immunophenotypic studies of B-CLL/SLL are as follows: SIgM+ (dim), SIgD+/–, CD19+, CD79a+, CD20+ (dim), CD23+,

Table 34-11 Comparison of the REAL Classification With the Kiel Classification*

Kiel Classification	Revised European-American Lymphoma Classification
B-lymphoblastic	Precursor B-lymphoblastic lymphoma/leukemia
B-lymphocytic, CLL†; B-lymphocytic, prolymphocytic leukemia; lymphoplasmacytoid immunocytoma	B-cell CLL/prolymphocytic leukemia/small lymphocyte lymphoma
Lymphoplasmacytic immunocytoma	Lymphoplasmacytoid lymphoma
Centrocytic†; centroblastic, centrocytoid subtype	Mantle cell lymphoma
Centroblastic-centrocytic, follicular†; centroblastic, follicular	Follicle center lymphoma, follicular (grade I, grade II, grade III)
Centroblastic-centrocytic, diffuse	Follicle center lymphoma, diffuse, small cell [provisional]
—	Extranodal marginal zone B-cell lymphoma (low-grade B-cell lymphoma of MALT type)
Monocytoid, including marginal zone†; immunocytoma	Nodal marginal zone B-cell lymphoma [provisional]
—	Splenic marginal zone B-cell lymphoma [provisional]
Hairy cell leukemia	Hairy cell leukemia
Plasmacytic	Plasmacytoma/myeloma
Centroblastic† (monomorphic, polymorphic, and multilobated subtypes); B-immunoblastic†; B-large cell anaplastic (Ki-1+)	Diffuse large B-cell lymphoma
—‡	Primary mediastinal large B-cell lymphoma
Burkitt's lymphoma	Burkitt's lymphoma
—	High-grade B-cell lymphoma, Burkitt-like [provisional]
? Some cases of centroblastic and immunoblastic	
T-lymphoblastic	Precursor T-lymphoblastic lymphoma/leukemia
T-lymphocytic, CLL type†; T-lymphocytic, prolymphocytic leukemia	T-cell chronic lymphocytic leukemia/prolymphocytic leukemia
T-lymphocytic, CLL type	Large granular lymphocytic leukemia T-cell type NK-cell type
Small cell cerebriform (mycosis fungoides, Sézary syndrome)	Mycosis fungoides/Sézary syndrome

Table 34-11 *Continued*

Kiel Classification	Revised European-American Lymphoma Classification
T-zone Lymphoepithelioid Pleomorphic, small T-cell Pleomorphic, medium-sized and large T-cell[†] T-immunoblastic	Peripheral T-cell lymphomas, unspecified [including provisional subtype: subcutaneous panniculitic T-cell lymphoma]
—	Hepatosplenic γ/δ T-cell lymphoma [provisional]
Angioimmunoblastic (AILD, LgX)	Angioimmunoblastic T-cell lymphoma
—[‡]	Angiocentric lymphoma
—	Intestinal T-cell lymphoma
Pleomorphic small T-cell, HTLV-I[+] Pleomorphic medium-sized and large T-cell, HTLV-I[†]	Adult T-cell lymphoma/leukemia
T-large cell anaplastic (Ki-1[+])	Anaplastic large cell lymphoma, T- and null-cell types

Abbreviations: CLL = chronic lymphocytic leukemia; MALT = mucosa-associated lymphoid tissue; NK = natural killer; HTLV = human T-cell leukemia virus.
*From Harris NL, Jaffe ES, Stein H, et al. A revised European-American classification of lymphoid neoplasms: a proposal from the International Lymphoma Study Group. *Blood.* 1994;84:1361–1392.
[†]When more than one Kiel category is listed, these compose the majority of the cases.
[‡]Not listed in classification, but discussed as rare or ambiguous type.

CD5+, CD43+, CD11c–/+ (dim), CD10–, CD25–/+. CD23 is especially useful in distinguishing this tumor from MCL, which is usually CD23–. In contrast to other mature B-cell neoplasms, CLL/SLL is frequently CD79b–.

Molecular and Cytogenetic Features
Immunoglobulin heavy (IgH) and immunoglobulin light (IgL) chain genes are clonally rearranged. Cytogenetic studies have shown trisomy 12 in 30% of patients, and abnormalities of 13q have been seen in 25% to 50% of patients (*see Table 34-1*).

34.6.2 B-Cell Prolymphocytic Leukemia (B-PLL)
Clinical Features
This is a disease of the elderly (men predominate) characterized by absolute peripheral lymphocytosis $\sim 100 \times 10^3/mm^3$ ($\sim 100 \times 10^9/L$) and striking splenomegaly without significant

Table 34-12 Small Lymphocytic B-cell Neoplasms: Characteristic Morphologic Features*

Lymphoma Type	Pattern	Small Cells	Large Cells
B-CLL/SLL	Diffuse proliferation centers (with pseudofollicles)	Round (may be cleaved)	Prolymphocytes, paraimmunoblasts
Lympho-plasmacytic lymphoma	Diffuse	Round (may be cleaved), plasma cells	Centroblasts, immunoblasts
Mantle cell lymphoma	Diffuse, vaguely nodular, mantle zone, rarely follicular	Cleaved (may be round or oval)	Usually none
Follicular lymphoma	Follicular with or without diffuse areas, rarely diffuse	Cleaved	Centroblasts
Marginal zone B-cell lymphoma	Diffuse, interfollicular, marginal zone, occasionally follicular (colonization)	Heterogeneous: round (small lymphocytes), cleaved (marginal zone/monocytoid B cells), plasma cells	Centroblasts, immunoblasts

*From Harris NL, Jaffe ES, Stein H, et al. A revised European-American classification of lymphoid neoplasms: a proposal from the International Lymphoma Study Group. *Blood.* 1994;84:1361–1392.

lymphadenopathy. There is often attendant anemia, thrombocytopenia, and neutropenia. The current French-American-British (FAB) criteria require that prolymphocytes compose greater than 55% of the leukemic infiltrate for a diagnosis of prolymphocytic leukemia to be made.

Morphology

Peripheral blood smears reveal marked lymphocytosis. The neoplastic prolymphocytes display round nuclei with moderately condensed chromatin, prominent central nucleoli, and moderate pale blue agranular cytoplasm. Splenic involvement is characterized by white pulp involvement with red pulp infiltration.

Immunophenotype

Immunophenotypic studies of B-PLL typically show sIg (bright), CD19+, CD20+ (bright), CD22+, FMC7+, CD5– (in contrast to B-CLL/SLL).

Table 34-13 Small Lymphocytic B-cell Neoplasms: Immunophenotypic Features

Lymphoma Type	CD5	CD10	CD23	CD43	CyD1	CD103
B-CLL/SLL	+	–	+	+	–	–
Lymphoplasmacytic	–	–	–	–/+	–	–
Mantle cell	+	–/+	–	+	+	–
Follicular	–	+/–	–/+	–	–	–/+
Marginal zone	–	–	–	–/+	–	–/+
Hairy cell leukemia	–	–	–	‡	*	+

Abbreviations: CyD1= cyclin D1; B-CLL/SLL = B-cell chronic lymphocytic leukemia/small lympho-cytic lymphoma; + = 90% positive; +/– = >50% positive; –/+ = <50% positive; – = <10% positive.
*Hairy cell leukemia may show over expression of CyD1 at the transcriptional (RNA) level, but usually not by immonophenotypic studies.
‡ = insufficient data available.
Source: Modified from Harris NL, Jaffe ES, Stein H, et al. A revised European-American classification of lymphoid neoplasms: a proposal from the International Lymphoma Study Group. *Blood.* 1994;84:1361–1392.

Molecular and Cytogenetic Features

IgH is clonally rearranged. The most common karyotypic abnormality is 14q+, with a breakpoint at the IgH locus often involving a reciprocal translocation with chromosome 11.

34.6.3 Lymphoplasmacytic Lymphoma (LPL)

Clinical Features

This is a rare lymphoma occuring in older patients. Involvement of the lymph nodes, spleen, and bone marrow is common, whereas that of peripheral blood or extranodal sites is less frequent. Most affected patients have monoclonal IgM and, when hyperviscosity symptoms are present, the findings are consistent with Waldenström's macroglobulinemia. As with B-CLL/SLL, LPLs have an indolent course and the disease is usually incurable with current chemotherapy.

Morphology

This lymphoma is characterized by proliferation of small lymphocytes, plasmacytoid lymphocytes, and plasma cells. However, it lacks the histologic features seen in B-CLL/SLL, mantle cell, or marginal zone lymphomas. The growth pattern of this lymphoma is often interfollicular.

Immunophenotype

Immunophenotypic studies reveal the following features: IgM+, IgD usually negative, CD19+, CD79a+, CD20+/–, CD22+, CD5–, CD10–, CD43+/–. CD25 or CD11c may be weakly positive in some cases. This tumor is distinguished from B-CLL/SLL by a lack of CD5 and the presence of strong cytoplasmic immunoglobulin.

Molecular and Cytogenetic Features

LPL has been associated with translocations involving band 9p13 and several different chromosomal partners, including the IgH locus at 14q32. The *PAX-5* gene has been implicated as the gene on 9p13, and it encodes a nuclear transcription factor known as "B-cell lineage specific activator protein" (BSAP). This gene is involved in the regulation of several B cell–specific genes and control of B cell development. Translocations involving the *PAX-5* locus are thought to interfere with the normal transcriptional regulation of B cell differentiation and development (*see Table 34-1*).

34.6.4 Mantle Cell Lymphoma

Clinical Features

The majority of patients with MCL are over the age of 60 and have stage III or IV disease. Up to 35% of patients have peripheral blood involvement at the time of diagnosis. There is frequent involvement of lymph nodes, spleen, gastrointestinal tract (multiple lymphomatous polyposis), and Waldeyer's ring. In contrast to other small lymphocytic neoplasms, MCL is not indolent and has a moderately aggressive course. At this time it is incurable with chemotherapy. The median survival time ranges from 3 to 5 years. A nodular or mantle zone pattern may be associated with a longer survival (5 years), but the blastoid variant is often associated with a poorer prognosis (median survival time, 3 years). In contrast to B-CLL/SLL, progression to large cell lymphoma is extremely rare.

Morphology

The morphologic pattern of MCL is vaguely nodular or diffuse. It comprises cells that are usually slightly larger than normal lymphocytes and have more dispersed chromatin, scant cytoplasm, and indistinct nucleoli. The nuclear contours are slightly irregular (**Images 34-2 to 34-4**), but in some cases the cells are round, resembling B-CLL/SLL. A blastic or lymphoblastoid variant and large cell type also may be seen. Scattered epithelioid histiocytes are often present. In MCLs, larger transformed cells are typically rare or absent.

Immunophenotype

Immunophenotypic studies reveal the following: SIgM+, SIgD+, CD19+, CD20+, CD22+, CD5+, CD10–/+, CD23–, CD43+, CD11c–, CD25–, nuclear cyclin D1+. In contrast to B-CLL/SLL, MCL shows stronger CD20 and CD19 expression by immunophenotypic studies. The lack of CD23 expression is a useful marker in distinguishing MCL from B-CLL/SLL. The presence of CD5 in MCLs is useful in distinguishing it from marginal zone lymphoma. Immunohistochemical demonstration of cyclin D1 expression in a small lymphocytic neoplasm is highly suggestive of MCL.

Molecular and Cytogenetic Features

Clonal IgH and IgL gene rearrangements are often present. The reciprocal chromosomal translocation t(11;14)(q13;q32), involving the putative proto-oncogene BCL-1, has been found in 40% to 95% of patients, depending on the technique used. The t(11;14) results in overexpression of a gene called *PRAD1*, which encodes cyclin D1.

34.6.5 Follicular Lymphoma

Clinical Features

Follicular lymphoma, together with large B-cell lymphoma, is the most common NHL in the United States (20% to 40%), but is less common in Asia and Africa (10%). The median age at presentation is 55 years. Most patients present with lymphadenopathy involving multiple sites, and more than 80% have stage III to IV disease. There may be a history of waxing and waning enlargement of the lymph nodes. The bone marrow is involved in 40% to 60% of cases (paratrabecular location), and peripheral blood involvement is common. The clinical course is indolent, and the disease is usually incurable with current therapy. Transformation to large B-cell lymphoma occurs in 50% of patients 5 to 10 years after diagnosis.

Morphology

Follicular lymphomas are composed of a mixture of centrocytes (cleaved follicle center cells) and centroblasts (large non-cleaved follicle center cells). In addition to the follicular pattern

(**Images 34-5** and **34-6**), diffuse areas also may be present. In the majority of patients, centrocytes predominate, but variable numbers of centroblasts are always present. Of the follicular lymphomas, the least common are those composed mainly of centroblasts. In the Working Formulation, the follicular lymphomas are divided into small, mixed small and large, and large cell types. The interobserver reproducibility of such a classification is poor. It is now recognized that instead of distinct subtypes there is a continuous gradation in the number of large cells. Grades I, II, and III have been proposed in the REAL/WHO classification.

The morphologic differential diagnosis includes reactive follicular hyperplasia, MCL with a nodular pattern, and marginal zone B-cell lymphoma.

Immunophenotype

Immunophenotypic studies reveal the following features: CD19+, CD79a+, CD20+, CD10+/–, CD5–, CD23–/+, CD43–, CD11c–, CD25–. The absence of CD5 and CD43 is helpful in differentiating follicular lymphoma from MCL, and the presence of CD10 may be helpful in distinguishing the disease from marginal zone B-cell lymphoma. BCL-2 protein expression is present in the majority of follicular lymphomas but absent from reactive follicles (**Images 34-7** and **34-8**). The expression of BCL-2 protein, however, is not useful in distinguishing follicular lymphomas from other lymphomas because BCL-2 is frequently expressed by other types of lymphomas.

Molecular and Cytogenetic Features

Clonal IgH and IgL gene rearrangements are often present. In more than 85% of follicular lymphomas, cytogenetic studies reveal t(14;18). This results in rearrangement of the *bcl*-2 gene. This abnormality can also be found in 30% of large B-cell lymphomas (*see Table 34-1*).

34.6.6 Follicular Lymphoma, Diffuse (Predominantly Small Cleaved Cell)

These extremely rare lymphomas are composed of small cleaved cells resembling centrocytes. It is assumed that most cases represent a sampling problem and are a diffuse counterpart of a follicular lymphoma. When larger biopsy specimens are obtained, follicular areas are usually seen.

34.6.7 Marginal Zone B-Cell Lymphoma (Mucosa-Associated Lymphoid Tissue Type)

Clinical Features

This is the most common type of primary extranodal lymphoma. Tumors usually occur in adults, with a slight predominance in women. There is often a history of autoimmune disorders, such as Sjögren's syndrome or Hashimoto's thyroiditis, or of *H pylori* gastritis. At presentation, the majority of patients have stage I or II extranodal disease with involvement of epithelial tissue at various sites. The most frequently involved organ is the stomach. Other affected organs include the salivary glands, thyroid gland, lung, orbit, breast, and skin. This lymphoma often remains localized to the primary extranodal site, but dissemination (sometimes following a long disease-free interval) may be seen in up to 30% of patients, sometimes involving two or more MALT sites synchronously or metachronously. When the disease is localized, it may be cured with local treatment (surgical resection, radiation therapy, or triple antibiotics in gastric MALT); when disseminated, the disease course is usually indolent and incurable with current chemotherapy. A high incidence (25%) of patients with gastric MALT lymphoma have other malignancies, especially carcinoma of gastrointestinal or urinary tracts. Transformation to large cell lymphoma ("high-grade MALT") occurs in some patients. It is controversial whether there is a significant difference in prognosis between high-grade MALT and other DLBCLs.

Morphology

This tumor is characterized by an infiltrate of marginal zone cells (**Images 34-9 to 34-12**). The cells have also been referred to as "centrocytelike", meaning small atypical cells resembling small cleaved follicle center cells, except with more abundant cytoplasm. In addition to the marginal zone cells, monocytoid B cells, small lymphocytes, and plasma cells are present in variable numbers. Reactive follicles are frequently seen, and the neoplastic marginal zone or monocytoid B cells occupy the marginal zone and/or the interfollicular region. "Follicular colonization" by the neoplastic cells also may be present. When the tumor involves epithelial tissues, the marginal zone cells infiltrate the epithelium, forming lymphoepithelial lesions. The morphologic differential diagnosis includes B-cell CLL/SLL, follicular lymphoma, and MCL.

Immunophenotype

Immunophenotypic studies reveal the following: CD19+, CD79a+, CD20+, CD22+, CD5–, CD23–, CD43–/+, CD11c+/–. A few cases of CD5+ marginal zone lymphoma have been reported.

Molecular and Cytogenetic Features   *H. pylori resistant to Therapy 50%*

The t(11;18) may represent the most frequent structural abnormality in MALT-type lymphomas. In this translocation, the *API2* gene on 11q21, which encodes an apoptosis inhibitor, is juxtaposed to the novel *MLT* gene on chromosome 18q21. Additionally, t(1;14), which juxtaposes the novel proapoptotic *BCL-10* gene on chromosome 1p22 to the IgH locus on 14q32, has been identified in a few cases of MALT-type lymphoma. Inactivating mutations or truncation of the *BCL-10* gene abolish the proapoptotic effect of the gene and provide a survival advantage to the lymphomatous cells. Recent studies have shown somatic mutations of the *Fas* gene in a subset of MALT-type lymphomas occurring in patients with autoimmune disorders. These discoveries may indicate that the structural aberrations involving genes in the apoptotic pathway may be important in the pathogenesis of MALT-type lymphomas. Abnormalities of chromosomes 3, 7, 12, and 18 have also been described. Although trisomy 3 was initially described in a high proportion of patients with MALT-type lymphomas, subsequent studies have failed to demonstrate that aberration as a consistent abnormality in these tumors (*see Table 34-1*).

Trisomy 3 60%

34.6.8 Nodal Marginal Zone B-Cell Lymphomas +/–
Monocytoid B-Cells (Monocytoid B-Cell Lymphoma)

Clinical Features

Most of the nodal marginal zone B-cell lymphomas are seen in patients with Sjögren's syndrome and are thought to represent nodal spread of a MALT-type lymphoma. However, there are patients in whom the disease appears to be confined to the lymph nodes. As with the extranodal marginal zone B-cell lymphoma (MALT), the nodal marginal zone lymphoma has an indolent course, but when disseminated it is usually incurable with current therapy.

Morphology

There is usually an interfollicular type of infiltrate of the monocytoid variant of centrocyticlike cells (**Image 34-13**).

Colonization of follicles by the tumor may be confused with follicular lymphoma. Such lesions also may be seen accompanying other NHLs, particularly follicular lymphomas.

Immunophenotype

Immunophenotypic studies reveal the following: CD19+, CD79a+, CD22+, CD10–, CD5–, CD23–, CD43–/+, CD11c+/–.

Molecular and Cytogenetic Features

IgH and IgL are clonally rearranged. BCL-1 and BCL-2 are in the germline configuration.

34.6.9 Splenic Marginal Zone B-Cell Lymphoma

Clinical Features

The most common presentation is that of splenomegaly and/or left upper quadrant pain. Peripheral lymphadenopathy is unusual. In contrast to other marginal zone B-cell lymphomas, the splenic type shows more widespread involvement (peripheral blood and bone marrow involvement up to 75%). The disease is usually indolent and, in the absence of massive splenomegaly, specific treatment is often not indicated.

Morphology

This entity overlaps with "splenic lymphoma with villous lymphocytes." There is increased white pulp with expansion of the marginal zones, producing a nodular pattern (**Image 34-14**). Central residual germinal centers may be seen. The characteristic pattern of white pulp involvement is a biphasic lesion, comprising a darker zone of small atypical lymphocytes surrounded by an expanded marginal zone with larger atypical lymphocytes with moderately abundant cytoplasm. Infiltration of the red pulp is common. The morphologic differential diagnosis includes follicular lymphoma.

Immunophenotype

Immunophenotypic studies reveal the following: CD19+, CD20+, CD22+, CD10–, CD23–, CD5–, CD3–, CD43–, CD25–, IgD+. As with other small B-lymphocytic neoplasms, BCL-2 protein is overexpressed in the tumor cells with immunohistochemistry.

Molecular and Cytogenetic Features

Clonal rearrangements of IgH and IgL are present. Trisomy 3 is present less frequently than in other marginal zone B-cell lymphomas.

34.6.10 Diffuse Large B-Cell Lymphoma

Clinical Features

The large B-cell lymphomas represent 30% to 40% of NHLs. They affect children and adults and may be nodal and/or extra-nodal at presentation. Primary extranodal large B-cell lymphomas account for 40% of cases, including those in skin, bone, gastrointestinal tract, genital tract, and central nervous system. The disease may be localized or disseminated. Although this tumor is aggressive, it may be curable.

Morphology

In the majority of cases, the predominant cell is either a centroblast (large noncleaved cell) or an immunoblast (**Images 34-15** and **34-16**). Frequently there is a mixture of centroblast-like and immunoblastlike cells. Also in this group are large cleaved or multilobated B-cell lymphomas and B-cell lymphomas with an anaplastic histology. The T cell–rich B-cell lymphoma (**Image 34-17**) is best classified as a DLBCL. The mediastinal (thymic) B-cell lymphoma, intravascular lymphoma, and primary effusion lymphoma have been identified as separate subtypes because of distinct clinical features. The morphologic differential diagnosis includes carcinoma, melanoma, seminoma/dysgerminoma, granulocytic sarcoma, and thymoma. Immunoperoxidase studies are very useful in the differential diagnosis of large cell tumors.

Immunophenotype

Immunophenotypic studies reveal the following: CD19+, CD20+, CD22+, CD79a+, CD45+/–, CD5–/+, CD10–/+.

Molecular and Cytogenetic Features

The IgH and IgL genes are clonally rearranged. The *bcl*-2 gene is rearranged in about 30% of patients. *BCL*-6 rearrangement may be seen in 30% of patients, and c-*myc* gene rearrangement is uncommon.

34.6.11 Primary Mediastinal (Thymic) Large B-Cell Lymphoma

Clinical Features

Primary mediastinal large B-cell lymphomas are most commonly seen in young adults with a male-female ratio of 1:2, but they also may be seen in children. As with other large cell lymphomas, the tumor is aggressive but may be curable.

Morphology

These tumors are composed of centroblasts, multilobated cells, or immunoblasts. A variable degree of compartmentalizing sclerosis is seen. Another common characteristic is the presence of abundant clear to pale cytoplasm with distinct cytoplasmic borders. The thymus is often involved. The differential diagnosis includes HL in addition to the other tumors mentioned under the large B-cell lymphoma classification. **Table 34-14** lists features useful in the differential diagnosis of mediastinal lymphomas.

Immunophenotype

Mediastinal large B-cell lymphoma characteristically shows a lack of surface immunoglobulin expression. Most cases show a CD10–, CD19+, CD20+, CD79a+, CD21–, CD22+, CD23–/+, CD45+/–, CD15–, CD30–/+ (weak) phenotype.

Molecular and Cytogenetic Features

Clonal IgH and IgL rearrangements are present. High-level amplifications of chromosome 9p involving the *REL* proto-oncogene have been demonstrated in a subset of cases.

Mal gene over expression

34.6.12 Intravascular Large B-Cell Lymphoma

Clinical Features

This is a rare lymphoma in which the tumor cells are confined to the lumen of blood vessels. The most common site is the central nervous system, but the tumor is seen in other sites as well. The symptoms and signs are often complex.

Morphology

In most cases, the tumor cells resemble centroblasts. Although the malignant cells are found in the lumen of blood vessels, they are rarely seen in peripheral blood smears.

Table 34-14 Useful Features in the Differential Diagnosis of Mediastinal Lymphomas*

Characteristic	PMLCL	LBL	HD
Histopathologic findings			
Cell morphology	Large cells	Blasts	Reed-Sternberg cells
Sclerosis	Present	Usually absent	Present
Immunophenotype			
CD20 (B cell)	Present	Usually absent	Usually absent
CD3 (T cell)	Absent	Usually present	Absent
CD15	Absent	Absent	Present
CD30	Absent	Absent	Present
TdT	Absent	Present	Absent

Abbreviations: PMLCL = primary mediastinal (thymic) large B-cell lymphoma; LBL = lymphoblastic lymphoma; HD = Hodgkin's disease; TdT = terminal deoxynucleotidyl transferase.
*From Piira T, Perkins SL, Anderson JR, et al. Primary mediastinal large cell lymphoma in children: a recent report from the Children Cancer Group. *Pediatr Pathol Lab Med.* 1995; 15:561–570.

Immunophenotype, Molecular, and Cytogenetic Features
The results are similar to those listed for large B-cell lymphomas. A few T-cell lymphomas have been identified.

34.6.13 Primary Effusion Lymphoma
Clinical Features
Most patients affected by this tumor have AIDS, and approximately 50% have had Kaposi's sarcoma. The pleural effusion generally is not associated with a tumor mass. The overall survival time is usually only a few months.

Morphology
Primary effusion lymphoma is usually composed of pleomorphic immunoblasts, sometimes with Reed-Sternberg–like features.

Immunophenotype
The malignant cells usually have a null cell immunophenotype: CD19–, CD20–, CD79a–, CD22–, CD45+, CD3–, CD5–, CD43–, CD30–. A few cases have been reported with B-cell or T-cell antigens.

Molecular and Cytogenetic Features

In most cases clonal B cell gene rearrangements can be demonstrated, and the tumor cells contain clonal EBV and human herpesvirus type 8 (HHV-8) genetic sequences.

34.6.14 Lymphomatoid Granulomatosis (LYG)

This group of tumors was previously classified within the group referred to as angiocentric lymphoma but is not currently listed among the B-cell neoplasms in the REAL or WHO classification. Although this disease may be considered within the spectrum of DLBCL, it is recommended that the term "lymphomatoid granulomatosis" be retained to reflect the unique characteristics of the disease.

Clinical Features

This is a disease of middle-aged patients and shows a predilection for extranodal sites, most frequently the lung, kidney, and central nervous system. It frequently shows bilateral nodular pulmonary involvement, and patients often present with hemoptysis, pleuritic chest pain, and fever without hilar lymphadenopathy. The natural history of LYG can vary from indolent to aggressive.

Morphology

These lesions are characterized by angioinvasion and foci of necrosis with karyorrhectic debris. The cellular infiltrate often comprises an admixture of reactive-appearing lymphocytes, plasma cells, and larger transformed neoplastic cells. Some authors have proposed that LYG may be graded (I to III) based on the proportion of large cells within the infiltrate, the extent of necrosis within the lesion, or the number of EBV-positive cells within a particular lesion.

Immunophenotype

In contrast to the nasal natural killer (NK)/T-cell "angiocentric" lymphomas, recent immunophenotypic studies have shown that the neoplastic cells in LYG are CD20+ B cells.

Molecular and Cytogenetic Features

The neoplastic B cells are consistently positive for EBV by in situ hybridization or other techniques. Thus this category of disorders is best conceptualized as an EBV-positive B-cell proliferation accompanied by an exuberant T-cell reaction. Histologic grade can be related to the relative proportions of EBV-positive large B cells within a lesion. Clonality studies have revealed clonal rearrangements of the IgH gene, while the T-cell receptor (TcR) genes yield a germline or polyclonal pattern in the majority of cases.

34.6.15 Burkitt's Lymphoma

Clinical Features

BL accounts for approximately 30% of childhood lymphomas. In adults, the tumor is often associated with immunodeficiency. In African cases, the jaw and other facial bones are commonly involved; in other cases the most common site is the abdomen, usually in the distal ileum, cecum, and/or mesentery. The tumor is highly aggressive but curable with aggressive therapy in approximately 60% of patients.

Morphology

This lymphoma is characterized by an infiltrate composed of monomorphic, medium-sized cells with round nuclei (small noncleaved cells), moderately clumped chromatin, multiple nucleoli, and moderately abundant basophilic cytoplasm. Imprints of tumor tissue are helpful in demonstrating nuclear and cytoplasmic lipid vacuoles (**Image 34-18**). A high mitotic index is seen, and a starry sky pattern is usually present.

The WHO classification recognizes endemic, sporadic, atypical (pleomorphic), and AIDS-associated variants of BL. The atypical variant includes some tumors that would be classified as "Burkitt's-like" lymphoma in the REAL classification. These atypical BLs show greater cellular pleomorphism and heterogeneity than classic BLs. Nevertheless, essentially 100% of the cells remain in cycle as determined by Ki-67 or MIB-1 reactivity. The WHO classification has included the Burkitt's-like lymphomas of the REAL classification within its DLBCL category because of the difficulty in reproducibly distinguishing this subgroup from some DLBCL and BL.

Immunophenotype

Immunophenotypic studies reveal CD19+, CD20+, CD79a+, CD22+, CD10+, CD5–, and CD23–. Bcl-6 +

Molecular and Cytogenetic Features

There are clonal rearrangements of the IgH and/or IgL chain genes. In most cases, there is translocation of c-*myc* from chromosome 8 to the IgH region on chromosome 14; t(8;14), and sometimes to IgL loci on chromosome 2 (Igκ); t(2;8) or 22 (Igλ), t(8;22). EBV genomes are detectable in the majority of endemic cases.

34.7 T-Cell and Putative Natural Killer–Cell Neoplasms

34.7.1 Precursor T-Cell Neoplasm: T-Precursor Lymphoblastic Lymphoma/Leukemia

Clinical Features

This tumor is most commonly seen in adolescent and young adult men; it constitutes 40% of childhood lymphomas and 15% of ALLs, when leukemia is defined as greater than 25% bone marrow lymphoblasts. The most common presentation is that of a mediastinal mass. If left untreated, the tumor terminates in acute leukemia, and central nervous system involvement is common. Although this tumor is highly aggressive, it is curable with intensive chemotherapy in approximately 60% of patients.

Morphology

The morphologic features of this tumor are very similar to those previously described for B-LBL (ALL). The infiltrating lymphoblasts have convoluted or round nuclei, a delicate chromatin pattern, indistinct nucleoli, and scant cytoplasm. Frequent mitotic figures are seen (**Image 34-19**). In the differential diagnosis, BL, granulocytic sarcoma, and lymphoblastoid variant of MCL should be considered.

Immunophenotype

Immunophenotypic studies generally reveal CD3+, CD7+, and variable expression of other T cell–associated antigens (T-cell antigen dropout). Many tumors show the presence of both CD4 and CD8 antigens. B cell–associated antigens CD19 and CD20 are negative. TdT is typically positive. A few tumors express the NK cell–associated antigens CD16 and CD57.

Molecular and Cytogenetic Features

Clonal rearrangements of TcR may be seen. A variable number of cytogenetic abnormalities have been reported.

34.7.2 Peripheral T-Cell Neoplasms

T-cell lymphomas account for less than 20% of lymphomas in the United States and Europe but are considerably more common in Asia. The peripheral T-cell neoplasms may be divided into peripheral T-cell lymphomas and peripheral T-cell leukemias. The peripheral (mature) T-cell leukemias refer to malignancies arising from clonal proliferation of mature (TDT–, CD1a–) T cells and typically present as a leukemia. The entities recognized in this category are T-cell prolymphocytic leukemia (T-PLL) and T-cell large granular lymphocyte leukemia (T-LGL).

34.7.3 T-Cell Prolymphocytic Leukemia

Clinical Features

As with B-PLL, patients have a high WBC count but also have cutaneous or mucosal involvement. This is usually an aggressive disease and incurable with current chemotherapy.

Morphology

In the majority of cases, the morphologic features of prolymphocytic leukemia are characterized by cells with prominent nucleoli, abundant cytoplasm, and nuclear irregularities. Histologically, there is diffuse infiltration of the splenic red pulp and/or white pulp. Lymph node involvement is characterized by a predominantly paracortical infiltrate of large cells with round to irregular nuclear contours and prominent central nucleoli. Skin involvement is often seen as nodular and perivascular/periadnexal infiltration by the neoplastic prolymphocytes.

Immunophenotype

Immunophenotypic studies reveal CD2+, CD3+, CD5+, CD7+, CD25–. TcR α/β is expressed in 80% of tumors, and CD4 is seen in approximately 60%. TdT is negative.

Molecular and Cytogenetic Features

The TcR genes are clonally rearranged. Cytogenetic studies show 75% of patients with inv 14 (q11;q32).

34.7.4 T-Cell Large Granular Lymphocytic Leukemia

Clinical Features

Patients with this disease usually have mild to moderate

lymphocytosis, often associated with neutropenia, rheumatoid arthritis or autoantibodies, and mild anemia.

Morphology

In the majority of patients, the clinical course is indolent. The morphologic features in the peripheral blood are lymphocytosis, the predominating cell having round nuclei with moderately condensed chromatin and abundant blue cytoplasm with azurophilic granules. Bone marrow infiltration is usually mild. Focal lymphoid aggregates are often present.

Immunophenotype

Immunophenotypic studies reveal CD2+, CD3+, CD5–, CD7–, CD4–, CD5+, CD8+, CD16+/–, CD56–/+, CD57+/–, CD25–.

Molecular and Cytogenetic Features

T-cell large granular lymphocytic leukemias have rearrangements of the TcRγ, TcRα, and TcRβ chain genes. The TcRδ genes are usually deleted.

34.7.5 Natural Killer Cell Large Granular Lymphocytic Leukemia (NK-LGL)

Clinical Features

This disease is more prevalent in younger Asian adults, and patients present with fever, hepatosplenomegaly, and/or lymphadenopathy. In most patients, the clinical course is highly aggressive, although rare indolent tumors have been reported.

Morphology

Peripheral blood smears reveal circulating abnormally large lymphocytes with prominent azurophilic granules.

Immunophenotype

Immunophenotypic studies reveal that the proliferating NK cells are typically CD2+, surface CD3–, CD4–, CD8+/–, CD16+, CD56+. There is also positive reactivity for cytotoxic proteins (eg, TIA-1).

Molecular and Cytogenetic Features

The TcR and IgH genes are in the germline configuration, and the EBV gene is frequently present in aggressive cases.

34.7.6 Mycosis Fungoides
Clinical Features

Mycosis fungoides (MF) is the most common of the cutaneous T-cell lymphomas. It presents as a scaly eczematous rash that progresses from a plaque stage to eventually form tumors in the skin. It is often misdiagnosed as psoriasis for months or years.

Morphology

Skin biopsies show an infiltrate composed of small and large cells with cerebriform nuclei in the upper dermis, frequently with infiltrates in the epidermis (epidermotropism or Pautrier's abscesses) (**Image 34-20**). Involvement of the peripheral blood and paracortex of the lymph nodes also may be seen.

Immunophenotype

Immunophenotypic studies reveal CD2+, CD3+, CD4+, CD5+, CD8–.

Molecular and Cytogenetic Features

The TcR genes are clonally rearranged.

34.7.7 Sézary Syndrome
Clinical Features

Most patients are adult men, although rare cases have been described in children. Sézary syndrome (SS) is characterized by exfoliative erythroderma, generalized lymphadenopathy, and malignant (Sézary cells) in the peripheral blood (*see Image 34-20*). Curiously, affected patients have a relatively high incidence of monoclonal gammopathy and secondary neoplasms (eg, carcinoma, NHL). There is also a reported association between MF/SS, HL, and lymphomatoid papulosis.

Morphology

The circulating atypical lymphocytes (Sézary cells) are intermediate to large in size with cerebriform nuclei, moderately condensed chromatin, and inconspicuous nucleoli. The cytoplasm is basophilic and agranular, with or without vacuolation. The predominance of larger Sézary cell forms is associated with progressive disease.

Immunophenotype

Sézary cells display a CD7–/+, CD2+, CD3+, CD4+, and

CD8– phenotype identical to that seen with MF. CD30 reactivity has been associated with transformation to a large cell lymphoma with anaplastic histology and may be a terminal event.

Molecular and Cytogenetic Features
The TcR genes are clonally rearranged.

34.7.8 Peripheral T-Cell Lymphomas (Unspecified)

Clinical Features
The majority of patients are adults with stage III or IV disease. The skin and lungs are frequently involved. The clinical course is usually more aggressive than that of B-cell lymphomas.

Morphology
Peripheral T-cell lymphomas are often composed of atypical small to medium-sized or large cells. Occasional Reed-Sternberg–like cells may be present. A variable number of eosinophils and/or epithelioid histiocytes are evident. Lymphoepithelioid lymphoma (Lennert's lymphoma) and T-zone lymphoma are classified as variants of this category.

Immunophenotype
Immunophenotypic studies reveal that the T cell–associated antigens are variably expressed: CD2+, CD3+, CD5+/–, CD7–/+; CD4 is seen more frequently than CD8. Aberrant loss of T cell–associated antigens is a characteristic feature.

Molecular and Cytogenetic Features
Clonal T cell gene rearrangements are common.

34.7.9 Angioimmunoblastic T-Cell Lymphoma

Clinical Features
Angioimmunoblastic lymphadenopathy with dysproteinemia (AILD) and angioimmunoblastic T-cell lymphoma represent a spectrum of malignant T-cell lymphomas. This disorder is characterized by generalized lymphadenopathy, fever, weight loss, skin rash, and polyclonal hypergammaglobulinemia. The disease process is moderately aggressive, but occasional responses to steroids may be obtained. In some patients, progression to large T-cell or (rarely) B-cell type lymphomas is seen.

Morphology

The lymph node architecture is effaced with patent subcapsular and trabecular sinuses. There is a characteristic proliferation of arborizing endothelial venules that are surrounded by proliferating follicular dendritic cells and irregular collections of homogeneous eosinophilic material. The germinal centers are often regressed or "burnt out." There are often aggregates of larger cells with abundant clear or pale cytoplasm (**Image 34-21**). Variable numbers of eosinophils, plasma cells, and epithelioid histiocytes also may be present.

Immunophenotype

The tumor cells are typically CD3+, CD4+ T cells.

Molecular and Cytogenetic Features

The TcR genes are clonally rearranged in the majority of patients. The IgH chain genes may be clonally rearranged in up to 10%. EBV also is detectable in some cases.

34.7.10 Extranodal NK/T-Cell Lymphoma, Nasal Type
Clinical Features

This group of tumors corresponds to lesions previously referred to as "polymorphic reticulosis", "lethal midline granuloma", or "angiocentric lymphoma". The most common clinical presentation is one of a destructive nasal or midline facial tumor. Recent studies have described nonnasal lymphomas exhibiting identical morphologic, phenotypic, and molecular features to the nasal lesions. It has been proposed that such lesions be designated "nasal-type" NK/T-cell lymphomas. Most studies indicate a poor prognosis.

Morphology

These lesions are characterized by angiocentric and angioinvasive infiltrates composed of atypical lymphoid cells with irregular nuclear contours and immunoblasts, together with a variable number of plasma cells and (less frequently) eosinophils and histiocytes. These neoplasms are also characterized by extensive necrosis that, in the past, was attributed to the high tumor propensity for angioinvasion. More recent studies, however, have shown that this necrosis may be mediated by chemokines such as Mig, IP-10, and TNF-α.

Immunophenotype

Immunophenotypic studies reveal CD2+, CD5+, CD7+. The

atypical cells may be CD4+ or CD8+ and frequently express CD56. These neoplasms commonly express cytotoxic granular proteins (TIA+, perforin+, granzyme B+). The tumor cells are typically CD4+ T cells.

Molecular and Cytogenetic Features

Results of studies for T-cell and B-cell rearrangement are usually negative. However, rare cases may show clonal TcR rearrangement. EBV has been consistently demonstrated in virtually all nasal NK/T-cell lymphomas by a variety of methods.

34.7.11 Enteropathy-Type T-Cell Lymphoma

Clinical Features

This disease is often associated with a history of gluten-sensitive enteropathy. The jejunum is involved most frequently, but the stomach and colon also may be affected. The disease is aggressive and characterized by multiple jejunal ulcers often associated with perforation.

Morphology

A variable mixture of small, medium, and large cells is seen. There are abundant intraepithelial T cells in adjacent mucosa (**Image 34-22**). The adjacent small bowel often shows villous atrophy associated with celiac disease. However, sporadic cases without clinical or histologic evidence of celiac disease have been described.

Immunophenotype

Immunophenotypic studies reveal CD3+, CD7+, CD8+/–, CD4–, CD103+. The tumor cells also express the cytotoxic associated proteins granzyme B, TIA-1, and perforin.

Molecular and Cytogenetic Features

TcR genes are clonally rearranged.

34.7.12 Adult T-Cell Lymphoma/Leukemia (ATL/L)

Clinical Features

This disease is most commonly seen in Japan but has also been described in the Caribbean, with smaller clusters of occasional cases seen in the southeastern United States. Several variants—acute, lymphomatous, chronic, smoldering, and Hodgkin's-like—have been described. The acute form appears to be most common, characterized by high WBC count, hepatosplenomegaly, hypercalcemia, and a median survival of less than 1 year. Other cases appear to be more chronic or smoldering in nature.

Morphology

A diffuse infiltrate, consisting of a mixture of small and large atypical cells with prominent nuclear pleomorphism, is seen in lymph nodes. Reed-Sternberg–like cells are present. In the peripheral blood, cells with hyperlobated nuclei (cloverleaf or flower cells) are characteristic. Bone marrow infiltration may be focal or diffuse.

Immunophenotype

Immunophenotypic studies reveal CD2+, CD3+, CD4+, CD5+, CD7–, CD25+.

Molecular and Cytogenetic Features

TcR genes are clonally rearranged. Human T-cell leukemia virus type I (HTLV-I) genomes are found in most cases.

34.7.13 Anaplastic Large Cell Lymphoma (T- and Null-Cell Types)

Clinical Features

This lymphoma has been reported in all age groups. There are two distinct forms of primary anaplastic large cell lymphoma (ALCL): a systemic form, which involves lymph nodes and extranodal sites, including skin, and a primary cutaneous form, without extracutaneous spread at the time of diagnosis. The primary cutaneous lymphomas occur predominantly in adults and may regress spontaneously.

Morphology

Morphologically, this lymphoma is characterized by an infiltrate of large pleomorphic cells, frequently with horseshoe-shaped (wreathlike) nuclei and prominent nucleoli (**Images 34-23** and **34-24**). Reed-Sternberg–like cells are often seen. The tumor cells frequently have a cohesive pattern and involve the lymph node sinuses similar to the involvement seen in metastatic carcinoma. In a small number of patients, the tumor cells are much smaller than typical ALCL cells; this has been referred to as a "small cell variant". Other variants, such as monomorphic, lymphohistiocytic, and Hodgkin's-related, also have been recognized.

Immunophenotype

Immunophenotypic studies usually reveal CD3+/–, CD15–, CD30+, CD43+/–, CD45+/–, EMA+/–, BNH9+, p80/ALK+.

Molecular and Cytogenetic Features

Classic ALCL is associated with a characteristic chromosomal translocation t(2;5)(p23;q35), which is seen in approximately 40% of patients. This translocation juxtaposes the anaplastic lymphoma kinase (ALK) gene at 2p23 to the nucleophosmin (NPM) gene at 5q35, resulting in a chimeric transcript, which plays a key role in ALCL pathogenesis. Overexpression of the ALK protein can be detected by immunohistochemistry and is one of the cardinal diagnostic features of ALCL. Sixty percent of patients have TcR rearrangement and 40% have no rearrangement of TcR or Ig genes. The nodal architecture, cellular morphology, and immunostaining (CD45– and CD45+) can make this entity difficult to distinguish from metastatic carcinoma.

34.7.14 Primary Cutaneous Anaplastic Large Cell Lymphoma

Clinical Features

This group includes lesions previously described as "primary cutaneous ALCL" and "lymphomatoid papulosis". Both entities are thought to represent a continuous clinical and histopathologic spectrum of related diseases. Lymphomatoid papulosis manifests as multiple papular lesions, usually less than 1 cm, distributed randomly on the extremities, trunk, and occasionally on the face or genitals. These lesions typically undergo spontaneous regression, leaving residual small scars over a period of a few weeks.

Morphology

The lesions are histologically composed of variable numbers of pleomorphic large lymphocytes (sometimes resembling Reed-Sternberg cells) admixed with smaller lymphocytes. Other inflammatory cells, including plasma cells and eosinophils, may be present. In cases with extensive alteration, there may be a marked neutrophilic infiltrate.

Immunophenotype

The atypical cells are CD3+/–, strongly 30+ (membrane and Golgi reactivity), CD15–, EMA–, and ALK–.

Molecular and Cytogenetic Features

Clonal rearrangements of the TcR genes are detected in about 60% of patients. The primary cutaneous lesions (ALCL and lymphomatoid papulosis) generally lack the t(2;5), in contrast to the classic nodal ALCL.

34.7.15 Subcutaneous Panniculitis-like T-Cell Lymphoma

The WHO proposal recognizes subcutaneous panniculitis-like T-cell lymphoma as a separate entity from other forms of panniculitis-like T-cell lymphomas.

Clinical Features

This disease typically presents as subcutaneous nodules affecting the extremities. A hemophagocytic syndrome is associated with most cases.

Morphology

Histologically, the lesions are largely confined to the subcutis and are composed of a monotonous infiltrate of atypical lymphocytes encircling fat lobules in a lacelike distribution. The tumor cells may appear deceptively benign or exhibit hyperchromatic or pleomorphic nuclei. Vacuolated macrophages containing ingested lipid and karyorrhectic nuclear material are often interspersed.

Immunophenotype

Immunophenotypic studies usually reveal a βF-1+, CD8+, T-cell phenotype. The neoplastic cells express the cytotoxic associated proteins perforin and TIA-1. It is believed that cases previously categorized as histiocytic cytophagic panniculitis represent subcutaneous panniculitis-like T-cell lymphoma.

Molecular and Cytogenetic Features

The TcR genes are clonally rearranged. Evidence of EBV has been consistently absent in subcutaneous panniculitis-like T-cell lymphoma.

34.7.16 Hepatosplenic γ/δ T-Cell Lymphoma

This is a very rare peripheral T-cell neoplasm. It is characterized by involvement of the sinusoidal areas of the liver, spleen, and (less frequently) bone marrow.

Clinical Features

This is a disease of young adults with a distinct male predominance. Patients present with marked hepatosplenomegaly without lymphadenopathy. The clinical course is often aggressive, with a median survival of about 3 years.

Morphology

Histologically, the neoplastic cells are of moderate size with slightly condensed nuclei, small nucleoli, and a pale cytoplasmic rim. There is a marked predilection for the sinusoids of the liver and spleen, with relative sparing of the portal triads and splenic white pulp.

Immunophenotype

Immunophenotypically, the neoplastic cells have a phenotype that resembles the normal γ/δ T cells: CD3+, CD4–, CD8–/+, βF1–, and γ/δ+. The neoplastic cells are also frequently TIA+ but perforin negative.

Molecular and Cytogenetic Features

Molecular studies have shown isochromosome 7q as a consistent abnormality.

34.8 Non-Hodgkin's Lymphoma in Children

Lymph node enlargement is a frequent finding in children, usually representing a transient response to localized infection. No single clinical feature allows a prediction of either benign or malignant lymphadenopathy. When supraclavicular or generalized lymphadenopathy with systemic symptoms is present, however, a lymph node biopsy is strongly recommended.

Children respond to antigenic stimuli with more pronounced lymph node hyperplasia than adults. Pathologists with little experience in evaluating lymph node biopsy specimens from children may mistake florid immunoblastic proliferations, often seen in

Figure 34-1 Frequency of non-Hodgkin's lymphoma in adults and children.

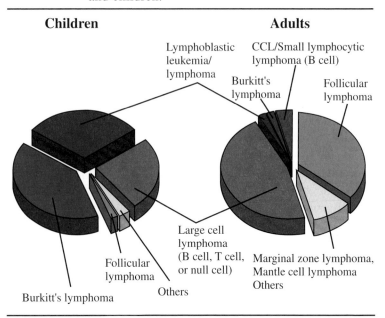

viral infections (such as infectious mononucleosis), for large cell lymphoma (see Chapter 25). A diagnosis of large cell immunoblastic lymphoma in a child or young adult should not be made without first considering the possibility of a viral infection.

Malignant lymphoma in children differs in many ways from that in adults and deserves separate attention (**Figure 34-1**). **Table 34-15** outlines the major differences between NHL in children and adults. Lymphomas with a follicular pattern, which in adults account for about 40% of all NHLs, are unusual in children. Small B-cell lymphomas such as B-CLL/SLL, MCL, follicular lymphoma, and marginal zone B-cell lymphoma are rare in children (*see Figure 34-1*). The majority of children have aggressive, disseminated disease at the time of diagnosis.

As seen in **Table 34-16**, the classification of NHL in children is mainly confined to lymphoblastic lymphoma (30%-40%), Burkitt's and atypical Burkitt's lymphomas (35%-50%), and large cell lymphoma (15%-25%). ALCL appears to represent a distinct entity, as it does in adults. The majority of ALCL cases are T-cell or null-cell lineage and ALK positive. **Table 34-17** presents a comparison of the major morphologic, cytochemical, and immunophenotypic features of childhood NHLs.

Table 34-15   Comparison of Non-Hodgkin's Lymphoma Features in Children and Adults

Children	Adults
Predominantly extranodal	Predominantly nodal
Rapidly proliferative (aggressive, high grade)	Often slowly proliferative (indolent, low grade)
Rarely follicular	Often follicular
Often leukemic	Rarely leukemic

Table 34-16   Classification of Non-Hodgkin's Lymphoma in Children

Lymphoblastic lymphoma (precursor T and B cell)
Burkitt's lymphoma
Atypical variant of Burkitt's lymphoma
Large-cell lymphoma (B and T cell, anaplastic large-cell lymphoma)
Others

There is a strong propensity for extranodal involvement in children, and a close relationship exists between the histologic types and the anatomic site of involvement. Thus, the lymphoblastic lymphomas are predominantly supradiaphragmatic, presenting with a mediastinal mass. Burkitt's lymphomas usually occur in the abdomen, particularly in the ileocecal region. Extranodal sites, such as soft tissues, bone, and skin, are more frequently involved in ALCL than in other histologic subsets.

Overall, the survival in NHL is considerably better in children than in adults. A survival rate of 60% to 85% is usually seen.

34.9 Diseases Simulating Malignant Lymphoma

A variety of disorders other than NHLs may not only cause enlargement of lymph nodes but may be mistaken on histologic examination for lymphoma (**Table 34-18**). These disorders are described in Chapter 25. It is important that the pathologist have an accurate clinical history and strong familiarity with the lymph node

Table 34-17   Comparison of Morphologic and Immunophenotypic Features in Childhood Non-Hodgkin's Lymphomas

Feature	Lymphoblastic	Burkitt's
Imprint cytology, Wright's stain	FAB L1 or FAB L2 blasts	FAB L3 blasts
Nuclear size	Smaller than macrophage nucleus	Approximates macrophage nucleus; nuclear monotony
Nuclear chromatin	Delicate	Coarsely reticulated
Nucleoli	Small, inconspicuous	Prominent
Mitotic index	High	High
Cytoplasm	Scant	Moderate
Cytoplasmic vacuoles	Inconspicuous	Prominent
TdT	Positive	Negative
Immunologic markers	Precursor T or B cell	B cell
Oncogene	NA	c-*myc*

Abbreviations: FAB = French-American-British acute leukemia classification; TdT = terminal deoxynucleotidyl transferase; NA = not applicable.

changes that may occur in a variety of benign reactive lymphadenopathies.

34.10 Diagnostic Approach

Management of a patient with NHL requires a team approach involving the primary care physician, the oncologist, the radiotherapist, the surgeon, the radiologist, and the pathologist. Good communication should be established among these participants in planning the evaluation and therapy of the patient.

Following a clinical history and physical examination, the workup of a patient with possible malignant lymphoma should proceed in the following fashion:

1. Tissue biopsy (required to diagnose malignant lymphoma).
2. Complete blood cell count, including evaluation of peripheral blood smear for circulating lymphoma cells.

Burkitt's-like	Large Cell
FAB L3 blasts	Variable, large transformed lymphocytes
Sometimes larger than macrophage nucleus; nuclear variability	Larger than macrophage nucleus
Coarsely reticulated	Clumped, vesicular
Prominent	Variable, often prominent
High	Variable
Moderate	Moderate to abundant
Variable	Inconspicuous
Negative	Negative
Usually B cell	Usually B cell; 20% T cell
c-*myc* occasionally present	p80, ALK-1 in ALCL

3. Bone marrow aspirate and biopsy examination.
4. Radiologic studies.
5. Liver and renal function assessment.
6. Cytologic examination of effusions, if present.

34.11 Tissue Biopsy

Because a tissue biopsy is required for the diagnosis of NHL and is the most important part of the diagnostic evaluation, it is discussed in a separate section. Histopathologic evaluation of a lymph node biopsy specimen is one of the most difficult problems in surgical pathology, and consultation from a hematopathologist is often desirable. The major reason for difficulty in interpretation is technical in nature and results from improper handling of the biopsy specimen.

An adequate specimen must be delivered to the pathologist intact immediately following removal. Before fixation, the tissue

Table 34-18   Causes of Lymph Node Enlargement Simulating
                 Malignant Lymphoma

Nonspecific reactive follicular hyperplasia
Infectious mononucleosis
Toxoplasmosis
Viral lymphadenitis (herpes, cytomegalovirus)
AIDS
Cat-scratch disease
Syphilis
Phenytoin lymph node hyperplasia
Rheumatoid arthritis
Dermatopathic lymphadenopathy
Giant lymph node hyperplasia (Castleman's disease)
Sinus histiocytosis with massive lymphadenopathy
Leukemia
Metastatic carcinoma
Metastatic melanoma

should be divided into multiple sections, as outlined in **Figure 34-2**, allowing a variety of studies to be performed. Not all of the procedures indicated in **Figure 34-2** may be necessary to make a correct diagnosis; however, samples for immunologic and possibly genotypic studies should be obtained routinely. A section of the tissue should regularly be snap-frozen for immunophenotypic and genotypic studies if histopathologic evaluation or immunophenotypic studies of paraffin sections are inconclusive.

When immunologic procedures cannot be performed in the hospital where the biopsy is performed, the specimen can be sent to a reference laboratory without compromising the immunologic and cytochemical investigations. Frozen tissue must be sent in dry ice, or sections of frozen tissue may be sent. Another method, which is simpler but may not work for all tumors, is to place intact tissue in refrigerated saline solution in a Styrofoam container with cold packs and immediately send it to the reference laboratory.

A diagnosis should never be made on the basis of immunologic or cytochemical studies alone; these results should always be correlated with the clinical and histopathologic features of the biopsy specimen. To provide the best morphologic features, the specimen to be used for histopathologic studies should be fixed in

Figure 34-2 Scheme for processing lymph node biopsy specimens.

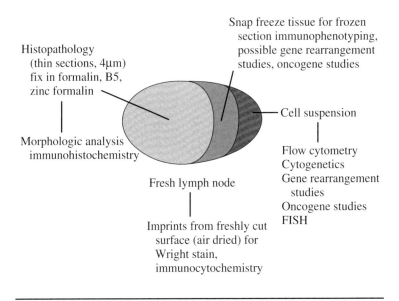

Snap freeze tissue for frozen section immunophenotyping, possible gene rearrangement studies, oncogene studies

Histopathology (thin sections, 4μm) fix in formalin, B5, zinc formalin

Cell suspension

Morphologic analysis immunohistochemistry

Flow cytometry
Cytogenetics
Gene rearrangement studies
Oncogene studies
FISH

Fresh lymph node

Imprints from freshly cut surface (air dried) for Wright stain, immunocytochemistry

a mercury-containing fixative such as B5, as well as in buffered formalin fixative. For adequate fixation in buffered formalin, the tissue should be fixed for at least 12 hours but not more than 24 hours. Postfixation in B5 after the tissue has been fixed in formalin often provides better morphologic results than formalin alone. The sections of the biopsy specimen must be thin (one cell thickness) and well stained.

The diagnosis and subclassification of malignant lymphoma should be made on the basis of the histopathologic features in the lymph node biopsy specimen before any treatment is initiated. The initial diagnosis should not be made on the basis of results of a bone marrow or liver biopsy alone, unless this is the only tissue involved. In true extranodal lymphomas, the diagnosis must be made from a biopsy specimen from the organ involved; however, every attempt should be made to find a suitable lymph node for biopsy.

Fine-needle aspiration (FNA), Tru-cut® needle (Travenol, Deerfield, Illinois) biopsy, or both are proven methods for obtaining samples of possible malignant tissue in the appropriate clinical setting. These techniques probably should not be used alone for the initial diagnosis unless it is impossible to obtain a lymph node biopsy specimen or appropriate extranodal biopsy specimen. Fine-needle aspiration may be very helpful in follow-up diagnosis. A liver biopsy specimen may be used to document the relatively common liver involvement of NHLs.

34.12 Hematologic Findings

The hematologic findings in NHLs are variable and depend on the type of lymphoma present. In some lymphomas, such as B-CLL/SLL, follicular lymphoma, MCL, and splenic marginal zone B-cell lymphoma, blood and bone marrow involvement are frequently present. On the other hand, in large cell lymphomas, the peripheral blood and bone marrow are usually not involved.

34.12.1 Blood Cell Measurements
The majority of patients who present with NHLs have normal blood counts. Anemia develops during the course of the disease in about 50% of patients. One or several of the following may be the cause of anemia: bone marrow insufficiency caused by bone marrow replacement by lymphoma or therapy-induced bone marrow hypoplasia, hypersplenism, autoimmune hemolytic anemia, and bleeding from lymphoma in the gastrointestinal tract or from a low platelet count.

34.12.2 Peripheral Blood Smear Morphology
Circulating lymphoma cells have been referred to as lymphosarcoma cell leukemia (see Chapter 33). This is not a specific clinical pathologic entity and may be found in many subtypes of NHL. The overall incidence is 10% to 25%. On rare occasions, the presenting feature of the lymphoma may be peripheral blood involvement. In follicular lymphoma, especially grade 1, the circulating lymphoma cells have scant cytoplasm with a characteristic notched or cleaved nucleus (**Image 34-25**). Similar features may be seen in MCL and splenic marginal zone B-cell lymphoma.

Confirmation that the circulating cells are malignant can usually be made using flow cytometry. The presence of circulating lymphoma cells in indolent NHL usually does not significantly affect the prognosis. In aggressive NHL, circulating lymphoma cells may be associated with a poor prognosis.

34.12.3 Bone Marrow Examination

Bone marrow aspiration and bone marrow biopsy should be done routinely in the staging of malignant lymphoma. A biopsy is usually more useful than an aspirate. Bilateral, posterior iliac crest biopsies increase the chance of detecting lymphoma. The overall incidence of bone marrow involvement in NHL is 30% to 50% but varies with different subtypes.

Bone marrow involvement at the time of diagnosis is seen in 60% of patients with follicular lymphoma and in fewer than 25% of patients with diffuse large cell lymphomas. It is associated with spread to the central nervous system in up to 35% of patients. "Bone marrow discordance" is frequently seen in patients with diffuse large cell lymphomas, where the bone marrow is infiltrated by a more indolent lesion, especially grade 1 follicular lymphoma. Survival rates in these patients are similar to those in patients with no bone marrow involvement and are better than those in patients with concordant bone marrow involvement (lymphoma in lymph node and bone marrow have the same histologic features).

The pattern of bone marrow involvement in NHL is usually focal (nodular) rather than diffuse. In B-CLL/SLL, the incidence of involvement is 80% to 90%, and the pattern may be focal, interstitial, or diffuse. In follicular lymphoma, the pattern is characteristically focal and paratrabecular (**Image 34-25**). In lymphoblastic and Burkitt's lymphomas, the pattern is often interstitial or diffuse. It is important that nodules of lymphoma in the bone marrow be differentiated from benign lymphoid nodules, which are commonly seen in older patients. Nodules of malignant lymphoma are usually not as well delineated as benign lymphoid nodules; in lymphoma, the infiltrate is frequently located adjacent to bone trabeculae (paratrabecular position). Sometimes, however, it is extremely difficult to differentiate a benign lymphoid nodule from a small B-cell lymphoma. In such instances, the term "atypical lymphoid aggregate" is often used to indicate uncertainty in the diagnosis.

Other Laboratory Tests

Test 34.1 Radiologic Studies

Various radiologic techniques are used to demonstrate NHL in the mediastinum, peritoneum, and bones. Mediastinal and hilar lymph nodes are demonstrated primarily with standard posterior-anterior and lateral chest radiographs. Computed tomography (CT) scans of the thorax may be helpful if abnormalities are found on the routine chest radiograph. Bipedal lymphangiography is the standard procedure for assessment of periaortic and pelvic lymph nodes, with an overall accuracy of 90%. Computed tomography is the technique of choice in the diagnosis of mesenteric, portahepatic, and splenic hilar nodal involvement; CT-guided biopsy may be useful in intra-abdominal masses. Magnetic resonance imaging (MRI) is used for defining lesions in the brain, spinal cord, and bone marrow.

Test 34.2 Renal and Liver Function Tests

The evaluation of renal and liver function with routine serum chemistries and urine analysis should be performed for every patient. The results may help detect disease in those organs and must be done as part of the workup before giving the patient chemotherapy, radiation therapy, or both. An elevated serum creatinine level indicates renal insufficiency, suggesting obstruction from a retroperitoneal NHL. Abnormal liver enzymes, bilirubin, and alkaline phosphatase may be an indication of liver or bone involvement.

Test 34.3 Laparotomy

Exploratory laparotomy and splenectomy are rarely performed and should be done only if the treatment decision depends on the identification of abdominal involvement. If a laparotomy is performed, a preoperative lymphangiogram should be done as a guide to direct surgical sampling of the lymph nodes.

Test 34.4 Cytology of Cerebrospinal Fluid and Serous Effusions

Of the NHLs, the most common types involving the central nervous system are lymphoblastic lymphoma, Burkitt's lymphoma, and large cell lymphoma. Indolent lymphomas such as follicular lymphoma, B-CLL/SLL, and marginal zone B-cell lymphoma rarely involve the central nervous system. Morphologically, lymphoblastic lymphomas affecting cerebrospinal fluid are similar in appearance to ALL. There is an increase in primary central nervous system lymphomas, which are particularly common in patients with cellular immune dysfunction, as seen in transplant patients and patients with AIDS. Large B-cell lymphoma and Burkitt's lymphoma are the most common types of lymphomas in these patients.

Pleural and peritoneal effusions are common in NHLs (especially in children), and cytologic examination of fluid specimens is an essential part of the clinical evaluation in such situations. The primary diagnosis may be made on such specimens. Effusion fluids are ideally suited for immunophenotypic analysis using flow cytometry to differentiate reactive from malignant effusions and to make the diagnosis. These studies are especially helpful in peritoneal effusions in patients who may have Burkitt's lymphoma or in a pleural effusion in a patient with lymphoblastic lymphoma involving the mediastinum.

Test 34.5 Fine-Needle Aspiration

In NHL, FNA of lymph nodes is best used to document recurrent disease, to demonstrate transformation to another type of lymphoma, or to obtain cells for immunophenotypic analysis in patients referred for treatment of NHL who were previously diagnosed with a tissue biopsy specimen. Most pathologists in the United States are reluctant to use FNA as the primary evaluation of NHL, partly because of problems with sampling errors if the lymph node is only partially involved with NHL or if there are few malignant lymphoid cells. This is especially problematic in ALCL, posttransplantation lymphoproliferative disorders, and T cell–rich B-cell lymphoma. The addition of immunophenotypic analysis with immunoperoxidase studies and/or flow cytometry increases the percentage of correct diagnoses (**Image 34-26**).

Chapter 25 provides more information regarding the FNA procedure.

34.13 Ancillary Tests

34.13.1 Cytochemistry

Cytochemical studies, such as the specific esterase stain (chloroacetate esterase), may be helpful in identifying immature granulocytic cells in granulocytic sarcomas and in differentiating such tumors from malignant lymphoma or undifferentiated carcinoma. Immunoperoxidase studies using an antibody to myeloperoxidase, however, are a more sensitive and reliable method for identifying granulocytic sarcomas.

The identification of TdT is very helpful in the diagnosis of lymphoblastic lymphoma (*see Image 34-19*) because this enzyme is not present in other malignant lymphomas. Identification of TdT can be done on imprints of tissue biopsy specimens, on cytocentrifuge preparations made from cell suspension of the biopsy specimen, on frozen sections, and on paraffin sections using an immunoperoxidase procedure.

34.13.2 Immunophenotypic Analysis

Immunohistochemistry has become available in most major pathology laboratories. A wide spectrum of immunologic markers is used in surgical pathology to aid the pathologist in the diagnosis of difficult cases. With the classification system used in this chapter, the diagnosis is made on the basis of histopathology and immunophenotypic analysis. Immunophenotypic studies may be used to rule out nonhematopoietic tumors (**Images 34-27** and **34-28**), to determine whether the lymphoid lesion is benign or malignant, to determine cell lineage, to indicate stage of differentiation of the tumor, to subclassify lymphoma, and sometimes to detect minimal residual disease.

Several approaches may be used for the immunophenotypic analysis of lymphoproliferative disorders. These approaches include flow cytometric analysis of cell suspensions from the tissue biopsy specimen, immunohistochemical studies of frozen tissue sections, immunohistochemical studies of paraffin-embedded tissue sections, and immunohistochemical analysis of cytocentrifuge smears prepared from cell suspensions of the biopsy specimen. Each of these procedures has advantages and disadvantages. The flow cytometric analysis gives the most information because the number of antibodies available for such procedures is considerably greater than those available for paraffin sections. Immunohistochemical analysis on paraffin-embedded tissue has several advantages because of superior morphologic characteristics, allowing better analysis of immunoreactivity in both malignant and reactive cell populations, and paraffin sections are much more readily available. When good techniques are applied in appropriately fixed tissue, reliable immunophenotypic analysis can be performed in more than 80% of cases using paraffin-embedded tissue sections. Unsuitable fixation of tissue is probably the most common cause of unsatisfactory results.

B5 is the fixative of choice for most hematopoietic antigens, but properly fixed buffered formalin tissue can also give satisfactory results. The immunoreactivity may sometimes be improved by protease digestion with pepsin, pronase, or trypsin. Antigen retrieval from formalin-fixed, paraffin-embedded tissues with microwave irradiation is frequently helpful and decreases the dependence of staining quality on the fixative used. This may be very helpful in consultation cases where the type of fixative used is unknown.

When using paraffin-embedded tissue sections for immunophenotypic analysis of lymphoproliferative disorders, many of the antibodies lack specificity, and knowledge of the immunoreactivity profile of each antibody is essential to making a correct diagnosis. A panel of antibodies should always be used, and the results should be correlated with the histologic appearance and clinical history before a diagnosis is rendered. A diagnosis should never be made on the basis of immunostaining alone. Also, attempts should always be made to obtain fresh or frozen tissue that may be needed for immunogenotypic analysis. In addition to phenotyping of paraffin sections, similar studies can be performed successfully on touch preparations (imprints) of the tumor.

Establishing monoclonality of a B lymphocyte proliferation is usually accomplished by the demonstration of light chain restriction. In small and medium malignant lymphoid cell populations, it is difficult to demonstrate surface immunoglobulin in paraffin sections. Microwave techniques are being improved so light chain restriction may now be demonstrated in many paraffin-embedded tissues as well. In difficult cases, immunogenotypic analysis is necessary. For T lymphocyte proliferations, clonality can be shown conclusively only by T lymphocyte receptor gene rearrangement studies. For frozen section immunophenotypic analysis, the most useful criteria in the diagnosis of T-cell neoplasia is the deletion of one or more of the pan T-cell antigens.

Table 34-19 presents a list of major reactivities of antibodies used in immunophenotyping malignant lymphomas in paraffin-

Table 34-19 Major Reactivities of Antibodies Used in Immunophenotyping of Malignant Lymphomas in Paraffin Sections*

Antibody	Reactivity	Comments†
CD45 (LCA)	Leukocytes	Immunoblastic, plasmacytoid, and lymphoblastic NHL, Ki-1 ALCL, and multiple myeloma are often negative; Reed-Sternberg cells and variants (except for L&H cells) are usually negative
B-Cell Associated		
CD20 (L26)	B cells	Reacts with 90% of B-cell NHL, rarely with T-cell NHL; reacts with 40% of precursor B-cell ALL/LBL; reacts with 80% of LPHL (L&H cells) and 10%-20% of NSHL and MCHL; no reactivity with nonhematopoietic tumors
CD45R (4KB5)	B cells	Reacts with 80% of B-cell NHL and 10% of T-cell NHL; immunoblastic B-cell NHL and plasma cell tumors are often negative; reacts with 20% myeloid tumors
Antihuman light chain Ig	B cells, plasma cells, immunoblasts	Used to identify light chain restriction in plasma cells (cytoplasmic); requires proteolytic digestion or pre-treatment; microwave difficult to demonstrate surface light chain expression consistently by paraffin immunohistochemistry; light chain restriction may also be identified in small and intermediate NHL and in L&H cells in LPHL
Antihuman heavy chain Ig	B cells, plasma cells, immunoblasts	Used to identify heavy chain Ig in B cells (surface) and plasma cells (cytoplasmic)
DBA-44	Hairy cell leukemia, B cells, mantle zone, monocytoid B cells	Useful in detecting hairy cell leukemia in bone marrow sections; CLL is usually unreactive; may react with follicular center lymphomas and high grade B-cell NHL
T-Cell Associated		
UCHL-1 (CD45RO)	T cells, some B cells, monocytes, myeloid cells	Reacts with 75% of T-cell NHL and <5% of B-cell NHL (large cell); reacts with <50% of T-cell ALL/LBL and 25% of AML; rarely positive in carcinomas
CD3 (anti-CD3)	T cells	Most specific T-cell antibody; reacts with 80% of T-cell NHL; unreactive with most B-cell NHL

Table 34-19 *Continued*

Antibody	Reactivity	Comments†
CD43	T cells, some B cells, myeloid cells, monocytes	Reacts with >80% of T-cell NHL; shows coexpression with CD20 in most small lymphoid NHL; such coexpression is usually not seen in benign proliferations; reacts with megakaryoblasts, granulocytic sarcomas, AML, most ALLs, plasmacytomas, and some nonhematopoietic tumors

Myeloid/Macrophage Associated

Myelo-peroxidase (MPO)	Granulocytes	Most specific antibody for myeloid leukemias and granulocytic sarcoma
CD68 (KP1)	Monocytes, macrophages, mast cells	Reacts with 50% of AML; positive with most FAB M4, M5; reacts with some B-cell NHL, hairy cell leukemia, Langerhans cell histiocytosis, mastocytosis, and SHML; occasionally reacts with nonhematopoietic tumors (melanoma)
S100	Macrophages, melanocytes, glial cells, Schwann cells, Langerhans cells	Reactive in Langerhans cell histiocytosis, SHML, melanomas, brain tumors, some carcinomas; stains blast cells in AML in 50% of cases, and in granulocytic sarcoma; rare reactivity in HL and NHL (ALCL)

Others

CD15 (Leu M1)	Granulocytes, Reed-Sternberg cells	Reacts with Reed-Sternberg cells in 85% of NSHL and MCHL and 20% of LPHL; reacts with 20% of T-cell NHL, 5% of B-cell NHL (large cell), and 50% of carcinomas
CD30 (Ber-H2) (Ki-1)	Activated B and T cells, Reed-Sternberg cells, granulocytes	Reacts with 90%, ALCL (Ki-1 lymphoma), Reed-Sternberg cells in 90% of NSHL and MCHL, and 10% of LPHL; reactivity may be seen in several low-, intermediate-, and high-grade NHLs; reactivity may also be seen in benign immunoblastic proliferations (infectious mononucleosis); reacts with 20% of plasma cell tumors, and rarely with nonhematopoietic tumors (germ cell)

Table 34-19   Continued

Antibody	Reactivity	Comments†
Bauhinia purpurea (BPA)	Reed-Sternberg cells, granulocytes, macrophages, germinal center lymphocytes	Reacts with Reed-Sternberg cells in >90% of NSHL and MCHL, and 75% of LPHL
CD34	Hematopoietic progenitor cells, leukemic blasts, vascular endothelial cells	Reacts with 30%-60% blasts in AML and ALL; nonreactive with NHL and HD; reacts with neoplasms of vascular origin, hemangiopericy-tomas, epithelioid sarcoma, dermatofibrosarcoma protuberans
CD61 (GPIIIa)	Platelets, megakaryocytes	Reacts with AML M7 and with erythroblasts in some cases of erythroleukemia
Factor VIIIR	Megakaryocytes, endothelial cells	Reacts with megakaryocyte proliferations and 70% of vascular tumors
Glyco-phorin A	Erythroid cells	Reacts with erythroid precursors; AML M6
Epithelial membrane antigen (EMA)	Epithelial cells	Reacts with 20%-30% of LPHL (L&H cells), 50% of Ki-1 ALCL, and most plasmacytic tumors; reacts with most epithelial cell tumors
BCL-2	*bcl*-2 proto-oncogene	Overexpressed in 60% of t(14;18) positive follicular lymphomas and other low-grade and some aggressive B-cell NHLs; constitutively expressed in T cells
BCL-1	*bcl*-1 (cyclin D1) proto-oncogene	Consistently overexpressed in t(11;14) positive mantle cell lymphoma; cyclin D1 overexpression may be histologically detectable in multiple myeloma; often detectable in epithelial cells and malignancies, mantle cell lymphoma
MIB-1	Ki-67 nuclear antigen	Indicator of proliferation rate in NHL
TdT	B- and T-cell precursors	Reactive with 90% of lymphoblastic lymphoma; negative in other NHL

Abbreviations: NHL = non-Hodgkin's lymphoma; ALCL = anaplastic large cell lymphoma; L&H = lymphocyte and histiocyte; ALL = acute lymphoblastic leukemia; LBL = lymphoblastic lymphoma; LPHL = lymphocyte-predominant Hodgkin's lymphoma; NSHL = nodular sclerosis Hodgkin's lymphoma; MCHL = mixed cellularity Hodgkin's lymphoma; CLL = chronic lymphoblastic leukemia; AML = acute myelogenous leukemia; FAB = French-American-British classification; SHML = sinus histiocytosis with massive lymphadenopathy; HL = Hodgkin's lymphoma; TdT = terminal deoxynucleotidyl transferase.
* Modified from Perkins SL, Kjeldsberg CR. Immunophenotyping of lymphomas and leukemias in paraffin-embedded tissues. *Am J Clin Pathol.* 1993;99:362–373.
† The reactivity percentages listed are approximate and depend on many technical factors.

Table 34-20   Applications of Immunophenotypic Analysis

Disorder	Antibody Panel
Rule out nonhematopoietic tumors (cell lineage determination)	CD45, keratin, S100, HMB45, vimentin, MPO, CD20, CD3
Reactive hyperplasia vs NHL	Light chains, CD5, CD43,* CD20,* bcl-2
Subclassification of NHL	CD45, CD20, CD43, CD3, CD30, EMA, TdT
NHL vs HL	CD45, CD20, CD43, CD3, CD30, CD15, EMA
NHL proliferation rate	MIB-1 (Ki-67), topoisomerase II

Abbreviations: CD45 = leukocyte common antigen; MPO = myeloperoxidase; CD20 = B-cell antigen; CD3, CD5, CD43 = T-cell antigen; NHL = non-Hodgkin's lymphoma; CD30 = (Ki-1); EMA = epithelial membrane antigen; TdT = terminal deoxynucleotidyl transferase; HL = Hodgkin's lymphoma.
*Coexpression of CD20 and CD43 favors a malignant lymphoma.

embedded tissue sections. **Tables 34-20 to 34-22** show the usefulness of immunophenotypic analysis in a number of NHLs.

In general, the T-cell NHLs appear to be more aggressive than B-cell types. High proliferative rates in NHL correlate with a poor prognosis. Immunohistochemical methods using antibody Ki-67 (frozen sections) or MIB-1 (paraffin sections) may be used to determine the proliferative index. A proliferative index greater than 80% has been associated with a very poor prognosis in aggressive NHL. Another marker that may prove useful is topoisomerase II.

34.13.3 Genotypic Analysis

During the course of their development, normal lymphoid cells undergo a series of rearrangements within their antigen receptor genes. The rearrangements effect shuffling of the various gene segments whose combinations account for the antigen specificity of the fully assembled immunoglobulin (Ig) or TcR molecules they encode. Thus, B and T lymphocytes have surface membrane antigen receptor proteins, Igs and TcRs, that are essential to their function. Monomeric immunoglobulins consist of two identical heavy chains adjoining with two identical light chains of either kappa or lambda type. TcRs exist in two forms: alpha-beta or gamma-delta heterodimers. Molecular assays for clonality are based on the premise that malignant lymphomas develop as clonal

Table 34-21 Undifferentiated Large Cell Neoplasm Antibody Panel for Paraffin Sections*

Disease	CD45	CD3	CD20	CD15	CD30	S100	Myeloperoxidase	Keratin	Vimentin
NHL	+	±	±	-	-/+	-/+	-	-	-/+
NLPHL	+	-	+	-	-	-	-	-	-
Classical Hodgkin's lymphoma	-	-	-	+	+	-	-	-	-
Carcinoma	-	-	-	-	-	-/+	-	+	-/+
Melanoma	-	-	-	-	-	+	-	-	+
Granulocytic sarcoma	-/+	-	-	-	-	-	+	-	-
Sarcoma	-	-	-	-	-	-	-	-	+

Abbreviations: ± = may be positive or negative depending on cell lineage (B or T); -/+ = less than 50% of cases positive; NHL = non-Hodgkin's lymphoma; NLPHL = nodular; lymphocyte predominance Hodgkin's lymphoma.
*CD45 may be negative in NHL, especially in immunoblastic and anaplastic large cell lymphoma. Rare carcinomas may express CD30. Keratin may be focally present in anaplastic large cell lymphoma. Myelomas are often CD45-, CD20-, CD43+, epithelial membrane antigen-positive, and sometimes keratin-positive.

Table 34-22 Immunophenotyping of Non-Hodgkin's and Hodgkin's Lymphomas in Paraffin Sections

Lymphoma	CD45*	CD20	CD43†	CD3	CD30‡	CD15§
NHL						
B cell +	+	+	–/+	–	–	–
T cell +	+	–	+	+/–	–/+	–
HL						
LPHL	+	+	–	–	–	–
Classical HL**	–	–	–	–	+	+

Abbreviations: NHL = non-Hodgkin's lymphoma; LPHL = lymphocyte predominant Hodgkin's lymphoma; HL = Hodgkin's lymphoma.
*CD45 is often negative in large cell lymphoma immunoblastic type, anaplastic large cell lymphoma, lymphoblastic lymphoma, and Reed-Sternberg cells in nodular sclerosis HL and mixed cellularity HL.
†Coexpression of CD43 and CD20 is common in low-grade small lymphoid neoplasms (small lymphocytic lymphoma, mantle cell lymphoma). This coexpression is usually not seen in reactive proliferations.
‡CD30 is often positive in immunoblasts in infectious mononucleosis.
§CD15 may be positive in cytomegalovirus-infected immunoblasts.
**CD20 or CD3 occasionally may be expressed in malignant cells in nodular sclerosis HL and mixed cellularity HL.
Source: Modified from Perkins SL, Kjeldsberg CR. Immunophenotyping of lymphomas and leukemias in paraffin-embedded tissues. *Am J Clin Pathol.* 1993;99:362–373.

expansions of a neoplastically transformed lymphocyte, that exhibits a specific antigen receptor gene rearrangement that is stably retained in its progeny (with a few exceptions), hence the term "monoclonal." By similar reasoning, reactive lymphoid populations are composed of a diverse group of lymphocytes, each with a unique antigen rearrangement, hence a "polyclonal" population. Thus, gene rearrangement studies are used to distinguish between malignant monoclonal cell populations and polyclonal benign proliferations.

Gene rearrangement analysis may be performed using the Southern blot hybridization or polymerase chain reaction (PCR) techniques. Unfixed cells in suspension from fresh or frozen tissue are the specimens of choice for such studies. Formalin-fixed tissue also may be used for PCR. B5-fixed tissue cannot be used. Almost all B-cell NHLs have a clonal IgH chain gene rearrangement. The vast majority of NHLs of T-cell lineage have clonal TcR gene rearrangements.

The Southern blot hybridization test for gene rearrangement is a sensitive method, capable of detecting clonal populations composing only 1% or 2% of the total DNA in a specimen. This may be advantageous in detecting a small number of neoplastic cells in specimens where histopathologic and immunophenotypic analysis is difficult. The major disadvantage of the Southern blot hybridization method is that the assay often takes 1 to 2 weeks to complete and is generally not available except in reference laboratories.

Recently, genotypic analysis has become available with PCR, which may not be as sensitive for detecting gene rearrangements. The advantages of PCR, however, are that the method requires only tiny amounts of DNA, and the results can be available within 1 to 2 days. PCR is especially valuable when the biopsy specimen contains only small amounts of lymphoid infiltrates (eg, cutaneous lymphoid infiltrates). A more detailed discussion of molecular techniques of diagnostic hematopathology is provided in Chapter 48.

Although clonal lymphoid proliferations are usually malignant, clonality cannot be equated with malignancy. Also, not all NHLs contain clonal antigen receptor gene rearrangement. One third of anaplastic large cell CD30+ lymphomas appear to lack clonal antigen receptor gene rearrangement. Only a small number of NK/T-cell lymphomas show TcR gene rearrangement. Thus, the results of genotypic analysis should always be interpreted together with the clinical, histopathologic, and immunophenotypic findings.

34.13.4 Cytogenetics

Although more than 90% of NHLs have cytogenetic abnormalities, conventional cytogenetic analysis currently has a limited value in routine diagnostics. Because conventional cytogenetic studies depend on viable cells, it is essential that the biopsy specimen be transported to the cytogenetic laboratory without delay. For metaphase cytogenetic analysis, a portion of the fresh biopsy material is mixed into a cell suspension. Chromosomes are harvested from direct preparations and short-term cultures.

In more than 90% of BLs, t(8;14)(q24;q32) or one of its variants—t(8;22)(q24;q11) and t(2;8)(p11;q24)—has been observed (*see Table 34-1*). Follicular lymphomas have t(14;18)(q32;q21) in 80% of patients. As mentioned previously, the t(11;14)(q13;q32) translocation has been found in up to 90% of mantle cell lymphomas. In anaplastic large cell lymphoma, CD30+ (Ki-1) t(2;5)(p23;q35) is frequently seen. In small lymphocytic lymphoma, trisomy 12 is seen in 30% of patients.

34.13.5 Serum and Urine Protein Electrophoresis and Immunoelectrophoresis

The NHLs may be associated with polyclonal or monoclonal gammopathy (usually IgM) and occasionally hypogammaglobulinemia.

34.13.6 Serum Chemistry

Serum lactate dehydrogenase (LDH) and serum β_2-microglobulin can be used as indirect indicators of tumor burdens and are independent prognostic factors. Serum calcium levels may be elevated in NHL, particularly in some of the peripheral T-cell lymphomas (adult T-cell leukemia/lymphoma), and uric acid levels may increase dramatically during treatment of fast-growing lymphomas such as Burkitt's lymphoma. Elevated levels of liver enzymes, bilirubin, and alkaline phosphatase may be signs of liver or bone involvement.

34.13.7 Prognostic Factors in Non-Hodgkin's Lymphoma

Despite recent advances in the therapy of malignant lymphomas, most indolent NHLs remain incurable, and more than half of patients with aggressive NHL die of their disease. This has necessitated the development of prognostic factor models that permit the assessment of patient risk and determine the adequacy of therapeutic regimens. In aggressive NHL in particular, the clinical indices that have been consistently associated with clinical outcome include the age at diagnosis, the presence or absence of B symptoms, performance status, the serum LDH concentration, the number of nodal and extranodal sites of disease, tumor size, and the distinction between localized disease (Ann Arbor stage I or II) and advanced disease (stage III or IV). These clinical characteristics have been included in the widely used International Prognostic Index (IPI) and are thought to reflect the following:

1. The tumor's growth and invasive potential (LDH, stage, tumor bulk, number of nodal and extranodal sites of disease, bone marrow involvement)
2. The patient's response to the tumor (performance status, B symptoms)
3. The patient's ability to tolerate intensive therapy (performance status, bone marrow involvement, and age)

Table 34-23 International Prognostic Index* of Parameters and Relative Risk

		Relative Risk
A. Patients of all ages		
Age	<60 years vs >60 years	1.96
LDH	<normal vs >normal	1.85
Performance status	0, 1 vs 2–4	1.80
Stage (Ann Arbor)	I/II vs III/IV	1.47
Extranodal involvement	≤1 site vs >1 site	1.48
B. Patients under 60		
Stage (Ann Arbor)	I/II vs III/IV	2.17
LDH	<normal vs >normal	1.95
Performance status	0, 1 vs 2–4	1.81

Abbreviation: LDH = lactate dehydrogenase.
*Although originally developed for aggressive non-Hodgkin's lymphomas, some studies indicate that the IPI may predict survival in indolent non-Hodgkin's lymphomas.
Adapted from Shipp MA. Prognostic factors in aggressive non-Hodgkin's lymphoma: who has "high-risk" disease? *Blood.* 1994;83:1165–1173.

These clinical characteristics serve only as surrogate indices for the actual molecular and cellular aberrations that are intrinsic to the pathogenesis and progression of these tumors. It is anticipated that the newer prognostic models will incorporate such molecular biologic parameters to improve the risk assessment and selection of appropriate therapeutic strategies for the individual patient. **Tables 34-22 to 34-27** present data on the IPI and several of the common prognostic factors in NHL.

34.14 Course and Treatment

Treatment of patients with NHL is based on the histopathologic features, the stage of the disease, and the clinical features (age and functional status of patient). The types of treatments used include surgery (rarely curative), cytotoxic chemotherapy, radiation therapy, biologic modifiers, and bone marrow transplantation. In general, patients with aggressive (intermediate and high-grade) disease are treated with the intent of curing the patient, whereas patients with indolent (low-grade) disease usually cannot be cured. Most patients with indolent NHLs, however, have a long median survival.

Table 34-24 International Prognostic Index*: The International Index and Age-Adjusted Index

Risk Group	Five-Year Survival Rate (%)		
	Age-Adjusted Index Applied to Patients >60 Years	International Index Applied to Patients of All Ages	Age-Adjusted Index Applied to Patients <60 Years
Low	56	73	83
Low-intermediate	44	51	69
High-intermediate	37	43	46
High	21	26	32

*Although the International Index was developed specifically to predict outcomes in patients with aggressive non-Hodgkin's lymphoma, it may also be useful in predicting outcomes in indolent lymphomas.
Adapted from Shipp MA. Prognostic factors in aggressive non-Hodgkin's lymphoma: who has "high-risk" disease? *Blood.* 1994;83:1165–1173.

Table 34-25 Histopathologic Prognostic Factors in Non-Hodgkin's Lymphomas

Histologic Category	Five-Year Overall Survival (%)	Five-Year Failure-Free Survival (%)
Follicular (all grades)	72	40
Mantle cell	27	11
Marginal zone B-cell, MALT	74	60
Marginal zone B-cell, nodal	57	29
Small lymphocytic	51	25
Lymphoplasmacytoid	59	25
Diffuse large B cell	46	41
Primary mediastinal large B cell	50	48
Burkitt's	44	44
Burkitt's-like	47	43
Peripheral T cell	25	18
Anaplastic large T cell/null cell	77	58

Abbreviation: MALT = mucosa-associated lymphoid tissue.
Adapted from The Non-Hodgkin's Lymphoma Classification Project. a clinical evaluation of the International Lymphoma Study Group Classification of non-Hodgkin's Lymphoma. *Blood.* 1997;89:3909–3918.

The majority of patients with indolent NHL (follicular lymphoma, B-CLL/SLL, and marginal zone B-cell lymphoma) survive for 5 or more years. Patients with follicular lymphoma have considerably longer survival times than those with B-CLL/SLL. The

Table 34-26 Cellular Prognostic Factors in Non-Hodgkin's Lymphomas

Prognostic Factors	Function	Comments
CD44	Lymphocyte adhesion to ECM and endothelial cells	High CD44 expression and serum levels correlate with advanced stage disease and decreased survival in aggressive NHLs
ICAM-1	Accessory molecule in immune recognition	Weak expression correlates with advanced disease in aggressive NHLs
Gelatinase B	Degradation of ECM components	High expression in DLCL is associated with shortened survival
VEGF	Endothelial cell specific mitogen and vascular permeability factor	A higher than median VEGF titer correlates with decreased overall survival
IL-6	Growth and differentiation factor for B and plasma cells	High levels of serum IL-6 in newly diagnosed DLCL are associated with the presence of B symptoms and poor outcome
TNF-α	Pleiotropic cytokine involved in lymphoid organ ontogeny	Higher than median plasma levels of TNF-α are associated with shorter overall survival

Abbreviations: ECM = Extracellular matrix; NHL = non-Hodgkin's lymphoma; ICAM = intercellular adhesion molecule; DLCL = diffuse large cell lymphoma; VEGF = vascular endothelial growth factor; IL-6 = interleukin-6; TNF-α = tumor necrosis factor-alpha.

optimal method of treatment for localized indolent NHL is radiation therapy, and many of these patients are long-term, disease-free survivors. Unfortunately, the majority of patients with indolent (low-grade) NHL have stage III or IV disease, and treatment for these patients remains controversial. A variety of chemotherapeutic approaches have been used, and many appear to be associated with complete remission; however, there is a very high relapse rate. Over a period of years, a number of patients with indolent disseminated NHL have their disease transform to an aggressive NHL, usually diffuse large cell lymphoma. This transformation is often manifested as a rapidly growing tumor in one or several sites.

In aggressive (intermediate and high-grade) localized NHLs, intensive therapy (chemotherapy and/or radiation therapy) is curable in approximately 60% of adult patients and in more than 80%

Table 34-27 Molecular Prognostic Factors in Non-Hodgkin's Lymphomas

Molecular Abnormality	Comments
bcl-1/JH	Cyclin D1 overexpression. Mantle cell lymphoma. Poor prognosis.
bcl-2/JH	BCL-2 protein overexpression, follicular lymphoma. The presence of the translocation does not predict survival in DLBCL; however, BCL-2 protein expression shows a strong association with disease-free overall survival.
bcl-6/JH	Although initial studies seemed to suggest that rearrangements delineate a subgroup of DLBCL with a favorable prognosis, more recent studies show similar outcomes in *BCL*-6/JH positive and *BCL*-6/JH negative DLBCL.
ALK/NPM	Anaplastic lymphoma kinase overexpression. Anaplastic large cell lymphoma, T cell/null cell. A small subset of DLBCL (good prognosis) overexpresses ALK without the translocation.
p53	Immunohistochemical detection correlates with the presence of mutations in most NHLs but not in HLs. Implicated in histologic progression from indolent to aggressive NHL. Immunohistochemical detection correlates with decreased overall survival in aggressive NHL.
p16	Deletions are associated with histologic progression. *p16* aberrations are associated with shortened survival.

Abbreviations: *bcl* = gene by convention; BCL = protein; JH = immunoglobulin heavy chain joining region; DLBCL = diffuse large B-cell lymphoma; ALK = anaplastic lymphoma kinase; NPM = nucleophosmin; NHL = non-Hodgkin's lymphoma; HL = Hodgkin's lymphoma.

of pediatric patients. In patients with disseminated aggressive NHL, combination chemotherapy is used, and 60% to 80% of patients with diffuse large cell lymphoma who achieve remission may be cured. However, the prognosis is poor in adult patients with aggressive NHL that relapses after combination chemotherapy.

Patients with lymphoblastic lymphoma are usually treated with intensive multiagent chemotherapy, similar to that given for ALL. In patients with Burkitt's lymphoma, surgical debulking of abdominal tumors, combination chemotherapy, and intensive metabolic support often provide remission. Approximately 80% of children with lymphoblastic lymphoma and Burkitt's lymphoma are curable. The prognosis is less favorable in adults.

Recently, bone marrow transplantation with peripheral blood stem cell or allogeneic bone marrow transplantation has improved the prognosis of patients with relapsed aggressive NHL from fatal to potentially curable.

Radiation therapy, especially combined with chemotherapy, and chemotherapy alone are associated with a number of serious side effects. The most common is myelosuppression associated with infection and/or hemorrhage. Other subsequent complications include infertility, second malignancies (especially myelodysplastic syndrome), and secondary leukemia. Elderly patients are more likely to develop these serious side effects than younger patients.

34.15 **References**

Armitage JO, Weisenburger DD. New approach to classifying non-Hodgkin's lymphomas: clinical features of the major histologic subtypes. *J Clin Oncol.* 1998;16:2780–2795.

Brunning RD, McKenna RW. Tumors of the bone marrow. *Atlas of Tumor Pathology.* 3rd series, fascicle 9. Washington, DC: Armed Forces Institute of Pathology; 1994.

Chan JKC. Peripheral T-cell and NK-cell neoplasms: an integrated approach to diagnosis. *Mod Pathol.* 1999;12:177–199.

Compton CC, Harris N, Ross DW. Protocol for the examination of specimens from patients with non-Hodgkin's lymphoma. *Arch Pathol Lab Med.* 1999;123:68–74.

Ferry JA, Harris NL. *Atlas of Lymphoid Hyperplasia and Lymphoma.* Philadelphia, Pa: Saunders; 1997.

Foucar K. Chronic lymphoid leukemias and lymphoproliferative disorders. *Mod Pathol.* 1999;12:141–150.

Frizzera G, Wu D, Inghirami G. The usefulness of immunophenotypic and genotypic studies in the diagnosis and classification of hematopoietic and lymphoid neoplasms. *Am J Clin Pathol.* 1999;111(suppl 1):S13–S39.

Harris NL, Isaacson PG. What are the criteria for distinguishing MALT from non-MALT lymphoma of extranodal sites? *Am J Clin Pathol.* 1999;111(suppl 1):S126–S132.

Harris NL, Jaffe ES, Stein H, et al. A revised European-American classification of lymphoid neoplasms: a proposal from the International Lymphoma Study Group. *Blood.* 1994;84:1361–1392.

Harris NL, Jaffe ES, Diebold J, et al. The World Health Organization Classification of Hematological Malignancies Report of the Clinical Advisory Committee Meeting, Airlie House, Virginia, November 1997. *Mod Pathol.* 2000;13(2):193–207.

Isaacson PG. Gastrointestinal lymphomas of T- and B-cell types. *Mod Pathol.* 1999;12:151–158.

Isaacson PG, Norton AJ. *Extranodal Lymphomas.* New York, NY: Churchill-Livingstone; 1994.

Jaffe ES. Hematopathology: integration of morphologic features and biologic markers for diagnosis. *Mod Pathol.* 1999;12:109–115.

Jaffe E, Harris NL, Diebold J, et al. World Health Organization classification of neoplastic diseases of the hematopoietic and lymphoid tissues: a progress report. *Am J Clin Pathol.* 1999;111(suppl 1):S8–S12.

Jeffers MD, Milton J, Herriot R, et al. Fine needle aspiration cytology in the investigation of non-Hodgkin's lymphoma. *J Clin Pathol.* 1998;51:189–196.

Mason DY, Harris NL (eds). *Human lymphoma: clinical implications of the REAL classification.* Springer-Verlag. London; 1999.

Shipp MA. Prognostic factors in aggressive non-Hodgkin's lymphoma: who has "high-risk" disease? *Blood.* 1994;83:1165–1173.

Swerdlow SH. Small B-cell lymphomas of the lymph nodes and spleen: practical insights to diagnosis and pathogenesis. *Mod Pathol.* 1999;12:125–140.

Warnke RA, Weiss LM, Chan JKC, et al. Tumors of lymph nodes and related organs. In: *Atlas of Tumor Pathology.* 3rd series, fascicle 14. Washington, DC: Armed Forces Institute of Pathology; 1995.

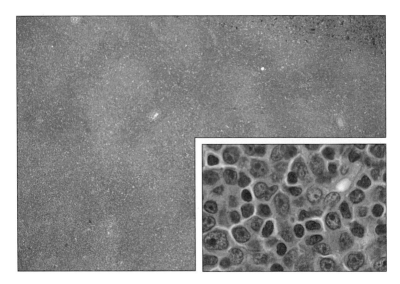

Image 34-1   B-cell chronic lymphocytic leukemia/small lymphocytic lymphoma. Low-power view shows vaguely delineated pale areas (proliferation centers), producing a nodular pattern in the lymph node. Inset shows a high-power view of a proliferation center consisting of prolymphocytes, immunoblasts, and small lymphocytes.

Image 34-2   Mantle cell lymphoma. High-power view shows cells that are slightly larger than normal lymphocytes and have more dispersed chromatin, indistinct nucleoli, and irregular nuclear contours. Inset shows mantle cells in the peripheral blood.

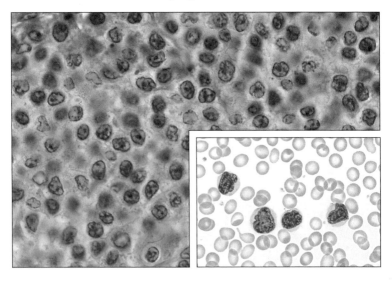

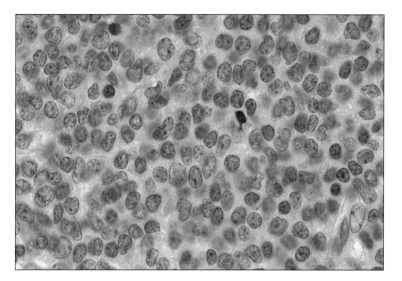

Image 34-3   Mantle cell lymphoma. High-power view shows the blastic variant of mantle cell lymphoma. The cells are slightly larger and have a fine chromatin pattern.

Image 34-4   Mantle cell lymphoma of the intestine (multiple lymphomatous polyposis). The lamina propria is diffusely infiltrated by mantle cells (left). Immunoperoxidase study shows the expression of nuclear cyclin D1 (right).

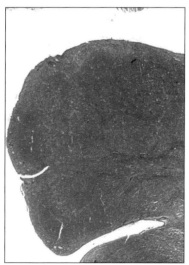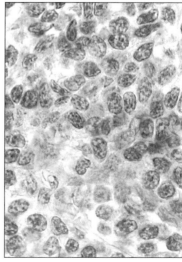

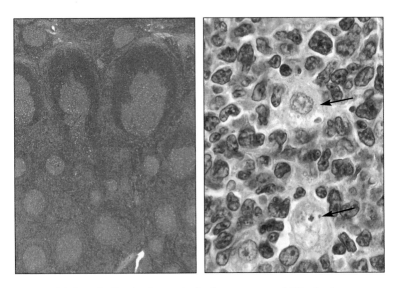

Image 34-5 Follicular hyperplasia. In contrast to follicular lymphoma (Image 34-6), the follicles are more widely dispersed (left). High power shows tingible body macrophages (arrows), centrocytes, and centroblasts (right).

Image 34-6 Follicular lymphoma. Low power shows multiple follicles in a back-to-back arrangement (left). Follicular lymphoma, grade 1, consists predominantly of centrocytes (right).

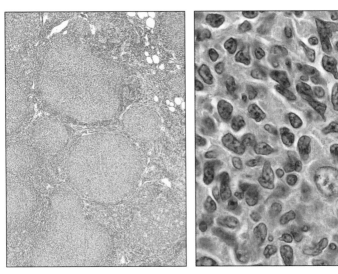

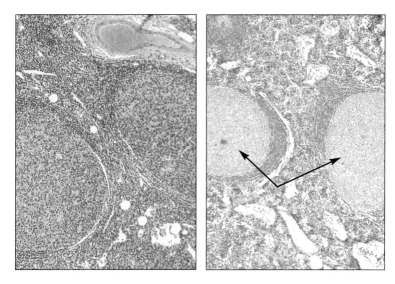

Image 34-7 Follicular hyperplasia. Medium power shows a characteristic heterogeneous population within follicle centers (left). Immunoperoxidase study shows BCL-2 protein expression within the mantle zone, but not in follicle centers (arrows), in contrast to follicular lymphoma (right; see Image 34-8).

Image 34-8 Medium power view of a follicular lymphoma, grade 1, shows a monotonous population of centrocytes within the follicles (left). Immunoperoxidase study shows expression of BCL-2 protein within follicular lymphoma (arrows).

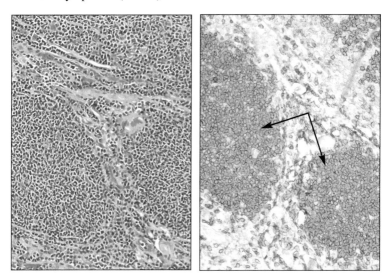

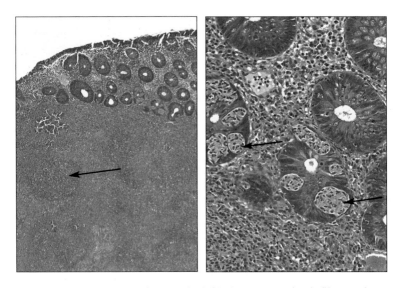

Image 34-9   Section of stomach (left) shows extensive infiltrate of lamina propria and contains reactive lymphoid follicle (arrow). Marginal zone cells have infiltrated the epithelium (right), forming lymphoid epithelial lesions (arrows).

Image 34-10   The variable morphologic characteristics that may be observed in marginal zone B-cell lymphomas: centrocyte-like cells (left) and monocytoid B cells (right) predominate.

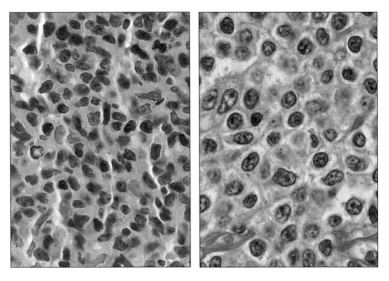

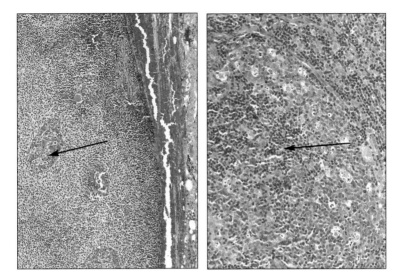

Image 34-11   MALT lymphoma in parotid gland (left). Low power shows large sheets of monocytoid B cells around and within epithelial structures (arrow). MALT lymphoma of the conjunctiva (right). Section shows a reactive follicle infiltrated by neoplastic marginal zone cells, producing "follicular colonization" (arrow).

Image 34-12   MALT lymphoma of the lung (left). A characteristic perivascular and peribronchial infiltrate is evident. MALT lymphoma of the thyroid gland (right).

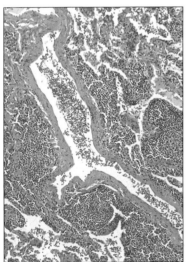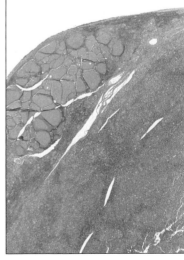

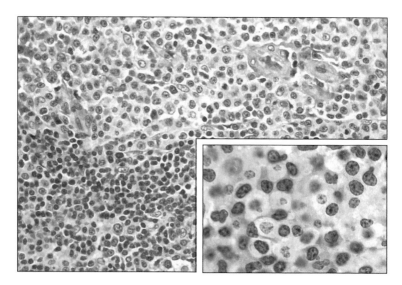

Image 34-13 Nodal marginal zone B-cell lymphoma (monocytoid B-cell lymphoma). The monocytoid B cells (upper half) are slightly larger than small lymphocytes (lower half) and have moderately abundant pale cytoplasm. Inset shows a high-power view of the monocytoid B cells.

Image 34-14 Splenic marginal zone B-cell lymphoma. Low power shows increased white pulp with expansion of the marginal zones (arrow), producing a nodular pattern. Infiltration of the red pulp is also seen (short arrows). Upper left inset shows a high-power view of a malignant infiltrate. Upper right inset shows involvement of the peripheral blood. Lower right inset shows a bone marrow infiltrate.

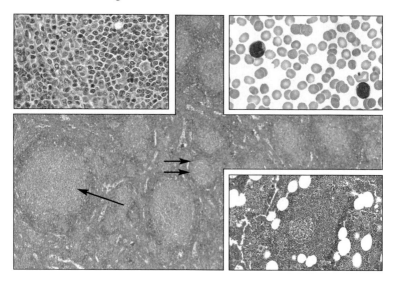

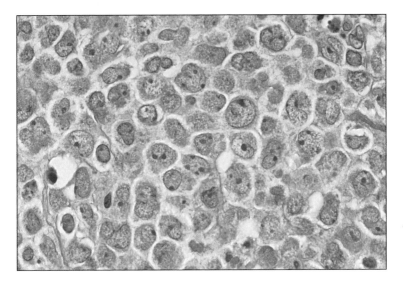

Image 34-15   Diffuse large B-cell lymphoma. A centroblastic-type lymphoma is shown.

Image 34-16   Diffuse large B-cell lymphoma. An immunoblastic-type lymphoma is shown. Inset shows an immunoperoxidase study with a strong expression of MIB-1.

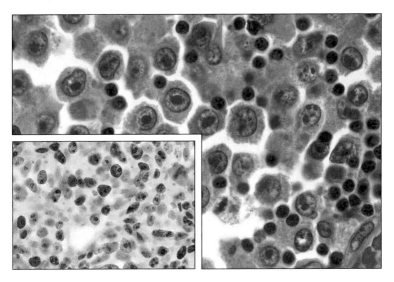

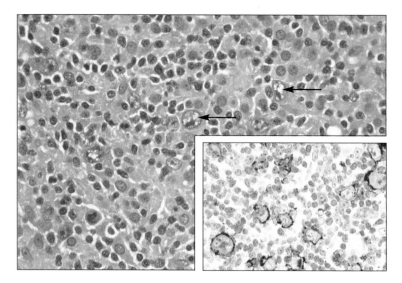

Image 34-17 Diffuse large B-cell lymphoma; T cell–rich B-cell lymphoma. A predominance of reactive small T lymphocytes are shown. The malignant cells (arrows) are larger but few in number. Inset shows an immunoperoxidase study with the large cells expressing CD20.

Image 34-18 Burkitt's lymphoma. An infiltrate of monomorphic, medium-sized cells with moderately abundant cytoplasm, moderately clumped chromatin, and several nucleoli is shown. Inset shows the imprint of tumor cells having characteristic cytoplasmic vacuoles.

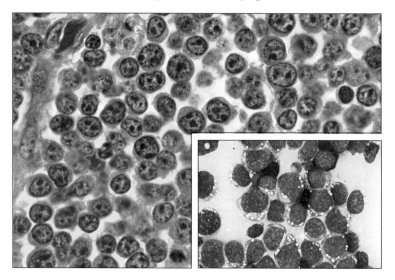

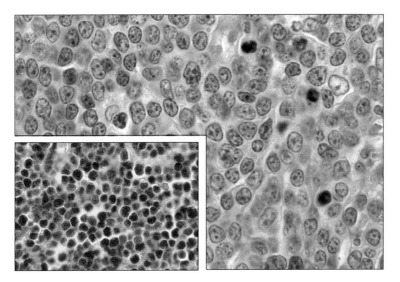

Image 34-19 T-precursor lymphoblastic lymphoma/leukemia. Medium-sized lymphocytes with scant cytoplasm, a finely dispersed chromatin pattern, and indistinct nucleoli are shown. Several mitotic figures are present. Inset shows an immunoperoxidase study with the cell nuclei expressing terminal deoxynucleotidyl transferase (TdT).

Image 34-20 Mycosis fungoides/Sézary syndrome. Section of a skin biopsy shows an infiltrate in the upper dermis and epidermis. Several Pautrier's abscesses are present (arrows). Inset shows a Sézary cell in the peripheral blood.

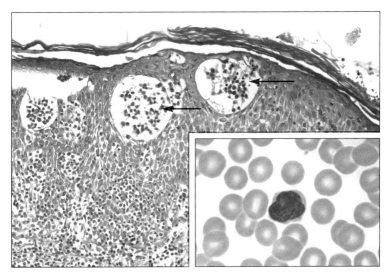

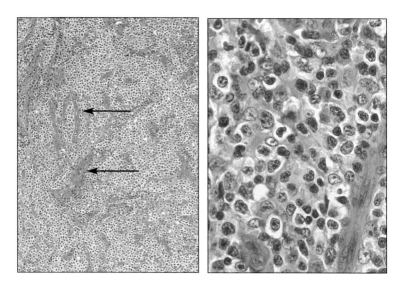

Image 34-21   Angioimmunoblastic T-cell lymphoma. A lymph node section shows a diffuse infiltrate of medium to large cells with a clear cytoplasm (left). The other striking feature is the presence of numerous arborizing, high endothelial venules, many of which show thickened hyalinized walls (arrows). High power shows a mixed population of atypical lymphoid cells (right).

Image 34-22   Enteropathy-type T-cell lymphoma. The mucosa and submucosa on the right side shows a diffuse cellular infiltrate. Left inset shows an immunoperoxidase study with the malignant cells expressing CD3. Right inset shows a high-power view of the malignant infiltrate.

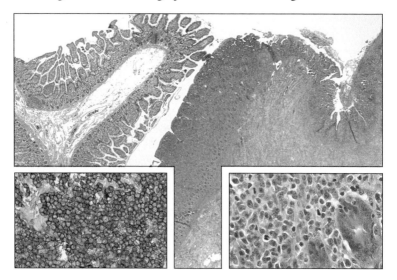

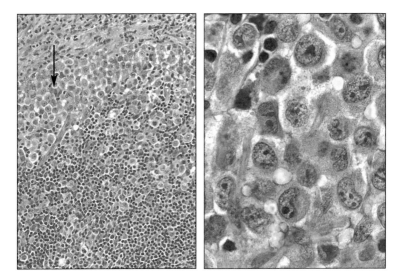

Image 34-23 Anaplastic large cell lymphoma. Medium-power view of a lymph node section shows a large cell infiltrate (arrow) within the distended sinuses (left). High-power view of anaplastic cells (right).

Image 34-24 Anaplastic large cell lymphoma. Immunoperoxidase study shows an expression of CD30 (left). Immunoperoxidase study shows nuclear and cytoplasmic expression of ALK-1 (right).

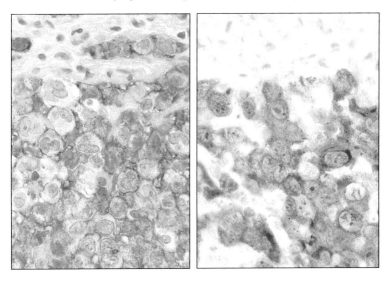

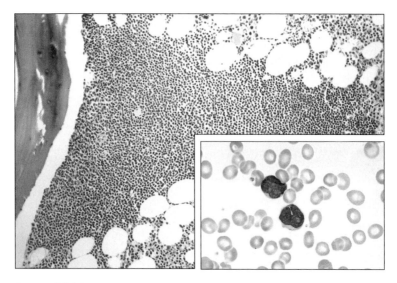

Image 34-25   Bone marrow biopsy section shows characteristic para-trabecular location of a follicular lymphoma. Inset shows peripheral blood with two circulating lymphoma cells having characteristic cleaved nuclei.

Image 34-26   Fine-needle aspirate. Cells aspirated from a lymph node with mantle cell lymphoma are shown. Upper inset is a high-power view of the mantle cells. Lower inset is an immunoperoxidase study showing expression of cyclin D1.

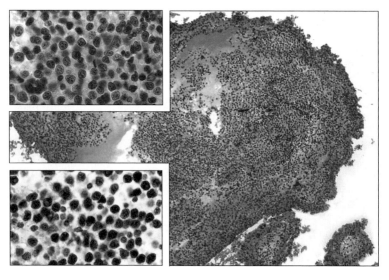

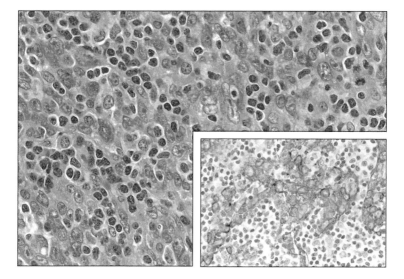

Image 34-27   Metastatic nasopharyngeal carcinoma in a lymph node biopsy. High-power view reveals a large cell infiltrate that could be mistaken for a large cell lymphoma. Inset shows an immunoperoxidase study with the large cells expressing keratin.

Image 34-28   Granulocytic sarcoma. High-power view of an ovarian tumor shows a diffuse infiltrate of large cells resembling large cell lymphoma. Inset shows an immunoperoxidase study with the malignant cells expressing myeloperoxidase.

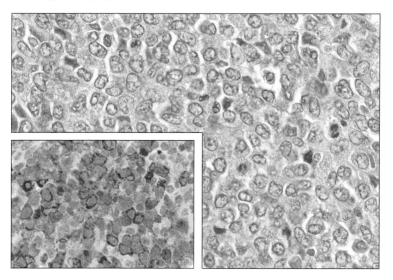

35   Hodgkin's Lymphoma

In 1832, Thomas Hodgkin first described seven patients with massive enlargement of the lymph nodes and spleen in a paper entitled, "On some morbid appearances of the absorbant [*sic*] glands and spleen." Hodgkin's lymphoma is characterized histologically by sparse numbers of large atypical multinucleate Reed-Sternberg (RS) cells (or their morphologic variants) in a background of reactive inflammatory cells. The consistent presence of this inflammatory infiltrate suggests that a complex interplay of immunologic processes is a significant component of the disease pathogenesis. In the 1990s, significant progress has been made in understanding this entity, including the determination that the characteristic RS cell and its variants are of lymphoid origin. The World Health Organization (WHO) classification of hematologic neoplasms proposes to recognize this discovery by appropriately changing the name from Hodgkin's disease to Hodgkin's lymphoma (HL). Accordingly, the proposed WHO terminology is used throughout this chapter.

35.1   Pathophysiology

Experimental evidence indicates that, in the vast majority of cases, the lymphocytic and histiocytic (L&H) cells of nodular lymphocyte predominance Hodgkin's lymphoma (NLPHL) and RS cells of classic HL are clonal proliferations of germinal center–derived B lymphocytes. Whereas the L&H cells of NLPHL are thought to be derived from antigen-selected germinal center B cells with productive rearrangements of the immunoglobulin heavy chain gene, the RS cells of classic HL are thought to arise from germinal center B cells that have suffered "crippling" nonsense or frameshift mutations of the immunoglobulin heavy chain variable region segment. There is also evidence that the RS cells of a subset of classic HL may arise from post–germinal center B cells, because they lack BCL-6 expression but consistently express CD138. Hence, although the L&H cells of NLPHL synthesize immunoglobulin J chain, mRNA, and protein, the RS cells of classic HL do not. Because crippled germinal center B cells are generally eliminated by apoptosis, an additional transforming event is necessary to permit continued survival of the RS cells that have lost their capacity for antigen receptor expression and selection. The frequent association of Epstein-Barr virus (EBV) in classic HL stimulates speculation that EBV may play a role in this regard, particularly because EBV expresses such genes as latent membrane protein 1 (LMP1) and Epstein-Barr nuclear antigen 1 (EBNA1), which are notable for their transforming capacity. In contrast to the story for B-cell derivation, evidence for T-cell origin in the RS cells of rare cases of HL is controversial. The predominant B-cell origin of the RS cells notwithstanding, the exact etiology of HL is unknown.

35.2 Clinical Findings

There are approximately 8000 new cases of HL in the United States each year, and the disease represents approximately 20% to 30% of all lymphomas in the United States and Europe. In Asians, HL accounts for only 10% of all lymphomas. HL has a bimodal age-specific incidence curve, with one mode in the 15- to 45-year-old group and another after the age of 50. The overall incidence of HL in economically underdeveloped countries is lower than that in developed countries, but the incidence before the age of 15 is higher.

The clinical presentation of HL is usually a progressive, painless enlargement of one or more lymph nodes in the neck. Occasionally, patients present with a mediastinal mass that may be discovered on a routine chest radiograph or on a radiograph obtained because of respiratory symptoms.

HL is more frequently (approximately 25% of patients) associated with constitutional "B" symptoms, such as fever, night sweats, pruritus, and weight loss, than is non-HL. Physical examination may reveal splenomegaly and hepatomegaly in addition to enlarged lymph nodes. In contrast to non-HL, primary extranodal disease is very unusual. HL usually spreads via contiguous lymph nodes.

35.3 Staging

Successful treatment of HL depends on accurate identification of all disease-bearing sites in the body. Compared to non-HL, patients with HL have less frequent involvement of Waldeyer's ring, the gastrointestinal tract, mesenteric lymph nodes, bone marrow, and skin. Generally, HL is initially detected in a less advanced stage than non-HL. In addition, patients with HL have more frequent involvement of the mediastinal lymph nodes than patients with non-HL. The procedures required to stage HL are outlined in **Table 35-1**. Once the pretreatment evaluation data are collected, the patient's disease is assigned a Roman numeral stage according to the criteria in **Table 35-2**. The stage is also assigned a substage designation depending on the presence (B) or absence (A) of significant systemic symptoms.

35.4 Classification

As stated previously, Hodgkin's disease is now recognized as a malignant lymphoma, and the term "Hodgkin's lymphoma" is used in the proposed WHO classification (**Table 35-3**). **Table 35-4** compares the Lukes and Butler classification, Rye modification of the Lukes and Butler classification, and the Revised European American Lymphoma (REAL)/proposed WHO classifications (which are identical as they relate to HL). The major difference, compared with the Rye modification, is the recognition in the REAL/WHO classifications of two fairly distinct disease entities: NLPHL and classic HL. The latter comprises nodular sclerosis, lymphocyte-rich, mixed cellularity, and lymphocyte depletion types.

Table 35-1   Staging Procedures in Hodgkin's Disease

Required procedures
    Clinical history and physical examination
    Lymph node biopsy
    Radiologic studies: chest roentgenogram; computed tomographic scan of
        chest and whole abdomen, including the pelvis; lymphangiography
    Laboratory tests: complete blood cell count; serum alkaline phosphatase
        and lactate dehydrogenase; liver and renal function tests, including uric
        acid and urinalysis; erythrocyte sedimentation rate
    Bilateral iliac crest bone marrow biopsies
Ancillary studies (when clinically indicated)
    Skeletal radiographic examination
    Gallium whole body scanning
    Laparotomy to include splenectomy, liver biopsy, and intra-abdominal
        lymph node biopsy (celiac, porta hepatis, mesenteric, para-aortic, iliac
        nodes), if information is likely to affect therapy

Table 35-2   The Cotswald Modification of the Ann Arbor Staging Classification for Hodgkin's Disease

Stage I	Involvement of a single lymph node region (I) or a single extralymphatic organ or site (IE)
Stage II	Involvement of two or more lymph node regions on the same side of the diaphragm (II) or localized involvement of an extralymphatic organ or site (IIE)
Stage III	Involvement of lymph node regions on both sides of the diaphragm (III) or localized involvement of an extralymphatic organ or site (IIIE) or spleen (IIIS) or both (IIISE)
III$_1$	With or without splenic hilar, celiac, or portal nodes
III$_2$	With para-aortic, iliac, or mesenteric nodes
Stage IV	Diffuse or disseminated involvement of one or more extralymphatic organs with or without lymph node involvement
A	No symptoms
B	Fever, drenching sweats, weight loss, pruritus
X	Bulky disease: >1/3 the width of the mediastinum >10 cm maximal dimension of nodal mass
E	Involvement of a single extranodal site, contiguous or proximal to a known nodal site

Modified from Lister TA, Crowther D, Sutcliffe SB, et al. Report of a committee convened to discuss the evaluation and staging of patients with Hodgkin's disease: Cotswald meeting. *J Clin Oncol.* 1989;7:1630–1636; *J Clin Oncol.* [erratum] 1990;8:1602.

Table 35-3 Proposed World Health Organization Classification of Hodgkin's Lymphoma

Nodular lymphocyte predominance Hodgkin's lymphoma

Classic Hodgkin's lymphoma
 Hodgkin's lymphoma, nodular sclerosis
 Hodgkin's lymphoma, lymphocyte-rich
 Hodgkin's lymphoma, mixed cellularity
 Hodgkin's lymphoma, lymphocytic depletion (includes some
  Hodgkin's-like anaplastic large cell lymphomas)

Table 35-4 Classification Schemes for Hodgkin's Lymphoma (Disease)

Lukes and Butler	Rye Modification	REAL/Proposed WHO*
Lymphocytic and/or histiocytic predominance Nodular Diffuse	Lymphocytic predominance	Nodular lymphocyte predominance
		Classic Hodgkin's lymphoma Lymphocyte-rich
Nodular sclerosis	Nodular sclerosis	Nodular sclerosis (grades I and II)
Mixed cellularity	Mixed cellularity	Mixed cellularity
Lymphocytic depletion	Lymphocytic depletion Diffuse fibrosis Reticular	Lymphocyte depletion

Abbreviations: REAL = Revised European American Lymphoma; WHO = World Health Organization.
*The REAL and proposed WHO classifications are identical as they relate to Hodgkin's lymphoma.

35.4.1 Nodular Lymphocyte Predominance Hodgkin's Lymphoma

The frequency of NLPHL is 5% to 10% of patients with lymphoma, and the disease has a single peak in the fourth decade of life. However, cases also may be seen in children and in the elderly. Patients usually present with localized disease of long duration and may have a history of a previous lymph node biopsy showing reactive hyperplasia. The mediastinum is rarely, if ever, involved in NLPHL. Late relapses are more common than in other types of HL. This does not, however, negatively affect survival. In 2% to 5% of patients, there is an association with or progression to large B-cell lymphoma.

The diagnosis of NLPHL is usually suspected on low-power examination. It has a characteristic nodular growth pattern, with or without diffuse areas (**Image 35-1**). It is controversial whether purely diffuse types exist. In rare cases, sclerosis may resemble nodular sclerosis. Classic diagnostic RS cells are usually not seen. A characteristic feature is the presence of L&H cells with multilobated (popcorn) nuclei and small nucleoli (**Image 35-1**). Within the nodules, the number of L&H cells vary from few to many and are often accompanied by epithelioid histiocytes, giving a mottled appearance to the lymph node section.

The immunophenotype of L&H cells is CD15–, CD30–/+, CD45+, CD20+/–. Most of the small lymphocytes within the nodules are B cells.

The differential diagnosis of NLPHL includes progressive transformation of germinal centers; nodular paracortical hyperplasia; classic HL; and non-HL such as small lymphocytic lymphoma/CLL, follicular lymphoma, and T-cell–rich B-cell lymphoma (**Table 35-5**). Immunohistochemistry is helpful in the differential diagnosis of classic HL; CD15 and CD30 positivity strongly favors classic HL.

35.4.2 Classic Hodgkin's Lymphoma

In classic HL, diagnostic RS cells are seen in a background of nodular sclerosis, lymphocyte-rich, mixed cellularity, or lymphocyte depletion. The immunophenotype (CD15+, CD30+, CD45–, negative T-cell/B-cell–associated antigens) is distinct and different from NLPHL. A variable number of reactive T cells are present in the background.

Hodgkin's Lymphoma, Nodular Sclerosis

Nodular sclerosis is by far the most common type of HL in the United States and Europe. It occurs with equal frequency in both sexes, whereas in all other types, men predominate. It is unusual in patients older than 50 years of age. Nodular sclerosis is usually associated with lower cervical, supraclavicular, and mediastinal lymph node involvement. It is the type that most commonly affects the lungs. The majority of patients have clinical stage II disease.

Nodular sclerosis HL has two distinct histologic features: the lymph node is divided into nodules by thick bands of collagen extending from the capsule, and RS cell variants are present in

Table 35-5   Differential Diagnosis of Hodgkin's Lymphoma

Nodular lymphocyte predominance
  Progressive transformation of germinal centers
  Nodular paracortical hyperplasia
  Lymphocyte-rich classic Hodgkin's lymphoma
  T-cell/histiocyte-rich large B-cell lymphoma
  Small lymphocytic lymphoma/classic lymphocytic lymphoma
  Follicular hyperplasia
  Follicular lymphoma

Lymphocyte-rich classic
  Nodular lymphocyte predominance
  Follicular lymphoma
  Mantle cell lymphoma
  Reactive hyperplasia

Nodular sclerosis
  Anaplastic large cell lymphoma
  Peripheral T-cell lymphoma
  Primary mediastinal (thymic) large B-cell lymphoma
  Mediastinal seminoma
  Metastatic neoplasms (eg, carcinoma, melanoma)
  Necrotizing granulomatous lymphadenitis (eg, cat scratch)

Mixed cellularity
  T-cell/histiocyte-rich large B-cell lymphoma
  Peripheral T-cell lymphoma
  Anaplastic large cell lymphoma
  Infectious mononucleosis
  Angioimmunoblastic lymphadenopathy

Lymphocyte depletion
  Nodular sclerosis, syncytial type
  Anaplastic large cell lymphoma
  Large cell non-Hodgkin's lymphoma

lacunar spaces (or lacunar cells) (**Image 35-2**). Extensive sheets of lacunar cells and atypical mononuclear cells are frequently present, but classic RS cells may be rare. Necrosis is not uncommon. A variant of nodular sclerosis—called "syncytial", "sarcomatous", or "monomorphic type"—is characterized by sheets of lacunar cells and atypical mononuclear cells (**Image 35-3**). The British National Lymphoma Investigation (BNLI) developed a system for grading nodular sclerosis (grades 1 and 2) based on the number and atypia of RS cells in the nodules. It has been suggested that patients with grade 2 disease may benefit from more aggressive therapy.

When a small biopsy specimen is obtained and fibrosis is evident, it may be extremely difficult to differentiate this type of HL from non-Hodgkin's large cell lymphoma, metastatic carcinoma, melanoma, or seminoma. Immunologic markers may be helpful in such instances. The presence of a high mitotic rate, extension through the capsule, prominent irregularity of the nucleus of small lymphocytes, and prominence of immunoblasts favors a diagnosis of non-HL over HL.

Lymphocyte-Rich Classical Hodgkin's Lymphoma (LRCHL)

Lymphocyte rich classical Hodgkin's lymphoma accounts for approximately 6% of cases of Hodgkin's lymphoma. There is a predominance of males. Patients usually present with early stage disease and lack B symptoms. Histologically, this subtype is characterized by RS cells within a background infiltrate that consists predominately of lymphocytes, with rare eosinophils and other inflammatory cells. Importantly, the characteristic L&H cells of LPHL are absent. LRCHL includes cases classified as "follicular" Hodgkin's lymphoma (FHL). In FHL, the lymph node exhibits a nodular architecture with regressed germinal centers and RS cells or variants distributed within the mantle zones and interfollicular regions. The RS cells in LRCHL exhibit the typical phenotypic characteristics of classic HL and are CD15+ and CD30+. Some cases of LRCHL may represent the so-called cellular phase of nodular sclerosis HL, or mixed cellularity HL.

Hodgkin's Lymphoma, Mixed Cellularity

Mixed cellularity composes 15% to 30% of HL and may be seen at all ages. The mediastinum is less commonly involved than in nodular sclerosis HL, and involvement of abdominal lymph nodes and the spleen is common.

The infiltrate is diffuse or vaguely nodular. Classic diagnostic RS cells (**Image 35-4**) are usually evident, and many mononuclear variants are often present. A variable number of eosinophils, plasma cells, and histiocytes are usually seen. There may be involvement of interfollicular regions.

This type of HL must be differentiated from various reactive lymphadenopathies (eg, infectious mononucleosis) and from certain types of non-HL, particularly the peripheral T-cell lymphomas (including so called "Lennert's lymphoma") and T-cell–rich large B-cell lymphoma (*see Table 35-5*).

Hodgkin's Lymphoma, Lymphocyte Depletion

Lymphocyte depletion HL is rare in the United States and Europe. Morphologically, it is characterized by a paucity of lymphocytes with increased numbers of abnormal mononuclear cells. RS cells are often numerous. Fibrosis and necrosis may be prominent. The patient is usually older, has stage III or IV disease, and is symptomatic. There is some doubt as to whether this entity exists. Most of the cases reported as lymphocyte depletion appear to have been non-HL (especially anaplastic large cell lymphoma) or HL, nodular sclerosis, syncytial variant.

It should be recognized that with the marked improvement in therapy for HL, the prognosis depends mainly on the stage of the disease and less on the histologic subclassification. The pathologist, however, must be able to accurately diagnose HL and be able to identify this disease in laparotomy specimens and biopsy specimens if relapse occurs.

35.5 Diagnostic Approach

Following a clinical history and physical examination, the workup of a patient with possible HL proceeds in the following fashion:

1. Tissue biopsy. The diagnosis and subclassification of HL should be made on the basis of histopathologic features in a lymph node biopsy specimen before initiating therapy. The initial diagnosis should not be made on the basis of a bone marrow biopsy or liver biopsy specimen alone. It is difficult to diagnose HL by fine-needle aspiration (FNA).
2. Complete blood cell count.
3. Bone marrow aspirate and biopsy specimen examination.
4. Radiologic studies.
5. Liver and renal function studies.
6. Laparotomy. Surgical laparotomy, which includes splenectomy, lymph node sampling, and liver biopsy, is rarely used because of advances of noninvasive techniques to obtain the necessary information, the efficacy of current therapies, and potential postsurgical complications.

35.6 Hematologic Findings

Unlike non-HL, significant abnormal hematologic findings are uncommon in HL. Despite this fact, examination of the peripheral blood and bone marrow should be done routinely as part of the staging procedure.

35.6.1 Blood Cell Measurements

A mild to moderate anemia is frequently present in patients with HL. It is usually normochromic and normocytic, with a low or normal reticulocyte count. In a small percentage of patients, autoimmune hemolytic anemia develops. One third of patients have leukocytosis caused by neutrophilia. The platelet count is normal or increased. In rare cases, severe anemia or pancytopenia may result from extensive involvement of the bone marrow or hypersplenism.

35.6.2 Peripheral Blood Smear Morphology

Neutrophilia, monocytosis, or eosinophilia are seen in 10% to 20% of patients, and lymphopenia may be present in patients with extensive disease.

35.6.3 Bone Marrow Examination

A bilateral posterior iliac crest bone marrow biopsy should be performed routinely in the staging procedure for patients with HL. Bone marrow involvement is unusual (less than 10% of patients) at time of diagnosis, especially in nodular lymphocyte predominance and nodular sclerosis subtypes. When the bone marrow is affected, the lesion is usually focal, is often associated with fibrosis, and may resemble a granuloma. Involvement of the marrow is usually recognized on low-power examination as an area containing a mixture of lymphocytes, plasma cells, eosinophils, histiocytes, and a variable number of atypical large cells. RS cells may be difficult to identify, and examination of multiple sections from the same biopsy may be necessary. The presence of mononuclear cells, with nuclear features of RS cells, in the characteristic cellular environment of HL should be regarded as consistent with bone marrow involvement, provided that a diagnosis of Hodgkin's disease has been made from a lymph node biopsy specimen.

Other Laboratory Tests

Test 35.1 **Tissue Biopsy**

A lymph node biopsy is required for the diagnosis of HL. Proper handling of the biopsy specimen is extremely important to make a correct diagnosis. See Chapter 34 for a detailed description of specimen handling. The histopathologic features observed in different types of HL were described earlier in this chapter.

Test 35.2 **Radiologic Studies**

The radiologic evaluation plays a crucial role in determining the extent of disease. It should start with routine chest radiographs. Computed tomography (CT) of the chest provides better definition of mediastinal, hilar, and paravertebral lymphadenopathy and pulmonary involvement, and should be done in all patients.

A bilateral lower extremity lymphangiogram is important to detect disease in the retroperitoneal lymph nodes. It should be noted that splenic, hilar, celiac, porta hepatis, and mesenteric nodes are not demonstrated by lymphangiography. The CT scan is particularly useful in the delineation of lymphadenopathy, which is not revealed on lymphangiography. A CT scan also may reveal tumor nodules in the spleen. Skeletal surveys or bone scans may be included to look for lytic or (less commonly) osteoblastic lesions in patients with bone pain. A gallium scan may be helpful in detecting disease in a variety of sites and may be used in patients unable to undergo lymphangiography; it is especially useful in evaluating response to therapy and in detecting recurrence after therapy.

Test 35.3 **Laparotomy**

Exploratory laparotomy is primarily a diagnostic procedure and includes a sampling of abdominal nodes, splenectomy, and open liver biopsy. It is not a routine procedure in staging HL and should only be done if the outcome will significantly alter therapy. It is occasionally used in patients with stage I, II, or IIIA disease after clinical examination and radiologic tests. The surgeon should obtain a biopsy specimen of all major lymph node groups regardless of the size and gross appearance of the nodes. Application of radiopaque clips at biopsy sites assists the radiotherapist in subsequent port design. The spleen and splenic hilar lymph nodes should be removed, and a wedge biopsy specimen should be taken from the liver.

The pathologist must carefully examine the removed spleen because excellent correlation exists between splenic involvement and the probability of hepatic involvement. It is extremely rare to have HL in the liver without splenic involvement. The spleen must be cut into thin sections and inspected carefully; multiple sections should be examined microscopically.

Approximately 20% of patients thought to have stage I or II disease are reclassified as having stage III disease after laparotomy. The value of the laparotomy needs to be weighed against the surgical risk.

35.7 Ancillary Tests

35.7.1 Immunophenotypic Analysis

Immunophenotyping and occasionally genotyping may facilitate the diagnosis of HL and help differentiate this disease from non-HL or metastatic nonhematopoietic neoplasms. Of the non-HLs that may simulate HL, anaplastic large cell lymphoma (Ki-1 lymphoma), peripheral T-cell lymphoma, T-cell–rich B-cell lymphoma, and primary mediastinal large B-cell lymphoma with sclerosis are especially noteworthy.

In the majority of cases, satisfactory immunophenotypic analysis can be done on paraffin sections, but fresh tissue should always be set aside (frozen) for possible gene rearrangement studies. This may be especially helpful when dealing with small mediastinal biopsy specimens, where the diagnosis may be uncertain.

Table 35-6 shows the common immunophenotypic findings in paraffin sections of different subtypes of HL. Nodular sclerosis and mixed cellularity have a similar immunophenotype (CD15+, CD30+/–, CD45–), but lymphocyte predominance is usually distinctly different (CD15–, CD30–/+, CD45+, CD20+/–). **Table**

Table 35-6 Immunophenotypic Features in Hodgkin's Lymphoma

Subtype	CD45	CD20	CD79a	J Chain	CD15	CD30	EMA	Fascin	BCL-6
NLPHL	+	+/–	+/–	+	–	–	+/–	–	+
cHL	–	–/+	–/+	–	+	+	–	+	–

Abbreviations: EMA = epithelial membrane antigen; NLPHL = nodular lymphocyte predominance Hodgkin's lymphoma; cHL = classic Hodgkin's lymphoma (includes lymphocyte-rich, mixed cellularity, nodular sclerosis, and lymphocyte depletion types); +/– = >50% of patients; –/+ = <50% of patients.

Table 35-7 Immunophenotypic Distinction of Hodgkin's Lymphoma from Non-Hodgkin's Lymphoma

Lymphoma	CD45	CD20	CD3	CD43	EMA	CD15	CD30	ALK/p80
NLPHL	+/–	+	–	–	+/–	–	–	–
cHL	–	–/+	–	–	–	+	+	–
T/HRBCL	+	+	–	–/+	–/+	–	–	–
ALCL, T/null	+/–	–	–/+	+/–	+	–	+	+
PTCL	+	–	+/–	+	–	–	–	–

Abbreviations: EMA = epithelial membrane antigen; ALK = anaplastic lymphoma kinase; NLPHL = nodular lymphocyte predominance Hodgkin's lymphoma; cHL = classical Hodgkin's lymphoma; T/HRBCL = T cell/histiocyte-rich large B-cell lymphoma; ALCL = anaplastic large cell lymphoma; PTCL = peripheral T-cell lymphoma; +/– = >50% of patients; –/+ = <50% of patients.

35-7 illustrates how immunophenotyping can be useful in distinguishing HL from anaplastic large cell lymphoma and some other non-HLs.

35.7.2 Epstein-Barr Virus

EBV is present in the RS cells of approximately one half of patients with HL, especially those with the mixed cellularity type. It is rarely seen in the lymphocyte predominance type. The presence of EBV can be demonstrated with polymerase chain reaction technique, with in situ hybridization for the detection of EBV RNA in tissue sections, and with immunohistochemistry for the EBV latent membrane protein. These studies are of interest regarding the pathogenesis of HL, but currently they are not useful in diagnosing the disease. Another interesting observation (although not diagnostically useful) is the expression of *bcl*-2 oncoprotein by Hodgkin's cells in approximately one half of patients studied.

35.7.3 Flow Cytometry

Although flow cytometry is rarely useful in diagnosing HL, it is an effective tool for diagnosing many of the entities in the differential diagnosis.

35.7.4 Gene Rearrangement Studies

Gene rearrangement studies may be helpful in difficult cases of distinguishing HL from non-HL when the immunophenotypic studies are equivocal. For the classic technique of Southern blot analysis, fresh or frozen tissue is required. Recently, polymerase chain reaction techniques have been developed that can use tissue from paraffin sections. The presence of B-cell or T-cell gene rearrangement favors a diagnosis of non-HL rather than HL. However, the failure to identify clonal gene rearrangement of immunoglobulin or T-cell receptor genes in HL may be due to the fact that RS cells often account for a very small part of the DNA extracted from the tissue biopsy specimen. Recently, supersensitive polymerase chain reaction techniques in combination with microdissection have demonstrated clonal B-cell gene rearrangements in some patients with lymphocyte predominance and clinical HL.

35.7.5 Cytogenetics

Karyotypic analysis of tissue with HL frequently (50% of cases) shows clonal hyperdiploid abnormalities. However, chromosome abnormalities specific for HL have not been described.

35.8 Course and Treatment

Approximately 75% of patients with HL can be cured. Factors that adversely affect the prognosis include stage III disease with involvement of lower abdominal lymph nodes, stage IV disease, old age, constitutional B symptoms, bulky mediastinal disease, extensive splenic involvement (more than four nodules), and the presence of multiple extranodal sites of involvement. The primary treatment of HL (stages I and II), which is confined to the lymph nodes, is extended-field radiation therapy or, in some geographic areas, combination chemotherapy. Patients with stage III or IV disease are treated with combination chemotherapy. Selected patients may be treated with both radiation therapy and chemotherapy. Bone marrow transplantation is used for selected patients with relapsed HL and unfavorable reactions such as pulmonary fibrosis. A number of complications, including a wide variety of secondary malignancies such as acute myeloblastic leukemia and non-HL, may follow therapy.

35.9 **References**

Aisenberg AC. Problems in Hodgkin's disease management: review article. *Blood.* 1999;93:761–779.

Ferry JA, Harris NL. *Atlas of Lymphoid Hyperplasia and Lymphoma.* Philadelphia, Pa: Saunders; 1997.

Harris NL. Hodgkin's disease: classification and differential diagnosis. *Mod Pathol.* 1999;12:159–176.

Harris NL, Jaffe ES, Stein H, et al. A revised European-American classification of lymphoid neoplasms: a proposal from the International Lymphoma Study Group. *Blood.* 1994;84:1361–1392.

Harris NL, Jaffe ES, Diebold J, et al. The World Health Organization Classification of Hematological Malignancies Report of the Clinical Advisory Committee Meeting, Airlie House, Virginia, November 1997. *Mod Pathol.* 2000;13(2):193–207.

Jaffe ES, Harris NL, Diebold J, et al. World Health Organization classification of neoplastic diseases of the hematopoietic and lymphoid tissue: a progress report. *Am J Clin Pathol.* 1999;111(suppl 1):S8–S12.

Kuppers R, Rajewsky K. The origin of Hodgkin and Reed/Sternberg cells in Hodgkin's diseases. *Annu Rev Immunol.* 1998;16:471–493.

von Wasielewski R, Mengel M, Fischer R, et al. Classical Hodgkin's disease: clinical impact of the immunophenotype. *Am J Pathol.* 1997;151:1123–1130.

Warnke RA, Weiss LM, Chan JKC, et al. Tumors of the lymph nodes and spleen. In: *Atlas of Tumor Pathology.* 3rd series, fascicle 14. Washington DC: Armed Forces Institute of Pathology; 1995.

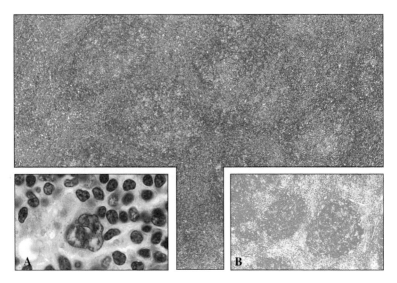

Image 35-1   Nodular lymphocyte predominance Hodgkin's lymphoma. Several poorly defined nodules have a characteristic mottled appearance. A high-power view (inset A) shows an L&H cell (popcorn cell) with a large, vesicular, lobated nucleus and indistinct nucleoli and scant cytoplasm (center). An immunoperoxidase study demonstrates expression of CD20 within the neoplastic nodules (inset B).

Image 35-2   Hodgkin's lymphoma, nodular sclerosis. Nodules of lymphoid tissue are surrounded by thick bands of collagen. A high-power view (inset) shows typical lacunar cells (arrows).

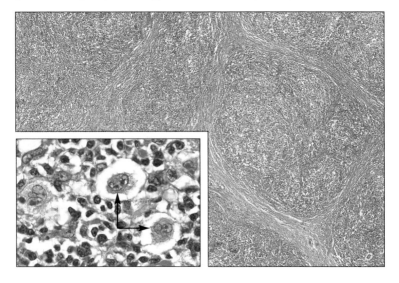

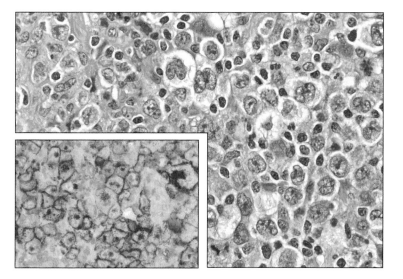

Image 35-3   Hodgkin's lymphoma, nodular sclerosis, syncytial variant. Sheets of large monomorphic cells and lacunar cells resemble non-Hodgkin's large cell lymphoma. An immunoperoxidase study demonstrates expression of CD15 in a typical membranous and Golgilike pattern (inset).

Image 35-4   Hodgkin's lymphoma, mixed cellularity. A classic binucleated Reed-Sternberg cell (arrow) is surrounded by small lymphocytes and occasional plasma cells. An immunoperoxidase study demonstrates CD15 expression within the Reed-Sternberg cell (arrow) (inset).

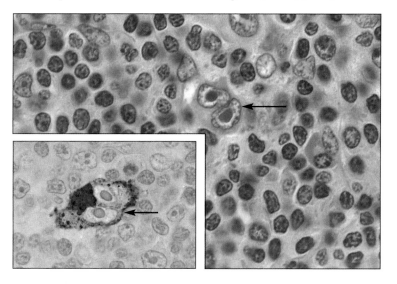

PART
X

Posttransplantation
Disorders

36 Disorders Associated with Organ Transplantation

Numerous disorders and sequelae associated with organ transplantation are well recognized. The immunosuppressive regimens of patients undergoing these procedures are responsible for many such processes, including posttransplantation lymphoproliferative disorders (PTLDs) and increased incidence of infections. Graft-versus-host disease (GVHD) is the major complication seen in allogeneic bone marrow transplant (BMT) recipients. In contrast to the PTLDs and infections, GVHD arises in patients with decreased immunosuppression. Organ rejection is a complex process that remains a significant cause of morbidity in solid organ transplant patients, and specialized texts offer descriptions of individual organ rejection.

36.1 Posttransplantation Lymphoproliferative Disorders

There is an increased incidence of lymphoproliferative disorders in solid organ and BMT recipients receiving intense immunosuppressive therapy. Among all transplant patients, there is approximately a 50 to 100 times greater prevalence of non-Hodgkin's lymphoma compared with the general population. The rate of occurrence of PTLDs appears to be related to the organ transplanted and the degree of immunosuppression.

Although first recognized in renal transplant recipients, PTLDs occur most commonly in heart (2%–10%) and heart/lung recipients (5%–9%) and least often in BMT patients (<1%). Patients receiving the potent immunosuppressive agent cyclosporin A and OKT3, an antibody against T-cells, are particularly at risk. Transplant recipients who are seronegative for Epstein-Barr virus (EBV) at the time of transplantation and subsequently become infected also have an increased risk of developing a PTLD.

36.1.1 Pathophysiology

The vast majority of all PTLDs are B-cell EBV-driven proliferations that arise in patients with immunosuppression. EBV is a ubiquitous double-stranded DNA herpes virus that predominantly infects B lymphocytes. The primary infection typically occurs via saliva exchange, and viral replication proceeds within the oropharynx. In very young children, the primary infection is usually subclinical. In older children and young adults, infectious mononucleosis is associated with fever, malaise, and cervical adenopathy. In a healthy host, the infection is abated by cytotoxic T cells. However, following the primary infection, the virus remains within the host in a latent form indefinitely.

During the latent stage of infection, the virus produces numerous viral proteins, including the cell surface latent membrane proteins (LMPs) and the Epstein-Barr nuclear antigens (EBNAs). In vitro studies suggest that these proteins are capable of transforming and immortalizing B cells and upregulating B-cell activation markers such as CD23. In an immunocompetent host, this upregulation of B-cell activation markers induces T-cell cytotoxicity and control of any EBV-induced B-cell proliferations. The CD8+ T cells exert their cytotoxic effect through class I human leukocyte (HLA) antigens.

During the latent phase of infection, the immune system maintains a balance between episodic viral shredding, B-cell activation and proliferation, and the destruction of the infected cells by cytotoxic T cells. Following organ transplantation, immunosuppressive regimens are used to deliberately suppress T-cell activity and prevent organ rejection. This suppression of T-cell function also disrupts the balance between EBV-induced B-cell proliferations and their destruction by cytotoxic T cells. The result is a decreased or absent cytotoxic T-cell response and uncontrolled B-cell proliferations. Initially, these proliferations are predominantly plasmacytic and polyclonal and contain evidence for multiple EBV infection events. However, from these polyclonal, plasmacytic expansions, oligoclonal and monoclonal populations with a single form of EBV can develop and proliferate. If such proliferation is followed by the activation of an oncogene or inactivation of a tumor suppressor gene, frank malignancy may develop.

36.1.2 Clinical Findings

The clinical presentation of patients with PTLDs can vary and often depends on the organ transplanted, the age of the patient, and the immunosuppressive regimen used. The presentation can be as mild as infectious mononucleosis–like symptoms—including fever, sore throat, and cervical adenopathy—to widespread multi-organ involvement with extensive lymphadenopathy. Three categories of presentation have been described. They include those patients who present with only mononucleosislike symptoms, those with gastrointestinal (GI) tract symptoms such as abdominal pain, and those who present with evidence of systemic and solid organ involvement. The first category typically includes younger patients who present within the first few months following transplantation. The latter category usually includes older patients with presentation of disease several years following transplantation. Treatment with cyclosporin A is associated with a higher frequency of GI tract involvement by PTLD.

36.1.3 Diagnostic Approach

The diagnosis of a PTLD typically requires the histologic examination of a tissue sample from the suspected site of involvement. This may represent a lymph node, GI tract, or solid tumor biopsy. The following steps to diagnosis should be considered:

1. Thorough review of the patient's history, including the date and type of transplantation, immunosuppressive regimen, and EBV status prior to transplantation.
2. Appropriate laboratory tests, including EBV serology as warranted. Imaging studies may be needed, depending on the patient's complaints and symptoms.

3. Physical examination with an emphasis on the presence of adenopathy, solid tumor masses, and GI and mononucleosis-like symptoms.
4. Biopsy and morphologic examination of tissue from the suspected site of involvement.
5. Appropriate adjunctive studies, including immunohistochemistry, in situ hybridization, and gene rearrangement analysis by Southern blot hybridization or polymerase chain reaction (PCR), as warranted.

36.1.4 Histologic Features

The PTLDs represent a spectrum of EBV-induced lymphoid disorders with variable histology. Although the morphologic appearance of these disorders can be diverse, they generally can be divided into three distinct categories: plasmacytic hyperplasias; polymorphic proliferations, including B-cell hyperplasias and B-cell lymphomas; and monomorphic proliferations, including immunoblastic lymphoma and multiple myeloma (**Table 36-1**). Because of their unpredictable response to treatment, many believe that these proliferations should be labeled PTLDs with specific reference to their general category of subtype and not outright lymphomas.

The plasmacytic hyperplasias are most commonly seen in the oropharynx and regional lymph nodes. They are characterized by a proliferation of plasma cells and plasmacytoid lymphocytes with occasional immunoblasts; the underlying architecture of the involved tissue or lymph node remains intact. The lymphoid cells are nearly always polyclonal and exhibit evidence of multiple EBV infection events.

The polymorphic proliferations, including polymorphic B-cell hyperplasias and polymorphic B-cell lymphomas, are grouped together because they share many similar features and are sometimes difficult to distinguish from each other. They frequently arise in extranodal sites, including the GI tract and lung, or within lymph nodes. They typically are monoclonal and contain a single form of EBV. Histologically, they exhibit diffuse effacement of the normal underlying architecture and are composed of a heterogeneous infiltrate of lymphoid cells, including small round or angulated cells, large centroblastlike cells, immunoblasts, and plasma cells. The polymorphic B-cell hyperplasias also exhibit single-cell necrosis but no atypical lymphoid cells. In contrast, the polymorphic B-cell lymphomas frequently exhibit geographic necrosis and large atyp-

Table 36-1 General Categories of Posttransplantation Lymphoproliferative Disorders

Category	Common Site Involvement	Histologic Features	Comments
Plasmacytic hyperplasia	Oropharynx and regional lymph nodes	Proliferation of plasma cells, plasmacytoid lymphocytes and rare immunoblasts Architecture maintained	Polyclonal with multiple EBV infection events
Polymorphic proliferations Polymorphic B-cell hyperplasia Polymorphic B-cell lymphoma	Nodal and extranodal sites (commonly lung and GI tract)	Heterogeneous proliferation of small and angulated cells, large centroblast-like cells, immunoblasts, and plasma cells Tissue architecture effaced	Monoclonal with a single form of EBV Polymorphic B-cell hyperplasia exhibits single-cell necrosis but no atypical cells Polymorphic B-cell lymphoma may have geographic necrosis and numerous atypical cells
Monomorphic proliferations* Immunoblastic lymphoma Multiple myeloma	Systemic or diffuse solid organ involvement	Histologic features similar to those seen in neoplasms in nonimmunocompromised patients	Monoclonal with single form of EBV Frequently contain abnormalities in oncogenes and/or tumor suppressor genes

Abbreviations: EBV = Epstein-Barr virus; GI = gastrointestinal.
*Other types of monomorphic lymphoid proliferations besides immunoblastic lymphoma and multiple myeloma may be seen.

ical mononuclear cells, some of which may resemble Reed-Sternberg cells (**Image 36-1**).

The monomorphic proliferations, such as immunoblastic lymphoma and multiple myeloma, exhibit histologic features similar to those seen in a nonimmunocompromised host. The immunoblastic lymphomas are always diffuse and composed of a relatively uniform population of neoplastic cells with prominent nucleoli. Similarly, the multiple myelomas are composed of a monotypic population of cytologically atypical plasma cells. This category of neoplasms is always monoclonal, usually presents with systemic disease, contains a single form of EBV, and often contains abnormalities in one or more tumor suppressor genes or oncogenes. Morphologic subtypes of monomorphic proliferations other than immunoblastic lymphoma and multiple myeloma have been described. They are typically high-grade neoplasms.

36.1.5 Ancillary Tests

Immunohistochemical stains to identify EBV latent membrane proteins and in situ hybridization studies such as EBER-1 (EBV early RNA) to document the presence of EBV genomic elements are typically used (**Image 36-2**). In addition, antigen receptor gene rearrangement studies by Southern blot hybridization or PCR may be indicated to determine clonality but are not predictable of biologic behavior. Correlation of the histologic findings with EBV serologic studies is recommended.

36.1.6 Course and Treatment

The initial treatment of PTLDs commonly involves the withdrawal of immunosuppression. This alone may result in complete regression of the lymphoid proliferation. Some clinicians also use antiviral therapy such as acyclovir and interferon-α. Frequently these regimens are most useful in treating the plasmacytic hyperplasias and polymorphic B-cell hyperplasias. The polymorphic and monomorphic lymphoma subtypes of PTLDs are more commonly treated with standard chemotherapeutic regimens, particularly if they fail to respond to withdrawal of immunosuppression.

The response to treatment varies greatly within each category of PTLD and among patients. Furthermore, the documentation of monoclonality does not definitively predict biologic behavior. In addition, it may not be feasible to reduce the amount of immunosuppression in some patients.

36.2 Graft-Versus-Host Disease

GVHD is a common complication of allogeneic bone marrow transplantation. It occurs in 20% to 50% of HLA identical and 70%

to 90% of nonidentical and unrelated allogeneic BMT recipients. Classically, GVHD has been divided into two forms, acute and chronic. Acute disease occurs within 100 days after transplantation, and chronic disease represents persistent acute disease or disease that occurs more than 200 days following transplantation. One third of the deaths within 6 months following allogeneic bone marrow transplantation can be attributed to GVHD.

36.2.1 Pathophysiology

The mechanism of GVHD is incompletely understood. It is generally accepted that donor T lymphocytes react against isoantigens in recipient host tissue. Prior to the development of GVHD, recipient target tissues increase their expression of HLA antigens and leukocyte adhesion molecules as a result of chemotherapeutic regimens, infections, and the presence of malignancy. The donor T lymphocytes, which are introduced into the recipient as a minor component of the BMT specimen, recognize the HLA antigens in recipient tissue. The donor T cells are activated, proliferate, secrete interleukin-2 (IL-2), and express IL-2 receptors on their cell surfaces in response to the recipient antigens. The secreted IL-2 stimulates donor mononuclear cells to secrete other cytokines, including IL-1, tumor necrosis factor, and interferon. These three cytokines are thought to be responsible for the tissue damage seen with GVHD. CD8+ cytotoxic T cells are believed to be the donor lymphocyte population involved in GVHD. Immunostaining of the lymphoid infiltrates seen in GVHD shows a predominance of these cells in established disease; however, early lesions may contain a mixture of CD4+ and CD8+ cells.

36.2.2 Clinical Findings

As already mentioned, GVHD can arbitrarily be divided into acute and chronic forms. Acute GVHD principally targets the skin and related appendages, the GI tract, and the liver. Initially, the skin is most commonly involved; an erythematous maculopapular rash develops on the palms, soles, and upper trunk. The rash then spreads to involve other areas, and occasionally the entire body is involved. Following rash formation, patients may develop bullous lesions and, if the disease is severe, desquamation of large patches of skin. Gastrointestinal tract involvement usually presents as nausea, abdominal pain, and diarrhea. The diarrhea may be profuse and is frequently bloody. Liver involvement is typically manifested by vomiting, nausea, and elevated liver function tests. Patients with GVHD commonly have oral involvement affecting the squamous mucosa and minor salivary glands. Oral GVHD is often associated with xerostomia. Chronic GVHD is characterized by autoimmunelike symptoms, wasting, recurrent infections, and prolonged immunodeficiency.

36.2.3 Diagnostic Approach

The diagnosis of acute GVHD based solely on clinical findings can be difficult. The clinical manifestations of drug reactions, chemotherapy effect, PTLDs, and infections (particularly viral) can mimic GVHD. Frequently, a skin, mucosal, minor salivary gland, or rectal biopsy is performed for histologic evaluation. The following steps to diagnosis should be considered:

1. Thorough review of the patient's history, including the date and type of transplantation, drug treatment, and previously diagnosed infections.
2. Appropriate laboratory tests and radiographic studies, as warranted.
3. Physical examination with emphasis on skin, oral mucosa, and GI signs and symptoms.
4. Skin, mucosa, minor salivary gland, and/or rectal biopsy to determine the etiology of the clinical findings.

36.2.4 Hematologic and Histologic Findings

Blood Cell and Chemistry Measurements

The peripheral blood cell counts and morphology can vary greatly and be nonspecific, depending on when the transplantation occurred. Frequently, affected patients may exhibit different degrees of cytopenia as a result of chemotherapeutic and irradiation regimens associated with the transplantation. Reactive changes may be seen if there is a concurrent infection.

Liver enzymes, including alanine aminotransferase (ALT), aspartate aminotransferase (AST), and lactate dehydrogenase (LDH), are often elevated with GVHD involvement of the liver. Veno-occlusive disease, another complication of allogeneic bone marrow transplantation, which is characterized by jaundice, hepatomegaly, and weight gain, also can result in increased liver enzymes.

Skin Biopsy

The histologic interpretation of skin biopsies in patients suspected of having GVHD can be difficult. Early in the disease process, the findings may be minimal, nonspecific, or variable. Lerner et al proposed a histologic grading schema of 0 to IV for skin biopsies based on the severity of the findings (**Table 36-2**). Grade I represents only very mild changes with focal or diffuse vacuolar degeneration of the acanthocytes or basal epithelial cells. In addition to the features seen in grade I disease, patients with grade II disease exhibit dyskeratosis and apoptotic degeneration of individual keratinocytes with associated spongiosis and edema of the overlying epithelium (**Image 36-3**). The apoptotic keratinocytes (**Image 36-3, inset**), which are commonly referred to as "eosinophilic bodies", are often surrounded by lymphocytes. Grade III disease involves grade II changes as well as splitting and degeneration of the acanthocytes and basal cells, resulting in cleft formation and separation of the dermal-epidermal junction. Grade IV disease is characterized by sloughing of the overlying epithelium. The designation grade 0 is reserved for biopsies without definitive evidence of GVHD.

There has been some controversy over the importance of a lymphocytic infiltrate being present in GVHD. It is generally agreed that there is commonly at least a mild to moderate infiltrate of lymphocytes within the superficial dermis that extends focally into the overlying epithelium. Definitive cases of GVHD, however, have been reported without evidence of a lymphocytic infiltrate.

The findings of GVHD seen in rectal biopsies are somewhat similar to those found in the skin. Early in the disease course there is flattening or atrophy of the overlying epithelium, which is often associated with degeneration and loss of crypts. Individual necrotic epithelial cells or apoptotic bodies with associated nuclear "dust" may be seen and are occasionally surrounded by lymphocytes (**Image 36-4**). With more severe disease, sloughing of the epithelium may be prominent. GVHD involving the minor salivary glands is divided into two grades characterized by abnormal periductal mononuclear infiltrates (grade I), which can be accompanied by ductal epithelial necrosis with dilation, and obliteration of the ducts (grade II).

Table 36-2 Histologic Grading of Graft-Versus-Host Disease (GVHD) in Skin Biopsies

Grade	Histologic Findings
0	No specific changes or features of GVHD as described below
I	Focal or diffuse vacuolar degeneration of the acanthocytes
II	Dyskeratosis and apoptotic degeneration of individual keratinocytes and spongiosis of overlying epithelium, in addition to grade I changes
III	Cleft formation and separation of the dermal-epidermal junction and acanthotic layer, in addition to grade II changes
IV	Sloughing and denudation of the overlying epithelium

Source: Lerner K, Kao G, Storb R, et al. Histopathology of graft-vs.-host reaction (GvHR) in human recipients of marrow from HLA-matched sibling donors. *Transplant Proc.* 1974;6:367–371.

36.2.5 Ancillary Tests

If classic clinical and histologic features of GVHD are not present, other diagnoses such as a drug reaction or infection must be entertained. In addition to Gram's, periodic acid–Schiff, and silver stains, immunohistochemical and in situ hybridization studies may be necessary to definitively document the presence of infection in these cases.

36.2.6 Course and Treatment

GVHD can be a life-threatening disorder in allogeneic BMT patients if left untreated. The key to successful treatment is the early identification and institution of appropriate therapy. Unlike the treatment for PTLD and infection, GVHD is frequently treated with increased systemic immunosuppression, which can include chemotherapeutic regimens, specific immunosuppressive agents, and steroids. Irradiation therapy also is used occasionally. The dichotomy in the treatment of GVHD as compared with that for PTLDs and infections emphasizes the need for a prompt and accurate diagnosis.

36.3 Additional Complications of Solid Organ and Bone Marrow Transplantation

36.3.1 Infection

Infection is a significant complication of organ transplantation and is responsible for substantial morbidity and mortality. Although improved antibiotics, prophylactic regimens, and detection systems have made great strides in the prevention and treatment of infections, they remain a major difficulty. A myriad of organisms can be responsible for infection in transplant recipients. They include the classic bacterial groups such as *Streptococcus* and *Staphylococcus* and more commonly opportunistic organisms such as viruses, atypical bacteria, fungi, and protozoa. Opportunistic infections commonly seen in transplantation patients are listed in **Table 36-3**. The patient's clinical history and a high index of suspicion can aid in detecting such infections. In addition to the morphologic detection of infections, special studies such as immunohistochemistry and in situ hybridization may be necessary (**Images 36-5** and **36-6**).

36.3.2 Nonengraftment

Allogeneic and autologous bone marrow transplantation is used to treat diverse malignant and nonmalignant conditions. Many of the common disorders treated with this procedure are listed in **Table 36-4**. Following bone marrow transplantation, it is customary for patients to undergo bone marrow biopsy at regular intervals to document engraftment. The morphologic evaluation of these specimens is necessary to ensure that appropriate trilineage engraftment has occurred. The lack of engraftment and single or bilineage engraftment can result in life-threatening cytopenias.

36.3.3 Rejection

Organ rejection is a complex process in which the transplant recipient's immune system identifies the transplanted organ as non-self or "foreign." The identification of non-self antigens on the transplanted organ evokes an immune response by the recipient involving both the humoral and cellular systems. The contribution of the humoral response to graft rejection is currently an area of intense investigation. It appears that the cellular immune response is more important in organ transplant rejection and is manifested

Table 36-3 Opportunistic Organisms Commonly Seen in Organ Transplant Recipients

Atypical bacteria
>   *Mycobacterium tuberculosis*
>   *Mycobacterium avium-intracellulare*
>   *Listeria monocytogenes*
>   *Nocardia*

Viruses
>   Epstein-Barr virus (EBV)
>   Herpes simplex virus
>   Cytomegalovirus

Fungi
>   *Candida*
>   *Aspergillus*
>   *Cryptococcus neoformans*
>   *Histoplasma capsulatum*

Protozoa
>   *Toxoplasma gondii*
>   *Pneumocystis carinii*

primarily by T lymphocytes and mononuclear cells. The activated recipient lymphocytes and mononuclear cells attack and destroy the transplanted organ.

The immunosuppressive regimens on which most transplant recipients are maintained help control the immune response and prevent transplant rejection. The balance between sufficient and insufficient immunosuppression is a challenge in caring for these patients. Matching the donor and recipient at specific HLA loci helps decrease the potential and severity of organ rejection. Specialized texts provide more specific and in-depth descriptions of specific organ transplant rejection.

36.4 Other Considerations

36.4.1 Growth Factor Effect

Cytopenias, including neutropenia, are common sequelae following intense chemotherapy administration. Many antineoplastic

Table 36-4 Disorders Commonly Treated With Bone Marrow Transplantation

Acute leukemia

Malignant lymphoma

Multiple myeloma

Myeloproliferative disorders, including chronic myelogenous leukemia

Myelodysplastic syndromes

Solid tumors, including breast carcinoma and neuroblastoma

Aplastic anemia

Paroxysmal nocturnal hemoglobinuria

Wiskott-Aldrich syndrome

Fanconi's anemia

---

drugs have direct toxic effects on the myeloid precursors within the bone marrow. In addition, during the early weeks and months following bone marrow transplantation, patients frequently remain pancytopenic until the bone marrow has had ample time for reconstitution. The neutropenia that results from chemotherapy administration or bone marrow transplantation is associated with an increased risk and incidence of infection. Infections are a major contributing factor to the morbidity and mortality of transplant patients.

The development and widespread use of recombinant cellular growth factors such as granulocyte-colony-stimulating factor (G-CSF) for the treatment of neutropenia has dramatically decreased neutropenia-associated side effects. The administration of G-CSF, however, is commonly associated with specific morphologic changes seen within the peripheral blood and bone marrow. These changes may be confused with other processes, so it is important to distinguish them. In addition, it is essential to inquire about any recent G-CSF therapy the patient may have been given, so this information may be used in interpretation.

36.4.2 Hematologic Findings

Blood Cell Measurements and Peripheral Blood Smear Morphology
The peripheral WBC counts of patients receiving G-CSF can

vary greatly. Factors influencing the WBC count include the dose of G-CSF administered, individual patient response, and where the patient is in the course of therapy. Frequently, the peak WBC count is achieved after 1 to 2 weeks of therapy and is elevated in the range of 20 to 50 × 10³/mm³ (20 to 50 × 10⁹/L). It can, however, approach 100 × 10³/mm³ (100 × 10⁹/L). The WBC differential count typically reveals greater than 80% to 90% granulocytes, with the majority being band forms and segmented neutrophils. It is common to see other myeloid precursors, including metamyelocytes, myelocytes, promyelocytes, and a rare myeloblast. The myeloid cells usually exhibit intense toxic granulation and/or Döhle's bodies (**Image 36-7**). Cytoplasmic vacuolization also may be seen.

Bone Marrow Examination

Similar to the peripheral WBC count following G-CSF therapy, the bone marrow cellularity can vary based on individual patient response and the therapy regimen. Examination of the bone marrow aspirate smear commonly reveals a myeloid hyperplasia. Depending on the stage of G-CSF therapy, the differential count also varies. Early in treatment, promyelocytes and myeloblasts often predominate, resulting in a morphologic appearance that may be confused with acute leukemia. Later in therapy, as the myeloid cells have time to mature, there is a spectrum of myeloid cells with many more mature forms (**Image 36-8**). At this stage, chronic myelogenous leukemia may be considered in the differential diagnosis if there is no history of G-CSF therapy. At all stages of therapy, the myeloid precursors typically exhibit prominent toxic granulation with Döhle's bodies and cytoplasmic vacuolization.

In patients with a history of acute myelogenous leukemia, G-CSF therapy often presents a challenging dilemma. Particularly early in the course of therapy, it may be difficult to distinguish growth factor effect from relapse. In these cases, it is often wise to err on the side of caution unless definitive evidence of residual or relapsed leukemia is seen. Repeated bone marrow examination in 1 to 2 weeks is often warranted to look for evidence of maturation of the myeloid cells as seen with G-CSF therapy. In addition, reexamination of the bone marrow following discontinuation of therapy may be helpful.

36.4.3 Notes and Precautions

It is of paramount importance to inquire about G-CSF therapy when examining peripheral blood and bone marrow specimens in transplant patients.

36.5 References

Craig F, Gulley M, Banks P. Posttransplantation lymphoproliferative disorders. *Am J Clin Pathol.* 1993;99:265–276.

Harris NL, Jaffe ES, Diebold J, et al. The World Health Organization Classification of Hematological Malignancies Report of the Clinical Advisory Committee Meeting, Airlie House, Virginia, November 1997. *Mod Pathol.* 2000;13(2):193–207.

Kerrigan D, Castillo A, Fourcar K, et al. Peripheral blood morphologic changes after high-dose antineoplastic chemotherapy and recombinant human granulocyte colony-stimulating factor administration. *Am J Clin Pathol.* 1989; 92:280–285.

Knowles DM, Cesarman E, Chadburn A, et al. Correlative morphologic and molecular genetic analysis demonstrates three distinct categories of posttransplantation lymphoproliferative disorders. *Blood.* 1995;85:552–565.

Kohler S, Henderickson M, Chao N, et al. Value of skin biopsies in assessing prognosis and progression of acute graft-versus-host disease. *Am J Surg Pathol.* 1997;21:988–996.

Kolbeck P, Markin R, McManus B. *Transplant Pathology.* Chicago, Ill: ASCP Press; 1994.

Lerner K, Kao G, Storb R, et al. Histopathology of graft-vs-host reaction (GvHR) in human recipients of marrow from HLA-matched sibling donors. *Transplant Proc.* 1974;6:367–371.

Schubert M, Sullivan K. Recognition, incidence and management of oral graft-versus-host disease. *NCI Monogr.* 1990;9:135–143.

Weiss L. *Pathology of Lymph Nodes.* New York, NY: Churchill-Livingstone; 1996.

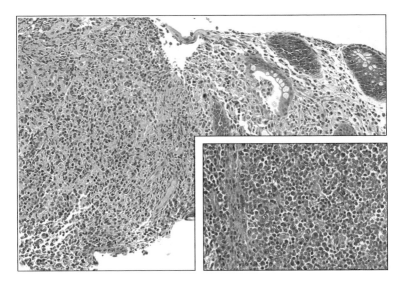

Image 36-1 Posttransplantation lymphoproliferative disorder, polymorphous B-cell lymphoma type, in the colon of a 4-year-old girl who underwent liver transplantation for biliary atresia. Inset shows a high-power view of the polymorphous lymphoid infiltrate, consisting of small round and angulated cells admixed with large atypical cells and plasma cells.

Image 36-2 Posttransplantation lymphoproliferative disorder, monomorphic B-cell lymphoma type, occurring in the lung. The disease has diffusely infiltrated and destroyed the normal pulmonary parenchyma. Inset shows results of an in situ hybridization study using an EBER-1 (EBV early RNA) probe to document the presence of Epstein-Barr virus infection.

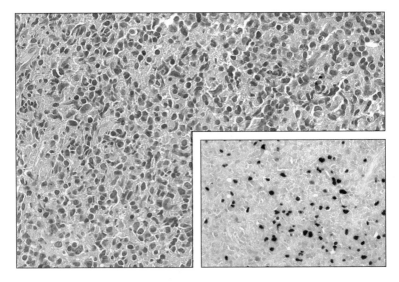

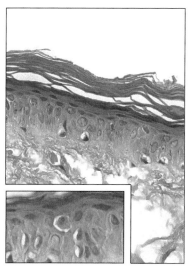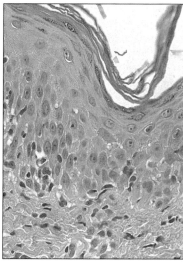

Image 36-3   Graft-versus-host disease, grade II. Left, Superficial skin biopsy with vacuolar degeneration of the basal epithelial cells and occasional apoptotic keratinocytes. Inset shows individual apoptotic keratinocytes. Right, A prominent lymphocytic infiltrate of the superficial dermis extending into the overlying epithelium. A scattered degenerating keratinocyte is evident.

Image 36-4   Rectal biopsy exhibiting graft-versus-host disease characterized by a mild lymphocytic infiltrate and necrosis of individual crypt cells with associated nuclear debris.

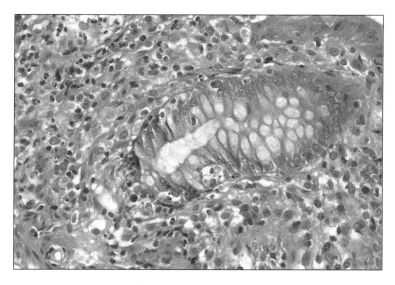

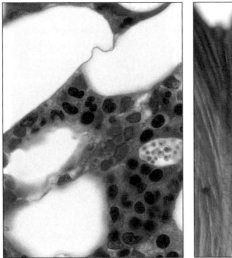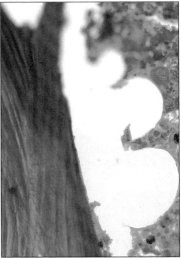

Image 36-5 Posttransplantation infection. Left, Bone marrow biopsy from a lung transplant patient with a history of recurring fevers. Numerous *Histoplasma capsulatum* organisms were identified. Right, Gomori's methenamine silver stain highlighting the presence of multiple aggregates of the organism.

Image 36-6 Esophageal biopsy from a liver transplant patient demonstrating numerous large and occasionally multinucleated cells with an associated inflammatory infiltrate. Inset shows herpes virus-infected cells detected by immunohistochemistry using a probe for herpes simplex virus 2.

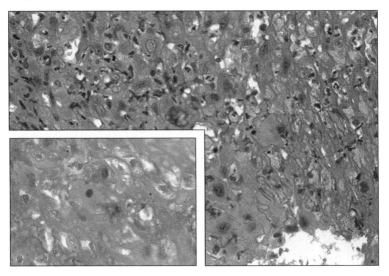

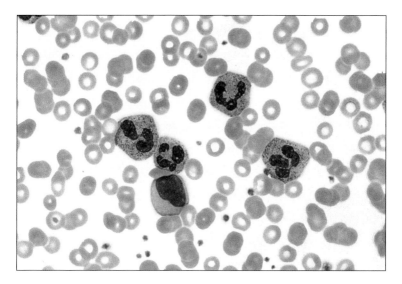

Image 36-7   Peripheral blood smear from a patient treated with granulocyte-colony-stimulating factor. Numerous band forms and segmented neutrophils with prominent toxic granulation and occasional Döhle's bodies can be seen.

Image 36-8   Bone marrow aspirate smear from a bone marrow transplant patient receiving granulocyte-colony-stimulating factor. Myeloid precursors in various stages of maturation with prominent cytoplasmic granulation constitute the majority of marrow elements.

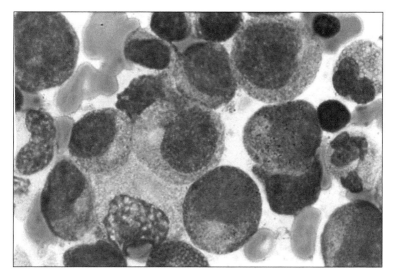

PART
XI

Immunoproliferative
Disorders

37 Multiple Myeloma and Related Disorders

The plasma cell dyscrasias comprise a group of diseases characterized by the proliferation of a single clone of immunoglobulin-producing cells usually recognized as plasma cells or lymphocytes. In these disorders, a single class or subunit of immunoglobulin is almost always secreted and can be detected as a monoclonal peak on electrophoresis of a serum or urine sample. The categories of plasma cell dyscrasias in the proposed World Health Organization (WHO) classification of hematologic malignancies include the following entities: multiple myeloma and variants, plasmacytomas, Waldenström's macroglobulinemia, the heavy-chain diseases, the immunoglobulin deposition diseases, and monoclonal gammopathy of undetermined significance (**Table 37-1**). Multiple myeloma is the focus of this chapter. Plasmacytomas, Waldenström's macroglobulinemia, primary amyloidosis, and the heavy-chain diseases also are discussed. Monoclonal gammopathy of undetermined significance and cryoglobulinemia are discussed in Chapter 38.

37.1 Pathophysiology

Multiple myeloma (plasma cell myeloma) is characterized by a neoplastic proliferation of plasma cells. The plasma cells prolifer-

Table 37-1 Proposed World Health Organization (WHO)
Classification of Plasma Cell Dyscrasias*

Multiple myeloma (plasma cell myeloma)

Myeloma variants
  Plasma cell leukemia
  Indolent myeloma
  Smoldering myeloma
  Osteosclerotic myeloma
  Nonsecretory myeloma

Plasmacytomas
  Solitary plasmacytoma of bone
  Extramedullary plasmacytoma

Waldenström's macroglobulinemia (lymphoplasmacytic lymphoma)

Heavy-chain disease
  γ heavy chain disease
  α heavy chain disease
  μ heavy chain disease

Immunoglobulin deposition diseases
  Systemic light-chain disease
  Primary amyloidosis

Monoclonal gammopathy of undetermined significance

*Harris NL, Jaffee ES, Diebold J, et al. World Health Organization classification of neoplastic diseases of the hematopoietic and lymphoid tissues: report of The Clinical Advisory Committee Meeting–Airlie House, Virginia, November 1997. *J Clin Oncol.* 1999;17:3835–3849.

---

ate throughout the bone marrow and frequently invade adjacent bone, causing widespread skeletal destruction. Other organs may be involved secondarily.

One of the major features of multiple myeloma is the secretion of monoclonal proteins (**Table 37-2**). The protein usually is a complete immunoglobulin molecule with electrophoresis of serum revealing monoclonal IgG or IgA heavy chains combined with κ or λ light chains. Monoclonal immunoglobulins of the IgG type are approximately two to three times more frequent than IgA. Mon-oclonal proteins of IgD or IgE type occur but are rare. In about 20% of patients, only the light-chain portion of the immunoglobulin molecule is present. Light chains are excreted in the urine and usually are detected as a monoclonal peak on urine electrophoresis. Many of the clinical manifestations of multiple myeloma, such as renal insufficiency, are related to the production of monoclonal proteins.

Table 37-2   Monoclonal Immunoglobulins in Malignant
Plasma Cell Dyscrasias

Disease Process	Monoclonal Immunoglobulin	Percentage of Cases
Multiple myeloma*	IgG	55
	IgA	22
	Light chain only	18
	IgD	2
	Biclonal	2
	Nonsecretory	1
	IgE	<1
	IgM	<1
Waldenström's macroglobulinemia	IgM	100
Heavy-chain (HC) diseases†	γ-HC fragment	25
	α-HC fragment	75
	μ-HC fragment	<5

*Kappa light chains are more common than lambda in all immunoglobulin types of myeloma except IgD.
†Percentages are approximate; reliable statistics are not available.

37.2 Clinical Findings

Bone pain, particularly in the back or chest, is the most common symptom of patients with multiple myeloma. Typically, the pain is localized and aggravated by movement. It often is associated with pathologic compression fractures of the thoracic or lumbar spine. Weakness and fatigue, often related to anemia, also are common. Bleeding tendencies, infections, or symptoms of renal failure or hypercalcemia are presenting features of some patients.

Pallor is the most common physical finding. Hepatosplenomegaly is present in 20% and splenomegaly in 5% of patients.

37.3 Approach to Diagnosis

The laboratory studies used to diagnose multiple myeloma are listed. The extent to which these evaluations are done depends on the level of suspicion of the diagnosis.

1. CBC count with leukocyte differential.
2. Bone marrow examination.
3. Serum and urine protein electrophoresis.
4. Serum and urine immunofixation.
5. Quantitation of serum and urine protein.
6. Radiographic skeletal survey.

37.4 Hematologic Findings

Different criteria have been proposed to diagnose multiple myeloma. The minimal criteria require at least 10% plasma cells in the bone marrow or the presence of a plasmacytoma plus one or more of the following:

1. Monoclonal protein in the serum (usually >3 g/dL [>30 g/L]).
2. Monoclonal protein in the urine.
3. Lytic bone lesions.

37.4.1 Blood Cell Measurements

Normochromic normocytic anemia is present in most patients with multiple myeloma at presentation. Leukopenia and thrombocytopenia are present in fewer than 20% of patients at diagnosis but are common in the later stages of the disease.

37.4.2 Peripheral Blood Smear Morphologic Features

Normochromic normocytic anemia is present in most patients at diagnosis. Leukopenia and thrombocytopenia are less common but often develop during the course of the disease. Rouleaux formation (**Image 37-1**) may be striking. The degree of rouleaux formation correlates with the magnitude of the monoclonal immunoglobulin and parallels the erythrocyte sedimentation rate. Occasional circulating plasma cells may be present.

37.4.3 Bone Marrow Examination

Bone marrow aspirate smears and trephine biopsy sections are essential for adequate evaluation for multiple myeloma. The plasma cells compose greater than 10% of the nucleated cells in the aspirate and usually average about 20% to 40%. The plasma cells vary from mature-appearing cells to those resembling blasts (**Image 37-2**). They vary in size with moderate to abundant basophilic cytoplasm. The nuclei often are larger than normal and the chromatin less condensed. Multinucleation may be present. Nucleoli often are prominent, and intranuclear inclusions may be apparent. Several types of cytoplasmic inclusions have been described in the plasma cells, including hyaline inclusions, crystalline inclusions, vacuoles, and granules. Patients with IgA myeloma tend to have strikingly pleomorphic plasma cells, including multinucleated cells, flaming plasma cells, and frequent intranuclear inclusions.

In trephine biopsy specimens, the plasma cell infiltrate is interstitial, focal, or diffuse. With diffuse involvement, large areas of normal hematopoietic tissue are replaced.

Plasma cells contain abundant cytoplasmic immunoglobulin and usually react strongly with antibodies to κ or λ light chains. This property can be used in immunohistochemical techniques to identify and quantify the number of plasma cells in bone marrow trephine biopsy sections and to evaluate a plasma cell population for clonality (**Image 37-3**). The plasma cells in myeloma exhibit a monoclonal pattern of reactivity with antibodies against κ or λ light chains. The ratio of the predominant light chain to the normal light chain is abnormal and usually is greater than 16:1. In reactive plasma cell proliferations, a mixture of κ- and λ-positive cells is present. This technique is especially useful when the percentage of plasma cells is low and in the rare cases in which no monoclonal protein is identified in the serum or urine sample.

37.5 Variants of Multiple Myeloma

37.5.1 Plasma Cell Leukemia

Plasma cell leukemia is the leukemic variant of multiple myeloma. Plasma cell leukemia is primary when it is diagnosed in the leukemic phase and secondary when it represents a leukemic transformation of previously diagnosed multiple myeloma. Plasma cell leukemia can be diagnosed when the peripheral blood contains greater than 20% plasma cells and the absolute plasma cell count is greater than $2.0 \times 10^3/mm^3$ (2.0×10^9/L) (**Image 37-4**). Patients with primary plasma cell leukemia tend to be younger than those with secondary plasma cell leukemia. They have hepatosplenomegaly and lymphadenopathy more often, fewer lytic lesions, and lower levels of monoclonal proteins. The prognosis for patients with plasma cell leukemia is very poor.

37.5.2 Smoldering and Indolent Multiple Myeloma

Smoldering multiple myeloma is the designation used to describe patients who meet the criteria for the diagnosis of multiple myeloma but have a stable disease course for months or years. They do not have anemia, bone lesions, renal insufficiency, or hypercalcemia. The patients have greater than 10% plasma cells in the bone marrow and a monoclonal protein in the serum or urine. The diagnostic criteria for *indolent multiple myeloma* are similar to those for smoldering multiple myeloma, but the patients may exhibit a few bone lesions and mild anemia. Overt multiple myeloma develops in most patients with the indolent variant in about 3 years.

37.5.3 Osteoslerotic Myeloma

Osteoslerotic myeloma is a component of a rare syndrome that includes polyneuropathy, organomegaly, endocrinopathy, monoclonal gammopathy, and skin lesions (POEMS syndrome).

37.5.4 Nonsecretory Multiple Myeloma

Nonsecretory multiple myeloma is a rare variant of multiple myeloma in which no monoclonal protein can be detected in the serum or urine. Other diagnostic features of multiple myeloma, including osteolytic lesions and bone marrow plasmacytosis, are present. Renal failure and hypercalcemia are absent. For diagnosis of multiple myeloma, a monoclonal protein should be identified in the plasma cells by immunostaining or other method.

Other Laboratory Tests

Test 37.1 **Serum Protein Electrophoresis**

Purpose. Serum protein electrophoresis should be done to evaluate for the presence of a monoclonal immunoglobulin whenever multiple myeloma or another plasma cell dyscrasia is suspected.

Principle. Proteins migrate in an electrical field. A monoclonal protein migrates to a single location, creating a dense discrete band on the agarose gel (**Figure 37-1**) or a narrow spike in the densitometric tracing.

Specimen. Serum.

Procedure. A high-resolution technique that provides clear separation of β-1 (transferrin) and β-2 (C3) bands is preferred. High-resolution agarose gel electrophoresis separates as many as 12 protein fractions and is sensitive for the detection of small monoclonal proteins. After electrophoresis the gels are fixed and stained, and the protein fractions are quantitated with densitometry.

Interpretation. Monoclonal immunoglobulins usually appear in the γ region but also can be found in the β or α_2-globulin area. Polyclonal increases in immunoglobulins produce broad bands or peaks and usually are limited to the γ region. Immunofix-ation should be performed whenever a band or peak is seen to identify the monoclonal protein. Hypogammaglobulinemia is characterized by a decrease in the γ component and is seen in about 10% of patients with multiple myeloma without a serum spike. Most of these patients exhibit monoclonal free light chains (Bence Jones protein) in the urine.

A small monoclonal protein may be present even when the total proteins and quantitative immunoglobulins are all within the reference ranges. Such proteins may be concealed in the normal β or γ components. In IgD myeloma, the monoclonal peak is small and also may be overlooked. Monoclonal light chains usually are too low to be detected. Immunofixation should be done whenever multiple myeloma or a related disorder is suspected.

Figure 37-1   High resolution serum protein electrophoresis
reveals a dense discrete band (M) in the γ region.
Control (C) specimen is below patient (P)
specimen. (Electrophoresis courtesy of D. Keren,
MD.)

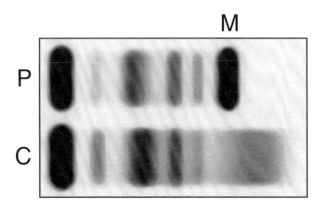

Test 37.2   **Urine Electrophoresis**

Purpose. Urine electrophoresis is done to determine the presence
or absence of a monoclonal protein in patients suspected of
having multiple myeloma or other plasma cell dyscrasia.
Classic heat precipitation tests for Bence Jones protein are not
reliable and should be abandoned.

Principle. As in serum, a monoclonal protein migrates as a band
on electrophoresis.

Specimen. A 24-hour collection of urine should be done, from
which the total protein excreted is determined. Then an aliquot
of the urine is concentrated for electrophoresis.

Procedure. Urine electrophoresis is performed and a densitometric scan done.

Interpretation. A urine monoclonal protein is seen on electrophoresis as a dense band strip or a narrow peak on the den-
sitometer tracing. The protein should be characterized further

by immunofixation. Measurement of the monoclonal protein is determined by multiplying the percentage of the monoclonal spike by the total protein in the 24-hour specimen. Occasionally, urine electrophoresis is positive for monoclonal protein when the serum is negative, and some cases have light chains in the urine and complete immunoglobulin or a mixture of light chains and complete immunoglobulin in the serum.

Test 37.3 Serum and Urine Immunofixation

Purpose. Immunofixation of serum and urine samples should be done when a dense band or sharp peak is noted with serum protein electrophoresis, when multiple myeloma or other plasma cell dyscrasia is suspected, or when the serum protein electrophoresis banding pattern changes in a patient previously diagnosed with a plasma cell dyscrasia. Immunofixation is the method of choice to identify monoclonal immunoglobulins. Immunofixation is critical for the differentiation of monoclonal from polyclonal increases in immunoglobulins. It is also helpful for detecting small monoclonal proteins or biclonal or triclonal gammopathies.

Principle. Proteins are separated in urine or serum by electrophoresis and then incubated with specific antisera against immunoglobulins of interest. Immune precipitates occur at the sites of antigen-antibody reaction.

Specimen. Serum or aliquot of a concentrated 24-hour urine specimen.

Procedure. The patient's serum or urine sample is placed in application slits on the electrophoretic gel, and the proteins are separated by electrophoresis. Following electrophoresis, specific antibody for each immunoglobulin is applied to the lanes. Precipitin bands that form at the site of antigen-antibody reactions are stained and analyzed.

Interpretation. A sharp narrow band indicates a monoclonal protein (**Figure 37-2**), whereas a broad blurred band is consistent with polyclonality.

About 90% of patients with multiple myeloma have a serum monoclonal protein at diagnosis. Approximately 80% have a urine monoclonal protein at diagnosis. Of patients with multiple myeloma, 99% have a monoclonal protein in the

Figure 37-2 Immunofixation of serum documenting an IgG κ monoclonal protein.

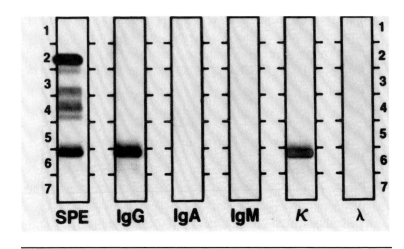

serum or urine at diagnosis. The incidence of the various mon-oclonal immunoglobulins in multiple myeloma is shown in **Table 37-2**.

Test 37.4 **Serum Immunoglobulin Quantitation**

Purpose. This procedure is to obtain objective and reproducible information about the quantity of the immunoglobulins present.

Principle. Rate nephelometry is the preferred method of immunoglobulin quantitation. The degree of turbidity produced by antigen-antibody interactions is measured with nephelometry.

Specimen. Serum.

Procedure. Specific antisera are mixed with serum in a series of fixed dilutions. A background measurement is taken when the patient's specimen is added, and the rate of increase in light scattered is measured. A microprocessor calculates the concentration of immunoglobulin.

Interpretation. Levels of monoclonal protein greater than 3 g/dL (30 g/L) usually indicate an overt multiple myeloma or macroglobulinemia. Levels of the uninvolved immunoglobulin classes almost always are reduced in multiple myeloma.

Quantification of the monoclonal protein is best accomplished by densitometric scan. Nephelometry quantitates the total isotype and not just the monoclonal protein.

37.6 Ancillary Tests

37.6.1 Immunophenotyping by Flow Cytometry

Plasma cells are mature B cells that lack surface immunoglobulin but express abundant cytoplasmic immunoglobulin. They also usually lack several B-cell antigens, including CD19 and CD20, and strongly express CD38. The combination of strong CD38 expression and monotypic cytoplasmic immunoglobulin is characteristic of multiple myeloma.

37.6.2 Tests of Renal Function

Serum creatinine is elevated in 50% of patients at diagnosis. The two major causes of renal insufficiency are myeloma kidney and hypercalcemia. Myeloma kidney is characterized by waxy laminated casts in the distal and collecting tubules and correlates with the amount of free light chain in the urine and the severity of the renal insufficiency. Amyloidosis (see "Primary Amyloidosis") occurs in 10% to 15% of patients with multiple myeloma and may cause renal insufficiency or nephrotic syndrome.

37.6.3 Bone Radiographs

Bone radiographs show osteolytic lesions, osteoporosis, or fractures in 80% of patients at diagnosis. The skull, ribs, vertebrae, and long bones are the most frequently involved. Bone scans do not demonstrate lytic lesions well, but computed tomographic scans may identify myeloma infiltrates when radiograph findings are normal in patients with severe bone pain.

37.6.4 Serum Viscosity

Serum viscosity should be determined when IgG or IgA levels are greater than 6.0 g/dL (60 g/L) or if IgM is greater than 4.0 g/dL (40 g/L) and for any patient in whom symptoms suggest a hyperviscosity syndrome. Symptoms of hyperviscosity are rare unless the value is greater than 4 centipoises, but the relationship between serum viscosity and symptoms is not precise.

37.7 Course and Treatment

Most patients with multiple myeloma have a progressive course with a median survival of about 3 years. Survival is related overall to the extent of disease at diagnosis. About 10% of patients with multiple myeloma, however, have a chronic course and survive for longer than 10 years; many of these patients have a smoldering or indolent myeloma. The most common cause of death is infection. Renal failure contributes to death in many patients. The standard therapy for symptomatic patients is alkylating agent chemotherapy. Melphalan or cyclophosphamide are used as single agents, combined with corticosteroids, or as components of multidrug chemotherapeutic regimens. Autologous and allogeneic bone marrow transplantations are being performed for an increasing number of patients.

37.8 Other Plasma Cell Dyscrasias

37.8.1 Plasmacytomas

Plasmacytomas fall into one of two general categories: (1) solitary plasmacytoma of bone and (2) extramedullary plasmacytoma.

Solitary plasmacytomas of bone are localized plasma cell tumors. The spine, long bones, and pelvis are the most common sites of involvement. The diagnostic criteria of a solitary plasmacytoma include the following: (1) bone lesion with monoclonal plasma cell infiltrate (**Image 37-5**), (2) absence of other lytic bone lesions, and (3) absence of plasma cell infiltrates in random bone marrow biopsy specimens. Myeloma eventually develops in most patients with solitary plasmacytoma.

Extramedullary plasmacytomas are plasma cell tumors that arise outside the bone marrow. The upper respiratory tract, including the nasal cavity, nasopharynx, and sinuses, is the most common location for these tumors (**Image 37-6**). Patients with extra-medullary plasmacytoma may have local recurrence. The rate of evolution to multiple myeloma is less than with solitary plasmacytoma of bone.

37.8.2 Waldenström's Macroglobulinemia (Lymphoplasmacytic Lymphoma)

Waldenström's macroglobulinemia is a lymphoplasmacytic lymphoma associated with the production of monoclonal IgM. The bone marrow is involved with the lymphoma in most patients, and lymphadenopathy and hepatosplenomegaly are common. The median age at diagnosis is about 60 years, and more than half of the patients are men. The most frequent symptoms include weakness, fatigue, and bleeding. Some patients suffer from hyperviscosity syndrome related to increased levels of the monoclonal proteins. Physical findings include pallor, lymphadenopathy, and hepatosplenomegaly. Retinal hemorrhages and venous congestion may be present. In contrast with multiple myeloma, lytic bone lesions usually are absent.

Most patients have a moderate to severe normochromic normocytic anemia with marked rouleaux formation. About 30% of patients have a leukemic blood picture consisting of lymphocytes, lymphoplasmacytoid lymphocytes, and occasional plasma cells. The malignant cells exhibit strong surface and/or cytoplasmic immunoglobulin and are CD19+, CD20+/–, CD22+, CD5–, and CD10–. Leukopenia and thrombocytopenia may be present.

The bone marrow aspirate specimen shows increased numbers of well-differentiated lymphocytes and plasmacytoid lymphocytes. The numbers of plasma cells, mast cells, and histiocytes almost always are increased. The extent of involvement in the biopsy specimens varies from small focal lesions to extensive bone marrow replacement. The pattern of infiltration is interstitial, focal, or diffuse. The infiltrating cells range from lymphocytes to plasma cells (**Image 37-7**). Intranuclear inclusions (Dutcher bodies) commonly are observed but are not specific for this disease.

Serum protein electrophoresis shows a tall peak or band, usually in the γ region. Immunoelectrophoresis characterizes the peak as IgM; 75% of IgM proteins have a κ light chain. The amount of uninvolved immunoglobulins is decreased in half the patients. A small amount of light chain often is present in the urine. Serum viscosity is increased in 90% of patients and may lead to clinical symptoms. Defects in platelet function and inhibition of coagulation factors often are related to the elevation in the IgM level and may be associated with a bleeding diathesis.

The median survival for patients with macroglobulinemia is 5 years. Treatment is aimed at ameliorating the hyperviscosity syndrome and treating the underlying lymphoma. Plasmapheresis often is used for patients who have symptoms from hyperviscosity syndrome.

37.8.3 Primary Amyloidosis

Amyloid is a fibrillary protein that is deposited in various tissues and may damage involved vital organs, such as the heart and kidneys. Systemic amyloidosis consists of three major types: primary amyloidosis (AL), secondary amyloidosis (AA), and familial amyloidosis (AF). Primary amyloidosis is the only one of these disorders associated with plasma cell dyscrasias and is discussed in this section.

In primary amyloidosis, the amyloid is derived from all or part of a monoclonal immunoglobulin light chain. About 20% of patients with primary amyloidosis have multiple myeloma; most of the remaining patients have plasmacytosis in the bone marrow, but the diagnostic criteria for myeloma are lacking.

Primary amyloidosis is rare. Most patients are between 60 and 70 years of age at diagnosis. Two thirds of the patients are men. Weight loss and fatigue are the most common presenting features. Symptoms related to congestive heart failure, peripheral neuropathy, nephrotic syndrome, and bleeding tendency also are relatively common.

A monoclonal protein can be identified in urine or serum in 80% to 90% of patients with primary amyloidosis. A monoclonal protein is found in serum in about two thirds of patients. Two thirds of patients have a monoclonal protein in the urine; λ chains are more common than κ chains at a ratio of about 3:1. The monoclonal spike often is small. It manifests as light chains only in the urine in about 20% of patients. The protein may be missed by screening with serum or urine protein electrophoresis; therefore, immunofixation of serum or urine should be done whenever amyloidosis is suspected. Evidence of nephrotic syndrome is present in about 35% of patients. The serum creatinine level is elevated in 20% to 25% of patients. Acquired coagulation factor X deficiency may be present secondary to binding of the factor to amyloid protein.

A diagnosis of amyloidosis is made by demonstration of amyloid in a biopsy specimen of an affected organ, such as the kidney or heart. Subcutaneous fat aspirate samples and rectal biopsy specimens each are diagnostic in about 80% of cases. Results of bone marrow biopsy specimens are positive in about 50% of cases. Amyloid stains pale pink with H&E stain. Its presence is confirmed with a Congo red stain that produces a characteristic apple-green birefringence when viewed with polarized light microscopy. Ultrastructurally, the amyloid consists of fine, linear, nonbranching fibrils.

Peripheral blood cell counts often are normal in patients with primary amyloidosis at diagnosis, but cytopenias are common in patients having concurrent multiple myeloma. Rouleaux formation may be increased in patients with a large monoclonal spike. About 20% of patients with primary amyloidosis have bone marrow findings that are diagnostic of multiple myeloma. In these patients, amyloid usually can be demonstrated in the bone marrow core biopsy section. Patients with primary amyloidosis but without myeloma frequently have increased numbers of plasma cells, but the plasma cells usually are less than 10% of the bone marrow cells. Immunostaining for κ and λ light chains reveals that the plasma cells often are clonal, even if the diagnostic criteria for myeloma are not present. In patients without multiple myeloma, amyloidosis is demonstrated in the bone marrow in fewer than 50% of the cases. When present in the bone marrow trephine biopsy section, the amyloid frequently is localized to the walls of blood vessels (**Image 37-8**). Rarely, the entire bone marrow core biopsy specimen is replaced with amyloid.

Treatment of primary amyloidosis is directed at controlling amyloid production. Alkylating agent therapy in combination with corticosteroids is the standard chemotherapeutic regimen. The overall survival rate for patients with amyloidosis, however, is poor. The median survival times range from 12 to 24 months from diagnosis. The most frequent causes of death include cardiac disease, renal failure, infection, and hemorrhage.

37.8.4 Heavy-Chain Disease

Heavy-chain diseases (HCDs) are rare malignant disorders characterized by the production of an incomplete monoclonal immunoglobulin heavy chain. The clinical picture in HCD differs from that in multiple myeloma. There are three types of heavy chain diseases: HCD, with features of lymphoplasmacytic lymphoma; HCD, characterized by a small bowel infiltrate that may cause malabsorption (immunoproliferative small intestinal disorder); and HCD, with features similar to chronic lymphocytic leukemia.

37.9 References

Anderson KC, Hamblin TJ, Traynor A. Management of multiple myeloma today. *Semin Hematol.* 1999;36:3–8.

Brunning RD, McKenna RW. Plasma cell dyscrasias and related disorders. In: *Atlas of Tumor Pathology: Tumors of the Bone Marrow.* Fascicle 9, 3rd Series. Washington, DC: Armed Forces Institute of Pathology; 1994:323–367.

Buxbaum J. Mechanisms of disease: monoclonal immunoglobulin deposition: amyloidosis, light chain deposition disease, and light and heavy chain deposition disease. *Hematol Oncol Clin North Am.* 1992;6:323–346.

Dimopoulos MA, Alexanian R. Waldenström's macroglobulinemia. *Blood.* 1994;83:1452–1459.

García-Sanz R, Orfão A, Gonzaléz M, et al. Primary plasma cell leukemia: clinical, immunophenotypic, DNA ploidy, and cytogenetic characteristics. *Blood.* 1999;93:1032–1037.

Gillmore JD. Amyloidosis: a review of recent diagnostic and therapeutic developments. *Br J Haematol.* 1997;99:245–256.

Greipp PR. Advances in the diagnosis and management of myeloma. *Semin Hematol.* 1992;29:24–45.

Harris NL, Jaffee ES, Diebold J, et al. World Health Organization Classification of Neoplastic Diseases of the Hematopoietic and Lymphoid Tissues: Report of the Clinical Advisory Committee Meeting - Arlie House, Virginia, November 1997. *J Clin Oncol.* 1999;17:3835–3849.

Hussong JW, Perkins SL, Schnitzer B, et al. Extramedullary plasmacytoma: a form of marginal zone cell lymphoma? *Am J Clin Pathol.* 1999;111:111–116.

Keren DF. Procedures for the evaluation of monoclonal immunoglobulins. *Arch Pathol Lab Med.* 1999;123:126–132.

Kyle RA. Sequence of testing for monoclonal gammopathies: serum and urine assays. *Arch Pathol Lab Med.* 1999;123:114–118.

Kyle RA, Gertz MA. Primary systemic amyloidosis. clinical and laboratory features in 474 cases. *Semin Hematol.* 1995;32:45–59.

Kyle RA, Greipp PR. Plasma cell dyscrasias: current status. *Crit Rev Oncol Hematol.* 1988;8:93–152.

Peterson LC, Brown BA, Crosson JT, et al. Application of the immunoperoxidase technique to bone marrow trephine biopsies in the classification of patients with monoclonal gammopathies. *Am J Clin Pathol.* 1986;85:688–693.

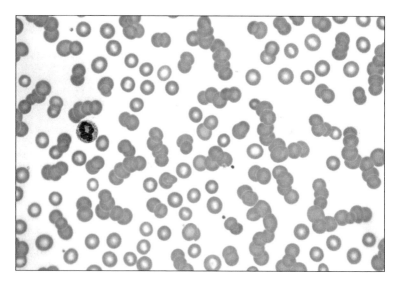

Image 37-1 Blood smear from patient with multiple myeloma shows marked rouleaux formation.

Image 37-2 Bone marrow aspirate specimen from a patient with multiple myeloma shows numerous plasma cells, many of which have nucleoli.

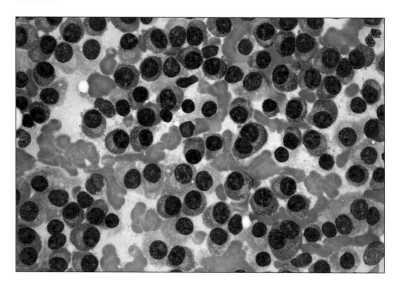

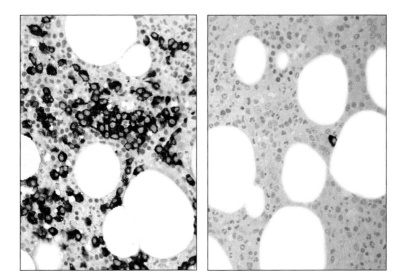

Image 37-3   Bone marrow biopsy specimen from a patient with multiple myeloma showing infiltration by plasma cells highlighted by immunostaining. The majority of the plasma cells are positive for κ light chains (left) and negative for λ light chains (right), confirming that they are monoclonal.

Image 37-4   Blood smear from patient with plasma cell leukemia. It is not unusual for the plasma cells in plasma cell leukemia to have a lymphoid appearance, as in this case.

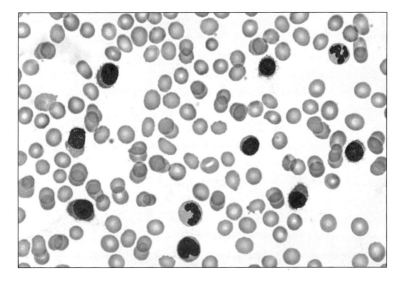

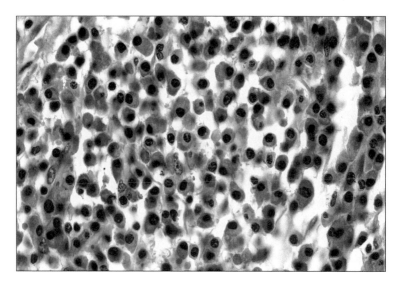

Image 37-5 Solitary plasmacytoma of bone presenting as a pathologic fracture of cervical spine. Bone marrow biopsy findings were negative for multiple myeloma.

Image 37-6 Extramedullary plasmacytoma from nasal cavity of a 20-year-old man. The plasma cells exhibited κ light-chain restriction.

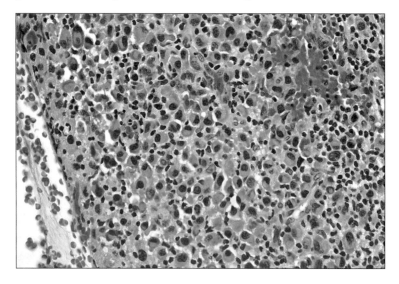

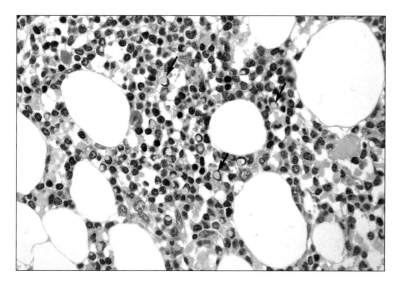

Image 37-7   Bone marrow biopsy specimen from a patient with Waldenström's macroglobulinemia showing a lymphoplasmacytic lymphoma. Dutcher bodies are prominent (arrows).

Image 37-8   Bone marrow biopsy specimen from patient with primary amyloidosis. Amyloid is deposited in the walls of the vessels. The surrounding bone marrow exhibits serous atrophy and hypocellularity secondary to amyloid involvement of the small bowel with malabsorption. The vessels were positive for Congo red with apple-green birefringence, and the surrounding bone marrow involved by serous atrophy was negative.

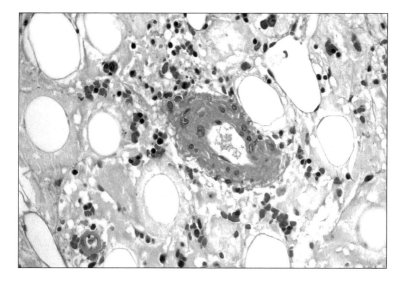

38 Monoclonal Gammopathy of Undetermined Significance and Cryoglobulinemia

Multiple myeloma and other neoplastic plasma cell dyscrasias are discussed in Chapter 37. Monoclonal gammopathy of undetermined significance (MGUS) is the focus of this chapter. Cryoglobulinemia is also discussed.

38.1 Pathophysiology

"MGUS" is the term used to describe the presence of a monoclonal immunoglobulin in serum, urine, or both without any diagnostic features of multiple myeloma, macroglobulinemia, or other related diseases. MGUS is the most frequent type of monoclonal gammopathy; it is far more common than the prototype malignant plasma cell dyscrasia, multiple myeloma (**Table 38-1**). The incidence of MGUS increases with age. MGUS is rare before the age of 40 years but increases with each succeeding decade. The overall rate of monoclonal proteins in most reports is approximately 1% in persons older than 50 years and 3% in persons older than 70 years. The incidence of monoclonal proteins is higher in the African American

Table 38-1 Approximate Incidence of Monoclonal
Gammopathies in the United States*

Condition	No. of Cases per Year
Monoclonal gammopathy of undetermined significance	>1,000,000
Multiple myeloma	13,000
Waldenström's macroglobulinemia	3000
Primary amyloidosis	2500
Solitary plasmacytoma	Rare
Heavy-chain disease	Rare

* Modified from Keren DF, Alexanian R, Goeken JA, et al. Guidelines for clinical and laboratory evaluation of patients with monoclonal gammopathies. *Arch Pathol Lab Med.* 1999;123:106-107.

population than in whites. The introduction of more sensitive techniques such as high-resolution serum protein electrophoresis and immunofixation to detect monoclonal proteins has increased the rate with which they are detected. A prevalence as high as 6% to 10% has been reported in persons older than 55 years. The majority of these monoclonal proteins are low concentration, usually less than 0.5 g/dL (5 g/L).

The paraprotein in MGUS is usually IgG but may be IgA or IgM. Occasionally, multiple monoclonal proteins are identified. The level usually is less than 3 g/dL (30 g/L). Monoclonal proteins in the urine are rare in MGUS. Most patients have stable or benign disease, but a malignant plasma cell dyscrasia such as multiple myeloma may evolve in a significant number of patients.

38.2 Clinical Findings

The median age of patients with MGUS is 64 years; 60% of the patients are men. Because of the advanced age of the patients, they frequently have underlying disorders unrelated to the gammopathy. No specific symptoms or physical findings are related to MGUS.

38.3 Approach to Diagnosis

It is important to differentiate MGUS from a malignant plasma cell dyscrasia, usually multiple myeloma. The following minimal studies in an asymptomatic patient with a normal physical examination are recommended:

1. CBC count with platelet count.
2. Serum calcium.
3. Serum creatinine.
4. Serum protein electrophoresis.
5. Serum immunofixation.
6. Quantitation of serum immunoglobulins.
7. Urinalysis (if positive for protein, a concentrated 24-hour urine specimen evaluated for a monoclonal protein is indicated).

If the serum protein is less than 2 g/dL (20 g/L) and results of the minimal studies are normal, a serum protein electrophoresis should be repeated in 6 months and, if stable, checked annually. If the monoclonal protein is greater than 2 g/dL (20 g/L) or other laboratory or clinical abnormalities support a diagnosis of malignant plasma cell dysplasia, the workup should be more extensive and may include a radiographic bone survey, bone marrow biopsy, and a 24-hour urine specimen for evaluation of a monoclonal protein.

38.4 Hematologic Findings

MGUS is characterized at diagnosis by the features shown in **Table 38-2**.

38.4.1 Blood Cell Measurements
When blood cell abnormalities such as anemia, leukopenia, or thrombocytopenia are present, they are unrelated to the MGUS.

38.4.2 Peripheral Blood Smear Morphologic Features
Rouleaux formation may be increased in patients with high levels of monoclonal immunoglobulin.

Table 38-2 Features of Monoclonal Gammopathy of Undetermined Significance

Serum monoclonal protein usually less than 3.0 g/dL (30 g/L)

Absent or small amount of Bence Jones protein in the urine

No anemia, renal failure, or hypercalcemia

No bone lesions

Fewer than 10% plasma cells and no plasma cell infiltrates in the bone marrow

38.4.3 Bone Marrow Examination

The percentage of plasma cells may be normal or slightly increased in the bone marrow, ranging from 1% to 10% but usually less than 5%. The appearance of the plasma cells usually is normal, but mild abnormalities, including nucleoli, may be present in some cases. The bone marrow core biopsy specimens generally are normocellular, and plasma cells are scattered throughout the bone marrow in an interstitial pattern. Focal plasma cell infiltrates are absent, and no other evidence of a lymphoproliferative disorder is present. Immunostaining for κ and λ light chains in the cytoplasm of plasma cells in MGUS usually shows a normal or only slightly skewed ratio of one light chain to the other.

Other Laboratory Tests

Test 38.1 Serum and Urine Protein Electrophoresis

Purpose, Principle, Specimen, and Procedure. See Tests 37.1 and 37.2.

Interpretation. A monoclonal spike is found on serum protein electrophoresis in most cases of MGUS. Monoclonal proteins in the urine usually are absent or present in small amounts.

Test 38.2 Urine and Serum Immunofixation

Purpose, Principle, Specimen, and Procedure. See Test 37.3.
Interpretation. The most common monoclonal protein in MGUS is IgG (74%), followed by IgM (16%) and IgA (10%). Occasionally, multiple monoclonal proteins are present. Monoclonal proteins in the urine are rare but may be present in small amounts.

Test 38.3 Serum Immunoglobulin Quantitation

Purpose, Principle, Specimen, and Procedure. See Test 37.4.
Interpretation. The monoclonal immunoglobulin level in patients with MGUS is usually less than 3 g/dL (30 g/L). Uninvolved immunoglobulins are decreased in about 25% of cases.

38.5 Course and Treatment

Treatment for MGUS is unnecessary. In most patients with MGUS, the monoclonal protein is stable with no evidence of progression to a malignant plasma cell dyscrasia. A minority, however, experience progression to an overt malignant plasma cell disorder.

In one long-term follow-up study (range, 22–38 years) of 241 patients with MGUS, the patients were placed into four groups (**Table 38-3**). In about 12% of the patients, the disease process was stable with no significant increase in the monoclonal protein, and the patients seemed to have a benign monoclonal gammopathy. In a small number of patients (10%), the monoclonal protein level increased to more than 3 g/dL (30 g/L), but multiple myeloma, macroglobulinemia, amyloidosis, or a related disorder did not develop. Approximately 52% of the patients died of seemingly unrelated causes without the occurrence of a malignant plasma cell dyscrasia. Finally, in about 26% of the patients, an overt malignant plasma cell dyscrasia developed. In the majority, multiple myeloma developed, but macroglobulinemia, amyloidosis, and other related disorders also were observed. The time from identification of the monoclonal protein to diagnosis of the serious disorders ranged from 2 to 29 years (median, 10 years). The risk of developing a

Table 38-3 Course of 241 Patients With Monoclonal Gammopathy of Undetermined Significance*

Group	Outcome†	Percentage of Patients
1	No significant increase in monoclonal protein	12
2	Increase of monoclonal protein to >3 g/dL (30 g/L)	10
3	Died of unrelated causes	52
4	Multiple myeloma, macroglobulinemia, or related diseases developed	26

* Adapted from Kyle RA. Monoclonal gammopathy of undetermined significance and solitary plasmacytoma: implications for progression to overt multiple myeloma. *Hematol Oncol Clin North Am.* 1997;11:71–87.
† Follow-up ranged from 22 to 38 years.

malignant plasma cell dyscrasia did not differ significantly among the immunoglobulin classes (IgG, IgA, IgM).

There is no single finding at diagnosis that differentiates patients with a benign, stable, monoclonal protein from patients in whom a malignant plasma cell dyscrasia will develop. Although a monoclonal protein level greater than 3 g/dL (30 g/L) usually is associated with myeloma, considerable overlap of immunoglobulin levels in multiple myeloma and MGUS exists. Levels of immunoglobulin not associated with the monoclonal protein usually are decreased in myeloma but also may be reduced in stable MGUS. Similarly, a monoclonal protein in the urine suggests a malignant process but may be identified in patients with stable MGUS. Nevertheless, Baldini et al identified a subset of patients who could be considered as having a "benign monoclonal gammopathy." These patients had a monoclonal protein level less than or equal to 1.5 g/dL (15 g/L), bone marrow plasma cell percentages less than 5%, no reduction in the level of polyclonal immunoglobulins, and absence of proteinuria.

Because it is not possible to accurately predict malignant conversion, patients with MGUS need long-term follow-up to avoid delayed diagnosis of overt disease. The most reliable way of distinguishing a benign from a malignant course is by serial measurements of the monoclonal protein. An increasing level of the serum monoclonal protein is the most reliable predictor of progression to a malignant plasma cell dyscrasia.

38.6 Cryoglobulinemia

Cryoglobulins are proteins that precipitate as serum is cooled below core body temperatures. They redissolve on rewarming. Simple or single-component cryoglobulins are monoclonal and contain only one isotype or subclass of immunoglobulin. Simple cryoglobulins are composed of IgM, IgG, IgA, or, rarely, Bence Jones (monoclonal light chains) proteins. Mixed cryoglobulins are composed of two different types of immunoglobulin, usually IgM (the antibody) and IgG (the antigen). Brouet et al defined simple cryoglobulins as type I and mixed cryoglobulins as type II when the antiglobulin is monoclonal and type III when it is polyclonal (**Table 38-4**).

Type I cryoglobulinemia is associated with multiple myeloma, Waldenström's macroglobulinemia, and other lymphoproliferative disorders. The most common disease associated with type II cryo-globulinemia is chronic active hepatitis C virus infection. Other diseases associated with type II cryoglobulinemia include autoimmune disease, Waldenström's macroglobulinemia, and other non-Hodgkin lymphomas. Type III cryoglobulinemia is associated with chronic infections and autoimmune diseases (**Table 38-4**).

Testing for cryoglobulinemia may be performed in two stages. The first involves screening the patient's serum for a cryoprecipitate that is primarily immunoglobulin and that resolubilizes on rewarming. The cryoglobulin may be quantitated at this stage. In the second stage, the cryoglobulin is characterized and typed by immunofixation; in the case of type I or type II cryoglobulins, performance of other testing for a monoclonal gammopathy should be considered.

Some patients have no symptoms related to the cryoglobulinemia, while others have cutaneous manifestations such as purpura, pain, Raynaud phenomenon, or ulceration. Arthralgias, nephritis, or neurologic symptoms also may be observed in patients with cryoglobulinemia. Corticosteroid administration is the usual therapy for cryoglobulinemia, although alkylating agents, plasmapheresis, and interferon-α have also been of benefit.

Table 38-4 Type of Cryoglobulin and Disease Associations

Cryoglobulin Type	Associated Disease
I	Multiple myeloma Waldenström's macroglobulinemia Other disorders with monoclonal proteins
II	Chronic hepatitis C virus infection Autoimmune disorders Non-Hodgkin lymphoma
III	Chronic infections Autoimmune disorders

38.7 References

Aguzzi F, Bergami MR, Gesparro C, et al. Occurrence of monoclonal components in general practice: Clinical implications. *Eur J Haematol.* 1992;48:192–195.

Baldini L, Guffanti A, Cesana BM, et al. Role of different hematologic variables in defining the risk of malignant transformation in monoclonal gammopathy. *Blood.* 1996;87:912–918.

Brouet JC, Clauvel JP, Danon F, et al. Biologic and clinical significance of cryoglobulins. *Am J Med.* 1974;57:775–788.

Chang KM, Rebermann B, Chisari FV. Immunopathology of hepatitis C. *Springer Semin Immunopathol.* 1997;19:57–68.

Harris NL, Jaffe ES, Diebold J, et al. The World Health Organization Classification of Hematological Malignancies Report of the Clinical Advisory Committee Meeting, Airlie House, Virginia, November 1997. *Mod Pathol.* 2000;13(2):193–207.

Kallemuchikkal U, Gorevic PD. Evaluation of cryoglobulins. *Arch Pathol Lab Med.* 1999;123:119–125.

Keren DF. Procedures for the evaluation of monoclonal immunoglobulins. *Arch Pathol Lab Med.* 1999;123:126–132.

Keren DF, Alexanian R, Goeken JA, et al. Guidelines for clinical and laboratory evaluation of patients with monoclonal gammopathies. *Arch Pathol Lab Med.* 1999;123:106–107.

Kyle RA. "Benign" monoclonal gammopathy: after 20 to 35 years of follow-up. *Mayo Clin Proc.* 1993;68:26–36.

Kyle RA. Monoclonal gammopathy of undetermined significance and solitary plasmacytoma: implications for progression to overt multiple myeloma. *Hematol Oncol Clin North Am.* 1997;11:71–87.

Kyle RA. Monoclonal gammopathy of undetermined significance (MGUS). *Baillieres Clin Haematol.* 1995;8:761–781.

Peterson LC, Brown BA, Crosson JT, et al. Application of the immunoperoxidase technique to bone marrow trephine biopsies in the classification of patients with monoclonal gammopathies. *Am J Clin Pathol.* 1986;85:688–693.

PART
XII

Bleeding Disorders

39 Diagnosis of Bleeding Disorders

39.1 Hemostatic Mechanisms

Hemostasis can be defined as that property of the circulation that maintains blood in the fluid state within the blood vessels and prevents excessive blood loss after vascular injury. Hemostasis depends on reciprocal and balanced interactions among three anatomic compartments—the tissues, especially the vascular endothelium; blood cells, especially platelets; and blood plasma containing the coagulation proteins. Other important hemostatic factors are the size and blood flow of the affected blood vessel.

In response to vascular damage, blood clots to seal the vessel and prevent leakage. Three major events are involved in blood coagulation—vascular constriction, platelet aggregation, and fibrin formation. They are intimately related and occur virtually simultaneously. Once the clot has formed and tissue repair has begun, digestion of the clot (fibrinolysis) begins, eventually leading to vascular patency.

The sequence of events leading to clotting is initiated by trauma to the vessel. Reflex vasoconstriction occurs, resulting in reduced blood flow. When the vascular endothelium is damaged, platelets adhere to subendothelial collagen fibers and microfibrils.

Tissue factor is exposed in the vessel wall to initiate clotting. The result of the coagulation mechanism is the generation of thrombin. In addition to aggregating platelets, thrombin converts fibrinogen to fibrin, which is incorporated into the platelet plug. With the cross-linking of fibrin strands by factor XIIIa and contraction of the platelet mass, a stable clot (thrombus) is formed. Thrombi formed in the arterial system are called "white thrombi" and are composed primarily of platelets. Red thrombi, found in the venous circulation, are composed of erythrocytes trapped in fibrin and contain few platelets.

39.2 Physiology and Biochemistry of Hemostasis

39.2.1 Platelets

Platelets are anucleated disc-shaped cytoplasmic fragments, 2 to 4 µm in diameter, normally found in the peripheral blood. In a Wright-stained blood smear, they are identified by their blue-gray cytoplasm and purplish granules. Platelets are formed in the bone marrow from giant (30- to 60-µm) polyploid cells called "megakaryocytes". Megakaryocytes mature by a series of nuclear replications within a common cytoplasm (endomitosis), leading to multilobar nuclei, and by differentiation of specific cytoplasmic granules. Following maturation, the megakaryocyte cytoplasm becomes demarcated into platelet subunits, and the platelets are released into the circulation through the marrow sinusoids. **Image 39-1** illustrates platelet and megakaryocyte morphology as seen in a Wright-stained blood smear and marrow aspirate, respectively. Ordinarily, each megakaryocyte, in its lifetime, produces approximately 1000 platelets. Platelets normally circulate for 9 to 10 days, and one third of the platelet mass is sequestered in a splenic pool that exchanges freely with the circulatory pool.

Platelets contain three types of secretory granules—lysosomes containing acid hydrolases; α-granules containing proteins; and (electron)-dense bodies (δ-granules) containing adenosine triphosphate, adenosine diphosphate, calcium, and serotonin. The α-granules contain platelet-specific proteins (platelet factor 4, β-thromboglobulin), as well as other proteins, such as platelet-derived growth factor (a mitogen for fibroblasts and smooth muscle cells) and coagulation proteins found in plasma (fibrinogen, von Willebrand's factor).

Adhesion of platelets to subendothelium initiates the platelet phase of hemostasis (primary hemostasis). Adhesion is mediated when von Willebrand's factor binds to subendothelial receptors and to glycoprotein Ib on platelets. Collagen fibers then induce platelets to aggregate by stimulating them to secrete intracellular granular contents (adenosine diphosphate) and to synthesize thromboxane A_2. These secreted substances mediate and further amplify aggregation. Thrombin formed by the soluble coagulation system also activates platelets.

Vasoconstriction is enhanced by the release of serotonin and thromboxane A_2. Platelet activation induces expression of binding sites for coagulation proteins; this activity has been termed "platelet factor 3". In addition to platelet–vessel wall interactions (adhesion), platelet-platelet interactions (aggregation) occur; the latter are mediated by fibrinogen, which links two platelets by the fibrinogen receptor, glycoprotein IIb-IIIa. The platelet plug formed is provisional and will not remain hemostatically effective unless a firm fibrin clot forms around it. Platelet actomyosin provides for clot retraction and consolidation.

39.2.2 Blood Coagulation

The process of blood coagulation represents the second phase of hemostasis, in which the soluble plasma protein (fibrinogen) is converted to an insoluble fibrin clot as a result of a series of enzymatic interactions leading to the formation of thrombin. These enzymatic interactions involve conversion of a zymogen (enzyme precursor) to a corresponding protease (active enzyme), which is responsible for activation of a subsequent zymogen.

The enzymatic pathways leading to fibrin formation can be initiated by two mechanisms (**Figure 39-1**). There is in vivo interdependence between the pathways, and important feedback-activation mechanisms occur. Formation of a normal blood clot requires several plasma coagulation proteins. There are four general categories of coagulation factors:

1. Serine endopeptidases (proteases). Factors II (prothrombin), VII, IX, X, XI, XII, and prekallikrein circulate in the zymogen form. Initiation of coagulation results in the activation of each factor. A lower case *a* indicates the active factor (eg, factor Xa).

Figure 39-1 The blood coagulation mechanism. In vivo coagulation is initiated by tissue factor expression; the tissue factor–factor VIIa complex activates factors IX and X. When small amounts of factor Xa are generated, tissue factor pathway inhibitor inhibits subsequent tissue factor activity. Thrombin generated by initial tissue factor activates factor XI to initiate intrinsic coagulation and additional thrombin formation. Thrombin generation is amplified by thrombin feedback activation of factors V and VIII. Factor XII initiation of coagulation is important when artificial surfaces are present, but not for in vivo coagulation. The initial fibrin generated by thrombin action on fibrinogen is soluble (fibrin$_s$); hemostatically effective insoluble fibrin (fibrin$_i$) is generated by factor XIIIa.

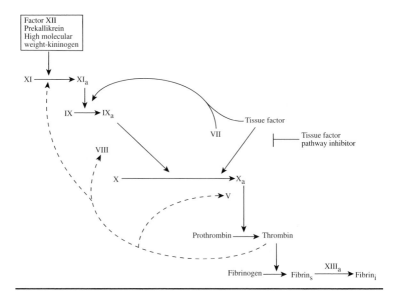

Prothrombin and factors VII, IX, and X are vitamin K–dependent, meaning that vitamin K is required for a posttranslational modification to synthesize fully active coagulation proteins that can bind calcium ions (**Table 39-1**).

2. Cofactors. Cofactors required for activation of some of the procoagulant proteins include high-molecular-weight (HMW)

Table 39-1   The Vitamin K-Dependent Procoagulant Proteins*

Prothrombin (factor II)

Factor VII

Factor IX

Factor X

*Following synthesis of these proteins by the liver, a posttranslational modification (γ-carboxylation of certain glutamic acid residues) occurs, resulting in functional coagulation proteins. This posttranslational modification requires vitamin K. In the absence of vitamin K (vitamin K deficiency) or in the presence of vitamin K antagonists (warfarin sodium [Coumadin]), nonfunctional coagulation proteins are synthesized.

kininogen and factors V and VIII. The two latter proteins have minimal activity until activated. Tissue factor also may be considered a cofactor, since factor VIIa is inactive unless complexed with tissue factor.

3. Fibrinogen. Factor I is a soluble protein that becomes the insoluble clot (fibrin) following cleavage by thrombin.

4. Factor XIII. This is a plasma transglutaminase, which, when activated to factor XIIIa, stabilizes the fibrin clot.

Activation of coagulation occurs by two mechanisms. Tissue factor initiates the extrinsic pathway of clotting (*see Figure 39-1*). High concentrations of tissue factor are present in skin, brain, lung, and placenta, as well as in monocytes and the adventitia of large blood vessels. In the basal, unperturbed state, blood is not in contact with tissue factor. Clotting is initiated only by induction of normally latent tissue factor or by exposure of blood to extravascular tissues expressing tissue factor.

Tissue factor initiates clotting by forming a complex with factor VIIa. Tissue factor–factor VIIa complex activates factor X; factor Xa, in the presence of the cofactor (factor Va), activates prothrombin and forms thrombin. Excessive activity of the tissue factor–factor VIIa complex is regulated by tissue factor pathway inhibitor. Prothrombin activation occurs on cellular surfaces of platelets, endothelial cells, smooth muscle cells, and monocytes, and requires calcium and factor Va. Prothrombin activation and thrombin cleavage of fibrinogen constitute the common pathway of coagulation.

Once thrombin is formed, clotting occurs. Thrombin cleavage of fibrinogen results in fibrin monomer formation. Polymerization of fibrin monomers and cross-linking of fibrin by thrombin-activated factor XIIIa lead to generation of the insoluble fibrin clot.

A variety of feedback-activation mechanisms are important in the amplification of coagulation. For example, thrombin activates factors V and VIII, markedly enhancing thrombin generation. Factor Xa also can activate factor VII to enhance factor X activation by the tissue factor–factor VIIa complex.

The second mechanism for initiating coagulation is the intrinsic pathway (*see Figure 39-1*). Traditionally it has been thought that exposure of subendothelial connective tissue, presumably collagen, activates factor XII. Factor XIIa then converts prekallikrein to kallikrein, which then converts more factor XII to factor XIIa, which in turn activates factor XI. These reactions require a cofactor protein, HMW kininogen. Factor XIa then converts factor IX to factor IXa. Factor XII, prekallikrein, and HMW kininogen are referred to as the contact proteins, because their activation occurs on contact with an abnormal surface (glass or kaolin).

Interdependence between the extrinsic and intrinsic pathways has been demonstrated; the tissue factor–factor VIIa complex can activate factor IX, providing a mechanism for bypassing the initial steps of the intrinsic pathway. Factor IXa activates factor X in a reaction that requires a cofactor (factor VIIIa) and calcium. Like factor V, factor VIII must be activated by thrombin to participate in factor X activation.

It is unclear how the intrinsic pathway of coagulation is actually initiated in vivo. Because patients with a deficiency of factor XII, prekallikrein, or HMW kininogen do not have abnormal bleeding, the importance of these factors in hemostasis is questionable. However, the physiologic importance of both pathways is indicated by the fact that patients lacking components of either the extrinsic (factor VII) or intrinsic (factors VIII, IX, and XI) pathways have hemorrhagic disease.

Thrombin feedback activation of factor XI has been proposed as a mechanism to explain how intrinsic coagulation might begin in the absence of the contact factors (ie, to explain why patients with contact factor deficiency do not have bleeding disorders). A current model for blood coagulation involves the following steps: First, tissue factor is expressed following vascular injury; complex formation with factor VIIa initiates clotting by activation of factors

X and IX. Tissue factor pathway inhibitor then prevents subsequent extrinsic activation of factor X. Thrombin formation is further amplified by feedback activation of factors V, VIII, and XI, leading to persistent activation of intrinsic coagulation. This model has the advantage of explaining both why patients with hemophilia (deficiencies of factors VIII, IX, or XI) bleed and why patients with contact factor deficiency do not.

A summary of the hemostatic events that occur immediately after vascular injury is presented in **Figure 39-2**. In the normal hemostatic response to vascular trauma, the processes of platelet function and blood coagulation are intimately related.

39.2.3 Fibrinolysis

Following hemostatic plug formation and cessation of hemorrhage, vascular repair begins with lysis of the fibrin clot. Local thrombin formation stimulates secretion of vascular endothelial cell tissue plasminogen activator (t-PA). Plasminogen and t-PA diffuse within the thrombus, where t-PA activates plasminogen to plasmin, a protease capable of degrading fibrin in a process called "physiologic fibrinolysis" (**Figure 39-3**). Fibrinolysis is restricted to the clot because inhibitors to t-PA and plasmin are present in blood (plasminogen activator inhibitors and α_2-antiplasmin, respectively).

39.3 Approach to the Bleeding Patient

In evaluating a patient with a putative bleeding disorder, answers should be obtained for the following questions as part of the patient history:

1. What is the duration of the bleeding tendency (is it inherited or acquired)?
2. Is there a family history of bleeding? If so, is it transmitted in a dominant or recessive fashion?
3. Is bleeding spontaneous, or is surgery or trauma required to elicit bleeding?
4. What is the location and type of bleeding?

The following questions should be addressed during the physical examination:

Figure 39-2 Summary of hemostatic events immediately following vascular injury. (1) Thromboresistant properties of the blood vessel wall (see Chapter 46) maintain blood in a fluid state. Platelets circulate in a nonadhesive state. (2) Immediately after vascular injury, exposure of subendothelial components, including collagen fibrils, induces platelet adhesion, mediated by the adhesive plasma protein, von Willebrand's factor (vWF), and its platelet receptor, glycoprotein (GP) Ib. (3) Platelet activation results from exposure to collagen, leading to thromboxane (Tx) A_2 generation, platelet secretion (release reaction), and formation of thrombin. These events lead to additional platelet recruitment into the platelet plug (aggregation). The platelet-platelet interaction results from fibrinogen binding to its platelet receptor, glycoprotein IIb-IIIa. (4) Tissue factor expressed by the subendothelium or by adventitial tissues generates thrombin; thrombin activity results in cross-linked fibrin strands that reinforce the platelet plug. Platelet actomyosin mediates clot retraction.

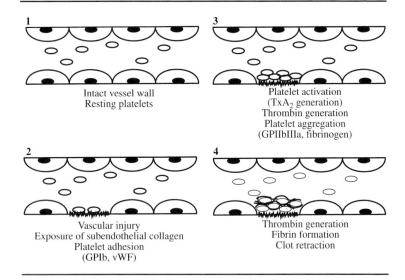

1

Intact vessel wall
Resting platelets

2

Vascular injury
Exposure of subendothelial collagen
Platelet adhesion
(GPIb, vWF)

3

Platelet activation
(TxA_2 generation)
Thrombin generation
Platelet aggregation
(GPIIbIIIa, fibrinogen)

4

Thrombin generation
Fibrin formation
Clot retraction

Figure 39-3 Physiologic fibrinolysis. Fibrin formation (*shaded area*) initiates secretion of vascular endothelial cell tissue plasminogen activator (t-PA). Plasminogen and t-PA assemble on fibrin to generate plasmin, an enzyme that degrades fibrin to fibrin degradation products (FDP). t-PA and plasmin activity are inhibited by plasminogen activator inhibitor and α_2-antiplasmin, respectively, if the active enzymes escape the confines of the clot.

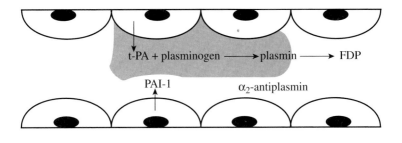

1. Is bleeding represented by petechiae or large soft tissue bruises?
2. Are hemarthroses present?
3. Are there telangiectasias?

Table 39-2 distinguishes the two major classes of bleeding disorders—platelet-vascular type and coagulation type—based on information obtained from the patient. Inherited bleeding disorders can be differentiated from acquired disorders by family history, age, and the presence or absence of an underlying disorder. Deficiency of factors VIII and IX (hemophilia A and B, respectively) are both X-linked recessive disorders among men. von Willebrand's disease is the most common bleeding disorder and is transmitted in an autosomal dominant fashion. Other inherited bleeding disorders (eg, factor VII deficiency, factor XI deficiency) are usually transmitted in an autosomal recessive manner.

Acquired bleeding disorders usually result from systemic disease, such as leukemia, sepsis, uremia, and liver disease. It is important to remember that abnormalities in blood vessels or their

Table 39-2 Clinical Manifestations in Patients with Bleeding
Disorders

Findings	Coagulation Disorders	Platelet or Vessel Disorders
Petechiae	Rare	Characteristic
Deep hematomas	Characteristic	Rare
Hemarthroses	Characteristic	Rare
Delayed bleeding	Common	Rare
Bleeding from superficial cuts	Minimal	Persistent
Patient gender	Most inherited disorders in men	Most inherited disorders in women
Mucosal bleeding	Minimal	Typical

supportive tissues may result in inherited or acquired bleeding (eg, hereditary hemorrhagic telangiectasia, scurvy).

Laboratory Screening

Coagulation tests are conducted primarily on plasma, which is the anticoagulated, acellular portion of the blood. Trisodium citrate (3.2% or 3.8%), which inhibits clotting by complexing free calcium, is used to anticoagulate the blood for laboratory screening. Consensus guidelines have recommended the use of 3.2% citrate anticoagulant. Most laboratories use silicone-coated glass tubes for collection. Unlike many clinical laboratory tests, sample quality is extremely important for coagulation testing. The correct ratio of citrate to plasma and the quality of venipuncture are important factors in the sample collection. Details of the various coagulation tests are given in the following sections, and **Table 39-3** summarizes test results in common bleeding disorders.

Test 39.1 **Prothrombin Time Assay**

Purpose. The prothrombin time (PT) assay is used to screen for inherited or acquired abnormalities in the extrinsic (factor VII)

Table 39-3   Results of Laboratory Tests for Common Bleeding Disorders

Disorder	PT	aPTT	Platelet Count	Bleeding Time
von Willebrand's disease	Normal	Normal or increased	Normal	Normal or increased
Hemophilia A or B	Normal	Usually increased	Normal	Normal
Thrombocytopenia	Normal	Normal	Decreased	Usually increased (test not usually indicated)
Vitamin K deficiency	Increased	Normal or increased	Normal	Normal

Abbreviations: PT = prothrombin time; aPTT = activated partial thromboplastin time.

and common (factors V and X, prothrombin, and fibrinogen) pathways (**Table 39-4**). It is also used to monitor the effect of oral anticoagulant therapy (see Chapter 47).

Principle. In this assay, clotting is initiated by a commercial tissue factor reagent called "thromboplastin". Plasma, thromboplastin, and calcium are mixed, and the clotting time is determined. The thromboplastin reagent contains phospholipid, so all activities of the extrinsic and common pathways are measured. The PT depends on the concentration of prothrombin; factors V, X, and VII; and fibrinogen. The assay is prolonged when factor levels are low, and normal when factor levels are borderline or normal. Because three of the five factors measured by the PT are vitamin K–dependent (prothrombin and factors VII and X), this assay is useful in identifying vitamin K deficiency (usually associated with liver disease or oral anticoagulant therapy). The PT assay does not measure the intrinsic factors (factors VIII, IX, and XI; contact factors) or factor XIII activity. Depending on the thromboplastin reagent used, the normal PT reference range may encompass 10 to 16 seconds.

Specimen. Citrated plasma obtained by clean venipuncture is used.

Procedure. The plasma sample is added to the thromboplastin reagent, which also contains calcium. The test is performed in duplicate and the clotting time average reported.

Interpretation. The large number of commercial thromboplastins in use in the United States and their variable sensitivity in

Table 39-4 Coagulation Factors Measured by aPTT and PT Assays

aPTT	PT	Both Tests
XII	VII	X
HMW-K	X	V
Prekallikrein	V	Prothrombin
XI	Prothrombin	Fibrinogen
IX	Fibrinogen	
VIII		
X		
V		
Prothrombin		
Fibrinogen		

Abbreviations: aPTT = activated partial thromboplastin time; PT = prothrombin time; HMW-K = high-molecular-weight kininogen.

detecting vitamin K deficiency has led to renewed awareness of the pitfalls of comparing results from PT assays using different thromboplastins. A prolongation of the PT usually indicates defective or decreased synthesis of the vitamin K–dependent clotting factors. The PT assay also is sensitive to a decrease in factor V and fibrinogen concentrations, which may occur in end-stage liver disease or in disseminated intravascular coagulation. Another variable affecting the PT reference range is the instrumentation used in the assay. If photo-optical instruments are used and plasma samples are turbid or icteric, the optical density change induced by clotting may not be detected, and the instruments will record the highest value of which they are capable.

Shortened PT values may be due to poor quality venipuncture, resulting in an activated sample. If this possibility is excluded, shortened values may be caused by chronic disseminated intravascular coagulation (in vivo activation).

An inherited deficiency of one of the factors affecting the PT assay is uncommon. The test may be prolonged due to the presence of antibodies to prothrombin (seen in patients with autoantibodies associated with the lupus anticoagulant) or to factor V, or with specimens from patients with certain abnormal fibrinogens (dysfibrinogenemias).

Notes and Precautions. If a normal plasma sample is left at cold temperatures for several hours, the PT of that sample may be shortened substantially. Contact (factor XII) activation of factor VII may be responsible for this phenomenon. Consensus guidelines recommend that 3.2% citrate be used to anticoagulate blood for coagulation testing (see Chapter 47).

Test 39.2 Activated Partial Thromboplastin Time

Purpose. The activated partial thromboplastin time (aPTT) assay is used to detect inherited and acquired factor deficiency of the intrinsic pathway, to screen for the lupus anticoagulant, and to monitor heparin therapy.

Principle. The aPTT is an assay of the intrinsic and common pathways. A platelet substitute (crude phospholipid) and a surface-activating agent such as micronized silica (to activate factor XII) are added to plasma. This achieves optimal contact activation. Calcium is then added and the clotting time is recorded. The aPTT assay measures all factors except factors VII and XIII (*see Table 39-4*). Depending on the reagent used, the aPTT reference clotting times may encompass 25 to 45 seconds. Because platelet-poor plasma is used, this assay is not influenced by quantitative or qualitative abnormalities in platelets.

Specimen. Citrated plasma obtained by a clean venipuncture is used.

Procedure. Patient plasma specimen is mixed with an aPTT reagent (containing phospholipid and contact activator), followed by the addition of calcium. The test is performed in duplicate, and the average clotting times are reported.

Interpretation. The aPTT reference range depends on two major variables—the aPTT reagent and the instrumentation used. The assay is prolonged when one or more of the factors measured is deficient. If the period of contact activation is greater than 2 to 3 minutes, the aPTT may not detect prekallikrein deficiency.

It must be realized that many commercial aPTT reagents are insensitive in screening for factor deficiency; mild deficiency (eg, a factor VIII level of 35%) is not detected with most reagents. In addition, reagents vary in detecting the lupus anticoagulant. When evaluating patients for this, it is important to ensure that aPTT plasma samples are prepared so they are platelet-poor. Heparin contamination must be considered in evaluating unexplained prolonged aPTT values, especially when these samples are obtained from patients in intensive care settings.

Specific inhibitors of clotting factors also may prolong the aPTT, the most common being factor VIII antibodies. Isolated prolonged aPTT values of unknown causes should be evaluated with a mixing study. The patient's plasma sample is mixed in equal volume with a normal plasma specimen, and the aPTT assay is run immediately (0 time) and 1 to 2 hours later. Correction of the prolonged aPTT value to the normal reference range with mixing at both intervals suggests factor deficiency as the cause of the prolonged aPTT value. Failure of the patient's prolonged aPTT value to correct suggests an inhibitor to coagulation, such as heparin, the lupus anticoagulant, or an antibody to a specific coagulation protein. If the patient's sample displays a markedly prolonged thrombin time but not reptilase time, heparin is present in the sample (discussed in the next section). If the mixing study results at 0 and 1 to 2 hours are similarly prolonged, the lupus anticoagulant is suspected, and corroborative tests for this antiphospholipid antibody can be performed (discussed later in this chapter). If the mixing study results demonstrate time-dependent prolongation, typically seen with protein-antibody interactions, an antibody to a specific coagulation factor is suggested, and specific factor assays can then be performed.

Shortened aPTT values may be due to poor-quality venipuncture, resulting in an activated sample. Excluding this possibility, two other causes of shortened aPTT values are marked elevation in factor VIII levels or chronic disseminated intravascular coagulation (in vivo activation).

Notes and Precautions. If plasma samples are turbid or icteric, the optical density change induced by clotting may not be detected, and photo-optical instruments will record the highest value of which they are capable. Similarly, if plasma samples have been activated and fibrin formation occurs during the instrument's lag period, the maximal clotting time will be printed. Whenever these maximum clotting time values are obtained on photo-optical instruments, the clotting assay should be repeated using a manual method. Consensus guidelines recommend that 3.2% citrate be used to anticoagulate blood for coagulation testing (see Chapter 47).

Test 39.3 **Thrombin Time**

Purpose. The thrombin time is used to screen for abnormalities in the conversion of fibrinogen to fibrin.

Principle. The addition of thrombin to plasma converts fibrinogen to fibrin, bypassing the intrinsic and extrinsic pathways. The time necessary for fibrinogen to clot is a function of fibrinogen concentration.

Procedure. In this test, thrombin (3 U/mL) is added to the patient's plasma sample and the clotting time measured.

Interpretation. A prolongation greater than 3 seconds over the control value is abnormal. Common causes of a prolonged thrombin time include fibrinogen deficiency (quantitative or qualitative), heparin, and fibrin degradation products. Less commonly, certain paraproteins may inhibit fibrin monomer polymerization and prolong the thrombin time. Hyperfibrinogenemia also may prolong the thrombin time, especially if fibrinogen levels are greater than 5 g/L.

Markedly long thrombin time values suggest the presence of heparin in the sample. The presence of heparin can be confirmed by using the reptilase time, which also measures the conversion of fibrinogen to fibrin but is insensitive to heparin. Thus, a prolonged thrombin time and normal reptilase time indicate the presence of heparin. Prolonged thrombin time values not due to heparin can be evaluated using assays for fibrinogen (functional and immunologic) and fibrin degradation products (see Chapter 43).

Notes and Precautions. The concentration of thrombin used in this assay determines the reference range for the test, as well as sensitivity. High concentrations of thrombin result in shorter clotting times and decreased sensitivity.

Test 39.4 **Platelet Count**

This test of hemostasis is performed routinely on almost all patients using particle counters as part of the routine complete blood count. The normal platelet count usually ranges from $150 \times 10^3/mm^3$ ($150 \times 10^9/L$) to $440 \times 10^3/mm^3$ ($440 \times 10^9/L$). Bleeding disorders may be associated with either thrombocytopenia or thrombocytosis; a bone marrow examination is frequently helpful in evaluating these two disorders.

Test 39.5 **Bleeding Time**

Purpose. The bleeding time should be used to screen patients for inherited platelet dysfunction (eg, von Willebrand's disease, qualitative platelet abnormalities).

Principle. The bleeding time is the time (in minutes) that it takes for bleeding to cease from a small, superficial wound made under standardized conditions. The bleeding time is mainly affected by primary hemostatic mechanisms (platelet number and function), but is also affected by a variety of other conditions.

Procedure. The Ivy bleeding time is the preferred method. A blood pressure cuff is placed around the patient's upper arm and the pressure is raised to 40 mm Hg. Two small punctures are made along the volar surface of the patient's forearm. The drops of blood issuing from the bleeding points are absorbed at intervals of 30 seconds into two filter paper disks—one for each puncture wound—until bleeding ceases. The average of the times required for bleeding to stop is taken as the bleeding time.

  Several modifications of this technique have attempted to standardize the skin puncture. Perhaps the best and least traumatic of these is a sterile disposable device (Simplate, General Diagnostics, Morris Plains, NJ) that makes two uniform incisions 5 × 1 mm using spring-loaded blades contained in a plastic housing. The device is placed firmly on the volar surface of the forearm without pressure and positioned so the incision is parallel to the fold of the elbow, with care taken to avoid superficial veins, scars, and bruises. The blade is then released by depression of the triggering device. The normal bleeding time with this method is less than 8 minutes.

Interpretation. Previous studies using the bleeding time indicated that this test might be an indicator of platelet function and therefore might be helpful in predicting bleeding in individual patients. More recent studies suggest that the bleeding time is determined not only by platelet function but also by hematocrit, certain components of the coagulation mechanism, skin quality, and testing technique. There is no evidence that the bleeding time can predict bleeding, and there is no correlation between a skin template bleeding time and certain visceral bleeding times. Consequently, the test is recommended to screen only patients who have a normal platelet count, hematocrit, and renal function for inherited platelet dysfunction (eg, von Willebrand's disease, qualitative platelet disorders).

An abnormal bleeding time in patients with a history of lifelong bleeding justifies further hemostatic testing for platelet dysfunction. Some patients with inherited platelet dysfunction may have normal bleeding times. Given the significant limitations of the bleeding time test, the author's preference is not to use it in evaluating patients, but rather to order specific tests to evaluate von Willebrand's disease and platelet dysfunction (see Chapter 41).

Antiplatelet drugs usually prolong skin bleeding times (but not necessarily visceral bleeding times). However, patients who are hemostatically normal usually have bleeding times within the normal reference range after aspirin ingestion. In contrast, patients with platelet dysfunction demonstrate marked prolongation of the bleeding time after taking aspirin. **Table 39-5** lists drug preparations containing aspirin.

Notes and Precautions. The bleeding time test may leave two small scars, and the patient should be so informed. The bleeding time test should not be performed on patients with moderate thrombocytopenia (platelet count $<50 \times 10^3/mm^3$ [$<50 \times 10^9/L$]), anemia, or uremia.

39.4 References

Broze GJ Jr. The role of tissue factor pathway inhibitor in a revised coagulation cascade. *Semin Hematol.* 1992;29:159–169.

Hougie C. Partial thromboplastin time (PTT) and activated partial thromboplastin time tests: one-stage prothrombin time. In: Williams WJ, Beutler E, Erslev AJ, Lichtman MA, eds. *Hematology.* 4th ed. New York, NY: McGraw-Hill; 1990:1766–1770.

Rapaport SI. Hemostatic mechanisms. In: *Introduction to Hematology.* Philadelphia, Pa: Lippincott; 1987:432–469.

Rapaport SI. Screening evaluation of hemostasis. In: *Introduction to Hematology.* Philadelphia, Pa: Lippincott; 1987:470–482.

Rodgers GM. The diagnostic approach to the bleeding disorders. In: Lee GR, Foerster J, Lukens JN, et al, eds. *Wintrobe's Clinical Hematology.* 10th ed. Baltimore, Md: Williams & Wilkins; 1998:1557–1578.

Rodgers RPC, Levin J. A critical reappraisal of the bleeding time. *Semin Thromb Hemost.* 1990;16:1–20.

Table 39-5   Aspirin-Containing Drugs*

Alka-Seltzer (extra strength)
Anacin (maximum strength)
Anodynos
APC
Arthritis pain formula
ASA
Ascriptin
  (regular or extra strength); A/D
Aspercin (extra)
Aspergum
Aspermin (extra)
Aspirbar
Aspirjen Jr
Aspirtab (maximum strength)
Azdone[†]
Azotal[†]
Bayer Aspirin (genuine; maximum;
  children's) delayed-release Enteric;
  extended-release 8-hour; plus buffered;
  plus extra strength buffered; therapy
Buffered (therapy)
Buff-A; Buff-A-Comp[†];
  Buff-A-Comp 3[†]
Buffaprin (extra)
Buffasal (maximum)
Bufferin (arthritis strength;
  extra strength; tri-buffered)
Buffex
Buffinol (extra)
Butalbital compound[†]
Cama arthritis pain reliever
Cope
Damason-P[†]
Darvon compound 65[†]
Doloral[†]
Duradyne
Easprin[†]
Ecotrin (maximum)
Empirin; with codeine (2,[†] 3,[†] 4[†])
Epromate[†]

Equagesic[†]
Equazine[†]
Excedrin (extra strength)
Fiorinal[†]; with codeine[†]
Genprin
Isollyl improved*
Lanorinal[†]
Lorprin[†]
Lortab ASA[†]
Magnaprin (arthritis strength)
Maxiprin
Measurin
Meprogesic Q[†]
Midol
Momentum
Norgesic[†]; Forte[†]
Norwich; extra strength
Orphenagesic[†]; Forte[†]
PAC revised formula analgesic
Palagesic
Percodan[†]; Demi[†]
Presalin
Rid-A-Pain with codeine[†]
Robaxisal[†]
Roxiprin[†]
Salecto
Salocol
Sedalgesic inserts[†]
Sine-Off tablets
Soma compound[†]; with codeine[†]
St. Joseph's aspirin
  (cold tablets for children)
Stanback powder (original formula)
Synalgos-DC[†]
Trigesic
Tri-Pain
Vanquish
Verin
Wesprin buffered
ZORprin[†]

*From Billups NF, ed. *American Drug Index 1994.* 38th ed. St Louis, Mo: Facts and Comparisons; 1994.
†Available through prescription only.

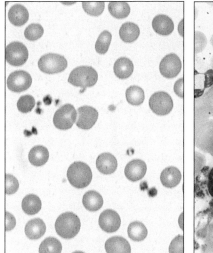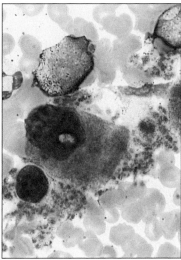

Image 39-1 Platelet and megakaryocyte morphology. The left panel is a peripheral blood smear showing approximately 10 platelets in the field (Wright's, × 50). The right panel is a bone marrow aspirate showing two megakaryocytes in the field (Wright's, × 50). One of the megakaryocytes is shedding platelets.

40   Thrombocytopenia

The typical clinical findings associated with thrombocytopenia include petechial hemorrhage, ecchymoses (bruises), and bleeding from mucous membranes (eg, epistaxis, gum bleeding, menorrhagia).

40.1 Pathophysiology

The causes of thrombocytopenia are summarized in **Table 40-1** (disorders are classified according to mechanism). Major mechanisms of thrombocytopenia include decreased marrow production, increased platelet destruction, and splenic sequestration. Occasionally, hemodilution results in thrombocytopenia.

Because splenic sequestration usually can be excluded easily by physical examination (palpable splenomegaly is almost always present), the typical evaluation for thrombocytopenia is to distinguish decreased platelet production from increased platelet destruction. If no obvious marrow insult can be identified (chemotherapeutic agents, ionizing radiation, toxic chemicals such as benzene, etc), a bone marrow examination is necessary to

Table 40-1   Causes of Thrombocytopenia

Failure of marrow production
  Reduced megakaryocytes
    Marrow infiltration with tumor, infection, or fibrosis
    Marrow aplasia (fatty replacement) due to drugs, chemicals, or radiation
    Congenital abnormalities (Wiskott-Aldrich syndrome, Fanconi's syndrome)
  Ineffective megakaryocytopoiesis
    Megaloblastic anemia
    Myelodysplasia
    Alcohol suppression
Increased platelet destruction
  Immune thrombocytopenia
    Autoantibody-mediated: systemic lupus erythematosus, lymphomas, drugs,
      infections, idiopathic (ITP)
    Alloantibody-mediated: posttransfusion purpura, fetal-maternal
      incompatibility
  Nonimmune thrombocytopenia
    Disseminated intravascular coagulation
    Thrombotic thrombocytopenic purpura
    Mechanical (prosthetic materials)
Splenic sequestration
Hemodilution
Spurious
  EDTA-pseudothrombocytopenia

Abbreviation: EDTA = ethylenediaminetetraacetic acid.

categorize the condition. If decreased megakaryocytes are present, the causative disorder should be identifiable, such as leukemia or solid tumor, infection (granuloma), fibrosis, or fatty infiltration, as may be seen in marrow aplasia. In rare cases, an inherited disorder of ineffective megakaryocytopoiesis may be present.

If increased megakaryocytes are present, peripheral platelet destruction is suggested. This categorization mandates distinguishing possible immune from nonimmune mechanisms by considering a variety of disorders, including disseminated intravascular coagulation (DIC), connective tissue diseases, lymphoproliferative disorders, infection, mechanical destruction, drugs, thrombotic thrombocytopenic purpura, and certain alloantibody-mediated thrombocytopenias. If consideration of the disorders associated with increased platelet destruction is nondiagnostic, the patient is diagnosed with idiopathic immune thrombocytopenic purpura (ITP).

Antibody-mediated thrombocytopenia may be associated with autoantibodies or alloantibodies to platelets. Autoantibodies are found in patients with connective tissue or lymphoproliferative diseases. In such cases, antibodies are elicited, which react with target platelet antigens, including platelet membrane receptors such as glycoprotein Ib and the glycoprotein IIb-IIIa complex. Virtually any drug may be associated with immune thrombocytopenia, especially sulfa drugs, quinidine, and heparin. In many cases, the drug acts as a hapten, combining with a serum protein to form an immunogenic complex. Antibody formation is induced against the drug-hapten complex; the antibodies then cross-react with platelets. Certain drugs, such as thiazide diuretics, may cause thrombocytopenia by suppressing platelet production. Antibodies to platelets may develop after viral or bacterial infection, resulting in thrombocytopenia. Regardless of the mechanism, antibody-coated platelets are removed from the circulation by macrophages of the reticuloendothelial system, predominantly in the spleen.

In posttransfusion purpura, patients lacking Pl^{A1} (a high-frequency platelet antigen) receive blood products containing this antigen and develop alloantibody-mediated thrombocytopenia 7 to 10 days later. For unknown reasons, the alloantibody interacts with the patient's own platelets as well, resulting in severe thrombocytopenia.

Neonatal thrombocytopenia may result from two mechanisms. Maternal platelet antibodies may cross the placenta to interact with fetal platelets. In this situation, the mother has underlying immune thrombocytopenia. Alternatively, fetal platelet antigens may immunize the mother to induce maternal platelet antibodies, similar to the situation of Rh hemolytic disease.

40.2 Clinical Aspects

Antecedent viral infections may occur in association with immune thrombocytopenia, especially in children. The acute form of immune thrombocytopenia may present with significant mucocutaneous (or visceral) hemorrhage, whereas chronic immune thrombocytopenia usually is more indolent and limited to bruising.

Splenomegaly usually is absent in immune thrombocytopenia. Idiopathic thrombocytopenic purpura is a diagnosis of exclusion; a search for potential underlying causes, including drugs, connective tissue disease, lymphoproliferative disease, and HIV or other infections, is important.

Inherited thrombocytopenic conditions are infrequent and include Fanconi's syndrome and thrombocytopenia with absence of radii, in which megakaryocytic hypoplasia is present. Wiskott-Aldrich syndrome is another inherited (X-linked) disorder characterized by thrombocytopenia, recurrent infections, and eczema.

40.3 Approach to Diagnosis

The widespread use of automated blood counters simplifies the diagnosis of thrombocytopenia. However, spurious thrombocytopenia may be observed, especially in blood specimens obtained from patients in whom ethylenediaminetetraacetic acid (EDTA) is used as the anticoagulant. A discrepancy is observed between the platelet count obtained using EDTA-anticoagulated blood and the platelet estimate on the peripheral smear, which reveals platelet clumping and/or satellitism (platelets adhere to neutrophils). A correct automated platelet count can be obtained in these cases by using citrate or heparin as the anticoagulant.

In addition to confirming the automated platelet count, a survey of the blood smear may provide clues to underlying disorders (eg, infection, leukemia) that may be associated with thrombocytopenia. **Figure 40-1** depicts an algorithm for evaluating patients with thrombocytopenia. If thrombocytopenia is confirmed on evaluation of the blood smear and there is no obvious reason for its presence, a bone marrow examination is helpful.

The presence or absence of megakaryocytes helps to categorize thrombocytopenia. If megakaryocytes are increased or normal, the marrow is otherwise normal, and splenomegaly is not present, specific disorders associated with platelet destruction should be evaluated. DIC should be excluded with a test for fibrinogen and D-dimer. Thrombotic thrombocytopenic purpura is a clinical diagnosis suggested by the presence of microangiopathic hemolysis and thrombocytopenia, the absence of DIC, and other appropriate clinical findings (eg, fever, neurologic abnormalities, renal dysfunction). A drug history is helpful, given the large number of

Figure 40-1 Algorithm for evaluation of thrombocytopenia. Abbreviations: DIC = disseminated intravascular coagulation; TTP = thrombotic thrombocytopenic purpura; SLE = systemic lupus erythematosus; ITP = idiopathic thrombocytopenic purpura.

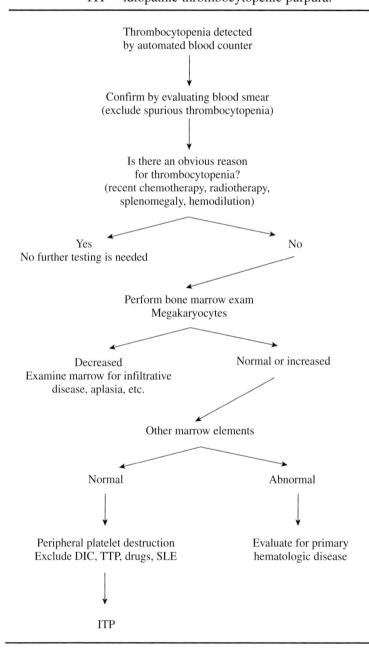

medications associated with immune thrombocytopenia. Tests for systemic lupus erythematosus (antinuclear antibodies, anti–double-stranded DNA) may uncover a systemic autoimmune disorder. Because immune thrombocytopenia may be associated with antiphospholipid antibodies, some investigators recommend assays for the lupus anticoagulant and anticardiolipin antibodies. The utility of evaluating the bleeding time in thrombocytopenic patients is marginal.

Clinically important thrombocytopenia (in the absence of platelet dysfunction) does not occur until the platelet count falls below $100 \times 10^3/mm^3$ ($100 \times 10^9/L$), usually less than $50 \times 10^3/mm^3$ ($50 \times 10^9/L$). Serious hemorrhage should not occur (again, in the absence of platelet dysfunction) unless the platelet count is less than $20 \times 10^3/mm^3$ ($20 \times 10^9/L$).

40.4 Hematologic Findings

40.4.1 Peripheral Blood Smear Morphology

In immune thrombocytopenia, the peripheral blood smear is unremarkable except for absent or decreased platelets that may be larger than normal. If significant hemorrhage has occurred, evidence of iron deficiency also may be present. Atypical lymphocytes suggest a viral origin, such as infectious mononucleosis or HIV infection. Left-shifted myeloid cells (eg, bands, metamyelocytes), together with features of neutrophil toxicity (eg, prominent granules, vacuoles, Döhle bodies), suggest the presence of bacterial infection. Immature cells (ie, myeloblasts, promyelocytes) indicate a leukemic process, whereas in aplastic anemia, neutropenia is present along with thrombocytopenia.

Fragmented RBCs (schistocytes, or helmet cells) indicate a microangiopathic hemolytic process such as DIC, thrombotic thrombocytopenic purpura, or hemolytic-uremic syndrome; these disorders are distinguished by results of coagulation tests for DIC and by the clinical picture. Oval macrocytes and hypersegmented neutrophils are seen in megaloblastic anemia (ie, vitamin B_{12} or folic acid deficiency). Thrombocytopenia seen in association with spherocytes, polychromasia, and an elevated reticulocyte count indicates immune hemolysis and thrombocytopenia (Evan's syndrome).

40.4.2 Bone Marrow Examination

This test is helpful in evaluating most cases of thrombocytopenia to exclude a primary hematologic disorder or a systemic disorder affecting the bone marrow. Disorders involving the marrow usually are apparent, whereas the marrow in immune thrombocytopenia is normal except for the possibility of increased megakaryocytes that may be more immature than those found in normal marrows. If the suspicion of marrow disease is low (ie, normal blood smear except for thrombocytopenia, no obvious systemic disease), a bone marrow aspirate without biopsy may be sufficient. Some physicians believe that a bone marrow examination is not always necessary for the diagnosis of ITP.

Other Laboratory Tests

Test 40.1 Bleeding Time

The bleeding time is expected to be prolonged in most cases of thrombocytopenia, and no useful clinical information is gained from performing the test.

Test 40.2 Prothrombin Time and Activated Partial Thromboplastin Time

These tests yield normal results for immune thrombocytopenia, unless the patient has an additional disorder (liver disease, systemic lupus erythematosus with a lupus anticoagulant, etc). The prothrombin time and activated partial thromboplastin time, fibrinogen, and D-dimer should be evaluated in all patients with unexplained thrombocytopenia to exclude DIC.

Test 40.3 Platelet Aggregation Studies

Platelet aggregation studies should not be performed routinely in evaluating thrombocytopenic disorders unless an inherited disorder is suspected. For example, patients with Bernard-Soulier syndrome, an inherited qualitative disorder affecting the von Willebrand's factor receptor, may have mild thrombocytopenia, and aggregometry identifies these patients. For the majority of patients with acquired thrombocytopenia, little additional clinically useful information is gained with this test.

Test 40.4 **Test for Heparin-Induced Thrombocytopenia**

Purpose. Thrombocytopenia may occur as a serious and diagnostically difficult complication of heparin therapy. Five to ten percent of patients receiving heparin may be affected, and a small number of these also have an associated arterial or venous thrombosis. Thrombocytopenia typically develops 6 to 10 days after initiation of heparin therapy, but may occur after only 2 days in patients who have received heparin therapy previously.

Principle. Serum samples from patients with heparin-induced thrombocytopenia initiate ^{14}C-serotonin release from labeled platelets at therapeutic but not high concentrations of heparin.

Specimen. Citrated whole blood is obtained from patients after the development of thrombocytopenia.

Procedure. Platelet-rich plasma is prepared and incubated with ^{14}C-serotonin, then the platelets are washed. The platelet count is adjusted. Test serum is then mixed with two separate heparin concentrations (0.1 U/mL and 100 U/mL final concentration) and with an aliquot of ^{14}C-serotonin–labeled platelets. After incubation and mixing, EDTA is added to terminate the release reaction. The mixture is then centrifuged, and an aliquot of the supernatant is counted in a scintillation counter. The percentage of serotonin release can be calculated from the values for background radioactivity, test sample release, and total radioactivity.

Interpretation. A positive test result occurs when there is more than 20% release at 0.1 U/mL of heparin and less than 20% release at 100 U/mL of heparin.

Notes and Precautions. This test is not routinely offered by most laboratories because it involves isotopes and is tedious to perform. A mechanism for developing heparin-associated thrombocytopenia that involves complex formation between heparin and platelet factor 4 has been described. Antibodies to heparin–platelet factor 4 form immune complexes that react with platelet Fc receptors, leading to thrombocytopenia and platelet activation. An enzyme-linked immunosorbent assay (ELISA) was described to identify these patients. This ELISA will likely replace the isotopic platelet aggregation method for routine evaluation of heparin-induced thrombocytopenia.

Test 40.5 Test for Platelet-Associated Immunoglobulins

Purpose. This test is used to measure IgG and IgM bound to the patient's platelets (direct test) or present in the patient's serum sample (indirect test). The direct test measures autoantibody on the surface of the platelet. It may be useful in distinguishing immune from nonimmune thrombocytopenia. The indirect assay is helpful in detecting the presence of alloantibodies, which may be found in posttransfusion purpura and also may be involved in drug-induced thrombocytopenia.

Principle. Monoclonal antibodies to antigenic determinants on IgG or IgM are obtained. These bind to their target antigen in a 1:1 ratio, and the amount of ligand may be determined by detection of a ^{125}I radiolabel previously attached to the monoclonal antibody. Patient platelets are used in the direct assay and are assayed for the amount of anti-IgG or anti-IgM bound. In the indirect assay, patient serum is first incubated with normal control platelets.

Specimen. The minimum sample required is 35 mL of whole blood collected in EDTA.

Procedure. The platelet count of the sample is determined, and platelet-rich plasma is prepared. A platelet pellet is isolated by centrifugation and then resuspended in buffer. The platelets are washed by the same procedure two more times. The platelets are recentrifuged, taken up in a small aliquot of buffer, and counted. A measured quantity of platelets is then mixed with ^{125}I-labeled anti-IgG (or anti-IgM) monoclonal antibody and incubated at 37°C. A measured quantity of these platelets is then layered over a phthalate oil support and microcentrifuged. The platelet pellet produced is then isolated and counted in a gamma counter. The number of IgG (or IgM) molecules on each platelet can be determined from the known quantities of the specific activity of the antibody, the molecular weight of the targeted immunoglobulin, the number of platelets, and Avogadro's number.

Interpretation. The results are reported as the number of immunoglobulin molecules per platelet. Significantly elevated levels may indicate the involvement of an immunologic process. However, the clinical utility of this test is uncertain, because increased amounts of platelet-associated antibody are not specific for immune thrombocytopenia.

Notes and Precautions. A newer method uses flow cytometry to quantitate platelet-associated antibody; however, whether this method is superior to existing methods is unproved. One advantage of the flow method is that isotopes are not required. Platelet antibody tests that measure IgG levels on individual platelet glycoproteins may prove to be more useful than current methods.

Test 40.6 **Thrombopoietin Level**

Purpose. Thrombopoietin is a recently described humoral mediator essential for normal thrombopoiesis. Some studies have suggested that measurement of thrombopoietin levels might indicate whether thrombocytopenia in a given patient is due to failure of marrow production of platelets or to peripheral platelet destruction.

Principle. Enzyme-linked immunosorbent assay methods have been described to measure thrombopoietin levels.

Specimen. Serum or plasma samples can be used for thrombopoietin measurement.

Procedure. Thrombopoietin standards (to generate a standard curve) or patient samples are incubated with microwell plates coated with an antibody to thrombopoietin. A second enzyme-linked antibody to thrombopoietin is added and, following washing, a substrate solution is added to the wells. Color develops in proportion to the amount of thrombopoietin bound initially, and color intensity is monitored spectrophotometrically.

Interpretation. Typically, thrombocytopenia due to peripheral destruction is associated with low thrombopoietin levels, whereas thrombocytopenia due to bone marrow failure is associated with elevated thrombopoietin levels.

Notes and Precautions. Thrombopoietin assays are relatively new, and their clinical utility is uncertain. A potential advantage of thrombopoietin measurement is that in thrombocytopenic patients who may have immune thrombocytopenia, a low thrombopoietin level might obviate the need for bone marrow confirmation.

40.5 Course and Treatment

Childhood immune thrombocytopenia is usually a self-limited disorder, and most patients recover with no treatment. Adult immune thrombocytopenia almost always requires treatment. Prednisone (1 mg/kg daily) is usually the initial therapy. If no response occurs or if thrombocytopenia recurs after taper of the prednisone dosage, splenectomy should be considered. Approximately 60% to 70% of patients have a complete response (normal platelet count) after splenectomy. Refractory immune thrombocytopenia can be managed by immunosuppression. Intravenous immunoglobulin is the treatment of choice for emergent bleeding associated with immune thrombocytopenia. Following IgG therapy, patients frequently respond to platelet transfusions.

The primary treatment of thrombocytopenia associated with decreased bone marrow production of platelets or ineffective megakaryocytopoiesis is platelet transfusion. Posttransfusion platelet counts should be obtained within 1 hour after transfusion to document efficacy of this expensive and potentially risky therapy. Patients with thrombocytopenia due to nonimmune platelet destruction (DIC) may not have significant responses to platelet transfusion until the underlying cause of thrombocytopenia has been treated. Platelet transfusion should be avoided in patients with thrombotic thrombocytopenic purpura.

40.6 References

Emmons RVB, Reid DM, Cohen RL, et al. Human thrombopoietin levels are high when thrombocytopenia is due to megakaryocyte deficiency and low when due to increased platelet destruction. *Blood*. 1996;87:4068–4071.

George JN, Woolf SH, Raskob GE, et al. Idiopathic thrombocytopenic purpura: a practice guideline developed by explicit methods for the American Society of Hematology. *Blood*. 1996;88:3–40.

Kelton JG, Murphy WG, Lucarelli A, et al. A prospective comparison of four techniques for measuring platelet-associated IgG. *Br J Haematol.* 1989;71:97–105.

Levine SP. Thrombocytopenia: pathophysiology and classification. In: Lee GR, Foerster J, Lukens JN, et al, eds. *Wintrobe's Clinical Hematology.* 10th ed. Baltimore, Md: Williams & Wilkins; 1998:1579-1582.

Visentin GP, Ford SE, Scott JP, et al. Antibodies from patients with heparin-induced thrombocytopenia/thrombosis are specific for platelet factor 4 complexed with heparin or bound to endothelial cells. *J Clin Invest.* 1994;93:81–88.

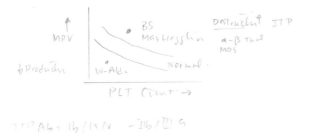

41 Qualitative Platelet Disorders and von Willebrand's Disease

The term "qualitative platelet disorders" refers to the group of bleeding disorders in which platelet dysfunction is associated with a normal platelet count. These disorders are characterized clinically by petechiae and purpura, and can be inherited or acquired.

41.1 Pathophysiology of Primary Hemostasis

When platelets are exposed to damaged endothelium, they adhere to the exposed basement membrane collagen and change their shape from smooth disks to spheres with pseudopodia. They then secrete the contents of their granules, a process referred to as the "release reaction". Additional platelets then form aggregates on those platelets that have already adhered to the vessel wall; this constitutes the primary hemostatic plug and arrests bleeding.

Shape change and release are induced readily in vitro by a variety of stimuli. Thrombin and adenosine diphosphate (ADP) are potent release and aggregation agents; the addition of relatively low concentrations of ADP to platelet-rich plasma induces primary aggregation of platelets, which is reversible. The secretion of ADP from dense bodies in platelets during the release reaction induces the secondary phase, or irreversible aggregation.

Arachidonic acid is formed from platelet phospholipids by the action of phospholipase A_2 whenever platelets are stimulated. Arachidonic acid, in turn, is converted by cyclooxygenase to labile endoperoxide precursors (prostaglandin G_2, prostaglandin H_2), which are converted by thromboxane synthetase to thromboxane A_2. Thromboxane A_2, which has a very short half-life, is a powerful platelet-aggregating agent and vasoconstrictor, and can induce the platelet release reaction. An important controlling mechanism for the release reaction is the concentration of cyclic adenosine monophosphate, which is derived from adenosine triphosphate by adenylate cyclase and is degraded by phosphodiesterase. Cyclic adenosine monophosphate activates a kinase that decreases the sensitivity of platelets to activating stimuli. Theophylline and dipyridamole (Persantine) inhibit phosphodiesterase, and prostacyclin stimulates adenylate cyclase. Both of these actions increase platelet cyclic adenosine monophosphate levels, thereby inhibiting the release reaction.

Prostaglandin synthesis also occurs in endothelial cells with formation of arachidonic acid and labile endoperoxides, but there is no thromboxane synthetase in endothelial cells, so prostacyclin is formed instead of thromboxane A_2. Aspirin irreversibly acetylates and inactivates cyclooxygenase in the platelets, resulting in decreased synthesis of thromboxane A_2 and inhibition of the release reaction. In endothelial cells, however, there is decreased prostacyclin synthesis, resulting in enhancement of the platelet release reaction. Because endothelial cells can synthesize more cyclooxygenase, the aspirin effect on them is relatively short-lived, whereas the effect on platelets is as long as the life span of the affected platelet (9 to 10 days).

The mechanisms for platelet adhesion and aggregation involve plasma adhesion molecules such as von Willebrand's factor (vWF) and fibrinogen, as well as platelet receptors for these adhesion molecules—glycoprotein Ib and the glycoprotein IIb-IIIa complex, respectively. Fibrinogen is required for normal platelet aggregation; vWF is essential for normal platelet adhesion. The fibrinogen receptor (glycoprotein IIb-IIIa) is deficient in the rare inherited qualitative platelet disorder, Glanzmann's thrombasthenia. The receptor for vWF (glycoprotein Ib) is deficient in an inherited platelet disorder known as "Bernard-Soulier syndrome".

The most common bleeding disorder is von Willebrand's disease (vWD), which may affect up to 1% of the population. It is characterized by the deficiency or functional abnormality of vWF, the plasma protein essential for normal platelet adhesion. This high-molecular-weight glycoprotein is synthesized by endothelial cells and megakaryocytes, and is present in the alpha granules of platelets and in the subendothelium. It circulates in the blood as a noncovalently linked complex with the procoagulant protein, factor VIII (previously known as factor VIII:C), which is present in only trace amounts. von Willebrand's factor stabilizes factor VIII and plays an important role in the interaction of platelets with the injured vessel wall. Electrophoresis of normal plasma in agarose gels, followed by incubation with ^{125}I–labeled antibody to vWF, reveals multiple bands with molecular weights (MWs) ranging from 1×10^6 to 20×10^6, reflecting the presence of large circulating polymers of a single subunit protein (MW 230,000); this technique is known as "multimeric analysis". Incubation of platelets with vWF and the antibiotic ristocetin results in platelet aggregation. It has been shown that the larger multimers of vWF are the most effective in this activity. Ristocetin may mimic the activity of a subendothelial constituent responsible for inducing platelet adhesion.

41.2 Clinical Findings

Most patients with inherited qualitative platelet disorders or vWD usually have a mild to moderate bleeding disorder in which there is excessive bleeding from the smallest cuts or wounds; a prolonged bleeding time; mucous membrane bleeding; and easy bruising, which occurs after trivial trauma or (apparently) spontaneously. However, some patients have no symptoms or significant history of bleeding. The ecchymoses are almost invariably superficial, and the deep-tissue hematomas and hemarthroses of severe hemophilia are rarely seen. These disorders are all transmitted in an autosomal manner, but there is an apparent predilection for women, because heavy menstrual bleeding focuses attention on the bleeding disorder. Normally, except in rare severe cases, the easy bruising and excessive bleeding from cuts are not significant enough to cause patients of either sex to seek medical attention. Many cases are so mild that symptoms manifest only when some precipitating factor, such as ingestion of aspirin or mild associated thrombocytopenia following an infection, is present. A careful history of recent medication use is essential, with special attention to aspirin or over-the-counter pain relievers containing aspirin. Patients frequently deny ingestion of aspirin or any medicines containing aspirin, yet on repeated questioning or after an abnormal result is obtained on platelet function testing, they recall taking an over-the-counter aspirin preparation (*see Table 39-5*).

Many other drugs also may interfere with platelet function; the most important of these are shown in **Table 41-1**. The thrombocytopenia that can accompany an infectious fever such as infectious mononucleosis may precipitate bleeding in a patient with a previously undiagnosed inherited qualitative platelet disorder or vWD.

41.3 Approach to Diagnosis

Figure 41-1 shows an algorithm for evaluating patients with suspected platelet-type bleeding disorders. Because patients with Bernard-Soulier syndrome and variant (type IIB) vWD may have mild thrombocytopenia, the presence of mild to moderate thrombocytopenia should not exclude such patients from consideration for platelet function disorders. von Willebrand's disease is suggested when a family history of bleeding compatible with an autosomal dominant disorder is found. Evaluation of vWD is considered initially because it is much more common than inherited platelet disorders. The tests used to diagnose vWD are discussed later in this chapter. Platelet aggregation studies should be reserved for patients in whom vWD has been excluded and who have the potential of an inherited qualitative platelet disorder. Platelet aggregation studies are rarely needed in the diagnosis of acquired disorders of platelet dysfunction (eg, uremia, myeloproliferative disorder).

41.4 Qualitative Platelet Disorders

Inherited platelet disorders may be classified on the basis of findings from platelet aggregation tests (**Tables 41-2** and **41-3**; **Figures 41-2** through **41-5**). They fall into three main groups: Bernard-Soulier syndrome, Glanzmann's thrombasthenia, and the throm-

Table 41-1 Drugs That Affect Platelet Function

Anesthetics
  Cocaine (local)
  Procaine (local)
  Volatile general anesthetics
Antibiotics
  Ampicillin
  Carbenicillin
  Gentamicin
  Penicillin G
  Ticarcillin
Anticoagulants
  Dextran
  Heparin
Anti-inflammatory agents and analgesics
  Aspirin
  Colchicine
  Ibuprofen (Motrin)
  Indomethacin (Indocin)
  Naproxen (Naprosyn)
  Phenylbutazone (Butazolidin)
  Sulfinpyrazone (Anturane)
Cardiovascular drugs (ie, vasodilators and antilipemic agents)
  Clofibrate
  Dipyridamole (Persantine)
  Nicotinic acid
  Papaverine (Myobid)
  Theophylline
Genitourinary drugs
  Furosemide (Lasix)
  Nitrofurantoin (Furadantin)
Psychiatric drugs
  Phenothiazines
  Tricyclic antidepressants: imipramine (Tofranil), amitriptyline (Triavil, Elavil)
Sympathetic blocking agents
  Phenoxybenzamine hydrochloride (Dibenzyline)
  Propranolol (Inderal)
Miscellaneous
  Antihistamines (diphenhydramine hydrochloride)
  Ethanol
  Glyceryl guaiacolate ether (cough suppressant)
  Hashish compounds
  Hydroxychloroquine sulfate
  Nitroprusside sodium

Reprinted with permission from Triplett DA, Harms OS, Newhouse P, et al. *Platelet Function: Laboratory Evaluation and Clinical Application.* Chicago, Ill: ASCP Press; 1978.

Figure 41-1 Algorithm for the diagnosis of qualitative platelet disorders or von Willebrand's disease. Evaluation of vWD is considered first because it is much more common than the inherited qualitative platelet disorders. Abbreviations: DIC = disseminated intravascular coagulation; vWf:Ag = von Willebrand's factor antigen; ADP = adenosine diphosphate. Reprinted with permission from Rodgers GM. Common clinical bleeding disorders. In: Boldt DH, ed. *Update on Hemostasis.* New York, NY: Churchill Livingstone; 1990:75–120.

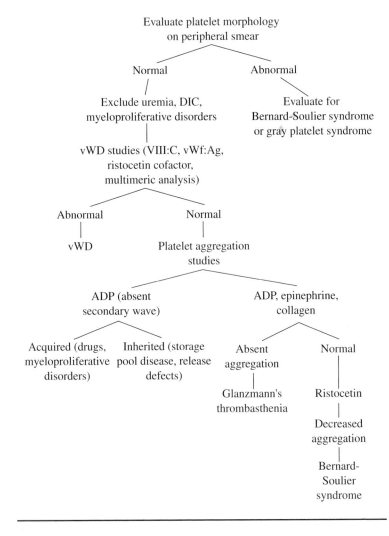

Table 41-2 Features of vWD and Inherited Qualitative Platelet Disorders

| | Aggregation Response | | | | |
| | ADP or Epinephrine | | | | |
Disorders	Primary	Secondary	Collagen	Ristocetin	Special Features
von Willebrand's disease	Normal	Normal	Normal	Absent or decreased	Patient's platelets aggregate with ristocetin in the presence of normal plasma
Bernard-Soulier syndrome	Normal	Normal	Normal	Absent	Large platelets seen on smear, clinically severe
Glanzmann's thrombasthenia	Absent	Absent	Absent	Normal	Clot retraction poor or absent; clinically severe
Storage pool disease	Normal or decreased	Absent	Normal or decreased	Normal	Decreased or absent dense granules on electron microscopy; platelet ATP:ADP ratio increased
Release defect (aspirinlike disorder)	Normal or decreased	Absent	Normal or decreased	Normal	Normal dense granules on electron microscopy
Intermediate type	Normal	Decreased	Normal or decreased	Normal	Bleeding time abnormal after aspirin ingestion; very mild

Abbreviations: ADP = adenosine diphosphate; ATP = adenosine triphosphate.

bopathies. Bernard-Soulier syndrome is characterized by the failure of platelets to aggregate with ristocetin in the presence of normal plasma; aggregation is normal with ADP, epinephrine, collagen, and thrombin (*see Figure 41-4*). Moderate thrombocytopenia may be present, and the platelets tend to be very large. The basic defect is an abnormality of a membrane-specific glycoprotein,

Table 41-3 Inherited Conditions Associated With Abnormal Platelet Aggregation

Glanzmann's thrombasthenia
Essential athrombia
Storage pool defect (decreased content of ADP)
    Chédiak-Higashi syndrome
    Thrombocytopenia with absent radii (TAR syndrome)
    Wiskott-Aldrich syndrome
    Hermansky-Pudlak syndrome
Aspirin-like defect
    Cyclooxygenase deficiency
    Thromboxane synthetase deficiency
Inborn errors of metabolism
    Homocystinuria
    Wilson's disease
    Glycogen storage disease, type I
Connective tissue abnormalities
    Ehlers-Danlos syndrome (collagen*)
    Pseudoxanthoma elasticum (collagen*)
    Osteogenesis imperfecta (collagen*)
    Marfan syndrome
    Constitutional abnormality of collagen (patient's collagen only*)
Afibrinogenemia
Bernard-Soulier syndrome (ristocetin*)
von Willebrand's disease (ristocetin*)
Gray platelet syndrome

*The abnormal aggregation patterns are obtained only when this aggregation reagent is used.
Reprinted with permission from Triplett DA, Harms CS, Newhouse P, et al. *Platelet Function: Laboratory Evaluation and Clinical Application.* Chicago, Ill: ASCP Press; 1978.
Abbreviations: ADP = adenosine diphosphate; TAR = thrombocytopenia-absent radius.

GPIb. Other similar conditions have been called "giant platelet syndromes" (May-Hegglin anomaly, Epstein syndrome). Bernard-Soulier syndrome is inherited in an autosomal recessive manner; it is very rare, and consanguinity is common among the parents of affected individuals. The hemorrhagic manifestations are severe.

Glanzmann's thrombasthenia is another rare condition in which there is no aggregation with any concentration of ADP, epinephrine, or collagen (*see Figure 41-3*); however, aggregation with ristocetin is normal. Clot retraction is poor or absent. The basic defect is an abnormality or absence of the platelet surface glycoprotein IIb-IIIa. The platelets, while failing to aggregate, undergo most of the normal changes, including the release reaction when

Figure 41-2 Platelet aggregation studies: normal tracings. Adenosine diphosphate, epinephrine, collagen, and ristocetin are used as agonists.

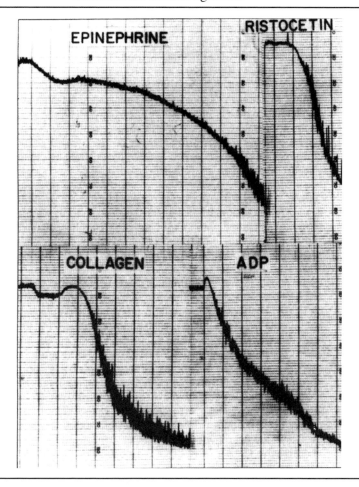

stimulated by collagen or thrombin. The platelets on the peripheral blood film are round and isolated but are otherwise unremarkable. Like Bernard-Soulier syndrome, Glanzmann's thrombasthenia is associated with severe bleeding manifestations and is inherited in an autosomal recessive manner.

Thrombopathies, characterized by abnormalities in the release reaction, are common, in contrast to Bernard-Soulier syndrome and Glanzmann's thrombasthenia. They can be divided into two subgroups: storage pool disease, in which there is a deficiency of

Figure 41-3 Platelet aggregation studies: Glanzmann's thrombasthenia. Note the absence of aggregation with epinephrine, collagen, and adenosine diphosphate, but normal aggregation with ristocetin.

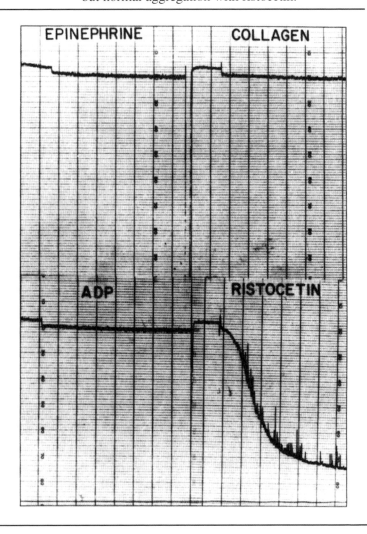

the specialized pool of ADP, and defects in the mechanism responsible for the release of the storage pool contents. Both of these subgroups are characterized by the absence of a secondary wave of aggregation with epinephrine or ADP; aggregation with ristocetin is normal (*see Figure 41-5*). Differentiation of the two subgroups requires special tests or procedures not usually available in most

Figure 41-4 Platelet aggregation studies: von Willebrand's disease (vWD). Note the absence of aggregation with ristocetin, but normal aggregation with epinephrine, collagen, and adenosine diphosphate. In milder cases, ristocetin aggregation is diminished but not absent. A similar pattern is seen in the inherited qualitative platelet disorder, Bernard-Soulier syndrome. Decreased ristocetin cofactor activity in vWD distinguishes it from Bernard-Soulier syndrome.

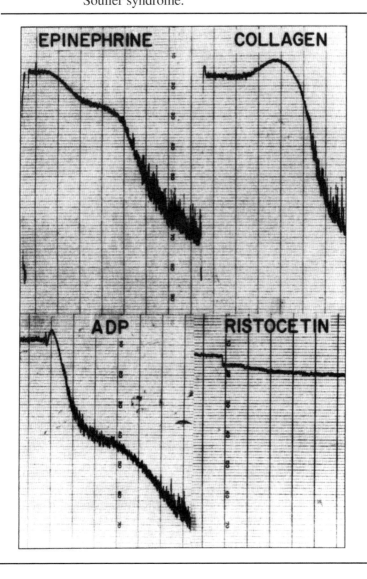

Figure 41-5   Platelet aggregation studies: storage pool disease. Primary aggregation waves are seen with epinephrine, collagen, and adenosine diphosphate, whereas secondary waves are absent. The response to ristocetin is normal. Similar tracings may be seen with aspirin ingestion or defects in the platelet release reaction (secretion).

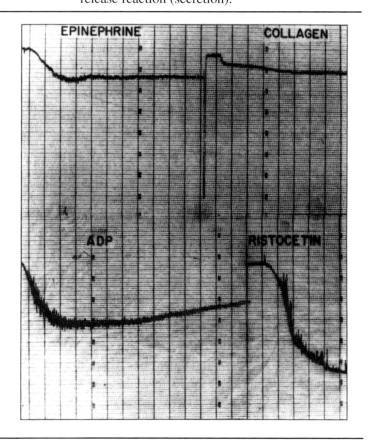

coagulation laboratories. In storage pool disease, electron microscopy shows a decrease in dense granules. In the second subgroup, the dense granules appear normal, but fail to release their constituents when the platelets are exposed to ADP, epinephrine, or collagen. This is by far the most frequently encountered type of inherited qualitative platelet abnormality, and the platelet defects closely resemble those seen after ingestion of aspirin. It has been pointed out recently that many patients with this condition have

normal to borderline bleeding times, which are significantly prolonged after aspirin ingestion; this type of case has been referred to
as an intermediate syndrome of platelet dysfunction. For conve-
nience, however, this condition may be considered a very mild type
of release defect. Its importance lies in the fact that postoperative
bleeding can be avoided in affected patients by abstinence from
drugs known to interfere with platelet function. The condition may
not be recognized with routine screening tests for hemostasis.

Qualitative platelet abnormalities have been reported in
patients with type I glycogen storage disease and Wilson's disease,
as well as in some patients with inherited connective tissue disorders, including Ehlers-Danlos and Marfan syndromes (*see Table
41-3*).

41.5 von Willebrand's disease

There are several variants of vWD. The majority of patients exhibit a quantitative deficiency of vWF. The activity of this protein as
determined by ristocetin cofactor activity is reduced in proportion
to the protein (vWF antigen) as measured with immunologic methods, usually by Laurell immunoelectrophoresis. In addition, factor
VIII coagulant activity in affected patients is reduced to a similar
extent.

The most frequently encountered type of vWD is referred to as
"type 1". Multimeric analysis reveals all polymeric forms for vWF,
but the intensity of the bands is decreased (**Figure 41-6**). Also, the
bleeding time is usually prolonged. Asymptomatic or mild forms
of this type of vWD are frequently found, in which the level of
vWF falls between 40% and 60%; in these patients, the bleeding
time is usually normal.

Another frequently encountered type is referred to as "type
2A". In this form, there is a qualitative defect of vWF, although the
amount of protein synthesized may be normal. The defect appears
to be a failure to form intermediate and large multimers, which is
revealed on multimeric analysis (*see Figure 41-6*) or on crossed-
immunoelectrophoresis. In type 2A, the bleeding time is usually
prolonged, and the factor VIII level is decreased or normal.

Other types of vWD appear to be less common. The recognition of type 2B is considered important because these patients may
not respond to desmopressin (1-desamino-8-D-arginine vasopressin

Figure 41-6   Multimeric analysis of von Willebrand's factor. Plasma was obtained from a normal subject (N), and from patients with various types of von Willebrand's disease (I, IIA, IIB, and III). Plasma was electrophoresed in an agarose gel, then von Willebrand's factor was identified using an immunoperoxidase method. The dark bands at the top of the gel (N) represent the high-molecular-weight multimers most important in platelet adhesion. Note the generalized decrease in band intensity characteristic of type I disease, the loss of intermediate and high-molecular-weight multimers in type IIA, the loss of only high-molecular-weight multimers in type IIB, and the virtual absence of all multimers in type III. This photograph is taken from an idealized drawing.

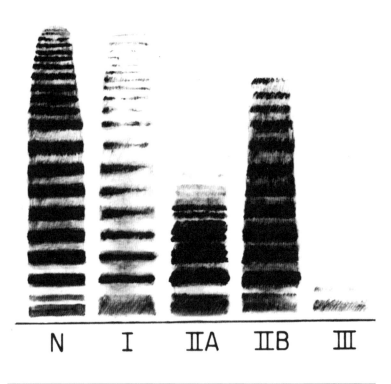

[DDAVP]). In this form of vWD, the bleeding time is prolonged, and vWF antigen is usually reduced, whereas the level of ristocetin cofactor activity is somewhat lower than that of the antigen. The diagnostic feature is a concentration of ristocetin that is too low to induce aggregation in normal platelet-rich plasma but does so in the patient's platelet-rich plasma. In this form of the disease, the largest multimers appear to be absent (*see Figure 41-6*), and it resembles another rare form (pseudo-vWD, or platelet-type vWD) in which there are abnormal platelet receptors for vWF. The laboratory findings for type 2B and platelet-type vWD are similar, showing enhanced responsiveness of platelet-rich plasma to lower-than-normal concentrations of ristocetin. Direct binding of vWF to the patient's platelets with aggregation in the absence of another agonist, however, has been demonstrated in platelet-type vWD.

Patients with type 3 vWD have a severe bleeding disorder resembling hemophilia A. These patients have very low levels of factor VIII:C, vWF antigen, and ristocetin cofactor activity. The laboratory features of vWD are summarized in **Table 41-4**.

Acquired forms of vWD have been reported. These disorders may result from development of an autoantibody to vWF appearing in a previously healthy individual without any apparent cause or in an individual with systemic lupus erythematosus. Acquired vWD also may occur with lymphoma or multiple myeloma due to the presence of an abnormal protein that in some way inhibits a physiologic counterpart of ristocetin.

Qualitative abnormalities of platelets are encountered in patients with myeloproliferative disorders (especially essential thrombocytosis) and, to a lesser extent, in those with polycythemia vera and myelofibrosis with myeloid metaplasia. Mild abnormalities are found in patients with uremia and cirrhosis. Certain acquired platelet function disorders are caused by in vivo platelet activation and result in an acquired storage pool defect (certain disorders associated with antiplatelet antibodies or immune complexes, disseminated intravascular coagulation, cardiopulmonary bypass, hairy cell leukemia) (**Table 41-5**). Evaluation of these disorders proceeds as follows:

1. Hematologic evaluation is conducted with particular attention paid to platelet number and morphology.
2. Screening tests for hemostasis, including the activated partial thromboplastin time (aPTT), prothrombin time (PT), and platelet count, are performed. In general, a coagulation-type

Table 41-4 Laboratory Features of von Willebrand's Disease*

	Type I	Type IIA	Type IIB	Type III	Platelet-type
Bleeding time	V	V	V	V	V
Factor VIII:C activity	D	D or N	D or N	D	D or N
Von Willebrand's factor antigen	D	N or D	N or D	D	D or N
Ristocetin cofactor activity	D	D	D or N	D	D
Ristocetin-induced platelet aggregation	D or N	D	I	D	I
Multimeric analysis	N	A	A	A	A

Abbreviations: I = increased; D = decreased; N = normal; A = abnormal; V = variable.
*The bleeding time may be normal or abnormal in vWD. Because patients with mild vWD may have borderline normal test results, repeated testing may be necessary to establish the diagnosis.

Table 41-5 Acquired Conditions Associated With Platelet Dysfunction

Myeloproliferative disorders
  Essential thrombocytosis
  Polycythemia vera
  Myelofibrosis
Lymphoproliferative disorders
  Waldenström's macroglobulinemia
  Myeloma
Other hematologic disorders
  Paroxysmal nocturnal hemoglobinuria
  Acute myeloid leukemia
  Sideroblastic anemia
  Immune thrombocytopenia
  Hairy cell leukemia
  Myelodysplasia
Cirrhosis
Uremia
Drug-induced dysfunction
Disseminated intravascular coagulation
Cardiopulmonary bypass
Connective tissue disorders

abnormality may be excluded if the aPTT and PT are normal. If results of one or both of these tests are prolonged, specific factor assays are performed (see Chapter 39).

3. von Willebrand's disease is evaluated by testing the three components of the von Willebrand's panel—factor VIII coagulant activity, vWF antigen, and ristocetin cofactor activity. Classification of vWD subtypes is performed using multimeric analysis.

4. Platelet aggregation tests, which are nonquantitative, are primarily used for the diagnosis of qualitative platelet disorders. Less commonly, some patients with vWD have a normal von Willebrand's panel but exhibit abnormal ristocetin-induced platelet aggregation. When this is the case, the patient has vWD or, rarely, Bernard-Soulier syndrome. A ristocetin cofactor activity test is then performed, using the patient's plasma specimen and freshly washed or formalin-fixed normal platelets. This test measures the vWF activity in the plasma specimen. It is normal in Bernard-Soulier syndrome, because normal platelets are used in the test; the defect in Bernard-Soulier syndrome resides in the platelets, whereas the plasma is normal. This is the reverse of vWD, in which the plasma ristocetin cofactor activity is reduced.

41.6 Hematologic Findings

General features are usually unremarkable and, apart from Bernard-Soulier syndrome in which giant platelets are seen, abnormal platelets are rarely seen on the smear. Occasionally, hematologic features may be consistent with iron deficiency anemia.

41.6.1 Peripheral Blood Smear Morphology

The number of platelets in the peripheral blood should be estimated and the presence of any large platelets noted. Unless there has been significant bleeding, the red and white blood cells will be normal. A direct platelet count should be performed.

41.6.2 Bone Marrow Examination

Characteristic changes in bone marrow are seen with acquired platelet defects secondary to myeloproliferative disorders or in association with lymphoproliferative disorders.

Other Laboratory Tests

Many of the laboratory tests described in this section are not routinely performed by most laboratories, and will be available only in reference coagulation laboratories.

Test 41.1 Platelet Aggregation Test

Purpose. Platelet aggregation tests are used to detect abnormalities in platelet function (*see Figures 41-2 through 41-5*). Such defects, which may be inherited or may result from the ingestion of certain drugs, can cause bleeding in certain patients.

Principle. When an aggregating agent is added to an initially turbid platelet-rich plasma specimen in the cuvette of an aggregometer, the specimen clears as platelets clump, permitting more light to pass through the plasma. The aggregometer is basically a photo-optical instrument; the amount of light transmitted through the cuvette is recorded.

Specimen. A platelet-rich plasma specimen is prepared from whole blood anticoagulated with sodium citrate. The responsiveness of the platelets to aggregating agents is influenced by the time elapsing from collection, and the tests should be completed within 1 to 3 hours of collection. The temperature at which the specimen is prepared, as well as the temperature at which the actual aggregation tests are carried out, have a significant influence on the rate and extent of aggregation. Platelets prepared at room temperature are more sensitive to ADP than are platelets stored at 37°C. Due to the large number of medications that can affect platelet function, it is recommended that all medications be discontinued at least 1 week prior to testing.

Procedure. Platelet-rich plasma is obtained by the slow centrifugation of whole blood anticoagulated with sodium citrate. This procedure is carried out in plastic tubes at room temperature, and at no time should the plasma be cooled. The supernatant (platelet-rich plasma) is pipetted off and retained. The remaining portion of anticoagulated blood is recentrifuged at high speed to obtain a platelet-poor plasma specimen. The platelet-rich plasma specimen is then mixed with the platelet-poor plasma specimen to obtain a final platelet count of $250 \times 10^3/mm^3$ (250×10^9/L). The aggregation agents used are ADP, collagen suspensions (which may be obtained commercially or prepared by homogenizing tissue obtained on site), epinephrine, and ristocetin (*see Figures 41-2 through 41-5*); some laboratories also use arachidonic acid or calcium ionophore. A blank value is obtained by using a platelet-poor plasma sample from the patient. The adjusted platelet-containing plasma sample is placed in the cuvette and warmed to 37°C, the aggregating agent is added, and the contents of the cuvette are stirred constantly by means of a small Teflon-coated stirring rod.

Interpretation. The results with each aggregation agent may be recorded as the slope of the curve, the absolute magnitude of the transmittance change, or the percentage change of the transmittance, or of the optical density. In most laboratories, however, the results are not reported in a quantitative manner, but merely in descriptive terms (normal vs abnormal aggregation), with a comment as to the type of abnormality.

The results depend on the concentration of the aggregating agents, which should be stated in the report. With relatively low doses of ADP (1 to 2 µg/mL), two waves of aggregation are seen. The first, or primary, wave is induced by the ADP added to the patient's plasma, whereas the secondary wave is attributed to the release of relatively large amounts of intrinsic ADP from the storage pool within the platelets (release reaction). With even lower concentrations of ADP (0.5 µg/mL), the release reaction does not occur, the platelets disaggregate, and only a primary wave is seen; with relatively large doses of ADP (10 to 20 µg/mL), a single broad wave is seen. A biphasic response occurs with epinephrine in up to 80% of healthy persons. However, 20% to 30% of healthy people exhibit abnormal epinephrine aggregation. Because collagen acts by inducing a release of ADP, a primary wave is not seen. In thrombasthenia, aggregation occurs with ristocetin, but not with any concentration of ADP, epinephrine, or collagen (*see Figure 41-3*). In storage pool disease and release defects (aspirinlike disorders), the secondary waves with ADP and epinephrine are absent (*see Figure 41-5*), and aggregation with collagen is reduced or absent; ristocetin aggregation is normal. More subtle changes may be clinically significant when ristocetin is used as the aggregating agent, and the slope should be compared with that of the control. A normal tracing with risto-cetin does not exclude a moderate vWF deficiency. Thus, when vWD is suspected, a quantitative ristocetin cofactor activity must be performed. In addition to the usual concentration of ristocetin, a lower concentration (0.5 mg/mL final concentration) also should be used in the platelet aggregation test to detect the rare type 2B of the disease. In this condition, aggregation occurs with the patient's platelet-rich plasma specimen and the lower concentration of ristocetin, whereas aggregation with the normal control platelet-rich plasma specimen and the low ristocetin concentration is not seen.

Notes and Precautions. Specimens left at room temperature for more than 4 hours may lose their ability to aggregate. Platelets stored at 0°C sometimes undergo spontaneous aggregation. Plasma should not be lipemic or icteric. Whenever an unexpectedly abnormal result is obtained, the test should be repeated on another specimen collected several days later. Numerous medications, including antibiotics, antidepressants, antihistamines, and so on, can markedly influence in vitro platelet function. Abnormal aggregation results in patients taking medications should be assumed to be due to antiplatelet drug effects. Whole blood aggregation methods that are less laborious than the method described here have been reported.

Test 41.2 von Willebrand's Factor–Ristocetin Cofactor Activity Test

Purpose. This test is used to measure the biologic activity of vWF.

Principle. The ability of the patient's plasma specimen to aggregate normal platelets in the presence of ristocetin is compared with that of a normal pooled plasma specimen.

Specimen. Plasma specimens used for the aPTT or PT tests are satisfactory; the specimens may be stored for several weeks at –70°C without losing activity.

Procedure. A standard curve is prepared by making serial dilutions of plasma in saline. An aliquot of each is then added to a fixed amount of a saline suspension of washed platelets in the cuvette of an aggregometer. Ristocetin is then added and the slope of the wave determined (maximum change in light transmittance). By plotting slope against the dilution of the plasma on log-log paper, a straight line is obtained. A dilution of the patient's plasma specimen is then tested, and the equivalent dilution of the normal plasma specimen that would give the same slope is read from the straight-line curve. For example, if a 1:5 dilution of the patient's plasma specimen gives the same slope as a 1:10 dilution of normal plasma specimen, the vWF activity in the patient's plasma specimen is 50% of normal.

Interpretation. A decrease in vWF parameters in a patient with a lifelong history of bleeding is diagnostic of vWD. Acquired deficiencies caused by antibodies to vWF and certain parapro-teins also may result in a decrease in vWF levels.

Notes and Precautions. The ristocetin cofactor assay already described is very time-consuming. Simpler methods based on enzyme-linked immunosorbent assay (ELISA), in which a monoclonal antibody recognizes a functional epitope of vWF, are now available.

Test 41.3 Laurell Immunoelectrophoresis Assay for von Willebrand's Factor Antigen

Purpose. The immunoelectrophoresis assay is used for the diag-nosis of vWD. In this disease, vWF antigen is usually decreased.

Principle. A precipitating rabbit antibody is used to quantitate vWF. The immunoassay is usually performed using the Laurell technique, which is an electroimmunodiffusion method for the quantitation of proteins in which rocket-shaped anodic immunoprecipitates are formed. The height of the rocket is proportional to the concentration of vWF.

Specimen. The patient's plasma or serum sample may be used, but the former is preferable. A plasma sample collected for the aPTT or PT test is satisfactory.

Procedure. The antibody is mixed with liquid agarose, which is then poured onto a plate and allowed to solidify by cooling. Holes are punched on one side of the plate, which is then placed in an electrophoresis chamber. Serial dilutions of nor-mal pooled plasma in saline (1:2, 1:4, 1:8, etc) are made to pre-pare the standard curve. The 1:2 and 1:4 dilutions of the plas-ma being tested are prepared and placed in the wells. Electrophoresis of the sample is then performed, and when the run is completed, the plate is examined. The rocket-shaped immunoprecipitates are sometimes difficult to see, but visibility can be increased by immersing the plates in tannic acid for a few minutes.

Interpretation. A value below 40% is consistent with vWD, and values between 40% and 60% are borderline. Both vWF antigen and ristocetin cofactor activity are increased by exercise, hepatitis, hormone replacement estrogen therapy, and pregnancy. Patients with vWD in one or more of these situations may have normal levels of vWF. Repeated testing may be necessary to diagnose vWD.

Notes and Precautions. The determination of vWF antigen, previously referred to as "factor VIII–related antigen", should be distinguished from the determination of the factor VIII antigen. The latter is the antigen corresponding to the factor VIII coagulant protein, which is decreased in at least 90% of patients with hemophilia A. The test to determine factor VIII antigen is currently available in some reference laboratories.

von Willebrand's factor antigen also can be measured using ELISA-based methods.

Test 41.4 von Willebrand's Factor Multimeric Analysis

Purpose. This test measures the qualitative (structural) aspects of vWF.

Principle. The patient's vWF is separated by gel electrophoresis and identified with immunologic methods. The patient's multimeric pattern is compared with those of normal patients.

Specimen. Plasma specimens used for the aPTT and PT assays are satisfactory. Plasma frozen at $-70°C$ for several weeks also may be used.

Procedure. An agarose gel (1% to 2%) is prepared, and patient and normal plasma samples are electrophoresed. The electrophoresed plasma proteins are then transferred to nitrocellulose paper and incubated with an antibody to vWF. Immunodetection of multimers can be performed with a ^{125}I label on the antibody, followed by autoradiography, or with the avidin-biotin-peroxidase technique.

Interpretation. Samples from patients with type 1 vWD have the full range of multimers, but in reduced quantities. Those from type 2A patients have no intermediate or high-molecular-weight bands, while those from type 2B patients do not exhibit the highest-molecular-weight bands. Type 3 patient samples show a virtual absence of all bands (*see Figure 41-6*).

Notes and Precautions. This is a laborious technique and is usually performed by coagulation reference laboratories.

41.7 References

Bennett JS. Platelet aggregation. In: Williams WJ, Beutler E, Erslev AJ, et al, eds. *Hematology.* 4th ed. New York, NY: McGraw-Hill; 1990:1778–1781.

Bennett JS, Shattil SJ. Congenital qualitative platelet disorders. In: Williams WJ, Beutler E, Erslev AJ, et al, eds. *Hematology.* 4th ed. New York, NY: McGraw-Hill; 1990:1407–1419.

Goodall AH, Jarvis J, Chand S, et al. An immunoradiometric assay for human factor VIII/von Willebrand factor (VIII:vWf) using a monoclonal antibody that defines a functional epitope. *Br J Haematol.* 1985;59:565–577.

Ingerman-Wojenski CM, Silver MJ. A quick method for screening platelet dysfunctions using the whole blood lumi-aggregometer. *Thromb Haemost.* 1984;51:154–156.

Rodgers GM, Greenberg CS. Inherited coagulation disorders. In Lee GR, Foerster J, Lukens JN, et al, eds. *Wintrobe's Clinical Hematology.* 10th ed. Baltimore, Md: Williams & Wilkins; 1998:1682–1732.

Zimmerman TS, Ruggeri ZM. von Willebrand's disease. *Hum Pathol.* 1987;18:140–152.

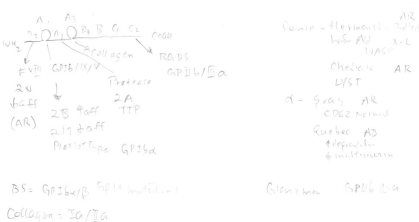

42   Inherited Coagulation Disorders

Inherited coagulation disorders result from quantitative deficiency or qualitative abnormality of a clotting factor. Deficiency of factors VIII or IX (hemophilia A or B, respectively) constitute the vast majority of patients with inherited coagulation disorders.

42.1 Pathophysiology

When a small vessel is punctured or cut, a hemostatic plug formed from aggregated platelets seals the leak, and the plug is subsequently reinforced by fibrin. When the formation of fibrin is abnormal, the hemostatic plug may be relatively weak and unstable, resulting in delayed bleeding, sometimes for several days following the injury. Based on the degree of symptom severity for the same level of reduced activity, factors VIII and IX appear to be the two most important procoagulant factors required for normal hemostasis. Factor XI deficiency yields mild or asymptomatic conditions; patients with deficiencies of factors V, VII, or X experience symptoms of intermediate severity. Deficiencies of the contact factors, other than factor XI, are not associated with any clinically important hemostatic abnormalities, which may be explained by the presence of bypass mechanisms (see Chapter 39).

42.2 Clinical Findings

The characteristic clinical features of a bleeding disorder caused by an abnormality of a blood clotting factor (features that distinguish them from platelet disorders) are outlined in *Table 39-2* (p 728).

The great majority of inherited coagulation-type disorders are relatively benign, and bleeding occurs only when the hemostatic mechanism is severely challenged. A history of easy bruising and excessive bleeding after minor surgery such as tonsillectomy or tooth extraction usually exists. Such bleeding is troublesome but rarely life-threatening. Hemarthroses are usually seen only in severe cases but may occur in mild cases following joint injury. The clinical differentiation of a coagulation-type disorder from a platelet-type disorder may be difficult, but a history of bleeding from a wound or injury starting after an interval of several hours or days suggests the former. The lifelong nature of the bleeding disorder is usually sufficient to permit its categorization as inherited rather than acquired. Acquired disorders of coagulation are discussed in Chapter 43.

42.3 Diagnostic Approach

Hemarthroses in a man may be considered the hallmark of a severe coagulation disorder. If this is sex-linked, the patient has either hemophilia A or hemophilia B; exceptions to this rule are rare. All that is then needed to establish the diagnosis is a specific assay of factor VIII and, if the results are normal, an assay for factor IX. Petechiae or purpura are rare in a coagulation disorder and suggest von Willebrand's disease (vWD), thrombocytopenia, or a qualitative platelet disorder.

Evaluation of inherited coagulation disorders proceeds as follows:

1. Hematologic evaluation is conducted to exclude thrombocytopenia and anemia.
2. Coagulation tests, including activated partial thromboplastin time (aPTT) and prothrombin time (PT), are performed. The necessity for and nature of subsequent studies depend on the results of these tests (**Tables 42-1** and **42-2**). If the diagnosis of an inherited coagulation disorder is uncertain, bleeding

Table 42-1 Results From aPTT and PT for Inherited Deficiencies of Clotting Factors

Factor	aPTT	PT
HMW-K, prekallikrein, XII, XI, IX, VIII	Increased	Normal
V, X, prothrombin, hypofibrinogenemia	Increased	Increased
VII	Normal	Increased
Dysfibrinogenemia	Increased or normal	Increased or normal
XIII deficiency	Normal	Normal
Alpha$_2$-antiplasmin	Increased or normal	Increased or normal

Abbreviations: HMW-K = high-molecular-weight kininogen; PT = prothrombin time; aPTT = activated partial thromboplastin time.

Table 42-2 Use of aPTT and PT Tests for Screening for Inherited Bleeding Disorders

aPTT	PT	Further Tests to Be Performed
Normal	Normal	Platelet aggregation studies, vWD studies, factor XIII screen, α_2-antiplasmin
Increased	Normal	Factor VIII:C assay; if normal, assays for factor IX, then factor XI; if Factor VIII is low, assays for vWF:Ag and ristocetin cofactor activity; exclude inhibitor/heparin
Increased	Increased	Thrombin time; if normal, assays for factors V and X and prothrombin; if thrombin time is prolonged, assay for fibrinogen by functional and antigenic methods; exclude heparin
Normal	Increased	Factor VII assay

Abbreviations: aPTT = activated partial thromboplastin time; PT = prothrombin time; vWD = von Willebrand's disease; vWF = von Willebrand's factor; Ag = antigen; VIII:C = factor VIII coagulant activity.

disorders such as vWD or qualitative platelet dysfunction should be considered (see Chapter 41).

3. An isolated prolonged PT suggests factor VII deficiency, which can be confirmed with a specific assay for factor VII.

4. An isolated prolonged aPTT in a patient with lifelong bleeding suggests deficiency of factor VIII, IX, or XI. vWD also should be considered, especially if the bleeding time is prolonged or if an autosomal dominant pattern of bleeding exists in the family history. Because deficiencies of factor XII, high-molecular-weight kininogen (HMW-K), and prekallikrein are not associated with excessive bleeding, their routine assay is not necessary to evaluate prolonged aPTT values in patients with bleeding disorders.

5. If both the aPTT and PT assays are prolonged, deficiency of prothrombin, fibrinogen, or factor V or X is possible. A prolonged thrombin time in such cases suggests hypofibrinogenemia or dysfibrinogenemia, and specific fibrinogen assays (functional and antigenic) can identify these patients. A normal thrombin time in such cases necessitates specific assays for factors V and X and prothrombin to identify the deficient factor. A mixing study should be performed to exclude an inhibitor to coagulation.

5. If the aPTT, PT, and thrombin time are normal, a test for clot solubility in 5 mol/L of urea should be performed to exclude factor XIII deficiency.

7. When the aPTT is prolonged and the PT is normal, the aPTT should be repeated using a mixture of equal parts of the patient's plasma and normal plasma. This test is called an "inhibitor screen", or "mixing study", and is useful to screen for antibodies or other inhibitors (eg, heparin). It is, however, relatively insensitive and nonspecific, and a specific test for the presence of an antibody to factor VIII should be performed for all patients with a known factor VIII deficiency. In patients with other types of inherited deficiencies, the development of an antibody specifically directed against the deficient factor is rare. Accordingly, unless there are unusual circumstances, such as a failure to respond to treatment with the appropriate concentrate or a positive aPTT inhibitor screen, a specific search for antibody is not part of a routine evaluation for hereditary deficiencies of clotting factors other than factor VIII.

8. In some patients with vWD, the bleeding time may be normal and the clinical and laboratory findings may mimic those seen in mild hemophilia (**Table 42-3**). It is therefore necessary to consider testing for vWD in all patients with decreased levels of factor VIII in whom there is no clear-cut sex-linked family history.

9. Patients with mild bleeding disorders may have normal results

Table 42-3   Distinguishing von Willebrand's Disease From Hemophilia A

Characteristic	von Willebrand's Disease	Hemophilia A
Inheritance	Autosomal dominant	Sex-linked recessive
Hemarthroses or joint damage	Rare	Present in most severe cases
Clinical severity	Usually mild and rarely dangerous or crippling	Mild to severe
Bleeding time	May be prolonged	Normal if performed correctly
Factor VIII:C level	Usually 6% to 50%	0% to 35%
vWF antigen	<50%	>50%
Ristocetin cofactor activity	Abnormal	Normal

Abbreviations: vWD = von Willebrand's disease; vWF = von Willebrand's factor; VIII:C = factor VIII coagulant activity.

on screening studies. If vascular disorders such as hereditary hemorrhagic telangiectasia are excluded, the following hemostatic disorders should be considered: vWD, carriers for factor VIII or IX deficiency, factor XI deficiency, dysfibrinogenemia, factor XIII deficiency, platelet dysfunction, and α_2-antiplasmin deficiency. It is important to remember that normal coagulation screening tests do not exclude a significant hemostatic defect.

10. Despite the advent of molecular biology techniques to identify genetic defects resulting in inherited coagulation disorders, these methods are not useful in the routine diagnosis of these disorders. This is because these bleeding disorders are due to genotypically heterogeneous mutations, which would require tedious mutation analysis. Consequently, the coagulation tests described in this chapter are preferred for initial diagnosis. On the other hand, if the molecular defect in a given patient is known, molecular techniques to identify carriers in the family and to determine whether a fetus would be affected are useful and are superior to coagulation tests.

Figure 42-1 summarizes one approach to evaluating isolated, prolonged aPTT values in patients with bleeding disorders. **Figure 42-2** depicts an algorithm for evaluating patients with a likely inherited bleeding disorder who have normal hemostasis screening studies.

Figure 42-1 Evaluation of a patient with bleeding and prolonged activated partial thromboplastin times. This algorithm refers only to patients with clinical bleeding who are candidates for an inherited disorder and who have isolated prolonged aPTT values. Abbreviations: PT = prothrombin time; aPTT = activated partial thromboplastin time. * = Patients with clinical bleeding but normal diagnostic studies should be evaluated further for lupus anticoagulants associated with either platelet dysfunction or thrombocytopenia.

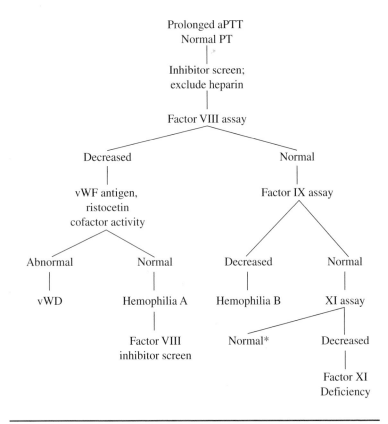

Figure 42-2 Algorithm to evaluate patients with a likely inherited bleeding disorder and normal screening studies. The type of bleeding (ie, soft tissue, mucosal, vascular) is used to determine the initial laboratory strategy. Abbreviations: PT = prothrombin time; PTT = partial thromboplastin time; vWD = von Willebrand's disease. Reproduced from Klein RR, Rodgers GM. Factor XIII deficiency: the laboratory evaluation of bleeding disorders associated with normal screening coagulation tests. *Check Sample Clinical Hematology No. CH 97-8.* Chicago, Ill: ASCP Press; 1997.

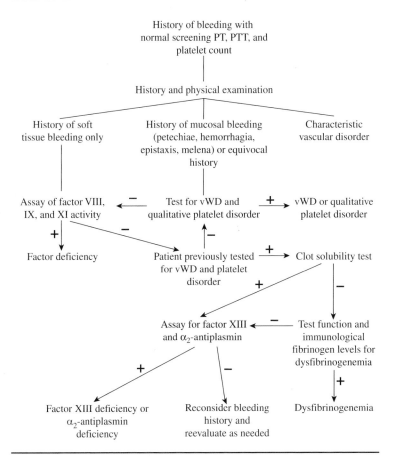

42.4 Hematologic Findings

Apart from the exclusion of anemia and thrombocytopenia, the morphology of the formed elements in the blood is usually unremarkable. Blood counts and red blood cell morphology may be consistent with chronic blood loss.

Other Laboratory Tests

Test 42.1 Assay for Factor VIII

Purpose. The determination of factor VIII level is necessary for the diagnosis of hemophilia A and vWD. The level usually correlates well with clinical severity. Assays also are used for monitoring response to therapy. Factor VIII is usually decreased in vWD in proportion to the level of von Willebrand's factor (vWF). Although hemophilia A carriers have decreased levels of factor VIII, their vWF antigen level is normal. Stress or pregnancy in hemophilia A carriers may cause factor VIII to rise to normal, but the ratio of vWF antigen to factor VIII activity remains increased. Factor VIII deficiency also must be considered in every patient who has an acquired coagulopathy with a prolonged aPTT and a normal PT.

Principle. The ability of dilutions of a sample of patient plasma deficient in factor VIII to correct the prolonged aPTT of commercially deficient plasma is compared with that of normal pooled plasma. For example, if a 1:20 dilution of normal plasma shortens the clotting time of deficient plasma to the same extent as a 1:5 dilution of the patient's plasma, the latter sample has 25% of normal activity.

Specimen. The plasma sample collected for the PT or aPTT assay is used. Factor VIII activity is fairly stable, and the test may be performed on a plasma sample frozen within 30 minutes of collection and stored at –30°C.

Procedure. The deficient plasma sample used is obtained from a patient known to have less than 1% factor VIII. It may be kept for several years if stored at –70°C. Dilutions of normal pooled plasma (1:5, 1:10, 1:20, 1:40, and 1:80) and the patient's plasma sample (1:5 and 1:10) in saline are prepared. One part of each dilution is added to one part of the deficient plasma, and an aPTT is performed in duplicate.

Interpretation. The 1:5 dilution of the normal pooled plasma sample is arbitrarily taken as 100% activity, the 1:10 as 50%, the 1:20 as 25%, and so forth. A line of best fit is obtained on log-log paper when clotting times are plotted against percentage concentration of normal plasma. The normal plasma concentrations that would give the same clotting times as the 1:5 and 1:10 dilutions of the patient's plasma sample are determined from the graph. The percentage concentration obtained with the 1:5 dilution is the actual concentration of factor VIII in the patient's plasma sample; the value obtained with the 1:10 dilution must be multiplied by two. The mean of the two values is reported. If the value with the 1:10 dilution is significantly higher than that of the 1:5 dilution, an inhibitor should be suspected, but the assay should be repeated to exclude an error in technique. The normal range for factors VIII and IX is approximately 60% to 150%.

Notes and Precautions. The activity of factor VIII may be increased significantly by trace amounts of thrombin that can form if the blood is collected too slowly or if mixing with the anticoagulant is incomplete. Factor VIII also is sometimes increased in low-grade disseminated intravascular coagulation (DIC), presumably owing to thrombin activation as well as exercise. Running for 5 minutes may double or even triple the level, which may remain high for several hours. Patients with chronic elevations of factor VIII >150% of normal may have a thrombotic risk (see Chapter 46).

Test 42.2 Assays for Other Factors Involved in Intrinsic Coagulation Only

Purpose. Assays for other factors (ie, factors, IX, XI, XII, prekallikrein, and HMW-K) involved in the intrinsic pathway may reveal the cause of a prolonged aPTT not attributable to factor VIII deficiency.

Principle. The principle is the same as that underlying the one-stage procedure for the factor VIII assay described previously. The relative ability of plasma to shorten prolonged aPTTs of commercially deficient plasma is compared with that of pooled normal plasma.

Procedure. The procedure is the same as that described for the factor VIII assay, using the appropriate factor-deficient plasma in place of factor VIII–deficient plasma. For the prekallikrein assay, the preincubation period in the aPTT test after addition of contact activator should not exceed 3 minutes; longer incubation periods cause the aPTT of prekallikrein-deficient plasma to approach the normal value. Accordingly, certain automated instruments in which the preincubation period exceeds 3 minutes cannot be used.

In the HMW-K assay, the 1:20 dilution of normal plasma may be as effective in shortening the aPTT of the HMW-K–deficient plasma as the 1:5 dilution. Therefore, in performing this assay, it is advisable to start at a 1:20 dilution and to continue up to a 1:640 dilution. The unknown is tested at 1:5 dilution up to a 1:20 dilution.

Interpretation. The normal range for prekallikrein and HMW-K is approximately 60% to 150%.

Notes and Precautions. The deficient plasma may be obtained from a commercial source. Prekallikrein- and HMW-K–deficient plasmas are rare, so few coagulation laboratories are able to perform these assays, although they are technically quite simple. In most instances, however, a provisional diagnosis of these two deficiencies may be made by a process of exclusion. Thus, if the patient has a prolonged aPTT, normal PT, normal levels of the relevant intrinsic factors (factors VIII, IX, and XI), and a negative bleeding history, a deficiency of factor XII, prekallikrein, or HMW-K should be considered. Prekallikrein-deficient plasma shortens progressively on incubation with kaolin (Celite) in an aPTT assay and may be normal after 8 minutes of preincubation, thereby distinguishing it from HMW-K deficiency or factor XII deficiency.

Test 42.3 Assays for Prothrombin and Factors V, VII, and X

Purpose. Assays for prothrombin and factors V, VII, and X are performed to determine the specific cause(s) of a prolonged PT.

Principle. The principle is the same as that for the assays described previously, but the PT is used instead of aPTT.

Specimen. Blood is collected in the same manner as for the factor VIII assay. The assay for factor V should be performed within 4 hours of collection because it is relatively labile. Assays for factor VII are best performed as soon as possible after collection because factor VII may increase in activity when the plasma is stored in the refrigerator (cold activation).

Procedure. The actual technique using plasma samples from patients deficient in prothrombin and factors V, VII, and X is simple; however, these deficient states are rare, and deficient plasma samples usually are prepared artificially and are commercially available. For example, factor V–deficient plasma is prepared by aging plasma at 37°C. The assays are performed in the same manner as the assays for the intrinsic factors (eg, factor VIII) using the PT instead of aPTT. The ability of the patient's plasma to shorten the prolonged PT of commercially deficient plasma is compared with that of normal plasma.

Interpretation. The normal range for prothrombin and factors V, VII, and X is approximately 60% to 150%. Elevated levels of prothrombin may be associated with a thrombotic risk (see Chapter 46).

Test 42.4 Inhibitor Screening Test

Purpose. The inhibitor screening test is used to detect clotting inhibitors, usually immunoglobulins or heparinlike substances.

Principle. The addition of plasma containing an inhibitor of a factor involved in intrinsic clotting prolongs the aPTT of normal plasma.

Specimen. The same plasma specimen for the aPTT test is used.

Procedure. One part of the plasma being tested is incubated with an equal part of normal plasma. The aPTTs of the mixture are determined immediately and after incubation at 37°C for 1 to 2 hours.

Interpretation. When one part of plasma that is congenitally deficient in a clotting factor such as factor VIII is mixed with an equal part of normal plasma, the aPTT of the mixture should be normal. Failure of the aPTT to correct to within the normal reference range suggests the presence of heparin or an antibody. The two most common types of inhibitors (excluding heparin) encountered by the coagulation laboratory are the lupus anticoagulant (antiphospholipid antibody) and antibodies to factor

VIII. In many cases, these two possibilities can be distinguished using the inhibitor screening test at two incubation times. The lupus anticoagulant frequently exhibits immediate prolongation of the aPTT (0 time) with similar values observed at the 2-hour incubation time. In contrast, antibodies to factor VIII exhibit time dependence, with increasing aPTT values seen in the 2-hour sample.

The presence of an inhibitor (especially the lupus anticoagulant) may result in spuriously low values of the intrinsic factors. Consequently, inhibitor screening should be considered a routine procedure in evaluating an isolated prolonged aPTT value.

Test 42.5 **Factor VIII Antibody Screening Test**

Purpose. Antibodies to factor VIII develop in up to 30% of patients with hemophilia A. The titer of antibody increases after infusions of factor VIII concentrates, and detection is important because the patient may become refractory to treatment. Factor VIII antibodies are an important cause of severe bleeding in previously healthy individuals; in patients with a background of immunologic disorders such as systemic lupus erythematosus, rheumatoid arthritis, and penicillin sensitivity; and in women following parturition. An antibody to factor VIII should be considered in every patient found during a preoperative workup to have an inhibitor. Although the vast majority of inhibitors are lupuslike (see Chapter 43) and do not give rise to excessive bleeding, surgery in a patient with a factor VIII inhibitor is dangerous and may be fatal.

Principle. If a plasma specimen suspected of containing a factor VIII inhibitor is incubated with an equal volume of normal plasma specimen, the factor VIII concentration of the mixture will be significantly decreased below normal after a period of incubation.

Specimen. The plasma specimen collected for the aPTT is used; the antibodies are remarkably stable and are present in both plasma and serum.

Procedure. One part of patient plasma is mixed with an equal volume of normal pooled plasma (used as the 100% standard). After incubation for 2 hours at 37°C, the mixture is diluted with saline in a 1:5 ratio and assayed for factor VIII.

Interpretation. If the factor VIII concentration of the mixture is 35% or more, the patient does not have an inhibitor or the inhibitor is too weak to be significant.

Notes and Precautions. To detect a low-titer inhibitor, it is advisable to obtain plasma specimens several days after, as well as before, replacement therapy.

Test 42.6 Factor VIII Antibody Titer

Purpose. Quantitation of the level of a factor VIII antibody is important in clinical treatment of hemophiliac patients.

Principle. Serial dilutions of a plasma specimen containing the inhibitor are incubated with a normal plasma specimen for a specified period, and the residual factor VIII is determined. Factor VIII inhibitor titers are commonly expressed in Bethesda units, which are defined as the amount that, when incubated with normal plasma for 2 hours, neutralizes half of the factor VIII activity.

Specimen. Blood is collected as for the aPTT test or factor VIII assay.

Procedure. Serial dilutions of the patient plasma sample in saline (1:2, 1:4, etc) are incubated with an equal volume of normal plasma for 2 hours at 37°C. The residual factor VIII in each of the incubation mixtures is determined. The inhibitor titer in Bethesda units is the reciprocal of the dilution of the test plasma sample that gives 50% inhibition; this may be determined by drawing a curve relating the activity of residual factor VIII to the reciprocal of the dilution or by a rough approximation made from inspection of the data.

Interpretation. A factor VIII antibody titer up to 5 Bethesda units is considered a low-titer inhibitor, whereas a value greater than 5 Bethesda units is considered a high-titer inhibitor. The clinical importance of quantitating the titer of a factor VIII antibody is that it may determine therapy. Low-titer inhibitors usually can be overcome by infusion of factor VIII, but this therapy is less effective in high-titer inhibitor patients.

There is considerable heterogeneity between the factor VIII antibodies of different patients. The antibodies seen in nonhemophiliacs may differ strikingly from those seen in hemophiliac patients. For example, some of the antibodies seen in nonhemophiliacs may neutralize only 80% of the available factor VIII in normal plasma over a period of 12 hours, reaching a plateau. Yet when the factor VIII concentration of the mixture is increased to 100% by addition of factor VIII concentrate, the level again falls to only 20%, indicating that the antibody was only partially neutralized. Moreover, if a factor VIII concentrate is given to a patient with a factor VIII antibody, the factor VIII level determined in the laboratory may not be a true reflection of the level at the time the plasma was drawn, because neutralization of factor VIII activity occurs in vitro between the time of collection and actual performance of the assay.

Other test systems with different unit definitions are used to assay factor VIII antibodies. The results obtained using different test systems are generally poorly correlated; however, each method gives useful information with respect to the relative potency of the antibody in any one patient over time. The standard Bethesda assay does not control pH, allowing variable low-level inactivation of factor VIII by nonimmunologic mechanisms. A modified assay, the Nijmegen modification, has been described for controlling pH and improving classification of positive and negative samples.

Test 42.7 Alpha$_2$-Antiplasmin Determination

Purpose. An α_2-antiplasmin determination is performed for patients with an acquired or inherited bleeding diathesis who have normal platelet function and normal levels of the known coagulation factors.

Principle. A known amount of plasmin is added to the patient's plasma specimen and, after a short interval, the amount of residual plasmin activity is measured. The method for determining the plasmin level is essentially the same as that used in the plasminogen assay, in which a fluorescent or chromogenic substrate is used (see Chapter 46). The percentage of plasmin inhibited provides a measure of the α_2-antiplasmin level, which also may be measured with immunologic methods.

Specimen. Citrated plasma is used for this test.

Procedure. Aliquots of a standardized and stable preparation of human plasmin are added to patient and control plasma samples and to a saline control sample. After exactly 1 minute, the mixture containing the plasmin is then added to a fluorescent or chromogenic synthetic substrate as described for the plasminogen assay (see Chapter 46). The residual plasmin is the difference between the values obtained for the plasma test sample and the control containing saline instead of plasma. A normal range has to be established for each laboratory and is usually 80% to 120%.

Interpretation. Heterozygotes with inherited α_2-antiplasmin deficiency at levels between 25% and 60% of normal may bleed excessively following surgery. In acquired deficiencies—which are seen with liver disease and thrombotic states, especially DIC—plasminogen activity is depressed concomitantly.

Notes and Precautions. Alpha$_2$-antiplasmin levels cannot be determined in patients who are receiving fibrinolytic inhibitors (eg, ε-aminocaproic acid [Amicar]).

Test 42.8 Factor XIII Screening Test

Purpose. Factor XIII deficiency is an uncommon bleeding disorder associated with normal screening tests of hemostasis.

Principle. Clots cross-linked by factor XIII resist denaturation by high concentrations of urea or acid. Factor XIII deficiency is associated with premature clot lysis.

Specimen. Citrated plasma is used in this test.

Procedure. Patient and control plasmas are recalcified separately to induce a clot. The clots are suspended in 5 mol/L urea (or trichloroacetic acid) for 24 hours. Clot stability is examined visually after 24 hours of incubation.

Interpretation. Clot lysis suggests factor XIII deficiency.

Notes and Precautions. This assay is a screening test. Abnormal results should be confirmed with a repeat assay, as well as a quantitative factor XIII assay. A mixing study using this assay should be done to exclude inhibitors to factor XIII.

42.5 Course and Treatment

The specific treatment for bleeding associated with inherited coagulation disorders is to raise the level of deficient or defective protein above the minimum concentration believed adequate for normal hemostasis (ie, approximately 30% to 50% of the mean normal level for most factors). To achieve this level with plasma alone in a patient with a very low baseline value is virtually impossible; therefore, concentrated forms of clotting factors are necessary. Monoclonal-purified factor VIII and IX preparations are available; these products, in addition to being highly purified, appear to be sterile regarding transmission of viral infections. Recombinant preparations of factors VIII and IX are also available. Concentrates to treat deficiencies of factors V, XI, or XIII are not yet available, so fresh-frozen plasma is used for affected patients.

A solvent-treated plasma product currently is available and appears to offer safety from viral infection. The dosage schedules depend on the half-life of the factor being replaced, which is roughly 12 hours for factor VIII and 24 hours for factor IX. Replacement therapy is indicated for life-threatening hemorrhages (eg, central nervous system or intraperitoneal bleeds), surgery, and the early treatment of hemarthroses and deep-tissue hematomas.

Almost all patients with mild hemophilia A and many patients with vWD (with the exception of those with the rare type 2B) respond well to intravenous or subcutaneous administration of desmopressin, a synthetic analog of vasopressin given as 0.3 µg/kg over a period of 15 to 30 minutes. This drug often increases factor VIII and vWF as much as twofold or threefold above the basal level, often without any side effects. Thus, plasma or plasma concentrates are rarely required by affected patients when they have minor bleeding. Desmopressin is also available as a nasal spray.

Epsilon-aminocaproic acid or tranexamic acid are sometimes useful for minor bleeding episodes associated with coagulation disorders and are very effective in the treatment of α_2-antiplasmin deficiency. Patients with vWD and significant bleeding or who require major surgery should receive sterile products that contain vWF activity, such as Humate-P.

42.6 References

Giddings JC, Peake IR. The investigation of factor VIII deficiency. In: Thomson JM, ed. *Blood Coagulation and Haemostasis: A Practical Guide.* New York, NY: Churchill-Livingstone; 1985:135–207.

Rodgers GM, Greenberg CS. Inherited coagulation disorders. In: Lee GR, Foerster J, Lukens JN, et al, eds. *Wintrobe's Clinical Hematology.* 10th ed. Baltimore, Md: Williams & Wilkins; 1998:1682–1732.

Santoro SA. Laboratory evaluation of hemostatic disorders. In: Hoffman R, Benz EJ, Shattil SJ, et al, eds. *Hematology: Basic Principles and Practice.* New York, NY: Churchill-Livingstone; 1991:1266–1276.

Verbruggen B, Novakova I, Wessels H, et al. The Nijmegen modification of the Bethesda assay for factor VIII:C inhibitors: improved specificity and reliability. *Thromb Haemost.* 1995;73:247–251.

43 Acquired Coagulation Disorders

The most common causes of acquired clotting factor deficiencies associated with hemorrhagic manifestations are decreased or abnormal synthesis of clotting factors caused by liver disease or disseminated intravascular coagulation (DIC). The latter is seen in many severe illnesses, including metastatic carcinoma and infectious diseases. Vitamin K deficiency is an important but less common cause of hemorrhagic diathesis. Although lupus anticoagulants are encountered frequently and are linked with abnormal coagulation tests, they are not associated with excessive bleeding. However, because lupus anticoagulants are associated with thrombosis and recurrent miscarriage, their laboratory identification is increasingly important. Antibodies to prothrombin and factors V, VIII, and XIII, although rare, may arise de novo in individuals with no previous hemorrhagic disorder and cause severe bleeding.

43.1 Pathophysiology

43.1.1 Liver Disease and Vitamin K Deficiency

The liver is the major site of clotting factor synthesis, and a hemorrhagic diathesis can occur in severe hepatitis or cirrhosis. In these conditions, the vitamin K–dependent procoagulant clotting factors (ie, prothrombin and factors VII, IX, and X; see Chapter 39), and the vitamin K–dependent anticoagulant proteins (ie, protein C and protein S; see Chapter 46) are usually the first to be reduced, followed by factor V. Factor VIII is not synthesized by hepatic parenchymal cells, and levels of this protein are actually increased in liver disease (acute-phase response). Similarly, von Willebrand's factor, synthesized in vascular endothelial cells, is elevated in liver disease. In addition to altered coagulation protein levels, other hemostatic defects exist with liver disease, including decreased clearance of activated clotting factors and increased levels of degradation products of fibrinogen and fibrin. Fibrin degradation products inhibit hemostasis by interfering with both platelet function and fibrin formation. Fibrinolysis also may be enhanced in liver disease.

Significant liver disease, with associated portal hypertension and splenomegaly, can result in mild to moderate thrombocytopenia. Hepatoma and cirrhosis also have been associated with synthesis of qualitatively abnormal fibrinogen (dysfibrinogen).

This description illustrates that the coagulopathy of liver disease is complex and affects global hemostasis, including platelet number and function, coagulation, and fibrinolysis. These defects usually result in a bleeding tendency.

Vitamin K is essential for the normal synthesis of the vitamin K–dependent clotting factors. In its absence, these factors do not bind calcium and, although synthesized in normal amounts, are inactive. Naturally occurring vitamin K is fat soluble, and bile is essential for its absorption from the gastrointestinal tract. In any condition in which the influx of bile into the gut is impeded, a hemorrhagic diathesis may ensue. The absorption of vitamin K occurs in the small intestine and may be deficient in such diseases of the intestinal wall as regional ileitis and nontropical sprue. Because bacterial flora play an important part in the synthesis of vitamin K in the gut, sterilization of the bowel resulting from the administration of antibiotics also may result in a coagulopathy.

43.1.2 Disseminated Intravascular Coagulation

The delicate hemostatic balance between the procoagulant factors and the natural inhibitors that is necessary for the maintenance of the fluidity of the blood may be disturbed in many disease states (**Table 43-1**). This may result in the uncontrolled generation of

Table 43-1   Causes of Disseminated Intravascular Coagulation

Excessive tissue factor activity
  Metastatic carcinoma (adenocarcinomas)
  Tissue injury (eg, brain tissue destruction, lung surgery)
  Extensive burn injury
  Heat stroke
  Promyelocytic leukemia
Infections
  Gram-negative endotoxemia
  Severe gram-positive septicemia
  Rocky Mountain spotted fever
  Viral infections
Obstetric disorders
  Amniotic fluid embolism
  Retained dead fetus
  Hypertonic saline abortion
  Placental abruption
Hemolytic transfusion reactions
Endothelial cell injury (vasculitis)
Giant hemangioma
Snakebites

thrombin in the blood, leading to formation of thrombi in the microcirculation, a process referred to as DIC. This term is usually used to include a paradoxical hypocoagulable state, which is the natural sequela of DIC and is attributable to the consumption of platelets, fibrinogen, and other procoagulant factors in the formation of the thrombi. Thrombi removal, essential for the survival of the patient, is accomplished by fibrinolysis, and this mechanism, although an appropriate secondary response and primarily protective, may aggravate the bleeding tendency. The formation of thrombin is believed to be essential to DIC. Its presence is presumed by the recognition of products of thrombin action on fibrinogen. These products include fibrinopeptides A and B, fibrin monomer, and D-dimer. Whereas some of the fibrin monomers polymerize and form fibrin, others form soluble complexes with native fibrinogen and with the degradation products that result from the lysis of formed fibrin. The fibrinopeptides have half-lives of only a few minutes, which limits their usefulness as an index of DIC. However, the soluble fibrin monomer complexes remain in the circulation for several hours. Fibrinolysis occurs as a consequence of thrombin generation and results in the formation of several fibrin degradation products, of which products D and E are the most stable and readily measured.

Fibrin is cross-linked by the action of factor XIIIa (transglutaminase). One of the major soluble degradation products is referred to as "D-dimer". Specific monoclonal antibodies to the cross-linked domains of this degradation product are used to detect D-dimer; such antibodies do not react with fibrinogen or fibrinogen degradation products because they lack the specific covalent bonds. Fibrinogen degradation products also are generated when urokinase or streptokinase is infused intravenously (fibrinolytic therapy) to convert plasminogen into plasmin and dissolve thrombi. The plasmin may not be neutralized completely by α_2-antiplasmin and can degrade fibrinogen, factor V, and other plasma proteins. If therapy is efficacious, the thrombus lyses and D-dimer is found, as are fibrinogen degradation products derived from the action of the plasmin on fibrinogen.

One of the consequences of intravascular fibrin deposition is the fragmentation of RBCs by strands of fibrin in the microcirculation, resulting in schistocytes or helmet cells. When associated with significant hemolytic anemia, this is referred to as microangiopathic hemolytic anemia. This process is prominent in a group of conditions called "thrombotic microangiopathies", which are characterized by hyaline microthrombi composed of fibrin and aggregated platelets in terminal arterioles and capillaries. The thrombotic microangiopathies include DIC, thrombotic thrombocytopenic purpura, and the hemolytic-uremic syndrome.

A common cause for many cases of DIC is tissue factor expression, either by tumor tissue (eg, promyelocytic leukemia, adenocarcinoma), damaged normal tissue (eg, obstetric emergencies, extensive burns), or activated monocytes and vascular endothelium (eg, gram-negative sepsis). Initiation of contact activation is not usually an important mechanism for DIC.

43.2 Clinical Findings

The bleeding found in thrombocytopenia and functional disorders of the platelets is purpuric, whereas the bleeding manifestations of acquired deficiencies of coagulation factors are of the coagulation type (*see Table 39-2*). In DIC, however, features of both types of bleeding may be present.

Hemorrhagic disease of the newborn caused by vitamin K deficiency has been virtually eliminated as a result of prophylactic vitamin K therapy. The bleeding typically occurs during the second to sixth day after delivery. Hemorrhagic disease of the newborn is an exaggeration of physiologic hypoprothrombinemia, a temporary state that reaches its maximum point of bleeding on the second or third day and usually returns to normal within 1 week. The onset of bleeding is usually abrupt, and the most common presenting symptoms include melena with hematemesis, umbilical bleeding, epistaxis, submucosal hemorrhage affecting the buccal cavity, intraventricular hemorrhage, and urethral and vaginal bleeding. The disease also may present as excessive bleeding at circumcision or persistent bleeding following a heel prick. Multiple ecchymoses may be found. Petechial hemorrhages are unusual and suggest thrombocytopenia. Premature infants are particularly prone to excessive bleeding, because immaturity of the liver cells results in decreased synthesis of vitamin K–dependent factors, which is enhanced by vitamin K deficiency.

43.3 Diagnostic Approach

43.3.1 Disseminated Intravascular Coagulation

If a patient with a severe illness, such as metastatic carcinoma or fulminant septicemia or viremia, develops purpuric manifestations, the likely cause is DIC (*see Table 43-1*). Fibrinogen is an acute-phase reactant protein, and the fibrinogen level may be very high in many conditions that can cause DIC. Therefore, a significant decrease in the concentration may not be apparent from a single fibrinogen determination, as it may be normal or high, depending on the baseline level. Serial fibrinogen determinations to follow the course of the process should therefore be performed. Factor VIII also is an acute-phase reactant protein and its level may remain above normal in DIC despite a significant fall. Thrombin is believed to activate factor VIII and also may cause a high factor VIII level. Factor V activity usually is decreased but rarely sufficiently to raise the prothrombin time (PT) by more than 1 or 2 seconds. Milder depressions of the other factor levels, such as that of factor XIII, also occur, but these changes are of little or no diagnostic value.

A falling platelet count is of considerable diagnostic and prognostic importance and is consistent with DIC. Probably the parameter used most often, however, is the presence of fibrin degradation products, of which the D-dimer appears to be the most specific. D-dimer is more helpful in diagnosing DIC than measurement of other fibrin (fibrinogen) degradation products, because the latter are elevated in both liver disease and DIC, but D-dimer is a specific marker for the presence of thrombin in blood. The presence of microangiopathic hemolytic anemia confirms a diagnosis of DIC, but many patients with DIC may not have morphologic evidence of RBC fragmentation.

43.3.2 Vitamin K Deficiency and Liver Disease

The PT response to the parenteral administration of vitamin K in patients who lack vitamin K–dependent factors is useful in differentiating hepatocellular diseases from other forms of vitamin K deficiency (malnutrition, biliary disease, etc). The PT remains prolonged in hepatocellular disease, but returns to normal in the other conditions unless some associated liver parenchymal damage is also present. In a previously healthy individual who has developed a bleeding diathesis, a prolonged PT with otherwise normal liver function test results often can be attributed to ingestion of warfarin sodium (Coumadin).

43.3.3 Antibodies to Coagulation Factors

The development of a coagulation-type bleeding disorder in an individual with previously normal hemostasis is often manifested by deep-tissue hematoma and suggests an antibody specifically directed against factor VIII, factor V, or, more rarely, one of the other clotting factors. Antibodies to specific factors are encountered far less frequently than the lupus anticoagulant (**Table 43-2**). The lupus anticoagulant results in a prolongation of the activated partial thromboplastin time (aPTT) and occasionally the PT. Patients with this nonspecific antibody rarely bleed excessively, even while undergoing major surgery. Because such an antibody was first found in a patient with systemic lupus erythematosus, it is referred to as the "lupus anticoagulant", even though lupus erythematosus is now known to be an uncommon cause. The lupus antibody may be seen in individuals who are taking certain drugs, such as quinidine, procainamide, and

Table 43-2   Acquired Coagulation Inhibitors

Type	Clinical Associations	Nature of Antibody	Clinical Findings and Course	Laboratory Findings
Specific antibodies to factor VIII	Previously healthy elderly persons; patients with autoimmune disorders; postpartum patients	IgG, monoclonal	May be persistent, especially in elderly patients; life-threatening bleeding can occur	Increased aPTT; normal PT; decreased factor VIII; positive mixing study
Specific antibodies to factor V	Usually preceded by streptomycin administration; may develop after massive blood transfusion	IgG or IgM, polyclonal	Bleeding tendency usually disappears in weeks or months	Increased aPTT; increased PT; decreased factor V; positive mixing study
Specific antibodies to prothrombin	Usually associated with lupus anticoagulant	IgG	Bleeding tendency usually disappears in weeks	Increased aPTT; increased PT; positive mixing study; decreased prothrombin; normal factors V, VII, and X
Specific antibodies to factor XIII or XIIIa	Therapy with isoniazid	IgG	Bleeding tendency usually disappears in weeks or months	Normal aPTT; normal PT; clot soluble in 5 mol/L of urea; positive clot solubility mixing study
Specific antibody to vWF	Myeloma; lymphoproliferative disorders; connective tissue disorders	IgG	Mild bleeding tendency	Increased bleeding time; decreased ristocetin cofactor activity; normal or decreased factor VIII
Lupus anticoagulant	Procainamide, chlorpromazine, quinidine, lupus erythematosus, pregnancy, HIV infection, no apparent disease	Usually IgG, sometimes IgM, or both	Bleeding tendency absent; patients may have thromboembolic events or recurrent abortions	Increased aPTT; usually normal PT; positive mixing study; positive DRVVT or KCT

Abbreviations: aPTT = activated partial thromboplastin time; PT = prothrombin time; vWF = von Willebrand's factor; DRVVT = dilute Russell's viper venom time; KCT = Kaolin clotting time.

chlorpromazine (often an IgM antibody), and after viral infections, such as HIV.

It also is commonly found in individuals in whom no causative factor can be determined (often an IgG antibody). The Venereal Disease Research Laboratory (VDRL) test may give a false-positive result in these patients. The lupus anticoagulant probably comprises a heterogeneous group of antibodies with different actions—IgG or IgM—that may be targeted against negatively charged phospholipid-protein complexes. When the lupus anticoagulant results in a marked prolongation of the aPTT, the aPTT of an equal part of both patient and control plasma usually exceeds that of the normal reference range. The coagulant activities of factors VIII, IX, XI, and XII appear reduced when assayed at a 1:5 dilution, but when assayed at higher dilutions, they usually increase significantly. This phenomenon is attributed to "diluting out the inhibitor." Factor VIII usually appears to be reduced the least and factors XI and XII the most. Weak lupus anticoagulants that result in only a slight prolongation of the aPTT are difficult to diagnose. In these cases, mixing studies may demonstrate correction of the prolonged aPTT, and additional specific tests for the lupus anticoagulant such as the dilute Russell's viper venom time (DRVVT) or the kaolin clotting time (KCT) may be necessary for diagnosis.

In rare cases, a lupus anticoagulant may be associated with a prothrombin deficiency and normal levels of factors V, VII, and X. This is attributable to another autoantibody that binds to but does not neutralize prothrombin, with rapid in vivo clearance of the antibody-prothrombin complex. Patients with this condition may develop a bleeding tendency. A lupus anticoagulant can develop in a patient with a preexisting congenital or acquired coagulation abnormality and give rise to diagnostic problems. Optimal detection of the lupus anticoagulant probably requires at least two phospholipid-dependent assays.

A rare cause of an acquired hemorrhagic diathesis that can result in severe bleeding is the acquired deficiency of factor X seen in primary amyloidosis. Evaluation of the acquired coagulation disorders proceeds as follows:

1. Hematologic evaluation is conducted, with particular attention paid to platelet number, RBC morphology indicative of DIC, and WBC count and differential.
2. Samples are screened for bleeding disorders using platelet count, aPTT, and PT. This battery of tests is useful in differen-

Table 43-3 Use of Screening Tests in Acquired Bleeding Disorders

Disorder	Platelet Count	aPTT	PT
Thrombocytopenic purpura*	Decreased	Normal	Normal
Liver disease	Normal or decreased	Normal or increased	Increased
Vitamin K deficiency	Normal	Normal or increased	Increased
Factor VIII antibody	Normal	Increased	Normal
Lupus anticoagulant	Normal (usually)	Increased	Normal or increased
DIC†	Decreased	Normal or increased	Increased

Abbreviations: aPTT = activated partial thromboplastin time; PT = prothrombin time; DIC = disseminated intravascular coagulation.
*See Chapter 40.
†Patients with low-grade chronic DIC may have normal screening test results.

tiating thrombocytopenic purpuras and the acquired diathesis caused by inhibitors, liver disease, vitamin K deficiency, or DIC (**Table 43-3**).

3. In all instances in which the aPTT is significantly prolonged, it is customary to perform inhibitor screening on a mixture of equal parts of normal plasma and patient plasma (sometimes referred to as a 50:50 mix). Failure of the addition of normal plasma to correct the prolonged aPTT is evidence of a circulating anticoagulant. This is in contrast to the finding in deficient states, in which the aPTT value of the 50:50 mix with normal plasma rarely exceeds the aPTT reference range. Correction, however, does not necessarily exclude the presence of an inhibitor. This is particularly applicable when the aPTT of the patient plasma alone is only a few seconds outside the upper limit of the normal range. If a plasma sample containing a potent lupus anticoagulant is diluted with a normal plasma sample to shorten the aPTT to approximately 40 seconds, it often is difficult to demonstrate the presence of a lupus anticoagulant in the resulting plasma mixture based solely on a failure to correct. In this instance, a specific test for the lupus anticoagulant, such as DRVVT or other phospholipid-dependent assays, may be helpful. In the case of some very slow-acting

factor VIII inhibitors, correction may be observed, particularly if the aPTT test is performed within a few minutes of preparing the 50:50 mix with normal plasma. However, the 1-hour incubation sample should indicate the presence of an antibody.

4. If an inhibitor is present or cannot be excluded on the basis of the aPTT of the 50:50 mix and the PT is normal, and the patient is bleeding, the presence of a factor VIII inhibitor must be excluded. One practice is to perform assays for factors VIII, IX, and XI routinely in all such cases when the patient has clinical bleeding. If the factor VIII level is normal, a factor VIII inhibitor can be excluded. However, if the factor VIII level is significantly decreased and does not appear to increase when tested at a higher dilution (eg, 1:20), a specific test for a factor VIII inhibitor is performed (see Chapter 42). When both the aPTT and PT are prolonged and neither is corrected in the 50:50 mix, a specific factor V inhibitor should be considered. If the PT prolongation is corrected in the 50:50 mix but the aPTT is not, specific assays for prothrombin and factors VII, V, and X should be performed. If they are all normal, the cause of the PT prolongation may be an unusual type of lupus anticoagulant. If prothrombin is the only factor whose level is decreased, a prothrombin inhibitor should be considered. The diagnosis of a lupus anticoagulant should be confirmed using DRVVT, the kaolin clotting time test, or other phospholipid-dependent assays.

5. Assay of D-dimer or fibrin monomer (using the protamine sulfate paracoagulation test), as well as serial fibrinogen determinations, are useful if DIC is suspected.

6. Serial PT assays after vitamin K therapy can confirm vitamin K deficiency due to warfarin sodium ingestion or malnutrition if the PT corrects.

43.4 Hematologic Findings

A platelet count is performed and the morphology of RBCs (schistocytes, etc) is evaluated by peripheral blood smear. If platelets are absent or markedly reduced, the patient is evaluated for thrombocytopenic purpura (see Chapter 40). A moderate to severe reduction, however, can be found in liver disease or DIC and may be associated with schistocytes (**Image 43-1**) and spherocytes in the peripheral blood smear for DIC.

Other Laboratory Tests

Test 43.1 Protamine Plasma Paracoagulation Test

Purpose. This test detects fibrin monomer in plasma and is used for the diagnosis of DIC.

Principle. Soluble complexes of fibrin monomer with fibrin (fibrinogen) degradation products or fibrin dissociate with the addition of protamine sulfate. The fibrin monomers then polymerize, forming a fibrin web.

Specimen. Platelet-poor plasma, as collected for the aPTT test, is used.

Procedure. Ten drops of plasma are placed in a small glass test tube warmed to 37°C. One drop of 1% protamine sulfate is added and, after gentle shaking, incubated for 20 minutes.

Interpretation. Fibrin webs or strands are considered an unequivocally positive result. A finely granular, noncohesive precipitate is usually interpreted as a weakly positive result.

Notes and Precautions. False-positive results may be obtained if there is difficulty with venipuncture or a delay in mixing the blood with anticoagulant because of the formation of small amounts of thrombin in vitro. A test should not be performed on oxalated or heparinized blood, but the administration of heparin to the patient does not interfere with the test. Many hospital laboratories have replaced the protamine sulfate test with the D-dimer test.

Test 43.2 Latex Particle Agglutination Tests for Fibrin or Fibrinogen Degradation Products; D-Dimer Test

Purpose. This test detects the presence of fibrin or fibrinogen degradation products (FDPs) and is used in the diagnosis of DIC.

Principle. Antibodies to fibrin (fibrinogen) degradation products are bound to latex particles, which clump in the presence of the antigen. If an antiserum to highly purified fibrinogen fragments D and E is employed in the FDP test, a positive result is obtained with fibrinogen and fibrinogen degradation products as well as with fibrin degradation products. In another version of the test—the D-dimer test—a highly specific monoclonal antibody to D-dimer (a cross-linked fibrin degradation product) is used, and positive results are obtained only with the D-dimer fragment.

Specimen. In some FDP tests, only serum samples may be used. The blood specimen must be obtained by careful and clean venipuncture and placed in a special sample collection tube that contains soybean trypsin inhibitor and thrombin or reptilase. After formation of a clot, the tube is incubated at 37°C for approximately 30 minutes before separating the serum by centrifugation. For the D-dimer test, either plasma or serum samples may be used, but the former is preferred.

Procedure. In the D-dimer test, the undiluted plasma (or serum) sample, a 1:2 dilution in buffer, and a 1:4 dilution in buffer are added to the suspension of latex beads on a glass slide. The suspensions are rotated on the slides for a precise number of minutes. The slide is then inspected for macroscopic agglutination. Known negative or positive controls are run with each test.

The procedure is almost identical in the FDP test, except for the use of 1:5 and 1:20 dilutions of serum in buffer. In the FDP test, the normal serum level of degradation products derived from fibrinogen or fibrin is less than 10 µg/mL, and the reagents are adjusted so a serum sample with less than this concentration will give no agglutination with either 1:5 or 1:20 dilutions of normal serum. In DIC, the level of FDPs exceeds 10 µg/mL and in most cases may exceed 40 µg/mL.

The normal plasma concentration of cross-linked FDPs containing the D-dimer domain is less than 200 ng/mL, and the reagents for this test are adjusted to give negative readings with this concentration. The concentration of D-dimer can be assayed semiquantitatively by preparing serial dilutions of the specimen and determining the highest dilution titer that remains positive. Quantitative methods for measuring D-dimer, including enzyme-linked immunosorbent assay (ELISA) methods, also are available. Most patients with clinically significant DIC have D-dimer values greater than 4 µg/mL.

Notes and Precautions. Degradation products of fibrinogen or fibrin may be incorporated into the clots formed in vitro during the preparation of the serum sample, thereby giving a normal (negative) result or a spuriously low value. The ability to use plasma is a significant advantage for the D-dimer test over FDPs. False-positive results may be seen with the FDP test in patients with dysfibrinogenemia when residual fibrinogen remains in the serum. For all these reasons, the D-dimer test is considered the better test. The D-dimer test cannot be used for monitoring fibrinolytic therapy (eg, streptokinase), in which it is desirable to assay fibrinogen degradation products as well as fibrin degradation products. Both types of tests may give positive results following surgical procedures or in patients with deep-vein thrombosis and pulmonary embolism (the quantitative D-dimer assay may be useful in the diagnosis of these disorders).

Because FDPs are cleared by the liver, patients with liver disease have elevated FDP levels. Consequently, the D-dimer assay is a better test to distinguish DIC from the coagulopathy of liver disease.

False-positive results can be seen with the D-dimer test in patients with rheumatoid factors (IgM molecules). However, D-dimer levels also can be assayed using ELISA-based methods. This method does not give false-positive results with samples containing rheumatoid factors (IgM), which may result with the latex agglutination method.

Test 43.3 Functional Fibrinogen Determination

Purpose. This test quantitates functional plasma fibrinogen levels and is most commonly used in the diagnosis of DIC. Less commonly, it is used to diagnose inherited fibrinogen disorders (eg, dysfibrinogenemia, afibrinogenemia).

Principle. A thrombin time–based clotting assay is used. Thrombin directly cleaves fibrinogen to fibrin monomer; fibrin monomers then polymerize. The clotting time is inversely proportional to the amount of fibrinogen in the sample when read off a standard curve.

Specimen. Citrated plasma sample, as collected for the PT or aPTT assay, is used.

Procedure. A calibration curve is constructed using serial dilutions of a fibrinogen reference preparation. Serial dilutions of patient plasma are prepared. Thrombin is added, and clotting times are measured in duplicate. Patient fibrinogen levels are determined from the standard curve.

Interpretation. The reference range for normal fibrinogen levels is 150 to 350 mg/dL (1.5 to 3.5 g/L). Fibrinogen is an acute-phase reactant with elevated levels occurring in liver disease and inflammatory diseases. Low levels are seen in end-stage liver disease, DIC, dysfibrinogenemias, and the inherited disorders, afibrinogenemia/hypofibrinogenemia.

Notes and Precautions. Large concentrations of heparin in the plasma sample or high levels of FDP may prolong the clotting time and falsely indicate low fibrinogen levels. When evaluating patients for dysfibrinogenemia, functional and antigenic fibrinogen levels should be tested on the same sample.

Test 43.4 Dilute Russell's Viper Venom Time

Purpose. The DRVVT test confirms the presence of the lupus anticoagulant in patients with positive findings on inhibitor screening or in patients with negative findings on inhibitor screening in whom the lupus anticoagulant is strongly suspected.

Principle. A modified PT assay is used in which clotting is initiated by a snake venom (Russell's viper venom) and dilute phospholipid. Russell's viper venom directly converts factor X to factor Xa. Factor Xa, factor V, and phospholipid convert prothrombin to thrombin. By diluting the venom and the phospholipid, the assay is more sensitive in detecting antiphospholipid antibodies that inhibit coagulation (lupus anticoagulant).

Specimen. Platelet-poor plasma, as collected for the aPTT assay, is used. Because platelets can neutralize antiphospholipid antibodies in these plasma samples, it is critical that measures be taken to ensure that the sample has a very low platelet count ($<10 \times 10^3$/mm^3 [$<10 \times 10^9$/L]). This can be achieved using centrifugation or filtration methods.

Procedure. Normal or patient plasma samples are mixed with a phospholipid source (eg, aPTT reagent) and the dilute Russell's viper venom reagent. Clotting times are then measured. If the patient's clotting time is prolonged, the clotting time test is repeated after mixing patient plasma sample with a normal pooled plasma sample. The DRVVT reference range in the author's laboratory is 26 to 35 seconds.

Interpretation. A prolonged DRVVT result in a plasma sample with a normal PT is suspicious for the lupus anticoagulant. A mixing study with a normal plasma sample that also results in a prolonged DRVVT is diagnostic of the lupus anticoagulant.

Notes and Precautions. Obtaining platelet-poor plasma samples is important in maintaining the sensitivity of this test. Samples with prolonged PT values (eg, from patients on oral anticoagulant therapy) exhibit prolonged DRVVT values even in the absence of the lupus anticoagulant. For patients who have prolonged PT values and in whom the lupus anticoagulant is suspected, anticardiolipin antibodies may be a helpful surrogate test. Alternatively, the kaolin clotting time or a dilute PT assay may be a useful test.

Some investigators recommend additional testing to demonstrate phospholipid neutralization of prolonged coagulation tests, definitively diagnosing the lupus anticoagulant. The choice of a "gold standard" coagulation assay to detect lupus anticoagulants is controversial. Many laboratories use the DRVVT assay. The kaolin clotting time appears to be more sensitive, and if this assay can be automated, it may represent the best test for diagnosing lupus anticoagulants.

43.5 Course and Treatment

Treatment for DIC is directed at the primary cause. For patients with significant thrombocytopenia and hypofibrinogenemia, platelet transfusion and cryoprecipitate may be helpful. Patients who have DIC and primarily thrombotic symptoms may benefit from heparin therapy. New therapies are being developed to inhibit thrombin and other coagulation proteases important in DIC.

Patients with the coagulopathy of liver disease and clinical bleeding rarely respond to vitamin K therapy owing to significant hepatocellular damage; these patients may benefit transiently from fresh-frozen plasma. Other disorders associated with vitamin K deficiency (eg, malnutrition, biliary obstruction, antibiotics, warfarin sodium ingestion) should reverse with vitamin K therapy.

Usually no treatment is required for the lupus anticoagulant, unless it is associated with significant thrombocytopenia, thrombosis or recurrent miscarriage. In these cases, anticoagulant therapy or immunosuppression (steroids) may be helpful. Antibodies to specific coagulation factors (especially factor VIII) are best treated with immunosuppression (steroids plus cyclophosphamide), because major bleeding is common in affected patients. Low-titer factor VIII antibodies may be overcome with factor VIII concentrate therapy, in amounts 2 to 3 times the usual 100% dosage. High-titer factor VIII antibodies can be treated with prothrombin complex concentrates, porcine factor VIII, or recombinant factor VIIa.

43.6 **References**

Brandt JT, Triplett DA, Alving B, et al. Criteria for the diagnosis of lupus anticoagulants: an update. *Thromb Haemost.* 1995;74:1185–1190.

Carey MJ, Rodgers GM. Disseminated intravascular coagulation: clinical and laboratory aspects. *Am J Hematol.* 1998;59:65–73.

Exner T, Burridge J, Power P, et al. An evaluation of currently available methods for plasma fibrinogen. *Am J Clin Pathol.* 1979;71:521–527.

Greenberg CS, Devine DV, McCrae KM. Measurement of plasma fibrin D-dimer levels with the use of a monoclonal antibody coupled to latex beads. *Am J Clin Pathol.* 1987;87:94–100.

Grosset ABM, Rodgers GM. Acquired coagulation disorders. In: Lee GR, Foerster J, Lukens JN, et al, eds. *Wintrobe's Clinical Hematology.*10th ed. Baltimore, Md: Williams & Wilkins; 1998:1733–1780.

Hougie C. Latex particle agglutination tests for fibrin or fibrinogen degradation products. In: Williams WJ, Beutler E, Erslev AJ, et al, eds. *Hematology.* 4th ed. New York, NY: McGraw-Hill; 1990:1770–1773.

Martin BA, Branch DW, Rodgers GM. Sensitivity of the activated partial thromboplastin time, the dilute Russell's viper venom time, and the kaolin clotting time for the detection of the lupus anticoagulant: a direct comparison using plasma dilutions. *Blood Coag Fibrinolysis.* 1996;7:31–38.

Thiagarajan P, Pengo V, Shapiro SS. The use of the dilute Russell viper venom time for the diagnosis of lupus anticoagulants. *Blood.* 1986;68:869–874.

Turkstra F, van Beek EJR, ten Cate JW, Buller HR. Reliable rapid blood test for the exclusion of venous thromboembolism in symptomatic outpatients. *Thromb Haemost.* 1996;76:9–11.

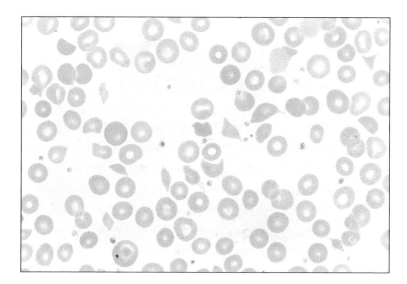

Image 43-1   Peripheral blood smear of a patient with disseminated intravascular coagulation. Numerous RBC fragments (schistocytes) are present. (Wright's stain, oil immersion). From Carey MJ, Rodgers GM. Disseminated intravascular coagulation. *Clinical Hematology Check Sample No.CH98-3.* Chicago, Ill: ASCP Press; 1998:33–47.

44 Laboratory Evaluation of the Patient With Bleeding

Chapters 39 through 43 discussed specific diseases and their laboratory tests. The purpose of this chapter is to synthesize this information into an overall approach to evaluate a patient with a bleeding disorder. **Table 44-1** summarizes the profiles of hemostasis screening tests for patients with bleeding and gives a differential diagnosis for each profile. A major assumption in this chapter is that the patient with bleeding has a hemostatic disorder and not structural bleeding (eg, esophageal varices), surgical bleeding due to a lacerated blood vessel, and so forth. Structural bleeding should always be considered before embarking on a potentially expensive hemostasis evaluation.

The appropriate confirmatory tests are suggested by the differential diagnosis. For example, an isolated prolonged prothrombin time (PT) is most commonly evaluated by liver function studies or by obtaining a history of warfarin use or malnutrition. An isolated prolonged activated partial thromboplastin time (aPTT) should be evaluated by an inhibitor screen and assays for factors VIII, IX, and XI, when heparin contamination is excluded. For patients with prolonged PT and aPTT values in whom disseminated intravascular coagulation is suspected, fibrinogen and D-dimer values should be obtained.

Table 44-1 Profiles of Hemostasis Screening Tests in Patients With Bleeding Disorders*

PT	aPTT	Platelet Count	Frequency	Differential Diagnosis
I	N	N	Common	Factor VII deficiency (early liver disease, early vitamin K deficiency, early warfarin therapy)
			Rare	Factor VII inhibitor, dysfibrinogenemia, inherited factor VII deficiency
N	I	N		Deficiency or inhibitor of factors VIII, IX, or XI; vWD; heparin; lupus inhibitor with qualitative platelet defect
I	I	N	Common	Vitamin K deficiency, liver disease, warfarin, heparin
			Rare	Deficiency or inhibitor of factors X or V, prothrombin, or fibrinogen; lupus inhibitor with hypoprothrombinemia; DIC; primary fibrinolysis; dysfibrinogenemia
I	I	D		DIC, liver disease, heparin therapy with associated thrombocytopenia
N	N	D	Common	Increased platelet destruction, decreased platelet production, splenomegaly, hemodilution
			Rare	Certain inherited platelet disorders (Wiskott-Aldrich syndrome, Bernard-Soulier syndrome)
N	N	I		Myeloproliferative disorders
N	N	N	Common	Mild vWD, acquired qualitative platelet disorders (eg, uremia, antiplatelet medications)
			Rare	Inherited qualitative platelet disorders; vascular disorders; fibrinolytic disorders; factor XIII deficiency; autoerythrocyte sensitization; dysfibrinogenemia; mild deficiency of factors VIII, IX, and XI

Abbreviations: PT = prothrombin time; aPTT = activated partial thromboplastin time; I = increased; D = decreased; N = normal; vWD = von Willebrand's disease; DIC = disseminated intravascular coagulation.
*This table addresses the differential diagnosis of hemostasis screening test results in patients with a history of bleeding. Patients with abnormal coagulation test results and no bleeding history are not included. Modified from Rodgers GM. Common clinical bleeding disorders. In: Boldt DH, ed. *Update on Hemostasis.* New York, NY: Churchill-Livingstone; 1990:75–120.

Patients with bleeding and normal findings on laboratory screening present a challenge, because normal test results do not exclude mild factor deficiency (eg, carriers of factors VIII or IX deficiency) or mild factor XI deficiency. In addition, many patients with mild von Willebrand's disease have normal results on screening. For these patients, extensive investigation may be required before a laboratory diagnosis is achieved.

44.1 **References**

Rodgers GM, Bithell TC. The diagnostic approach to the bleeding disorders. In: Lee GR, Foerster J, Lukens JN, et al, eds. *Wintrobe's Clinical Hematology.* 10th ed. Baltimore, Md: Williams & Wilkins; 1998:1557–1575.

Santoro SA. Laboratory evaluation of hemostatic disorders. In: Hoffman R, Benz EJ, Shattil SJ, et al, eds. *Hematology: Basic Principles and Practice.* New York, NY: Churchill-Livingstone; 1991:1266–1276.

45 Preoperative Hemostasis Screening

The use of screening coagulation tests in preoperative patients is controversial. Large amounts of money are routinely spent to obtain a low yield of positive results. However, the outcome of major surgery in a patient with an unknown hemostatic defect may be catastrophic. One sensible approach is to balance the financial costs of preoperative testing with the extent of surgery to be done and with the amount of bleeding that can be tolerated safely. This approach places critical importance on obtaining a thorough hemostasis history. Patients scheduled for minor procedures (eg, oral surgery, skin biopsy) do not need routine screening tests if they have a negative history. Patients undergoing neurosurgery or procedures that may induce a hemostatic defect (eg, cardiothoracic surgery with a bypass pump) and those with a positive bleeding history need a hemostasis evaluation by the laboratory.

Table 45-1 summarizes Rapaport's suggested guidelines for evaluating preoperative patients. Based on the patient's bleeding history and the type of planned surgery, four levels are identified. Based on these levels of concern, recommendations are made as to the intensity of suggested hemostasis evaluation. Assays for factors VIII, IX, and XI are suggested in the level IV evaluation, because most aPTT reagents are insensitive in detecting mild factor deficiency; factor levels of 20% to 30% may not be detected, and these

Table 45-1 Guidelines for Preoperative Hemostasis Evaluation

Level	Bleeding History	Surgical Procedure	Recommended Hemostasis Evaluation
I	Negative	Minor	None
II	Negative	Major	Platelet count, aPTT
III	Equivocal	Major, involving hemostatic impairment	PT, aPTT, platelet count, factor XIII assay, ECLT
IV	Positive	Major or minor	Level III tests; if negative, then factors VIII, IX, and XI assays, thrombin time, α_2-antiplasmin assay; consider vWD and platelet aggregation testing

Abbreviations: aPTT = activated partial thromboplastin time; PT = prothrombin time; ECLT = euglobulin clot lysis time (a screen for abnormal fibrinolysis); vWD = von Willebrand's disease.

patients would bleed with surgery. The thrombin time screens for dysfibrinogens, and the α_2-antiplasmin assay screens for deficiency of this fibrinolysis inhibitor.

45.1 **Reference**

Rapaport SI. Preoperative hemostatic evaluation: which tests, if any? *Blood.* 1983;61:229–232.

PART
XIII

Thrombotic Disorders

46 Inherited Thrombotic Disorders

Thrombosis is defined as the formation of a blood clot in the circulatory system during life. Arterial thrombi, especially those in the smallest vessels, are composed primarily of platelets, whereas fibrin is the predominant component of venous thrombi. "Hypercoagulability" is a much-abused term and should be used only to refer to changes in the blood associated with an abnormal tendency toward thrombosis. It should never be used to refer to conditions in which clotting time is shortened or procoagulant factor levels are increased, unless these changes are known to be associated with an abnormal tendency toward thrombosis.

46.1 Pathophysiology

Hemostasis is a complex process in which the vascular endothelial cell surface plays a pivotal role in maintaining the fluidity of the blood. The coagulation cascade is modulated by many regulatory mechanisms. **Figure 46-1** summarizes the anticoagulant properties of endothelium. One of the regulatory mechanisms shown is the protein C pathway, which consists of two vitamin K–dependent

Figure 46-1 Antithrombotic properties of the blood vessel wall.
The major antithrombotic properties are depicted.
Heparinlike glycosaminoglycans (GAG) present
on the luminal surface catalyze inactivation of
coagulation proteases, including thrombin, by
antithrombin III (AT III). Complex formation of
the endothelial cell membrane protein (thrombomodulin) with thrombin generates activated
protein C (APC). Binding of APC to endothelial
cell–bound protein S promotes proteolysis of
factors Va and VIIIa, resulting in inhibition of
coagulation. Tissue plasminogen activator (t-PA) is
secreted by endothelial cells to initiate fibrinolysis.
Vascular endothelium also secretes two antiplatelet
substances—prostacyclin (PGI_2) and nitric oxide
(not shown). Endothelial cells also express CD39,
an ADPase with antiplatelet properties (not
shown). Modified with permission from Rodgers
GM. Hemostatic properties of normal and per-
turbed vascular cells. *FASEB J.* 1988;2:116–123.

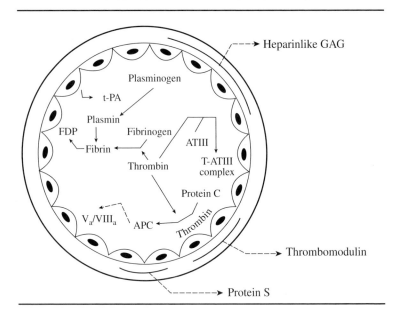

Table 46-1   Features of Vitamin K–Dependent Anticoagulant Proteins

	Protein C	Protein S
Activation	Zymogen activated by thrombin-thrombomodulin complex	None required
Function	Inactivation of factors Va and VIIIa	Cofactor of APC; binds to C4b-binding protein
Inactivation	APC inhibitor	Thrombin cleavage

Abbreviation: APC = activated protein C.

plasma proteins—protein C and protein S (**Table 46-1**). Both of these proteins are potent anticoagulants. Protein C is converted to an active form (APC); this activation is mediated by a receptor, thrombomodulin, which is present on endothelial cell surfaces. Thrombomodulin forms a stoichiometric complex with thrombin on the endothelial cell surface, and this complex activates protein C, which in turn inactivates factors Va and VIIIa. Protein S binds to the endothelial cell surface, providing a receptor for APC. Protein S circulates in the blood in a free form that exhibits anticoagulant activity and a form bound to C4b-binding protein, which has no anticoagulant activity. A factor V mutation (factor V Leiden) that results in thrombosis due to the inability of APC to degrade the abnormal factor Va molecule (APC resistance) has recently been described. Both protein S and factor V promote activation of protein C.

Antithrombin III is another naturally occurring plasma protein with anticoagulant activity. It irreversibly binds to and inactivates certain activated clotting factors such as factor Xa and thrombin. This inactivation is catalyzed (enhanced) by heparinlike glycosaminoglycans on the endothelial cell surface (*see Figure 46-1*) or by commercial heparin used in therapy.

The formation of fibrin is essential in wound healing as well as in hemostasis, but its removal, as soon as it has served its purpose, is equally important. This removal is accomplished by the fibrinolytic mechanism, which, like the coagulation system, is composed of activators and inhibitors in a delicate balance. Moreover, this system, which is part of the overall hemostatic mechanism, functions cooperatively with the coagulation system. Both may be triggered in the same way, and the formation of fibrin greatly enhances fibrinolysis activation.

Well-characterized components of the fibrinolytic system (**Table 46-2**) include the active serine endopeptidase plasmin, which is derived from the inactive zymogen, plasminogen; α_2-antiplasmin, an inhibitor that neutralizes free plasmin almost instantaneously; tissue-plasminogen activator (t-PA); and the major plasminogen activator inhibitor (PAI-1).

The fibrinolytic system may be initiated by the coagulation cascade or by tissue injury. As soon as fibrin is formed, it binds plasminogen, plasminogen activators, and α_2-antiplasmin. Plasminogen activation occurs in the fibrin clot, but any plasmin formed may be neutralized by α_2-antiplasmin, which is present in the clot at the equivalent molar concentration as the fibrin-bound plasminogen. The state of equilibrium is such that when clots are formed in vitro, they do not lyse under normal conditions. In the circulation, however, plasminogen activators are released from the endothelial cell surface in contact with the clot and are absorbed into the thrombus so the equilibrium then favors fibrinolysis (*see Figure 46-1*). In congenital or acquired states in which the activity of the fibrinolytic inhibitor α_2-antiplasmin is decreased, excessive clot lysis occurs at a site of injury, and the hemostatic plugs break down prematurely, resulting in bleeding.

Fibrin plays an integral role in the interplay between t-PA, plasminogen, and α_2-antiplasmin. Tissue plasminogen activator has little effect on plasminogen in the absence of fibrin. The affinity of plasminogen for fibrin is attributable to lysine-rich binding sites and is inhibited by lysine, ε-aminocaproic acid (Amicar), and tranexamic acid. Even a hundredfold increase of free t-PA activity such as occurs in good responders after strenuous exercise does not result in the presence of free plasmin in the blood. Kallikrein formed during the initial contact phase of blood coagulation converts precursor urinary plasminogen activator or urokinase (which is present in plasma) from a single-chain form to a more active two-chain form.

Of the classic triad of Virchow (ie, the risk factors predisposing to thrombosis—endothelial cell damage, stasis, and hypercoagulability), endothelial cell damage is by far the most important factor in arterial thrombosis. Because platelets adhere to damaged endothelium, thrombosis may be considered the natural sequela of arterial disease; the most common cause of this is atherosclerosis.

Table 46-2 Components of the Fibrinolytic Mechanism

Protein	Site of Synthesis	Comments
Plasminogen	Liver	Precursor of plasmin
t-PA	Endothelial cells	Most inactivated by PAI-1; high concentrations released from endothelial cells by occlusion, exercise, epinephrine, etc
PAI-1	Endothelial cells, platelets	t-PA inhibitor
Alpha$_2$-antiplasmin	Liver	Potent plasmin inhibitor

Abbreviations: t-PA = tissue plasminogen activator; PAI-1 = plasminogen activator inhibitor-1.

Thrombotic episodes, usually arterial and involving the smaller vessels, are frequent in myeloproliferative disorders, especially in polycythemia vera and essential thrombocytosis when the platelet count is very high. The vessel wall regulates platelet activation and aggregation by secreting two mediators, prostacyclin (PGI$_2$) and nitric oxide, as well as expressing an endothelial cell protein, CD39, an ADPase that can inhibit platelet activation. However, the clinical importance of these mediators in preventing arterial thrombosis in vivo is uncertain.

In contrast to arterial thrombosis, in which underlying vascular disease is of major importance, stasis and hypercoagulability are critical factors in venous thrombosis. Thus, even in normal individuals, venous thrombosis in the lower extremity occurs with surprising frequency whenever the leg is immobilized for a number of hours (eg, during a long plane journey), but the fibrinolytic system almost always lyses the thrombi. Abnormalities or decreases in the activity of natural anticoagulants, protein C, protein S, or antithrombin III, or the presence of the factor V Leiden mutation, may be associated with an increased incidence of primarily venous thrombosis, whereas the therapeutic infusions of antifibrinolytic agents or activated clotting factors have resulted in massive venous thrombosis. This may explain why altering the equilibrium between procoagulants and anticoagulants using anticoagulant drugs is generally more useful in the treatment of venous thrombosis than of arterial thrombosis.

46.2 Clinical Findings

The symptoms of arterial thrombosis or embolism depend on the size of the vessel, the state of the vessel wall, the degree and length of time of occlusion, the adequacy of a collateral circulation, and the organ involved. If the thrombus or embolus occludes the retinal artery, permanent loss of sight may result; however, occlusion of a small branch of a renal artery may be asymptomatic. The consequences of venous thrombosis usually are not as severe as those of arterial thrombosis. Thus, thrombi in the lower calf veins are often asymptomatic. Because deep venous thrombosis is so frequently asymptomatic, a high index of suspicion is usually required for its recognition, and the differential diagnosis is often difficult. The diagnosis is best established by objective testing, such as ultrasonography or venography. The utility of quantitative D-dimer testing in the diagnosis of venous thromboembolism is under investigation.

46.3 Summary of the Inherited Thrombotic Disorders

Table 46-3 classifies the inherited thrombotic disorders and briefly describes their prevalence, inheritance patterns, and clinical features. Abnormalities of the protein C pathway (protein C, protein S, APC resistance, thrombomodulin) constitute almost half of all cases of inherited thrombosis. In general, inherited disorders are transmitted in an autosomal dominant manner, and venous thromboembolism is the common clinical feature. The prevalence of abnormal fibrinolysis is uncertain because few studies have used optimal assay methods for t-PA and PAI-1. When optimal assays were used, abnormal fibrinolysis was observed in approximately 30% of cases. However, it has not been established whether abnormal fibrinolysis is inherited. Therefore, the importance of inherited t-PA deficiency or excess PAI-1 activity is uncertain.

A recently described inherited thrombotic disorder is the prothrombin mutation; this disorder may account for up to 10% of patients with recurrent thrombosis. Some patients with this mutation have elevated plasma prothrombin levels.

Homocysteinemia (homocystinuria) is a metabolic disorder associated with thrombosis. The prevalence of homocysteinemia in patients with inherited thrombosis is uncertain because this

Table 46-3 A Summary of the Inherited Thrombotic Disorders

Classification and Disorders	Inheritance	Estimated Prevalence*	Clinical Features
Deficiency or qualitative abnormalities of inhibitors to activated coagulation factors			
AT III deficiency	AD	1%–2%	Venous thromboembolism (usual and unusual sites), heparin resistance
TM deficiency	AD	1%–5%	Venous thrombosis
Protein C deficiency	AD	5%–6%	Venous thromboembolism
Protein S deficiency	AD	5%–6%	Venous and arterial thromboembolism
APC resistance	AD	20%–50%	Venous and arterial thromboembolism
Abnormality of coagulation zymogen or cofactor			
Prothrombin mutation	AD	5%–10%	Venous thromboembolism
Elevated factor VIII	Unknown	10%–20%	Venous thromboembolism
Impaired clot lysis			
Dysfibrinogenemia	AD	1%–2%	Venous thrombosis > arterial thrombosis
Plasminogen deficiency	AD, AR	1%–2%	Venous thromboembolism
t-PA deficiency	AD	?	Venous thromboembolism
Excess PAI-1 activity	AD	?	Venous thromboembolism and arterial thrombosis
Metabolic defect			
Homocysteinemia	AR	1 in 335,000 live births; 25% of patients with recurrent thrombosis	Arterial and venous thrombosis (homozygous patients); premature development of coronary and cerebral arterial thrombotic disease (heterozygous patients)

Abbreviations: AT III = antithrombin III; APC = activated protein C; t-PA = tissue plasminogen activator; PAI-1 = plasminogen activator inhibitor-1; TM = thrombomodulin; AD = autosomal dominant; AR = autosomal recessive; ? = uncertain prevalence of abnormal fibrinolysis.
*Prevalence data are estimated by pooling information from studies in which large groups of patients with thrombosis were screened for these disorders. Results are expressed in terms of a percentage that each disorder might constitute of the total patient population with inherited thrombosis. (DNA-based assays for the prothrombin mutation and TM mutations are not widely available.)

diagnosis has not been considered routinely. Although pediatric patients present clinically with the homozygous defect, adult patients heterozygous for homocysteinemia have primarily premature arterial disease. Heterozygous homocysteinemia may account for a significant number of patients with premature vascular disease in the absence of traditional risk factors (eg, tobacco use, hypertension, hyperlipidemia). It has been estimated that 1% to 2% of the general population has heterozygous homocysteinemia. The association of homocysteinemia with venous thromboembolism is increasingly recognized.

Another recently described inherited risk factor for thrombosis is elevated factor VIII activity levels. Although factor VIII is an acute-phase reactant, studies indicate that 10% to 20% of patients with recurrent thrombosis have elevated factor VIII levels as their only risk factor. However, the genetic basis for this risk factor is not understood.

46.4 Diagnostic Approach

Obesity, diabetes, smoking, hyperlipidemia, and hypertension are associated with an increased risk of atherosclerosis and of arterial and venous thrombosis. Venous thrombosis is particularly common after surgical procedures associated with tissue injury, after fractures of the neck of the femur, and in the postpartum period; immobilization of the lower limbs in these situations also is an important causative factor. When one or more of these conditions is present, a special hemostasis workup is rarely indicated. However, when there is no predisposing cause, the venous thrombosis occurs at a very early age or an unusual site (eg, axillary vein), there have been several episodes, or there is a family history of venous thrombosis, the possibility of an inherited or primary hypercoagulable state should be considered. Six key points to address in the laboratory evaluation of these patients include:

1. The laboratory evaluation should be deferred until 2 to 3 months after the acute thrombotic event when the patient is clinically well and preferably has not been receiving anticoagulant therapy for 2 weeks. Thrombosis induces an acute-phase response that may make interpretation of certain test results difficult. Optimal data are obtained in the absence of anticoagulants, because these drugs alter levels of important

factors to be assayed. If anticoagulants cannot be discontinued, symptomatic family members who are not receiving anticoagulants can be tested. However, if DNA-based tests (for the factor V Leiden or the prothrombin mutations) are used, these are unaffected by acute phase changes of thrombosis. Similarly, homocysteine testing will not be affected by anticoagulant therapy. Factor VIII activity testing should be deferred until 6 months after the thrombotic event.

2. The likelihood of obtaining positive results is increased if the patient population being evaluated is restricted to young patients with recurrent thrombosis or patients under 50 years of age with a single event and a positive family history.

3. Functional coagulation assays are preferable to immunologic assays. Functional assays detect patients with either quantitative deficiency of the protein or qualitative abnormality of the protein. However, functional assays are affected more than immunologic assays by anticoagulant therapy.

4. Assay for components of the protein C pathway should be performed initially, because abnormalities of these components (protein C, protein S, APC resistance) are found in at least half of the patients with inherited thrombosis.

5. If fibrinolytic assays are to be performed, optimal assays are critical.

6. Heterozygous homocysteinemia should be considered as a cause for thrombosis in middle-aged patients with premature vascular disease. These patients are best evaluated by a methionine-loading test, usually assayed by the chemistry laboratory by directly measuring blood levels of homocysteine. Immunoassays for this metabolite are now available.

Establishing a specific diagnosis of inherited thrombosis is important, because it allows a single test to be performed on the patient's siblings and children who also may be at risk for thrombosis, since most disorders are transmitted in a dominant fashion.

46.5 Strategy for Laboratory Evaluation of Inherited Thrombosis

Patients with arterial thrombosis should be evaluated initially by assays for PAI-1 or homocysteinemia, depending on their age (**Figure 46-2**). In contrast, patients with venous thromboembolism

Figure 46-2 Suggested algorithm for evaluation of inherited arterial thrombosis. It is assumed that common acquired etiologies for arterial disease (hyperlipidemia, diabetes, myeloproliferative disease, lupus anticoagulants, etc) have been excluded. Possible etiologies for inherited arterial thrombosis include abnormal fibrinolysis, homocysteinemia, activated protein C (APC) resistance, and protein S deficiency. Up to 30% of patients have no identifiable cause of thrombosis, whereas others may have two or more abnormalities (eg, APC resistance and heterozygous homocysteinemia).

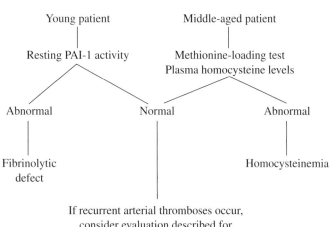

are initially evaluated by assays of the protein C pathway (protein C, protein S, APC resistance); if these are normal, other causes of inherited thrombosis (eg, prothrombin mutation, homocysteinemia, antithrombin III deficiency, dysfibrinogenemia, abnormal fibrinolysis) can be considered. **Figure 46-3** summarizes one approach to the laboratory evaluation of these patients. The exact sequence of test ordering may vary, depending on test availability in a given laboratory, whether the patient is on anticoagulant therapy, and so forth. Factor VIII activity levels should be deferred for many (at least 6) months, to minimize any acute-phase effects.

Laboratory Tests

Test 46.1 **Antithrombin III Determination**

Purpose. Antithrombin III determinations are usually performed to detect a hypercoagulable state associated with venous thrombotic episodes. This assay also may be useful for evaluating patients who appear to be resistant to heparin therapy, or who have thrombosis in an unusual location (intra-abdominal thrombosis).

Principle. A known amount of thrombin is added to a patient plasma sample, and the residual thrombin activity is determined. Antithrombin III antigen levels also may be measured by the Laurell immunoelectrophoresis or radial diffusion methods using specific antibodies, but the functional assay is preferred.

Specimen. Citrated plasma is used in synthetic substrate methods. In clotting assay methods, either citrated plasma or serum may be used, but plasma should be defibrinated.

Procedure. A known amount of thrombin is added to the plasma sample in the presence of heparin; after a timed interval, an aliquot is removed and added to a specific synthetic chromogenic or fluorescent thrombin substrate. In the chromogenic method, colored p-nitroaniline is liberated from the colorless substrate by the thrombin and measured spectrophotometrically.

Figure 46-3 Suggested algorithm for evaluation of patients with inherited venous thrombosis. In this approach, patients with an appropriate personal and family history are tested several weeks after the acute thrombotic event, preferably at a time when they are not taking anticoagulants. Patients with venous thromboembolism who have negative findings on studies of protein C, activated protein C (APC) resistance, protein S, antithrombin III, and dysfibrinogenemia should be considered for testing for homocysteinemia, the prothrombin mutation, and abnormal fibrinolysis. Because APC resistance is common in patients with inherited thrombosis, consideration should be given to assaying for this disorder in the initial evaluation. DNA-based assays can be done for the factor V Leiden mutation in lieu of clotting assays for APC resistance. Assays for elevated factor VIII activity can be performed 6 months after the thrombotic event when anticoagulant therapy has been discontinued. Modified with permission from Rodgers GM, Chandler WL. Laboratory and clinical aspects of inherited thrombotic disorders. *Am J Hematol.* 1992;41:113–122.

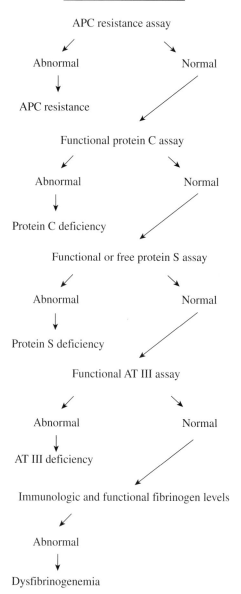

Venous Thromboembolism

APC resistance assay

Abnormal → APC resistance

Normal →

Functional protein C assay

Abnormal → Protein C deficiency

Normal →

Functional or free protein S assay

Abnormal → Protein S deficiency

Normal →

Functional AT III assay

Abnormal → AT III deficiency

Normal →

Immunologic and functional fibrinogen levels

Abnormal → Dysfibrinogenemia

In the fluorescence method, a fluorescent compound is released and measured in a fluorometer. This assay is automated.

Interpretation. The normal range appears to be relatively narrow (82% to 114% based on a normal pool). The level is slightly decreased by oral contraceptives; it is also decreased in the last trimester of pregnancy, but the levels rarely fall below 75% of normal. Such minor decreases may have no clinical relevance. Prolonged use of heparin can result in marked decreases in antithrombin III; such decreases also may occur following a thrombotic event or in association with disseminated intravascular coagulation (DIC). Low values are also seen with liver disease. In inherited deficiency states, the levels are usually in the 40% to 65% range. The antigen level may be normal in approximately 10% of patients with antithrombin III deficiency, so a functional measurement should be performed, at least initially, to exclude these variants.

Notes and Precautions. Serum samples give values approximately 30% lower than plasma samples. Long-term warfarin therapy may increase plasma antithrombin III levels in certain patients. One disadvantage of functional antithrombin III assays is that the presence of heparin cofactor II in the plasma may result in overestimation of antithrombin III activity. Assays using bovine thrombin and lower heparin concentrations (3 U/mL) may minimize thrombin inhibition by heparin cofactor II. Assays based on inhibition of factor Xa rather than thrombin yield more accurate results.

Test 46.2 Protein C Determination

Purpose. This test is performed to detect hypercoagulable states associated with protein C deficiency. The functional assay can detect both quantitative and qualitative abnormalities in protein C.

Principle. Protein C in plasma is most commonly activated by a specific snake venom (Protac). The APC is then assayed by its ability to prolong the aPTT of normal plasma (clotting assay) or to cleave a specific synthetic substrate. Specific antibodies are commercially available, and antigenic determinations can be performed using Laurell immunoelectrophoresis or the enzyme-linked immunosorbent assay (ELISA).

Specimen. A citrated plasma sample is used.

Procedure. The protein C in the plasma sample is activated directly with Protac. The APC is then assayed using either a clotting method or an amidolytic method with a chromogenic substrate.

Interpretation. The normal range in adults is 70% to 130%; however, the normal range is age-dependent for younger patients. The level is reduced in patients with hepatocellular disease, and even a moderate disturbance of liver function may reduce the level to as low as 30%. Heterozygotes have levels of 30% to 65%. Homozygotes are born with DIC (neonatal purpura fulminans) and protein C levels less than 5% of normal; their parents are heterozygotes. A normal antigenic level does not exclude heterozygosity, because in rare variants there is synthesis of an abnormal protein. Because protein C is a vitamin K–dependent protein with a very short half-life, it is depressed early during oral anticoagulant therapy, leading to a transient hypercoagulable state. The ratio of protein C activity to protein C antigen is reduced by warfarin therapy, even in the absence of an inherited abnormality of protein C. The protein C level is reduced in DIC and is lower in serum than in plasma. Newborn infants have physiologically low levels of protein C that rise slowly after birth; the levels are even lower in premature infants. Acute thrombosis also may result in low protein C levels.

Protein C can be assayed in patients receiving stable oral anticoagulation; however, identification of protein C deficiency in patients receiving warfarin therapy requires comparison of these patients' laboratory values with those of patients who receive warfarin and do not have protein C deficiency. Most commonly, ratios of protein C activity to prothrombin activity are compared.

Notes and Precautions. Disadvantages of the Protac functional protein C assay include the inability of chromogenic substrate assays to measure all functional aspects of protein C activity in patients receiving oral anticoagulants. Clot-based functional protein C assays have the advantage of measuring complete biologic functions of APC. However, clotting assays are hampered by acute elevations in plasma factor VIII activity, which result in false low protein C values, and by heparin treatment. Therapeutic heparin levels do not affect the functional chromogenic substrate assay.

Test 46.3 Protein S Determination

Purpose. This test is performed to detect hypercoagulable states associated with protein S deficiency. The functional assay can detect both quantitative and qualitative abnormalities in protein S.

Principle. Protein S acts as a cofactor for APC. Protein S deficiency should be considered in patients evaluated for an inherited disorder of thrombosis.

Specimen. Citrated plasma is used for this determination.

Procedure. Immunologic methods are currently used, including ELISA and Laurell immunoelectrophoresis. A functional assay is based on aPTT with activated factor V as a substrate for APC. Protein S–deficient plasma is mixed with a reference or test plasma sample. Factor Va and APC are added prior to recalcification.

Interpretation. Heterozygotes with protein S levels between 30% and 60% of the normal range may have recurrent venous thrombotic episodes. The functional protein S assay detects quantitative deficiency and qualitative abnormality of protein S.

Notes and Precautions. Spuriously low protein S values may be obtained in patients with APC resistance who are tested using the functional assay. Low protein S levels are seen in acute thrombosis, because C4b-binding protein is an acute phase reactant, whose elevated levels suppress protein S activity. Because protein S is a vitamin K–dependent protein, liver disease and warfarin therapy also reduce protein S levels.

Test 46.4 APC Resistance Assay

Purpose. APC resistance appears to be the major cause of inherited venous thrombosis. This disorder can be diagnosed using clotting assays or molecular diagnostics. This section discusses clotting assays.

Principle. APC is an anticoagulant. When added to normal plasma, clotting times are prolonged; when added to plasma from a patient with the factor V Leiden mutation, clotting times are less prolonged.

Specimen. Citrated plasma is used.

Procedure. Both aPTT- and PT-based assays are available. They are performed with and without APC. Reference range values are determined with a normal population. If the patient's baseline aPTT value is normal (no lupus anticoagulant or anticoagulant therapy), a normalized ratio (aPTT + APC/aPTT) is sufficient. For patients with lupus anticoagulants or those on anticoagulant therapy, PT- or aPTT-based assays in which the patient sample is diluted in factor V–deficient plasma have been described.

Interpretation. In affected patients, the APC-dependent clotting time is prolonged less than the mean minus 2 standard deviations of the normal population.

Notes and Precautions. Because patients with APC resistance may have spuriously low functional protein S levels, APC resistance should be considered in protein S–deficient patients who were diagnosed with a functional assay. Because APC resistance appears to be the most common cause of inherited thrombosis, this disorder should be evaluated initially. A polymerase chain reaction–based assay that detects most patients with APC resistance (discussed later in this chapter) has been described. If the laboratory has large numbers of samples from patients taking heparin or warfarin therapy, this DNA-based test may be a more appropriate assay. It is not usually necessary to do both the APC resistance clotting assay and the factor V Leiden DNA test.

Test 46.5 **Plasminogen Determination**

Purpose. In addition to identifying inherited plasminogen deficiency, this test is also used to distinguish inherited from acquired deficiencies of α_2-antiplasmin. In inherited deficiencies, plasminogen is normal, but in acquired states (eg, liver disease, DIC), plasminogen and α_2-antiplasmin are reduced proportionately.

Principle. Plasminogen is converted to its active form, plasmin, by the addition of an activator. The plasmin is then assayed by the release of a chromophore or fluorescent molecule from a small synthetic peptide substrate. Specific antibodies are commercially available, and immunologic assays may be used.

Specimen. Citrated plasma is used.

Procedure. Streptokinase is usually added to the plasma sample, converting inactive plasminogen to plasmin. The plasmin is then assayed by removing an aliquot and adding a small synthetic peptide substrate bound either to a fluorescent molecule or to a p-nitroanilide compound. The release of fluorescence is measured by a fluorometer; the release of the colored p-nitroanilide compound from the colorless substrate is followed by measurement of optical density at 405 nm in a spectrophotometer.

Interpretation. The normal plasminogen level is 2.4 to 4.4 CTA (Committee on Thrombolytic Agents) U/mL. Striking decreases are found in primary and secondary fibrinolysis (DIC). Plasminogen levels are decreased in liver disease and may be very low or absent following treatment with t-PA, urokinase, or streptokinase.

Notes and Precautions. The test cannot be performed on patients who have received fibrinolytic inhibitors (eg, ε-aminocaproic acid) or on plasma samples containing these types of inhibitors. Antigenic assays give higher values than functional methods, probably because of the action of natural inhibitors in the latter. Several different substrates such as fibrin or casein may be used, but these have been almost completely replaced in routine coagulation laboratories by methods using synthetic chromogenic or fluorescent substrates. Methods to measure α_2-antiplasmin levels are described in Chapter 42.

Test 46.6 Tissue Plasminogen Activator Determination

Purpose. This test is used to identify a fibrinolytic disorder associated with inherited thrombosis.

Principle. Functional assays for t-PA use a plasminogen-chromogenic substrate assay. Total t-PA antigen (free t-PA and t-PA complexed with PAI-1) is measured using an ELISA. Assays for t-PA need to take into consideration the sample collection and timing issues necessary for optimal results.

Specimen. Activity of t-PA is unstable in normal plasma. For optimal measurements, citrated blood must be acidified immediately and the RBCs rapidly removed. Acidification prevents neutralization of t-PA by PAI-1 and prevents PAI-1 from interfering in the assay. Citrated plasma can be used to measure t-PA antigen levels. Because there is diurnal variation in fibrinolysis, samples should be obtained between 8:00 AM and 9:00 AM Some investigators recommend obtaining postvenous occlusion samples for optimal identification of normal individuals from patients with abnormal fibrinolysis.

Procedure. Citrated blood must be acidified with 0.5 M acetate buffer, pH 4.2 (0.5 mL blood:0.25 mL acetate buffer), mixed, and centrifuged. The acidified plasma is collected immediately. For the assay, acidified plasma is incubated with plasminogen, cyanogen-bromide cleaved fibrinogen fragments, and a chromogenic substrate for plasmin. The change in absorbance at 405 nm is proportional to the t-PA activity in the sample; a standard curve is prepared using purified single-chain t-PA.

Interpretation. Low t-PA levels indicate diminished fibrinolysis and may represent a risk factor for thrombosis. Elevated t-PA levels have been associated with excessive fibrinolysis and a bleeding tendency.

Notes and Precautions. As previously mentioned, optimal results require attention to sample collection and timing. Otherwise, it may be difficult to correctly classify patients who may have abnormal findings on fibrinolysis assays. A literature survey by Prins and Hirsh evaluated the evidence for an association between venous thromboembolism and abnormal fibrinolysis. The authors concluded that the published evidence does not prove such an association except in the postoperative setting. Therefore, the association remains unestablished, and the utility of routinely testing patients with inherited thrombosis for fibrinolytic defects remains uncertain.

Test 46.7 Plasminogen Activator Inhibitor–1 Determination

Purpose. Elevated levels of PAI-1 have been linked to recurrent thrombosis, and abnormal fibrinolysis has been suggested as a common cause for thrombosis.

Principle. PAI-1 activity is measured using a back-titration method with t-PA. PAI-1 antigen levels can be measured using ELISA.

Specimen. Citrated plasma can be used to measure PAI-1 activity and antigen levels. Acidification of plasma is not necessary. Some investigators suggest obtaining postvenous occlusion samples to optimally distinguish normal individuals from patients with abnormal fibrinolysis.

Procedure. PAI-1 activity is measured by using multiple dilutions of citrated plasma to which a standard amount of purified single-chain t-PA is added. After incubation, the plasma samples are acidified (to inhibit α_2-plasmin inhibitor), and residual t-PA activity is measured as described previously, using the chromogenic substrate assay.

Interpretation. Elevated PAI-1 levels may be associated with thrombosis.

Notes and Precautions. Sample collection and timing are important variables in fibrinolysis assays. Because an association between inherited thrombosis and abnormal fibrinolysis has not been demonstrated conclusively, the routine use of these assays in evaluating patients for inherited thrombosis is not recommended.

Test 46.8 Homocysteine Measurement

Purpose. The metabolic disorder heterozygous homocysteinemia is a common risk factor for arterial and venous thrombosis.

Principle. Various methods have been described to measure homocysteine levels, including high performance liquid chromatography (HPLC) and fluorescence polarization immunoassay.

Specimen. Most methods use a fasting plasma or serum sample. The most sensitive method to identify heterozygous homocysteinemic patients uses serum measurements before and after oral methionine loading. It is preferable that the collected blood sample be placed on ice. Plasma or serum must be separated promptly from the RBCs.

Procedure. Details of the biochemical measurement of homocysteine are provided in the review articles cited in the references. This assay is typically performed in a clinical chemistry reference laboratory. A common method treats the plasma sample with a reducing agent to reduce homocystine to homocysteine. Perchloric acid is added to remove disulfide-bound homocysteine from protein. Next, a fluorographic reagent is added, chromatography is performed, and total homocysteine is quantitated by a fluorescence detector.

Interpretation. Reference ranges in the author's laboratory are 4 to 12 mmol for men and 4 to 10 mmol for women. The risk for vascular disease (arterial or venous) increases progressively with homocysteine concentration.

Notes and Precautions. A routine fasting homocysteine level may not identify 40% of patients with heterozygous homocysteinemia; these patients are best identified by homocysteine measurements before and after oral methionine loading. Less expensive and easier assays to measure plasma homocysteine levels are under evaluation in the United States; both fluorescent polarization enzyme immunoassay and a microtiter enzyme immunoassay are being studied. These methods will likely replace the HPLC methods.

In evaluating patients for venous thrombosis, the author typically reserves the evaluation of homocysteinemia for patients who test negative for APC resistance, protein C, protein S, antithrombin III deficiency, and the prothrombin mutation.

Test 46.9 Molecular Diagnostic Testing for Inherited Thrombosis

Molecular diagnostic methods have not been clinically relevant for the general evaluation of hemostatic and thrombotic disorders because most of these disorders (von Willebrand's disease, the hemophilias, protein C and S deficiencies, etc) are genetically heterogeneous. However, with the discovery of APC resistance and the prothrombin mutation, each of which is due to highly conserved point mutations in the factor V or prothrombin gene, respectively, these methods have become more useful. This is especially true for the laboratory evaluation of thrombosis in patients receiving anticoagulant therapy, because standard clotting assays are less reliable in diagnosing these patients.

Test 46.10 Factor V Leiden Mutation Detection

Purpose. The factor V Leiden mutation is the most common cause of APC resistance and the most common etiology for inherited thrombosis. Patients on anticoagulant therapy can be evaluated reliably by this DNA-based method.

Principle. Several polymerase chain reaction–based assays have been used to diagnose the factor V Leiden mutation ($Arg^{506} \rightarrow Gln$). In the original method described by Bertina et al, the restriction enzyme *Mnl* was used to digest a 267-bp amplified fragment of patient DNA. Normal DNA digestion results in three fragments, whereas the factor V Leiden mutation results in two fragments. A variety of modifications for detecting this mutation also have been reported (see review by Florell and Rodgers).

Specimen. A blood specimen anticoagulated by ethylenediaminetetraacetic acid (EDTA) is used. The sample should be refrigerated if DNA isolation cannot be done promptly.

Procedure. Details of DNA isolation and PCR methodologies can be found in the references and in Chapter 48.

Interpretation. If DNA isolation and amplification as well as restriction enzyme digestion are successful, three results are possible:

1. Negative. The patient does not have the factor V Leiden mutation (the major cause of APC resistance).
2. Heterozygous. The patient has one allele positive for the factor V Leiden mutation.
3. Homozygous. The patient has two alleles positive for the factor V Leiden mutation.

A negative test result for the factor V Leiden mutation does not exclude APC resistance due to other genetic defects (~5% of patients with APC resistance).

Notes and Precautions. This DNA-based test costs more than the clotting assay for the disorder. Before genetic testing is done, consideration should be given to counseling the patient and obtaining informed consent, particularly because genetic tests have implications for patients and their families. It is not usually necessary to do both the APC resistance clotting assay and the factor V Leiden DNA test.

46.6 **References**

Bertina RM, Koeleman BPC, Koster T, et al. Mutation in blood coagulation factor V associated with resistance to activated protein C. *Nature.* 1994;369:64–67.

Chandler WL, Trimble SL, Loo SC, et al. Effect of PAI-1 levels on the molar concentrations of active tissue plasminogen activator (t-PA) and the t-PA/PAI-1 complex in plasma. *Blood.* 1990;76:930–937.

Comp PC. Measurement of the natural anticoagulant protein S: how and when. *Am J Clin Pathol.* 1991;92:242–243.

de Ronde H, Bertina RM. Laboratory diagnosis of APC-resistance: a critical evaluation of the test and the development of diagnostic criteria. *Thromb Haemost.* 1994;72:880–886.

Florell SR, Rodgers GM. Inherited thrombotic disorders: an update. *Am J Hematol.* 1997;54:53–60.

Hirsh J. Congenital antithrombin III deficiency: incidence and clinical features. *Am J Med.* 1989;87(suppl 3B):34–38.

Koster T, Blann AD, Briët E, et al. Role of clotting factor VIII in effect of von Willebrand factor on occurrence of deep-vein thrombosis. *Lancet.* 1995;345:152–155.

Marcus AJ, Broekman MJ, Drosopoulos JHF, et al. The endothelial cell ecto-ADPase responsible for inhibition of platelet function is CD39. *J Clin Invest.* 1997;99:1351–1360.

Marlar RA, Adock DM. Clinical evaluation of protein C: a comparative review of antigenic and functional assays. *Hum Pathol.* 1989;20:1040–1046.

Nguyen G, Horellou MH, Kruithof EKO, et al. Residual plasminogen activator inhibitor activity after venous stasis as a criterion for hypofibrinolysis: a study in 83 patients with confirmed deep vein thrombosis. *Blood.* 1988;72:601–605.

Ohlin A-K, Norlund L, Marlar RA. Thrombomodulin gene variations and thromboembolic disease. *Thromb Haemost.* 1997;78:396–400.

Poort SR, Rosendaal FR, Reitsma PH, et al. A common genetic variation in the 3'-untranslated region of the prothrombin gene is associated with elevated plasma prothrombin levels and an increase in venous thrombosis. *Blood.* 1996;88:3698–3703.

Prins MH, Hirsh J. A critical review of the evidence supporting a relationship between impaired fibrinolytic activity and venous thromboembolism. *Arch Intern Med.* 1991;151:1721–1731.

Rees MM, Rodgers GM: Homocysteinemia: association of a metabolic disorder with vascular disease and thrombosis. *Thromb Res.* 1993;71:337–359.

Rodgers GM, Chandler WL. Laboratory and clinical aspects of inherited thrombotic disorders. *Am J Hematol.* 1992;41:113–122.

Rosendaal FR. Venous thrombosis: a multicausal disease. *Lancet.* 1999;353:1167-1173.

Svensson PJ, Dahlback B. Resistance to activated protein C as a basis for venous thrombosis. *N Engl J Med.* 1994;330:517–522.

Ueland PM, Refsum H, Stabler SP, et al. Total homocysteine in plasma or serum: methods and clinical applications. *Clin Chem.* 1993;39:1764–1779.

PART
XIV

Anticoagulant Therapy

47 Laboratory Monitoring of Anticoagulant and Fibrinolytic Therapy

Anticoagulant therapy is designed to inhibit the formation of thrombi and to prevent the extension and propagation of existing thrombi. The goal of fibrinolytic therapy is to dissolve or lyse a recent thrombus. Antiplatelet therapy is a form of anticoagulant therapy aimed at reducing the ability of platelets to adhere to one another (aggregate) or to adhere to the damaged endothelium and thereby inhibit thrombosis.

47.1 Pathophysiology

Endothelial cell damage is the most important factor in arterial thrombosis. Because this damage is almost always induced by atherosclerosis, measures designed to reverse or halt this process may be considered antithrombotic. Platelets adhere to the damaged endothelial cell lining, forming the foundation for a thrombus; platelets also can form aggregates in the circulation that may be large enough to block a small artery. In contrast to arterial thrombosis, endothelial cell damage is not an essential component in venous thrombosis. Stasis is relatively more important because it hinders the flowing blood from removing activated coagulation proteases from the site of the thrombus. Thus, immobilization of the lower limbs, particularly in bedridden patients or following surgery or childbirth, may precipitate venous thrombosis.

The oral anticoagulants comprise derivatives of coumarin and include warfarin (Coumadin) and a closely related compound used in Europe, phenindione (Dindevan). These drugs inhibit the synthesis of vitamin K–dependent proteins by the liver. The vitamin K–dependent proteins involved in coagulation are the procoagulants; factors II (prothrombin), VII, IX, and X; and the anticoagulant proteins C and S. Vitamin K is essential for a posttranslational event in which glutamic acid residues are carboxylated, allowing the protein to bind calcium and to phospholipid of cell surfaces. Because the half-lives of the various vitamin K–dependent factors differ, their levels decrease at different rates after warfarin is started. Factor VII and protein C have half-lives of less than 10 hours and are the first to decrease with therapy and to reappear on cessation, while prothrombin has the longest half-life (3 days) and is the last to decrease and reappear.

The other type of widely used anticoagulant is heparin, a heterogeneous substance consisting of glycosaminoglycans of widely varying but high average molecular weight. Several low-molecular-weight heparins also are available. Heparin, which is negatively charged, binds to antithrombin III and sterically modifies this molecule so that its ability to bind to and inactivate thrombin and factors IXa and Xa is greatly enhanced. Heparin is rapidly neutralized by protamine sulfate, which is positively charged. Administration is usually intravenous and may be subcutaneous, but is never intramuscular.

Unlike anticoagulant therapy with either oral anticoagulants or heparin, fibrinolytic agents (also called "thrombolytic agents") have a relatively rapid action. Treatment with fibrinolytic agents, which include urinary plasminogen activator (u-PA) or urokinase, streptokinase, and tissue plasminogen activator (t-PA), may result in bleeding from sites at which venipuncture was performed some days earlier, indicating dissolution of the hemostatic plugs and the effectiveness of these agents.

When the degree of anticoagulation with oral medications exceeds a toxic level, hematuria is almost inevitable, and purpura is a frequent complication. Similarly, a patient receiving heparin is likely to bleed from an open wound. Despite the hemorrhagic complications associated with these drugs, their efficacy in preventing or treating thrombotic disease is well established, and they are among the most commonly used in treating hospitalized patients. The advent of low-molecular-weight heparin also allows anticoagulation of patients in the outpatient setting.

47.2 Clinical Indications

Heparin is currently used for the prophylaxis and treatment of venous thromboembolism, unstable angina, acute myocardial infarction, and chronic disseminated intravascular coagulation (DIC). It is also used in hemodialysis and cardiac bypass surgery and to maintain catheter patency. Warfarin is used in the treatment and prophylaxis of venous thromboembolism and in the prevention of systemic embolism in the settings of tissue heart valves, mechanical heart valves, acute myocardial infarction, and atrial fibrillation.

Common indications for fibrinolytic therapy include acute myocardial infarction, massive venous thrombosis or pulmonary embolism, peripheral arterial thromboembolism, and restoration of catheter patency.

Indications for aspirin and other antiplatelet drugs include primary and secondary prophylaxis of arterial vascular disease.

47.3 Administration Methods

Anticoagulant therapy in patients with acute venous thrombosis initially consists of heparin administration. Heparin is best given intravenously, starting with a bolus of 5000 or 10,000 units followed by a constant infusion of at least 1300 units/hour. After therapeutic anticoagulation with heparin has been achieved (preferably within the first 24 hours), oral warfarin is started, usually at dosages of 5 to 10 mg/day. There should be at least a 5-day overlap of heparin and warfarin so the patient remains anticoagulated until attaining therapeutic vitamin K deficiency with warfarin. When heparin is used prophylactically, the usual regimen is 5000 units, given subcutaneously, every 8 to 12 hours.

A low-molecular-weight heparin (enoxaparin [Lovenox]) is available to treat acute deep venous thrombosis. This drug is given subcutaneously at a dosage of 1 mg/kg every 12 hours, and as discussed in the next section, does not require laboratory monitoring. Fibrinolytic agents are administered intravenously. Streptokinase and urokinase are given in bolus form, followed by continuous infusion over 12 to 72 hours; t-PA is given in a shorter intravenous infusion.

47.4 Laboratory Monitoring

With the increasing use of anticoagulant drugs in treating thrombotic disease, accurate laboratory methods to monitor anticoagulant intensity is an important issue. Recognition of laboratory variables that may result in inaccurate monitoring has led to attempts to standardize these assays. Consensus guidelines for monitoring heparin therapy and warfarin therapy have been published.

47.4.1 Monitoring Heparin Therapy

The effect of heparin can be monitored by a variety of assays, but the standard method is the activated partial thromboplastin time (aPTT) test. Heparin should be given in doses sufficient to prolong the aPTT from 1.5 to 2.5 times the mean laboratory control aPTT (mean of the therapeutic range). This recommendation assumes that the aPTT reagent is responsive to heparin so that plasma heparin levels of 0.2 to 0.4 U/mL (measured by protamine titration) or 0.35 to 0.7 U/mL (measured by anti–factor Xa activity) result in the aPTT being prolonged in the suggested range. However, because aPTT reagents may vary widely in terms of heparin responsiveness, each laboratory should establish its own therapeutic range so it corresponds to the plasma heparin levels given here. The most appropriate method for determining the therapeutic range is direct comparison of the aPTT with heparin concentrations in plasma samples from patients receiving heparin. Details of College of American Pathologists consensus guidelines on the standardization of aPTT assays have been summarized by Olson et al.

The timing and type of sample collected for monitoring heparin therapy is important. The aPTT should be checked 4 to 6 hours after heparin bolus or after a change in infusion rate so steady-state levels are measured. Samples drawn from indwelling lines may give nonrepresentative results. If prophylactic subcutaneous heparin or low-molecular-weight heparin is used, laboratory monitoring is usually not necessary.

Heparin (or low-molecular-weight heparin) monitoring also can be done using heparin levels (anti–factor Xa activity). This assay is not routinely used in monitoring but is usually reserved for patients receiving heparin in whom the aPTT assay is not reliable (eg, lupus anticoagulant) or for patients receiving low-molecular-weight heparin who accumulate the drug abnormally (eg, renal failure). Platelet counts should be monitored during heparin administration, because decreasing counts are common and heparin-induced thrombocytopenia is a rare but potentially serious complication. Heparin-induced thrombocytopenia is much less likely with low-molecular-weight heparin.

47.4.2 Monitoring Warfarin Therapy

All patients receiving warfarin (or other oral anticoagulants) should be monitored using the prothrombin time (PT) assay with calculation of the international normalized ratio (INR). Only recently has there been any measure of agreement as to an efficacious or therapeutic range at which the PT should be maintained; controversy arose from the absence of a uniform or standard way of performing the one-stage PT test (see Chapter 39). The reason is that different tissue extracts, or "tissue thromboplastins," can give different PT values with different pathologic plasma samples, although the normal control times may be the same. Even extracts prepared by the same method from the same tissue do not always give identical results with a pathologic plasma, although the differences are minimized. In general, human brain extracts, now rarely used, give longer clotting times than rabbit brain extracts. When the test was first devised by Quick, it was believed to measure prothrombin specifically, provided the concentration of fibrinogen was above a certain critical level, and the results were often recorded in percentage of prothrombin activity. With the subsequent discovery of factors V, VII, and X, which are also measured by the test along with prothrombin, this method of reporting became invalid. In addition laboratories traditionally used a variety of reporting methods to quantify oral anticoagulation intensity. These differences in assays and reporting methods resulted in inadequate anticoagulation or excessive anticoagulation with adverse consequences.

An important advance was the adoption of a World Health Organization (WHO) international reference thromboplastin preparation. Each new batch of thromboplastin can be calibrated against the primary WHO reference material by using each batch to determine the PTs of plasma samples from different patients whose conditions have been stabilized with long-term oral anticoagulant therapy. The unknown preparation of thromboplastin is found to give PT values that are the same as, longer (higher ratios), or shorter (lower ratios) than those obtained with the standard thromboplastin, but a consistent and reproducible pattern is obtained. These results are used to calculate the relative sensitivity of the unknown preparation compared with the standard (International Sensitivity Index [ISI]). **Figure 47-1** illustrates how ISI values are derived. From this value, an INR, defined as the PT ratio that would have been obtained if the WHO international reference thromboplastin had been used, can be determined for any ratio obtained with the unknown thromboplastin (INR = [PT ratio]^{ISI}) (**Figure 47-2**).

The manufacturer should calibrate each new lot of thromboplastin, and a table enabling conversion to the equivalent INR should be included in the product insert. This table is valid only for the particular instrument-reagent combination used by the manufacturer. The laboratory report should always state the PT value in seconds, as well as the PT ratio and the INR. Only then can a result be interpreted by a physician at another institution without having to first consult the pathologist performing the test. In the past, many physicians endeavored to maintain the PT ratio at 2, but with some reagents, this represented an excessive degree of anticoagulation and resulted in a relatively high incidence of hemorrhagic manifestations; with other reagents, this ratio provided relatively little protection against thrombosis. **Table 47–1** summarizes the guidelines issued by a consensus conference (American College of Chest Physicians–National Heart Lung and Blood Institute, November 1998); the therapeutic ranges in terms of INR are shown. Prothrombin time ratios are less useful because the ISI values of thromboplastins used in the United States still differ dramatically. With the exception of treating patients with high-risk prosthetic (metal) heart valves or patients with recurrent embolism, standard warfarin therapy is targeted at an INR of 2.0 to 3.0. Many investigators prefer to treat thrombosis associated with antiphospholipid antibodies using high-intensity warfarin (INR 2.5 to 3.5).

Figure 47-1   Derivation of an International Sensitivity Index (ISI) value for a thromboplastin preparation. Log prothrombin time (PT) values are determined using a reference thromboplastin reagent and the commercial laboratory thromboplastin reagent. Patients receiving stable oral anticoagulants are tested, as are a group of normal volunteers. The best-fit line is determined, and the slope of this line multiplied by the ISI of the reference thromboplastin reagent is the ISI value for the commercial thromboplastin reagent.

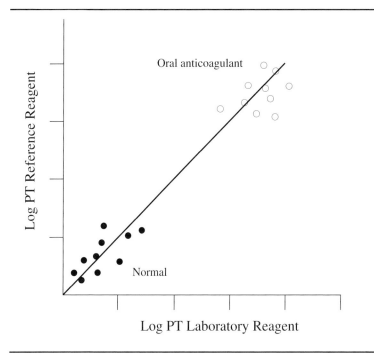

With more widespread use, limitations in using the INR format have been reported. Manufacturers of thromboplastin reagents do not provide ISI values derived for all instrument-reagent combinations. Consequently, the thromboplastin ISI package insert is not accurate for all laboratories. Less sensitive thromboplastins (higher ISI values) yield INR results with greater variability than do

Figure 47-2 Relationship between the prothrombin time (PT) ratio and the International Normalized Ratio (INR) for thromboplastin reagents over a range of International Sensitivity Index (ISI) values. The example shown is for a PT ratio of 1.3 to 1.5 for a thromboplastin preparation with an ISI value of 2.3. From the formula, INR = PT ratio^{ISI}, the INR is calculated as $1.3^{2.3}$ to $1.5^{2.3}$, or 1.83 to 2.54. Reprinted, with permission, from Hirsh J. Oral anti-coagulant drugs. *N Engl J Med.* 991;324:1865–1875. (Copyright © 1991 Massachusetts Medical Society. All rights reserved.)

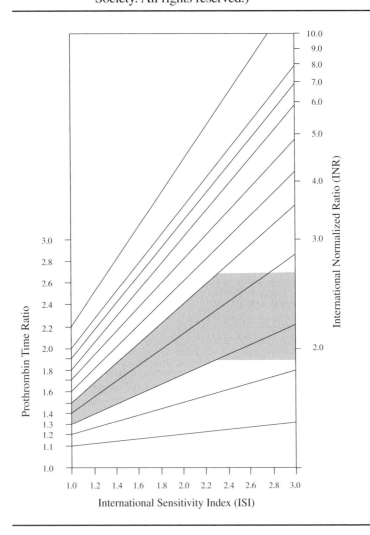

Table 47-1   Recommended Therapeutic Range for Warfarin
Therapy

Indication	International Normalized Ratio
Treatment of venous thrombosis Treatment of pulmonary embolism Prevention of systemic embolism Tissue heart valves Acute myocardial infarction Atrial fibrillation	2.0–3.0 (low intensity)
Recurrent embolism Mechanical heart valves (high-risk) Antiphospholipid antibodies*	2.5–3.5 (high intensity)

*Many investigators believe that antiphospholipid antibodies are an indication for high-intensity warfarin therapy.
Source: From a consensus conference report published in *Chest*. 1998;114(suppl):445S–469S.

more sensitive thromboplastins (lower ISI values), because determination of PT results using less sensitive thromboplastins is associated with higher coefficients of variation. More optimal INR values are obtained if the coagulation laboratory uses a sensitive thromboplastin (ISI 1.0 to 1.5) and ensures that the ISI value is correct, either by calibrating the reagent or by using a thromboplastin whose ISI is appropriate for the laboratory's instrumentation. Many manufacturers now provide sensitive thromboplastins, and recombinant thromboplastins with ISI values of 1.0 also are available. Unfractionated heparin therapy may variably affect the PT/INR values. This latter effect results from some, but not all, thromboplastin manufacturers including heparin-neutralizing substances (such as polybrene) in their reagents.

Many other drugs or medical conditions, particularly liver disease, inhibit or enhance the effect of oral anticoagulants. Recent ingestion of such a drug or the presence of one of these illnesses should be suspected whenever the PT changes unexpectedly in a patient whose condition was previously stabilized (**Table 47-2**). For individuals with marginal dietary vitamin K intake, sterilization of the gut by an antibiotic can result in increased sensitivity to

Table 47-2 Drugs and Medical Conditions Affecting the Potency of Warfarin

Drugs	Conditions
Increased	
Antibiotics	Age
Aspirin	Liver disease
Cimetidine	Malabsorption
Allopurinol	Congestive heart failure
	Malnutrition
Decreased	
Barbiturates	Excess dietary vitamin K
Vitamin K	Nephrotic syndrome

oral anticoagulants; this is perhaps the most common adverse interaction that occurs with warfarin.

Warfarin also affects the metabolism and blood levels of many common prescription medications. Reassessment of dosages and therapeutic levels of these other medications may be required after starting warfarin therapy.

Alternative methods to monitor oral anticoagulant therapy, including fingerstick-monitor devices, have been investigated. A recent study found some of the fingerstick devices to be problematic for monitoring warfarin therapy. If these devices are to be used, the laboratory must validate them against a reference PT method to ensure their reliability. Consensus guidelines have been published on laboratory monitoring of oral anticoagulation using PT methods and fingerstick-monitor devices. These recommendations include (1) using 3.2% citrate as the anticoagulant for coagulation testing, (2) processing and testing PT specimens within 24 hours for room temperature storage, (3) using a thromboplastin with a low ISI value (~1.0), (4) using thromboplastin reagents with known reagent-instrument ISI relationships, and (5) being aware that lupus anticoagulants and heparin may affect the PT/INR.

47.4.3 Monitoring Fibrinolytic Therapy

The systemic intravenous infusion of streptokinase has been used for at least three decades to dissolve arterial or venous clots. Streptokinase, however, is a bacterial product derived from streptococci and, because many individuals have significant titers of antistreptokinase antibodies as a result of a previous streptococcal infection, this complicates therapy and may result in severe side effects. Until recently, urokinase and t-PA were derived only from human sources, making them scarce and expensive; however, these drugs are now available as recombinant products.

Fibrinolytic drugs can be administered systemically to treat venous thromboembolism or myocardial infarction, or infused locally to lyse catheter clots. Local infusions do not require routine laboratory monitoring. However, when these agents are used systemically, it is useful to ensure that a "lytic effect" is achieved. This is especially true for streptokinase therapy, because some patients may have neutralizing antibodies to this bacterial antigen. The lytic state is most easily monitored using the thrombin time assay; prolongation of the thrombin time to values between two and five times over baseline indicates the presence of the lytic state. Since there is no correlation between efficacy of therapy and changes in coagulation or fibrinolytic assays, no additional testing is necessary if an appropriate increase in the thrombin time occurs. For patients with myocardial infarction who receive short-term t-PA infusion, laboratory monitoring may not be necessary. If the patient receives concomitant heparin therapy, the thrombin time will not be a useful test, and the reptilase test or fibrinogen assays should be considered as assays to monitor the lytic state.

47.4.4 Aspirin and Other Antiplatelet Therapy

Aspirin is now used extensively to treat arterial thromboembolic disease and to prevent occlusion of arterial grafts and formation of thrombi on prosthetic heart valves. It reduces thromboxane production for the life of the platelet, thereby decreasing platelet aggregation. However, it also diminishes the production of prostacyclin by the endothelium, albeit for a relatively shorter time, thereby enhancing aggregation. Extensive studies have been performed to evaluate the possibility of using low-dose aspirin therapy selectively to inhibit platelet thromboxane synthesis without affecting vascular prostacyclin formation. In recent clinical trials, the daily dose has varied from 80 mg ("baby aspirin") to 650 mg. Antiplatelet therapy is not monitored by laboratory testing.

Other antiplatelet therapies currently used include an antibody to the platelet fibrinogen receptor (abciximab, Reo-Pro), as well as a variety of peptide inhibitors to this receptor. Inhibitors to the platelet ADP receptor such as ticlopidine and clopidogrel are also in use.

Laboratory Tests

Test 47.1 **Heparin Level**

Purpose. Occasionally it is necessary to determine plasma heparin levels to monitor heparin anticoagulation in patients for whom the aPTT is not a reliable assay (those with lupus anticoagulant).

Principle. The ability of dilutions of patient plasma to inhibit factor Xa is compared with that of standard concentrations of heparin in normal pooled plasma.

Specimen. Citrated plasma collected during stable heparin infusion is used. Blood specimens should not be drawn from indwelling catheters.

Procedure. The manual (fibrometer) method for assaying heparin levels is tedious. Dilutions of heparin are made in saline and normal pooled plasma. Calcium, the aPTT reagent, and factor Xa are added and clotting times measured. Control and patient plasma standard curves are constructed, and a best-fit line is drawn. Plasma heparin levels are determined from these curves.

Interpretation. The therapeutic heparin level from this assay is 0.35 to 0.7 U/mL. The heparin used to construct laboratory standard curves should be the same brand as that for which the sample is being tested.

Notes and Precautions. Automated methods to measure heparin levels are available from a variety of manufacturers. In these methods, a chromogenic substrate assay is used to quantitate inhibition of bovine factor Xa by heparin–antithrombin III. With the increasing use of low-molecular-weight heparins (LMWH), some patients with renal failure who receive these drugs require monitoring using this assay. A calibrated LMWH should be used to establish the standard curve for the assay to measure LMWH. The target concentration for the peak LMWH level in platelets treated with twice-daily dosing (ie, enoxaparin) for acute deep-vein thrombosis should be 0.5-1.1 U/mL.

47.5 **References**

Fairweather RB, Ansell J, van den Besselaar AMHP, et al. College of American Pathologists Conference XXXI on Laboratory Monitoring of Anticoagulant Therapy: laboratory monitoring of oral anticoagulant therapy. *Arch Pathol Lab Med.* 1998;122:768–781.

Foulis PR, Wallach PM, Adelman HM. Performance of the Coumatrak system in a large anticoagulation clinic. *Am J Clin Pathol.* 1995;103:98–102.

Hirsh J. Oral anticoagulant drugs. *N Engl J Med.* 1991;324:1865–1875.

Hirsh J. Heparin. *N Engl J Med.* 1991;324:1565–1574.

Hirsh J, Dalen JE, Anderson DR, et al. Oral anticoagulants: mechanism of action, clinical effectiveness, and optimal therapeutic range. *Chest.* 1998;114(suppl):445S–469S.

Hirsh J, Poller L. The international normalized ratio: a guide to understanding and correcting its problems. *Arch Intern Med.* 1994;154:282–288.

Laposata M, Green D, Van Cott EM, et al. College of American Pathologists Conference XXXI on Laboratory Monitoring of Anticoagulant Therapy: the clinical use and laboratory monitoring of low-molecular-weight heparin, danaparoid, hirudin and related compounds, and argatroban. *Arch Pathol Lab Med.* 1998;122:799–807.

Ng VL, Valdes-Camin R, Gottfried EL, et al. Highly sensitive thromboplastins do not improve INR precision. *Am J Clin Pathol.* 1998:109:335–345.

Olson JD, Arkin CF, Brandt JT, et al. College of American Pathologists Conference XXXI on Laboratory Monitoring of Anticoagulant Therapy: laboratory monitoring of unfractionated heparin therapy. *Arch Pathol Lab Med.* 1998;122:782–798.

Rodgers GM. Thrombosis and antithrombotic therapy. In: Lee GR, Foerster J, Lukens JN, et al, eds. *Wintrobe's Clinical Hematology.* 10th ed. Baltimore, Md: Williams & Wilkins; 1998:1781–1820.

Shojania AM, Tetreault J, Turnbull G. The variations between heparin sensitivity of different lots of activated partial thromboplastin time reagent produced by the same manufacturer. *Am J Clin Pathol.* 1988;89:19–23.

PART
XV

Special Techniques

48 Special Techniques: Flow Cytometry, Molecular Diagnostics, Fluorescent In-Situ Hybridization and Cytogenetics

The diagnosis of hematopoietic neoplasms requires the integration of numerous pieces of data for a final interpretation. Although histologic examination remains the gold standard by which diagnoses are made, numerous ancillary techniques are readily available to support or confirm the histologic impression. Flow cytometry, molecular diagnostics, fluorescent in situ hybridization (FISH), and conventional chromosome metaphase spread analysis are the most commonly used adjunctive studies in the diagnosis of hematopoietic tumors. These techniques often provide diagnostic information beyond that seen with routine light microscopy. Although useful and often necessary, the use of these techniques is not needed in the diagnosis of many common hematopoietic disorders. In addition, many of these specialized tests are relatively expensive and should be used judiciously.

Because many of the adjunctive tests used in the workup of hematopoietic neoplasms require a fresh tissue sample, it is important to plan ahead and anticipate which ancillary studies may be needed. Often the patient's clinical presentation and medical history provide insight into the potential need for these studies. Such preparation ensures that an adequate specimen is obtained and processed to avoid returning to the patient for additional specimens.

This chapter discusses many of the most common and readily available specialized tests used in hematopathology. The basic principles of each technique as they relate to hematopoietic disorders are presented in a simplified overview. Specialized texts and the references at the end of this chapter may provide more complete and in-depth descriptions and discussions of these techniques. Each of the techniques described here has its own specific utility and specimen requirement. Although more than one of these tests may be indicated for any given specimen, they often are performed in different laboratories by specialized personnel with each requiring a separate sample. The tests are described individually to highlight their unique advantages and disadvantages as well as specific indications and requirements.

48.1 Flow Cytometry

Flow cytometry is a rapid and reliable technique for immunophenotyping hematopoietic cells. Because of the lack of cohesiveness of these cells, they are ideally suited for study by flow cytometry, which allows quick analysis of large numbers of cells and quantification of their biologic parameters. Flow cytometry has a broad range of uses in the evaluation of hematopoietic processes. One of the most common is immunophenotyping of peripheral blood, lymph node, and bone marrow samples to establish the presence of clonality or leukemia. Flow cytometry, however, has many other uses, including determining CD4/CD8 ratios and absolute counts, establishing the presence of congenital immunodeficiencies, determining the ploidy and S-phase of tumors, and evaluating RBCs for specific defects associated with paroxysmal nocturnal hemoglobinuria (PNH). This chapter concentrates on the use of flow cytometry in evaluating clonality of lymphoid cells and diagnosing leukemias. Its use in the diagnosis of PNH is discussed in Chapter 11.

48.1.1 Purpose

Hematopoietic cells express a wide range of cell surface antigens. The detection of these antigens by flow cytometry allows identification of normal and abnormal expression patterns.

48.1.2 Principle

Flow cytometry is the process of passing cells singly in a fluid stream through a beam of light (**Figure 48-1**). The light source is typically a laser and as the cells pass through the laser beam, photons of light are emitted and scattered. These photons are separated and collected by forward and side light scatter detectors. The detected light signal is converted into a digital signal with the aid of photomultiplier tubes. The digital signal generated by each cell is proportional to its light emission and is plotted on a histogram. One of the most important requirements of flow cytometry is the passage of single cells through the light source. This is achieved by forcing an isotonic (sheath) fluid through a cylindrical nozzle to create a laminar flow. The sample, also suspended in isotonic fluid, is introduced simultaneously into the nozzle. The differential pressure under which the sample and the sheath fluid are forced into the nozzle results in the hydrodynamic focusing of the cells in the center of the fluid stream, in which they pass singly through the light source (**Figure 48-2**).

All cells have intrinsic properties that cause light to scatter 360 degrees when exposed to a beam of light. In flow cytometry, scattered light is typically detected in two axes: forward light scatter, which is parallel to the laser beam, and side light scatter, which is detected at a 90-degree angle to the laser beam. Forward light scatter roughly corresponds to the size of the cell; side light scatter corresponds to the nuclear complexity and cytoplasmic granularity of the cell. For example, mature lymphocytes, which are relatively smaller cells with round nuclei and little cytoplasmic granulation, exhibit low forward and low side light scatter. In contrast, granulocytes, which are larger in size with abundant cytoplasmic granulation, exhibit increased forward and increased side light scatter. These differences in forward and side light scatter allow identification of lymphocytic, monocytic, and granulocytic cell populations. Abnormal cell populations also can be detected by their light scatter patterns.

In addition to the intrinsic light scattering properties of hematopoietic cells, flow cytometry uses numerous fluorochrome-conjugated antibodies that can tag individual cells to further delineate their antigenic profile. The fluorochromes typically used in clinical flow cytometry have specific and distinct excitation and emission spectra. The argon laser is the most commonly used light source for clinical hematopoietic flow cytometry. It produces a 488-nm excitation wavelength, which is able to excite many

Figure 48-1 Schematic representation of a flow cytometer. As cells pass through the laser light source, light is scattered and recorded by forward, side, and fluorescence light detectors.

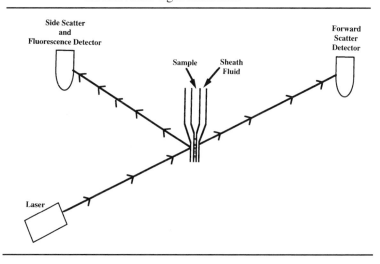

different fluorochromes. Two of the most widely used fluorochromes that can be excited by this wavelength are fluorescein isothiocyanate (FITC) and phycoerythrin (PE) (**Table 48-1**). These fluorochromes are commonly used simultaneously because they can both be excited by the same light source yet have different spectra of light emission. It is their difference in light emission that allows them to be detected as separate signals and wavelength groups. Texas red (TR) and cyanine 5 (Cy5) are two other fluorochromes that can be coupled with PE to produce tandem conjugate fluorochromes. When TR or Cy5 are conjugated with PE, excitation can take place at 488 nm (with an argon laser), followed by energy transfer from the excited PE molecules to the TR or Cy5 molecules. The emitted light is at 613 nm and 667 nm, respectively, which can be detected as separate and distinct third signals or "colors." Thus the use of three separate fluorochromes or fluorochrome conjugates, each attached to different monoclonal antibodies, allows simultaneous detection of three separate parameters or signals on a single cell (three-color flow cytometry).

Newer flow cytometers contain two lasers or four detectors that can simultaneously excite and detect four or more fluorochromes (four-color flow cytometry) on a single cell. Propidium

Figure 48-2 A typical flow chamber by which the sample and sheath fluid are introduced into the cytometer. Cells from the sample are forced into the middle of the fluid stream by hydrodynamic properties and past the laser beam in single file.

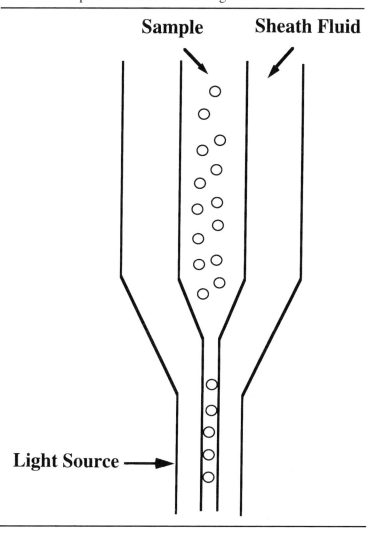

Sample   **Sheath Fluid**

Light Source

iodide (PI), a DNA-staining fluorochrome that is excited at 488 nm, is commonly used in DNA S-phase and ploidy studies. Because PI is excited at the same wavelength as FITC and PE, the same argon laser can be used for DNA analysis testing.

Table 48-1 Fluorochromes Commonly Used in Flow Cytometry

Fluorochrome	Laser Used	Wavelength of Excitation (nm)	Peak Emission Wavelength (nm)
Fluorescein isothiocyanate	Argon	488	520
Phycoerythrin	Argon	488	575
Tandem conjugates			
PE-TR	Argon	488	613
PE-CY5	Argon	488	667
Propidium iodide	Argon	488	620

Numerous monoclonal antibodies that recognize various cell surface antigens on hematopoietic cells are currently available. These antigens are recognized and referred to by their antigen cluster designation (CD). **Table 48-2** provides a list of the most common and well-recognized monoclonal antibodies for hematopoietic cells. Many companies now supply monoclonal antibodies that are preconjugated to FITC and PE or to fluorochrome conjugates. When hematopoietic cells are mixed and incubated with these fluorochrome-conjugated antibodies, the antibodies bind to those cells that express the corresponding antigen on their surface. After incubation and removal of excess unbound antibody and fluorochrome by washing, the cells are then analyzed or "counted" by the flow cytometer. As cells with antibody-bound fluorochrome pass through the laser beam, there is excitation of the fluorochrome, followed by light emission. The light emission from the fluorochrome has a specific wavelength, as noted previously. This light emission results from the fluorochrome-conjugated antibody that has bound to its corresponding antigen on the cell surface, indicating cellular expression of that specific antigen. The "positive" light emission signal is converted to a digital signal and plotted on a histogram. A series of dichroic mirrors and filters allow the separation of the emitted light into different wavelength groups and detection by multiple fluorescence detectors.

Because any given cell expresses multiple antigens on its surface, it is possible and common for a cell to exhibit positivity for multiple antigens. When two or more antigens are expressed by the same cell, they are referred to as "coexpressed antigens". The coexpression of antigens may be normal, as seen with the expression of CD3 and CD5 by mature lymphocytes, or abnormal, as seen when

Table 48-2 Commonly Used Monoclonal Antibodies by Cluster Designation

CD	Common Names	Activity
CD1	T6, Leu-6, OKT6	Immature thymocytes, Langerhans' cells
CD2	T11, Leu-6, OKT11	Pan-T cells, NK cells
CD3	T3, Leu-4, OKT3	Pan-T cells
CD4	T4, Leu-3, OKT4	Helper T cells, monocytes, macrophages
CD5	T1, Leu-1, OKT1	Pan-T cells, rare B cells, B-CLL, MCL
CD6	T12	Pan-T cells
CD7	Leu-9, OKT16	T cells, NK cells
CD8	T8, Leu-2, OKT8	Suppressor T cells, some macrophages, monocytes
CD9	FMC8	Early B cells, activated T cells, platelets
CD10	T5, CALLA	Early B cells, early T cells, germinal center cells, neutrophils
CD11b	Mol, Leu-15	Monocytes, neutrophils, NK cells
CD11c	Leu-M5, BLY6	Monocytes, activated lymphocytes, granulocytes, HCL
CD13	My7, Leu-M7	Myeloid cells, monocytes
CDw14	Mo2, MY4, Leu-M3	Monocytes, immature granulocytes
CD15	MY1, Leu-M1	Granulocytes, monocytes, RS cells, eosinophils
CD16	Leu-11	NK cells, neutrophils, monocytes
CD19	B4, Leu-12	Pan-B cells, not plasma cells
CD20	B1, Leu-16, L26	Pan-B cells, not plasma cells
CD21	B2, CR2	Blood B cells, follicular dendritic cells
CD22	B3, Leu-14, HD39	Pan-B cells
CD23	B6, Leu-20	Activated B cells, activated monocytes, eosinophils
CD24	BA-1	Pan-B cells, granulocytes, plasma cells
CD25	IL2R	Activated B and T cells, HCL, monocytes
CD30	Ki-1, Ber-H2	Activated B and T cells, RS cells, ALCL
CD33	MY9, Leu-M9	Early myeloid cells (granulocytes), monocytes
CD34	MY10	Hematopoietic stem cells, blasts
CD38	OKT10, Leu-17	Early B and T cells, activated B and T cells, plasma cells
CDW41	Gp IIb/IIIa	Megakaryocytes, platelets
CD45	LCA, Hle	Leukocytes, plasma cells (dim to absent)
CD56	NKH1, Leu-19	NK cells, subset of T cells
CD57	Leu-7	NK cells, subset of T cells
CD61	Y2/51	Platelets, megakaryocytes
CD68	KP-1	Macrophages
CD71	OKT9, T9	Activated T and B cells
CD103	BLY7	HCL, activated T cells
	HLA-DR	B cells, activated T cells, monocytes, early myeloid cells
	PCA-1	Plasma cells
	Kappa	B cells
	Lambda	B cells
	TdT	Cortical thymocytes, B- and T-cell precursors, some AMLs
	Glycophorin	Red blood cells
	MPO	Myeloid cells
	FMC7	Some B cells
	TcR α/β	Most mature T cells
	TcR γ/δ	A subset of mature T cells

Abbreviations: NK = natural killer; B-CLL = B-cell chronic lymphocytic leukemia; MCL = mantle cell lymphoma; HCL = hairy cell leukemia; RS = Reed-Sternberg; ALCL = anaplastic large cell lymphoma; AML = acute myelogenous leukemia.

CD19 and CD5 are coexpressed. Abnormal coexpression assists in the detection of neoplastic processes. In general, normal B cells and T cells express either CD19 or CD5; however, neoplastic cells such as B-cell chronic lymphocytic leukemia/small lymphocytic lymphoma and mantle cell lymphoma coexpress both of these antigens simultaneously (**Figure 48-3**). B-cell neoplasms also show light chain restriction.

Although the majority of antigens detected on hematopoietic cells by flow cytometry are cell surface antigens, intracytoplasmic and nuclear antigens also can be studied. This procedure is somewhat more difficult to perform and interpret because of the need to permeabilize the cell membrane. The permeabilization step provides the mechanism by which the fluorochrome-conjugated antibodies can enter the cell so binding can take place. Many antibodies are available to study intracytoplasmic and nuclear antigens by flow cytometry. Two of the more commonly used are myeloperoxidase (MPO) and terminal deoxynucleotidyl transferase (TdT). Many others, including cyclin D-1 and intracytoplasmic light chains, are also available.

48.1.3 Specimen

Fresh peripheral blood or bone marrow aspirate samples anticoagulated with heparin (green top), acid citrate dextrose (yellow top), or ethylenediaminetetraacetic acid (EDTA) (lavender top) are acceptable. Heparin is the preferred anticoagulant, but only heparin sodium—not heparin lithium—should be used. Lymph node or other tissue samples should be submitted fresh (not fixed) in transport medium or an isotonic salt solution. If a bone marrow aspirate cannot be obtained, as is commonly the case with hairy cell leukemia or marrow fibrosis, a fresh bone marrow core biopsy may be submitted as described for lymph node samples. Body fluids such as pleural and peritoneal fluids can be submitted fresh but should be anticoagulated if they are contaminated with blood. Specimens in heparin lithium, fixatives such as formalin, B5, Bouin's and alcohol solutions are unacceptable for analysis.

Specimens should be kept at ambient temperature and analyzed within 24 hours of collection, although up to 72 hours may be acceptable, depending on sample type and laboratory conditions. If analysis will not occur within 24 hours, specimens may be refrigerated. Frozen specimens are unacceptable.

Approximately 5 mL of peripheral blood (depending on WBC count), 1 to 2 mL of bone marrow, and 500 mg of lymph node or

Figure 48-3 Histogram demonstrating CD19 and CD5 coexpression (right upper quadrant) in a peripheral blood sample from a patient with chronic lymphocytic leukemia. CD19 is labeled with fluorescein isothiocyanate and CD5 is labeled with phycoerythrin.

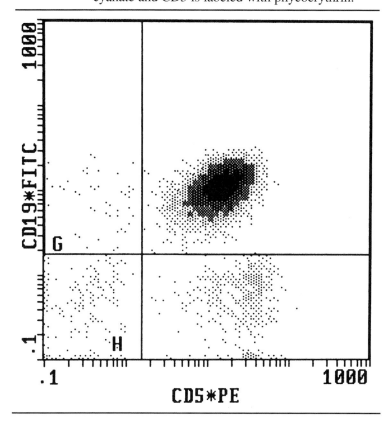

other tissue are minimum requirements for adequate analysis. Thus, a tissue sample approximately the size of a pencil eraser is typically sufficient. If the lymphoid infiltrate is scant or has a patchy distribution or if the WBC count or percentage of cells of interest is low, a larger sample may be required.

48.1.4 **Procedure**

As previously described, single cell suspensions are required for analysis by flow cytometry. Anticoagulation is all that is needed to achieve this for peripheral blood and bone marrow aspirate samples. Lymph nodes or other solid tissue specimens must be dissociated into single cell suspensions. This is typically accomplished by pressing the tissue through a metal mesh. A syringe needle can be used to tease and dislodge hematopoietic cells from the trabecular bone if a bone marrow core biopsy is submitted. If a sample contains numerous RBCs or erythroid precursors, it is desirable to remove them prior to flow cytometric analysis of the leukocytes. A number of RBC lysing solutions such as ammonium chloride are readily available.

Once a single cell suspension is obtained, the cells are washed several times with phosphate buffered saline and/or dilute detergent solutions. The cells are then resuspended in a buffered saline solution and mixed with a series of antibody-conjugated fluorochromes or tandem conjugates. The number of different antibody-conjugated fluorochromes or tandem conjugates added per tube of cells depends on the capabilities of the flow cytometer. Most laboratories use two- or three-color flow cytometers, but some use four-color or more. Many laboratories use CD45 (leukocyte common antigen) as one of the antigens in all tubes to ensure that the cellular events analyzed are hematopoietic cells and not nonhematopoietic tumor cells. Reed-Sternberg cells are notable exceptions—they are CD45 negative. This technique also allows better separation of lymphocytes, monocytes, and granulocytes on the histogram, particularly with bone marrow aspirate samples (**Figure 48-4**).

Only combinations of antibody-conjugated fluorochromes or tandem conjugates with different emission spectra can be analyzed simultaneously. The number of cells to be admixed with the fluorochrome conjugates and the amount of conjugate to be used are typically recommended by the manufacturer. Furthermore, each laboratory must make adjustments based on its particular cytometer and laboratory conditions. After the cells and antibody-conjugated fluorochromes are admixed, they are allowed to incubate in the dark for various lengths of time, usually 10 to 20 minutes.

At this stage, some laboratories fix the cells in dilute formalin, which preserves the cells for longer periods of analysis and kills potential infectious agents in the sample. The cell suspensions are then analyzed by the flow cytometer, tube by tube, and histograms of detected signals are produced.

48.1.5 Interpretation

The sample type, patient's clinical history, and histologic evaluation provide guidance as to which antigens may need to be

Figure 48-4 CD45 vs log side scatter histogram from a peripheral blood sample. Note the clean separation of the lymphocytic (B), monocytic (C), and granulocytic (D) cell populations.

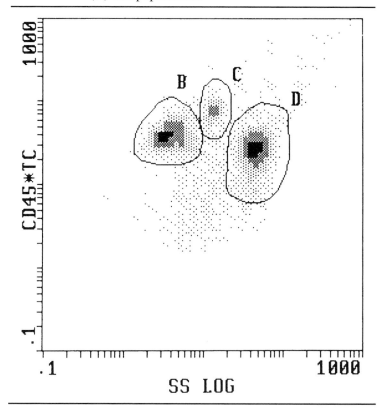

studied. Most laboratories have standard panels of antibodies they use for specific disease processes or groups of disease processes such as acute leukemias, chronic leukemias, or lymphomas. As preliminary results are obtained on a specific case, additional antibodies may need to be added to further characterize the hematologic process. Many lymphomas and leukemias have specific, characteristic antigen expression patterns that aid in their diagnosis. Frequently, however, a nonspecific or aberrant pattern of antigen expression is observed that requires careful correlation with the histologic impression. The typical antigenic expression patterns of many B-cell and T-cell neoplasms are summarized in **Tables 48-3** and **48-4**. The ability to detect light chain restriction in B-cell

Table 48-3 Common Antigen Expression Patterns of B-Cell Neoplasms

	CD19	CD20	CD22	CD23	CD25	CD5
B-CLL	+	+ (D)	–	+	–/+	+
HCL	+	+ (B)	+	–	+	–
MCL	+	+ (B)	+	–	–/+	+
MZL	+	+	+	–	–	–
FL	+	+	+	–/+	–/+	–
Plasma cell dyscrasias*	–	–	–	–	–	–
B-PLL	+	+	+	–	+/–	–

Abbreviations: B-CLL = B-cell chronic lymphocytic leukemia; HCL = hairy cell leukemia; MCL = mantle cell lymphoma; MZL = marginal zone lymphoma; FL = follicular lymphoma; B-PLL = B-cell prolymphocytic leukemia; D = dim; C = often cytoplasmic; B = bright; + = positive; +/– = often positive; –/+ = occasionally positive; – = negative.
*Plasma cell dyscrasias also commonly express CD56 with dim or absent CD45.

Table 48-4 Common Antigen Expression Patterns of T-Cell Neoplasms

	CD2	CD3	CD4	CD5	CD7	CD8	CD16	CD25	CD56	CD57
T-LGL	+	+	–	–	–	+	+	–	–	+
NK-LGL	+	–	–	–	+/–	–/+	+	–	+	–/+
T-CLL	+	+	+	+	+	–	–	–	–	–
Mycosis fungoides (SS)	+	+	+	+/–	–/+	–	–	–	–	–
ATLL	–/+	+	+	+	–	–	–	+	–	–

Abbreviations: T-LGL = T-cell large granular lymphocyte leukemia; NK-LGL = natural killer cell large granular lymphocyte leukemia; T-CLL = T-cell chronic lymphocytic leukemia; SS = Sézary syndrome; ATLL = adult T-cell leukemia/lymphoma; + = positive; +/– = often positive; –/+ = occasionally positive; – = negative.

neoplasms often facilitates a definitive diagnosis of clonality in this group of tumors. The flow cytometric detection of T-cell neoplasms can be more difficult unless specific expression or deletion patterns are observed. Correlation with morphology and T-cell gene rearrangement studies is often necessary (discussed in a later section).

Table 48-3 *Continued*

CD10	CD11c	CD38	CD79b	CD103	HLA-DR	Cyclin D-1	Light Chain Restriction
−	+/−	−	−	−	+	−	+ (D)
−	+	−	+	+	+	−/+	+ (B)
−	−	−	+	+	+	+	+ (B)
−	+	−	+	−/+	+	−	+
+	−	−	+	−/+	+	−	+ (B)
−	−	+	−	−	−	−/+	+ (C)
−	−	−	+/−	−	+	−	+ (B)

Table 48-5 Common Antigen Expression Patterns of Acute Myelogenous Leukemias

	CD13	CD14	CD15	CD33	CD34	HLA-DR	TdT	Comments
M0	+	−	−	+	+	+	−/+	Occasionally express CD7 or CD4
M1	+	−	−/+	+	+	+	−	Occasionally express CD4
M2	+	−	+/−	+	+/−	+	−	Occasionally express CD19 or CD56
M3	+	−	+	+	−	−	−	Occasionally express CD2
M4	+/−	+	+	+	−/+	+	−	Occasionally express CD2
M5	+/−	+	+	+	−/+	+	−	May express CD56
M6	+	−	−	+/−	+	+	−	May express glyco-phorin and CD71
M7	−/+	−	−	+/−	+	−/+	−	Often express CD41 and CD61

+ = positive; +/− = often positive; −/+ = occasionally positive; − = negative.

The expression patterns of acute leukemias are listed in **Tables 48-5** and **48-6**. Flow cytometry is particularly useful in determining lineage, which often has a great impact on treatment. The diag-

Table 48-6 Common Antigen Expression Patterns of Acute Lymphoblastic Leukemias

	CD1	CD2	CD3	CD4	CD5	CD7	CD8
B Cell							
B-precursor ALL							
Pre-B ALL							
B-ALL							
T Cell							
T-ALL	+	+	+ (C)	+	+	+	+

Abbreviations: SIg = surface immunoglobulin; ALL = acute lymphoblastic leukemia; C = usually cytoplasmic; + = positive; +/– = often positive; –/+ = occasionally positive; – = negative.

nosis of chronic myelogenous leukemia (CML) by flow cytometry can be challenging, and samples typically exhibit a predominance of myeloid cells in various stages of maturation. Such specimens are commonly studied to enumerate the blast count in a patient suspected of progressing to an accelerated or transformation phase of the disease.

48.1.6 Notes and Precautions

Although flow cytometry is often sensitive in detecting clonality among B-cell neoplasms, it is much less sensitive in detecting malignant T-cell processes. In addition, Hodgkin's and T-cell rich B-cell lymphoma typically are not detected due to the small number of malignant cells admixed with many benign, reactive hematopoietic cells. Flow cytometry is less sensitive than Southern blot hybridization and polymerase chain reaction (PCR) in detecting clonality and minimal residual disease. It is, however, a quicker method of analysis and provides more extensive antigen expression information.

48.2 Molecular Diagnostics

Molecular diagnostic tests such as Southern blot hybridization and PCR have rapidly emerged as leading adjunctive technologies that aid in the diagnosis of hematopoietic neoplasms. They are

Table 48-6 *Continued*

CD10	CD19	CD20	CD22	CD24	CD34	TdT	DR	SIg
+/–	+	–/+	–	+	+	+	+	–
+	+	+/–	–/+	+	+	+/–	+	–
+/–	+	+	+	+	–	–	+	+
+/–					–/+	+	–/+	

particularly useful in determining clonality of B-cell and T-cell neoplasms and in establishing tumor lineage. In addition, these techniques can be used to detect certain chromosomal translocations, mutations in clotting factors such as factor V Leiden, and the presence of microorganisms.

Southern blot hybridization and PCR offer some distinct advantages over flow cytometry, including the more reliable determination of B-cell clonality in neoplasms that do not express surface immunoglobulin and T-cell clonality. In addition, molecular diagnostic techniques are more sensitive in detecting neoplastic populations that represent only a minor component of the lymphoid cells. The use of Southern blot hybridization and PCR in establishing T-cell and B-cell clonality and in the detection of specific chromosomal translocations are reviewed in the following sections.

48.3 Southern Blot Hybridization

48.3.1 Purpose

Southern blot hybridization allows the identification of clonal B-cell and T-cell populations through the detection of antigen receptor gene rearrangements. Certain chromosomal translocations also can be identified.

48.3.2 Principle

B lymphocytes and T lymphocytes express specific antigen receptor proteins that aid in the function of these cells. For B cells, the antigen receptor proteins are the immunoglobulins, and for T cells, they are the T-cell receptors. The genes that encode these antigen receptor proteins have been studied extensively. Although much is still unknown, it is clear that as B cells and T-cells develop, they undergo rearrangement or assembly of specific gene segments or regions, resulting in a complete antigen receptor gene locus. Although the process is basically the same for both B-cell and T-cell antigen receptor gene formation, there are differences, including gene organization.

The B-cell antigen receptor proteins, or immunoglobulins, are composed of two subunits. These include an immunoglobulin heavy chain (IgH) and light chain (IgL). The light chains can be either kappa (κ) or lambda (λ) type, but not both. Two identical heavy chain subunits combine with two identical light chain subunits to form an intact immunoglobulin molecule. The gene for the IgH is located on the long arm of chromosome 14 and the genes for κ and λ light chains are located on the short arm of chromosome 2 and the long arm of chromosome 22, respectively.

The intact T-cell receptor is a heterodimer composed of two different subunits. The subunits comprise four possible types, including alpha (α), beta (β), gamma (γ), or delta (δ). α Subunits combine only with β subunits, γ subunits combine only with δ subunits, and vice versa. Therefore, the T-cell receptor located on the cell membrane is either an α/β or a γ/δ heterodimer. The majority of T cells contain an α/β heterodimer on their cell membranes. The gene that codes for the α and δ subunits is located on the long arm of chromosome 14. Those that code for the β and γ subunits are located on the long and short arms of chromosome 7, respectively. The general structure of all lymphocyte receptor genes is similar, although there are individual differences. They are composed of three or four different types of gene segments, including variable (V), diversity (D), joining (J), and constant (C) regions. All antigen receptor genes contain a V, J, and C region, whereas only the IgH and β and δ T-cell receptor genes contain a D region. Each antigen receptor gene has different and variable numbers of each region. The general features of the B-cell and T-cell antigen receptor genes are summarized in **Table 48-7**.

Although this is an oversimplification, gene rearrangement occurs during lymphocyte development such that there is random

Table 48-7 Lymphocyte Antigen Receptor Genes

Gene	Location	Subunit Regions
IgH	14q32	V, D, J, C
Kappa	2p12	V, J, C
Lambda	22q11	V, J, C
TcR-α	14q11	V, J, C
TcR-β	7q34	V, D, J, C
TcR-δ	14q11	V, D, J, C
TcR-γ	7p15	V, J, C

Abbreviations: IgH = immunoglobin heavy chain; TcR = T-cell receptor; V = variable; D = diversity; J = joining; C = constant.

selection and combination of V, J, and C regions. As stated earlier, the IgH and β and δ T-cell receptor genes also combine with a D region. It is this random rearrangement of lymphocytes that allows them to respond to different external stimuli and pathogens. Lymphocytes that escape apoptosis or are actively replicating can give rise to multiple progeny with the same gene rearrangement pattern. Molecular diagnostic tests such as Southern blot hybridization and PCR take advantage of the fact that all B cells and T cells undergo gene rearrangements. These tests are able to detect populations of clonal lymphoid cells that have the same antigen receptor gene rearrangement pattern or chromosomal translocation.

48.3.3 Specimen

Fresh whole blood (anticoagulated with EDTA or heparin sodium), bone marrow, body fluid, or unfixed tissue samples are acceptable for Southern blot hybridization. As an anticoagulant, EDTA is preferred over heparin. Whole blood, bone marrow, and tissue samples frozen at –20°C or –70°C are acceptable as long as any associated RBCs are lysed prior to freezing. If samples will not be analyzed within 24 hours, they should be refrigerated (at 2°C to 8°C) or frozen. Refrigerated blood and bone marrow samples may be stored for up to 1 week. Frozen blood, bone marrow, and tissue samples can be stored at –20°C or –70°C for 2 weeks or 1 to 2 years, respectively, prior to analysis.

Approximately 5 to 7 mL of whole blood, 1 to 2 mL of bone marrow, or 2 mm^3 of tissue is required. Thus, a tissue sample approximately the size of a pencil eraser is typically adequate. If the lymphoid infiltrate is scant or has a patchy distribution, a larger sample may be required.

48.3.4 Procedure

DNA is isolated from specimens by phenol-chloroform extraction and precipitation with ethanol. Isolated DNA is cut into small fragments by restriction enzymes that cleave the DNA at specific base pair sequences. The most commonly used restriction enzymes for hematopoietic testing are *Bam*HI, *Eco*RI, and *Hin*dIII. The cut DNA fragments are run on an agarose gel, denatured into single strands, and transferred onto a nitrocellulose membrane. The membrane containing the sample is then incubated with the radioisotope-labeled probe of interest and followed by autoradiography or incubated with a probe attached to a chemiluminescence detection system (**Figure 48-5**). The latter systems are commercially available as detection kits. Bands containing the DNA segment or gene of interest are detected by labeled DNA probes.

For detection of gene rearrangements associated with malignant lymphomas, probes to the joining region of the immunoglobulin heavy chain (J_H), the constant region of the light chains (C_κ, C_λ), and the β or γ region of the T-cell receptor (T_β and T_γ) are commonly used. Placental tissue or normal lymphocytes should be examined simultaneously to serve as normal controls. A normal control sample exhibits a nonrearranged germline band, but not a rearranged band. The germline band represents alleles of lymphocytes that have not undergone rearrangement or nonlymphoid cells. The germline band is typically located near the top of the gel. A positive control sample that is known to have a rearranged band as well as a negative control sample should be included in the analysis.

48.3.5 Interpretation

All B cells and T cells undergo gene rearrangement. In a heterogeneous population of lymphoid cells, essentially all of the

Figure 48-5 Schematic of the Southern blot hybridization procedure. Extracted DNA is electrophoresed on an agarose gel, denatured, transferred to a nitrocellulose membrane, and labeled with detection probes.

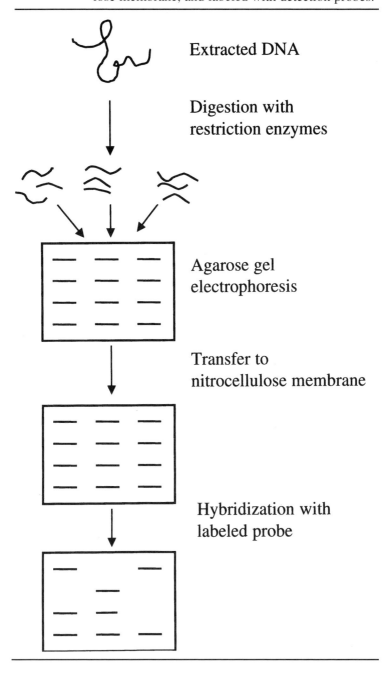

Extracted DNA

Digestion with restriction enzymes

Agarose gel electrophoresis

Transfer to nitrocellulose membrane

Hybridization with labeled probe

lymphoid cells rearrange their antigen receptor genes differently. In a clonal proliferation of lymphoid cells, all cells from that clone undergo an identical antigen receptor gene rearrangement. Therefore, in a nonclonal lymphoid population, digestion with restriction enzymes and probing results in a visible germline band only. The rearranged antigen receptor genes from this nonclonal lymphoid population are of different sizes and undetectable as a discrete band. In clonal lymphoid populations, digestion with restriction enzymes results in DNA fragments of the same size because all cells derived from that clone have the same antigen receptor gene rearrangement. After electrophoresis and probe hybridization, a distinct rearranged DNA band is detected in addition to the germline band (**Figure 48-6**). If the band is detected with the J_H probe, this indicates a clonal B-cell process. If the band is detected with either the TcR β or γ probe, this suggests a clonal T-cell process. It is conventional to cut each DNA sample with three different restriction enzymes, such as those already listed, and require the detection of a rearranged band in at least two of the three preparations, using the same probe (*see Figure 48-6*).

Chromosomal translocations such as the t(8;21) seen in acute myelogenous leukemia (AML) M2 also can be detected by Southern blot hybridization analysis. Due to the translocation, there are changes in the restriction enzyme cutting sites. Following cutting of the DNA by the restriction enzymes, altered lengths of DNA fragments result. However, all of the cells from the translocation have the same size fragments. Probing the translocation region with specific probes for that site detects a distinct rearranged band in the clonal population of cells with the translocation.

48.3.6 Notes and Precautions

It is important that both positive and negative controls are run with each sample analyzed. Samples with degraded DNA can provide false-negative results. Incompletely cut or digested DNA samples can result in a false-positive interpretation. The conditions and procedures used for Southern blot analysis and PCR studies are not standardized among laboratories, and individual methodologies may affect results and interpretation. This should be kept in mind when reviewing and analyzing individual patient results.

In addition, the presence of a clonally rearranged band does not definitively indicate malignancy. Rearranged antigen receptor bands have been detected in many nonneoplastic conditions such

Figure 48-6 Schematic of the Southern blot hybridization procedure using the J_H probe. In addition to germline bands, rearranged bands are seen in the positive control (+C) and the patient (P) sample using each of the three restriction enzymes. The negative control (-C) contains only a germline band. These results indicate the presence of a clonal B-cell population in the patient sample.

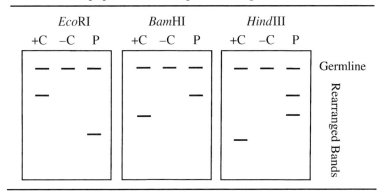

as AIDS, autoimmune disease, reactive gastritis, and systemic Castleman's disease. Also, the lack of detection of a clonally rearranged band does not entirely exclude its presence. One distinct disadvantage of Southern blot hybridization compared to flow cytometry is the longer turnaround time, which can be several days to a few weeks.

48.4 Polymerase Chain Reaction

48.4.1 Purpose

PCR is an in vitro method of amplifying specific segments of DNA using enzymes. It is a highly sensitive technique with the potential to detect a single copy of DNA within a specimen.

48.4.2 Principle

PCR is the process of replicating specific DNA sequences of interest. In hematopathology, this procedure is primarily used to detect chromosomal translocations as well as B-cell and T-cell antigen receptor gene rearrangements. The detection of DNA sequences that span a translocation site, such as t(15;17) seen in AML-M3 or t(14;18) associated with follicular lymphoma, provide diagnostic and prognostic information regarding a specific neoplastic process. Negative PCR results are often followed by Southern blot hybridization analysis because the latter is more sensitive. (See section on Southern blot hybridization.)

48.4.3 Specimen

For PCR studies, sample types similar to those recommended for Southern blot hybridization are generally acceptable. Ethylenediaminetetraacetic acid is the preferred anticoagulant; heparin should not be used. Although fresh unfixed samples are preferred, tissue samples fixed in formalin are acceptable. Mercury-based fixatives such as B5 should not be used. Refrigerated blood and bone marrow samples may be stored for about 1 week as long as the RBCs have been removed or the WBC component has been isolated. Frozen samples may be stored at –20°C or –70°C for up to 1 year following removal of the RBCs. Fresh tissue samples should be snap frozen in liquid nitrogen and can be stored at –70°C for 1 to 2 years.

Approximately 1 mL of blood, 0.5 mL of bone marrow, or 0.5 mm^3 of tissue is required.

48.4.4 Procedure

PCR involves the repetition of three reactions: DNA denaturation, primer annealing, and DNA extension (**Figure 48-7**). Each of these reactions takes place within the same test tube but at different temperatures. The discovery of the heat-stable Taq DNA polymerase has allowed automation of this procedure. DNA polymerase, primers, excess nucleotides, and the isolated DNA from the sample of interest are admixed. Double-stranded DNA is denatured at 90°C to 95°C into two single-stranded segments. Short complementary DNA sequences that flank the target location serve as primers and are annealed to the single-stranded DNA segments at 45°C to 55°C. For the detection of clonality of lymphoid neoplasms, primer sequences are available for the IgH and TcR γ and δ genes. Primer sequences that flank some specific translocation segments also are available.

Figure 48-7 Simplified illustration of the polymerase chain reaction procedure. Double-stranded DNA is denatured, and primers complementary to regions flanking the DNA segment to be replicated are annealed to the single-stranded DNA template. Polymerase en-zymes catalyze the extension of the DNA segments by adding nucleotides, resulting in two identical copies of the DNA segment.

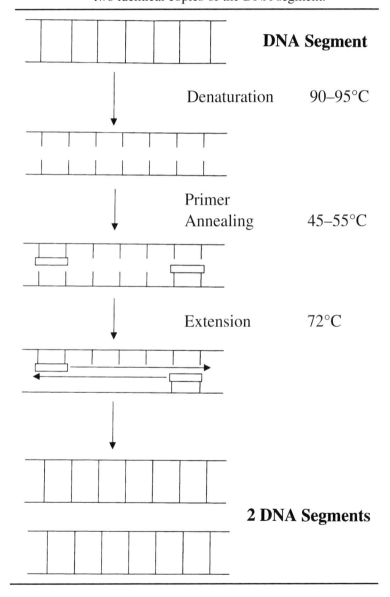

DNA Segment

Denaturation   90–95°C

Primer
Annealing   45–55°C

Extension   72°C

2 DNA Segments

Following annealing of the primers, the Taq polymerase catalyzes the extension of the DNA segment, at approximately 72°C, to form two identical DNA molecules. This process is repeated approximately 30 times to yield up to 1 million copies of the DNA segment; automated PCR machines that can perform these repeated cycles are readily available. The DNA PCR product is then electrophoresed, and if a clonal gene rearrangment or translocation is present, it shows up on the gel as a discrete band after ethidium bromide staining (**Image 48-1**). If the sample contains only polyclonal lymphocytes or does not contain the targeted translocation, the amplification product is not detected as a discrete band on the gel after electrophoresis and staining.

One major limitation of this technology is the fact that a primer to the specific DNA segment of interest is required. In addition, if the DNA segment is extemely long, as with some translocation sites, conventional PCR amplification cannot occur. In these cases, reverse transcriptase polymerase chain reaction (RT-PCR) procedures may be used in which RNA is first converted to DNA prior to PCR. An intact segment of DNA is always necessary to begin the PCR process.

48.4.5 Interpretation

Interpretation requires the identification of an amplified DNA product of the expected size following PCR. This is detectable as a discrete band after electrophoresis and staining. It is important to size the band to be sure it is of the expected size and not a nonspecifically amplified DNA segment. Further confirmation that the PCR product is the one of interest can be obtained by performing autoradiography or chemiluminescence detection with the corresponding probe.

48.4.6 Notes and Precautions

PCR is a highly sensitive and efficient process. It is important to have stringent PCR amplification procedures and conditions in place to prevent contamination of the product and ensure amplification. Intact DNA is a requirement for the process. As with Southern blot hybridization, detection of a clonally rearranged band by PCR does not definitively indicate malignancy. Such bands have been detected in reactive processes such as chronic gastritis and autoimmune disorders. In addition, it is important to interpret the result and its significance in connection with the morphology and clinical history. Occasionally, very small populations of minimal residual disease are detected by PCR, but they have little or unknown clinical significance and do not predict relapse.

48.5 Cytogenetics

Cytogenetic analysis has become an integral part of the workup and diagnosis of many hematopoietic disorders. It is particularly important in the evaluation and classification of leukemias, lymphomas, and myelodysplastic and myeloproliferative syndromes. Traditional cytogenetic analysis, or karyotyping, evaluates chromosome metaphase preparations to detect structural and numeric abnormalities. Such abnormalities are detected in more than 50% of patients with acute leukemias. A number of disorders have been associated with specific chromosomal abnormalities, including t(15;17) in acute promyelocytic leukemia, t(14;18) in follicular lymphoma, and inversion of chromosome 16 in AML-M4 with eosinophilia.

Although cytogenetic analysis is often necessary and frequently essential in diagnosing hematopoietic neoplasms, the need for viable tumor cells and the relatively long turnaround time are major disadvantages. Often a morphologic impression must be rendered before the cytogenetic results are available. More recent techniques such as FISH, particularly interphase FISH analysis, have allowed specific cytogenetic questions to be answered more quickly. Traditional G-banded chromosome metaphase spread analysis and FISH are reviewed in the next sections.

48.6 Conventional Chromosome Metaphase Spread Analysis

48.6.1 Purpose
Chromosome metaphase spread analysis is used to detect structural and numeric chromosomal abnormalities. This information is used in the diagnosis and prognostication of many hematopoietic disorders.

48.6.2 Principle

The acquisition of chromosomal abnormalities is frequently associated with the development of neoplasms. The mechanism by which such cytogenetic alterations induce disease is often due to the activation or inactivation of specific oncogenes. Many hematopoietic tumors exhibit chromosomal abnormalities such as translocations, deletions, and inversions. Although these chromosomal alterations occasionally are nonspecific, they are frequently characteristic for specific disorders. New or additional chromosomal abnormalities are commonly associated with disease progression.

48.6.3 Specimen

Approximately 2 to 3 mL of fresh bone marrow or peripheral blood anticoagulated with sodium heparin is necessary. A bone marrow sample is preferable if available, but peripheral blood is acceptable. The specimen should be kept at ambient temperature and transported to the laboratory within 24 hours. Frozen samples or those exposed to extreme temperatures are unacceptable.

48.6.4 Procedure

Fresh bone marrow or peripheral blood samples are placed in short-term cultures, which are often supplemented with growth factors or mitogens. Once the cells are growing in culture, they are exposed to a mitotic inhibitor such as colchicine, which arrests the cells in metaphase. They are then exposed to a hypotonic solution that causes them to swell and the chromosomes to spread apart. The cells are fixed with methanol and glacial acetic acid and dropped onto glass slides. The slides are then exposed to a denaturation procedure (heat or protease), which is followed by Giemsa staining (G-banding). The G-banding induces differential staining along the length of the chromosomes, enabling identification of each chromosome by photography or microscopy.

48.6.5 Interpretation

The production and interpretation of chromosome metaphase spreads is a complex and specialized procedure. Highly skilled and experienced personnel use the differential staining patterns produced by G-banding to identify individual chromosomes.

Chromosomal abnormalities such as the loss or gain of an entire chromosome, partial deletions, inversions, and translocations can be identified by the characteristic size and staining patterns of the long and short arms of individual chromosomes. **Image 48-2** demonstrates a classic G-banded metaphase spread (karyotype) from a patient with CML exhibiting the t(9;22)(q34;q11) or Philadelphia chromosome. **Tables 48-8** and **48-9** list common cytogenetic findings in leukemias and lymphomas, respectively.

48.6.6 Notes and Precautions

Metaphase spread analysis requires a specimen containing viable cells capable of mitotic division. In addition, because these samples must be grown in culture, it is important that they be acquired under sterile conditions.

48.7 Fluorescent In Situ Hybridization

48.7.1 Purpose

FISH is used to detect numeric and structural chromosomal abnormalities within intact cells or metaphase spreads. It is particularly useful in the detection of specific chromosomal translocations.

48.7.2 Principle

FISH takes advantage of the double-stranded and complementary sequence arrangement of DNA. Fluorescently labeled probes consisting of single-stranded DNA sequences can bind complementary denatured DNA segments to identify specific chromosomes or gene sequences in intact cells. Depending on the information sought, different types of probes are used. The fluorescent reporting molecule can be directly attached to the DNA sequence or be attached to an antibody that detects the DNA sequence through an indirect reporter system. Centromeric, telomeric, and repeat sequence probes are commonly used to identify chromo-

Table 48-8 Common Cytogenetic Findings Associated With Acute Leukemias, Chronic Leukemias, and Myelodysplastic/Myeloproliferative Syndromes

Condition	Clinical Findings
Acute myelogenous leukemias	
M0	No consistent finding
M1	No consistent finding
M2	t(8;21)(q22;q22)
M3	t(15;17)(q22;q12–21)
M4	inv(3)(q21;q26)
M4E	inv(16)(p13;q22)/t(16;16)
M5	t(9;11)(p22;q23)
M6	No consistent finding
M7	t(1;22)(p13;q13)
Acute lymphoblastic leukemias	
B-precursor ALL	t(9;22)(q34;q11)
B-precursor ALL	t(1;19)(q23;p13)
B-ALL	t(8;14)(q24;q32), also t(2;8) and t(8;22)
T-ALL	t(11;14)(p13;q11), t(10;14)(q24;q11), t(8;14)(q24;q11), t(1;14)(p32;q11)
Chronic leukemias	
HCL	+14,-6q
B-CLL	+12, -13q, +14(q32)
B-PLL	t(11;14)(q13;q32)
T-PLL	t/del 14q11
T-CLL	inv(14)(q11;q52)
Others	
CML	t(9;22)(q34;q11)
MDS	–5, –7, –12p, –20q
5q- syndrome	–5q

Abbreviations: ALL = acute lymphoblastic leukemia; HCL = hairy cell leukemia; CLL = chronic lymphocytic leukemia; PLL = prolymphocytic leukemia; CML = chronic myelogenous leukemia; MDS = myelodysplastic syndrome.

somes and detect the loss or gain of a particular chromosome (numeric abnormalities). Unique sequence probes such as cosmid and yeast artificial chromosome (YAC) probes are used to locate a specific DNA sequence. Unique sequence probes are useful in the identification of chromosomal translocations.

Table 48-9   Common Cytogenetic Findings Associated With Malignant Lymphomas

SLL	–14(q22–24), t(11;18)(q21;q21), –6q
FL	t(14;18)(q32;q21)
MCL	t(11;14)(q13;q32)
MZL	+3, t(11;18)
DLBL	t(3;14)(q27;q32), t(3;22)(q27;q11)
LPL	No consistent finding
ALCL	t(2;5)(p23;q35)
Burkitt's	t(8;14)(q24;q32), t(2;8)(p12;q24), t(8;22)(q24;q11)
MF	–6q, +14
ATLL	–6q, +14q
MM	1q abnormalities

Abbreviations: SLL = small lymphocytic lymphoma; FL = follicular lymphoma; MCL = mantle cell lymphoma; MZL = marginal zone lymphoma; DLBL = diffuse large B-cell lymphoma; LPL = lymphoplasmacytic lymphoma; ALCL = anaplastic large cell lymphoma; Burkitt's = Burkitt's lymphoma; MF = mycosis fungoides; ATLL = adult T-cell lymphoma/leukemia; MM = multiple myeloma.

48.7.3 Specimen

Bone marrow and peripheral blood samples anticoagulated with sodium heparin are both acceptable, but bone marrow samples are preferable to whole blood samples. Samples should be transported to the laboratory at ambient temperature within 24 hours. Formalin-fixed tissue samples are acceptable for interphase FISH analysis. Neither Bouin's solution nor B5 should be used. For metaphase FISH analysis, only viable cell samples are acceptable.

48.7.4 Procedure

For interphase analysis, intact cells or formalin-fixed tissue samples are affixed to a glass slide. The specimen is treated with heat and formamide to denature the double-stranded DNA and divide it into single strands. The denatured DNA is hybridized to single-stranded labeled probes.

To assess for chromosomal translocations, two separate and different colored probes are used. Each probe is complementary to specific DNA sequences located on one or the other of the two chromosomes at sites near the involved area of translocation. The unbound, nonhybridized probe is removed by washing. The bound probe may be directly attached to the fluorescent dye or to a hapten such as biotin, which must then be reacted with an antibody-tagged fluorescent dye. The sample is then visualized using a fluorescence microscope.

When metaphase analysis is performed, the cells in question must first be grown in culture. Therefore only a fresh, uncontaminated sample must be provided to the laboratory. Fixed tissue is unacceptable. Metaphase spreads are prepared, and then the procedure continues similar to that for interphase analysis.

48.7.5 Interpretation

The signal detected depends on the probe and fluorescent dye used. A positive signal is detected as a single colored dot observed under the fluorescence microscope. If specific sequence probes are used to look for a translocation, two separate colored signals are detected if the translocation is not present. If the translocation is present, a single third fusion colored dot or signal is detected (**Image 48-3**). If numeric probes are used, the number of signals detected per cell equals the number of the particular chromosome present. Chromosome losses or gains can be detected in this manner.

48.7.6 Notes and Precautions

The cells to be analyzed must be spread evenly over the surface of the slide so incorrect interpretation does not result from overlapping cells. Metaphase analysis is not possible if viable cells are unavailable or if the cells do not grow in culture. Interphase FISH analysis is significantly quicker than traditional G-banding metaphase analysis because the cells do not need to be grown in culture. It has the disadvantage of not allowing the entire chromosomal pattern to be analyzed, potentially missing some useful information.

48.8 References

Association for Molecular Pathology. Recommendations for in-house development and operation of molecular diagnostic tests. *Am J Clin Pathol.* 1999;111:449–463.

Coleman WB, Tsongalis GJ. *Molecular Diagnostics for the Clinical Laboratorian.* Totowa, NJ: Humana Press; 1997.

Dierlamm J, Stul M, Vranckx H, et al. FISH and related techniques in the diagnosis of lymphoma. *Cancer Surv.* 1997;30:3–20.

Fan H, Gulley M, Gascoyne R, et al. Molecular methods for detecting t(11;14) translocations in mantle-cell lymphomas. *Diagn Mol Pathol.* 1998;7:209–214.

Frizzera G, Wu CD, Inghirami G. The usefulness of immunophenotypic and genotypic studies in the diagnosis and classification of hematopoietic and lymphoid neoplasms. *Am J Clin Pathol.* 1999;111(suppl 1):S13-S39.

Gersen SL, Keagle MB. *The Principles of Clinical Cytogenetics.* Totowa, NJ: Humana Press; 1999.

Harris N, Jaffe E, Stein H, et al. A revised European-American classification of lymphoid neoplasms: a proposal from the International Lymphoma Study Group. *Blood.* 1994;84:1361–1392.

Jennings CD, Foon KA. Recent advances in flow cytometry: application to the diagnosis of hematologic malignancy. *Blood.* 1997;90:2863–2892.

Keren DF, Hanson CA, Hurtubise GJ. *Flow Cytometry and Clinical Diagnosis.* Chicago, Ill: ASCP Press; 1994.

Knowles DM. *Neoplastic Hematopathology.* Baltimore, Md: Williams & Wilkins; 1992.

Scarpa A, Tognon M. Molecular approach in human tumor investigation: oncogenes, tumor suppressor genes and DNA tumor polyomaviruses. *Int J Mol Med.* 1998;1:1011–1023.

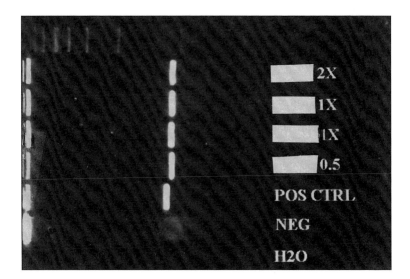

Image 48-1 A rearranged band detected at various dilutions of the patient's DNA sample (0.5 to 2 times) following polymerase chain reaction, electrophoresis, and ethidium bromide staining. Consensus primers to the V and J regions of the IgH were used for the PCR step. Positive and negative control samples were also included in the analysis.

Image 48-2 G-banded chromosome metaphase spread demonstrating the classic t(9;22)(q34;q11) Philadelphia chromosome in a 37-year-old man with CML (arrows). The karyotype is otherwise unremarkable, 46XY. (Karyotype provided by Dr Zhong Chen, MD, Cytogenetics Laboratory, University of Utah Health Sciences Center, Salt Lake City.)

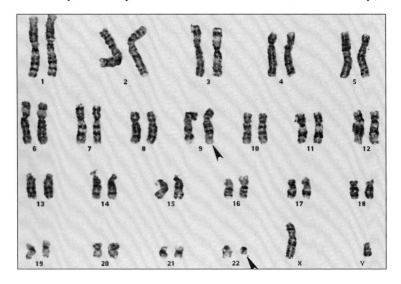

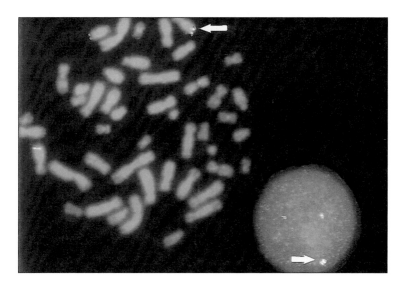

Image 48-3 Detection of the t(8;14)(q24;q32) by fluorescent in situ hybridization. The *IgH*/c-*myc* fusion gene was detected using a 14qter telomeric probe (Oncor Inc, Gaithersburg, Md) and a combination of two YAC probes (I2 and P72) spanning the c-*myc* locus localized to 8q24. The normal chromosome 14 is identified by a red signal and the normal chromosome 8 is identified by a green signal. The deriviative chromosome 8 of the t(8;14) rearrangement shows the red/green fusion signal (arrows) in both the metaphase spread (upper left) and the interphase nucleus (lower right). (The YAC probes were provided by Dr Maria Luisa Veronese, PhD, Jefferson Medical College, Philadelphia, Pa. Photograph courtesy of Dr Marilyn L. Slovak, PhD, City of Hope National Medical Center, Duarte, Calif.)

APPENDIX

Hematology Reference Values

Table 1 Hematology Reference Values in Adults for Common Tests[*]

Test	Men	
	Conventional Units	SI Units
Hemoglobin	13–18 g/dL	130–180 g/L
Hematocrit	40%–52%	0.40–0.52
Red blood cell count	$4.4–5.9 \times 10^6/mm^3$	$4.4–5.9 \times 10^{12}/L$
White blood cell count	$3.8–10.6 \times 10^3/mm^3$	$3.8–10.6 \times 10^9/L$
MCV	$80–100\ \mu m^3$	80–100 fL
MCH	26–34 pg	26–34 pg
MCHC	32–36 g/dL	320–360 g/L
Platelet count	$150–440 \times 10^3/mm^3$	$150–440 \times 10^9/L$
Reticulocyte count	0.8%–2.5%	0.008–0.025
Reticulocyte count	$18,000–158,000/mm^3$	$18–158 \times 10^9/L$
Sedimentation rate[†]	0–10 mm/h	0–10 mm/h
Zeta sedimentation rate	40–52	40–52

Abbreviations: MCV = mean corpuscular volume; MCH = mean corpuscular hemoglobin; MCHC = mean corpuscular hemoglobin concentration.

[*]Modified from: Wintrobe MM. *Clinical Hematology*. 8th ed. Philadelphia, Pa: Lea & Febiger; 1984: Henry JB. *Clinical Diagnosis and Management by Laboratory Methods*. 17th ed. Philadelphia, Pa: WB Saunders Co; 1984. Miale JB. *Laboratory Medicine: Hematology*. 6th ed. St Louis, Mo: CV Mosby; 1982. Williams WJ, Beutler E, Erslev AJ, Lichtman MA. *Hematology*. 3rd ed. New York, NY: McGraw-Hill Book Co; 1983.

[†]May be age dependent, according to method.

Women	
Conventional Units	SI Units
12–16 g/dL	120–160 g/L
35%–47%	0.35–0.47
$3.8–5.2 \times 10^6/mm^3$	$3.8–5.2 \times 10^{12}/L$
$3.6–11.0 \times 10^3/mm^3$	$3.6–11.0 \times 10^9/L$
80–100 µm^3	80–100 fL
26–34 pg	26–34 pg
32–36 g/dL	320–360 g/L
$150–440 \times 10^3/mm^3$	$150–440 \times 10^9/L$
0.8%–4.0%	0.008–0.04
$18,000–158,000/mm^3$	$18–158 \times 10^9/L$
0–20 mm/h	0–20 mm/h
40–52	40–52

Table 2   Automated Hematology Reference Values in Normal Men at 4,500 ft[*]

| Test | Coulter S+ STKR (80 Men) | |
	Mean	Central 95% Range
White blood cells ($\times 10^3$/mm^3)	6.6	3.5–9.8
Platelets ($\times 10^3$/mm^3)	280	147–412
Red blood cells ($\times 10^6$/mm^3)	5.4	4.76–6.04
Hemoglobin (g/dL)	16.4	14.7–18.1
Hematocrit (%)	48.7	43.7–53.6
MCV (μm^3)	90.3	83.3–97.2
MCH (pg)	30.5	28.1–32.9
MCHC (g/dL)	33.8	33.0–34.6
RDW	12.4	11.5 13.4
Mean platelet volume	8.4	6.8–10.0

Abbreviations: MCV = mean corpuscular volume; MCH = mean corpuscular hemoglobin; MCHC = mean corpuscular hemoglobin concentration; RDW = red cell distribution width.

[*]Data are based on measurements from healthy male medical students, age range 23–31 years, at an altitude of 4500 ft. From *Wintrobe's Clinical Hematology*. 9th ed. Philadelphia, Pa: Lea & Febiger; 1993.

Table 3   Effect of Altitude on VPRC in Normal Men[*]

| Altitude | | No. of Subjects | VPRC (L/L) |
Feet	Meters		
0	0	721	0.47
4400	1340	744	0.495
7457	2280	100	0.51
12,240	3740	40	0.54
14,900	4540	32	0.61
17,800	5430	10	0.69

Abbreviation: VPRC = volume packed red cells.

[*]Mean values in males. From *Wintrobe's Clinical Hematology*. 9th ed. Philadelphia, Pa: Lea & Febiger; 199.

Technicon HI (64 Men)	
Mean	Central 95% Range
6.7	4.4–8.2
285	147–422
5.54	4.87 6.20
16.2	14.6–17.8
48.7	43.6–53.8
88.0	80.9–95.2
29.3	27.0–31.7
33.3	32.1–34.6
12.8	12.0–13.6
8.9	7.6–10.2

Table 4 Manual White Blood Cell Differential Count, Reference Values in Adults

	Conventional Units	
Cell Type	Relative	Absolute Counts
Segmented neutrophils	50%–70%	2400–7560/mm^3
Bands	2%–6%	96–648/mm^3
Lymphocytes	20%–44%	960–4752/mm^3
Monocytes	2%–9%	96–972/mm^3
Eosinophils	0%–4%	0–432/mm^3
Basophils	0%–2%	0–216/mm^3

Table 5 Automated Leukocyte Differential Counts, Reference Values in Normal Male Adults[*]

	Coulter S+ STKR (80 Men)	
Percentage	Mean	Central 95% Range
Lymphocytes	36.1	22.3–49.9
Monocytes	4.1	0.7–7.5
Granulocytes	59.7	45.5–74.0
Neutrophils	—	—
Eosinophils	—	—
Basophils	—	—
LUC	—	—
Absolute Numbers		
Lymphocytes ($\times 10^3$/mm^3)	2.4	1.2–3.5
Monocytes ($\times 10^3$/mm^3)	0.3	0.0–0.5
Granulocytes ($\times 10^3$/mm^3)	4.0	1.4–6.6
Neutrophils ($\times 10^3$/mm^3)	—	—
Eosinophils ($\times 10^3$/mm^3)	—	—
Basophils ($\times 10^3$/mm^3)	—	—
LUC ($\times 10^3$/mm^3)	—	—

Abbreviation: LUC = large unstained cells.
[*]Data are based on measurements from healthy male medical students, age range 23–31 years, at an altitude of 4,500 ft. From *Wintrobe's Clinical Hematology*. 9th ed. Philadelphia, Pa: Lea & Febiger; 1993.

SI Units	
Relative	Absolute Counts
0.5–0.7	$2.40–7.56 \times 10^9$/L
0.02–0.06	$0.10–0.65 \times 10^9$/L
0.2–0.44	$0.96–4.75 \times 10^9$/L
0.02–0.09	$0.10–0.97 \times 10^9$/L
0.0–0.04	$0.00–0.43 \times 10^9$/L
0.0–0.02	$0.00–0.22 \times 10^9$/L

Technicon HI (64 Men)	
Mean	Central 95% Range
31.3	18.3–44.2
5.5	2.6–8.5
—	—
58.8	45.5–73.1
1.9	0.0–4.4
0.7	0.2–1.2
1.8	0.0 4.9
2.06	0.9–3.22
0.37	0.12–0.62
—	—
4.01	1.31–6.71
0.13	0.00–0.30
0.05	0.01–0.09
0.12	0.00–0.31

Table 6 Hematologic Reference Ranges in Racial and Ethnic Subgroups (2.5th to 97.5th Percentiles) in Men[*]

	Range	
	White	Black
Test		
	(n = 181)	(n = 172)
WBCs ($\times 10^3$/mm^3)	3.7–10.4	3.5–9.6
RBCs ($\times 10^6$/mm^3)	4.3–5.8	4.0–5.8
Hemoglobin (g/dL)	13.0–17.3	11.9–16.7
MCHC (g/dL)	32.4–35.4	32.1–35.2
Platelets ($\times 10^3$/mm^3)	176–372	167–408
MPV (μm^3)	7.7–1.2	7.5–12.4
Hematocrit (%)	38–49	36–48
MCV (μm^3)	81.6–96.6	71.8–99.8
MCH (pg)	27.2–33.4	23.3–33.9
RDW (%)	11.9–14.3	12.1–16.2
Three-part differential cell count		
	(n = 106)	(n = 114)
Lymphocytes ($\times 10^3$/mm^3)	1.26–3.05	1.20–3.17
Monocytes ($\times 10^3$/mm^3)	0.13–0.66	0.14–0.77
Granulocytes ($\times 10^3$/mm^3)	1.78–7.72	1.49–6.56
Manual differential cell count		
	(n = 80)	(n = 72)
Segmented neutrophils ($\times 10^3$/mm^3)	1.51–7.00	1.11–6.70
Band cells ($\times 10^3$/mm^3)	0.00–0.07	0.00–0.07
Lymphocytes ($\times 10^3$/mm^3)	0.65–2.80	0.97–3.30
Monocytes ($\times 10^3$/mm^3)	0.00–0.51	0.02–0.83
Eosinophils ($\times 10^3$/mm^3)	0.00–0.42	0.00–0.47
Basophils ($\times 10^3$/mm^3)	0.00–0.16	0.00–0.16

Abbreviations: MCHC = mean corpuscular hemoglobin concentration; MPV = mean platelet volume; MCV = mean cell volume; MCH = mean corpuscular hemoglobin; RDW = red cell distribution width.

[*]From Saxena S, Wong ET. Heterogeneity of common hematologic parameters among racial, ethnic, and gender subgroups. *Arch Pathol Lab Med*. 1990;114:715–719.

	Range	
	Latino	Asian
	(n = 141)	(n = 72)
	4.1–11.5	3.4–11.5
	4.4–5.6	4.0–6.2
	13.7–17.0	12.5–17.0
	32.5–35.6	32.1–35.3
	176–397	223–422
	7.4–11.3	7.4–10.9
	40–50	36–50
	82.0–96.5	67.3–96.3
	26.7–33.2	21.6–33.4
	12.1–14.7	11.8–14.6
	(n = 101)	(n = 46)
	1.12–3.36	1.03–3.38
	0.14–0.68	0.08–0.77
	2.41–8.33	1.51–7.26
	(n = 48)	(n = 43)
	2.40–7.59	2.02–5.50
	0.00–0.21	0.00–0.06
	0.94–4.22	0.90–3.50
	0.00–0.68	0.00–0.53
	0.00–0.80	0.00–0.32
	0.00–0.17	0–0.14

Table 7 Hematologic Reference Ranges in Racial and Ethnic Subgroups (2.5th to 97th Percentiles) in Women[*]

	Range	
	White	Black
Test	(n = 482)	(n = 525)
WBCs ($\times 10^3/mm^3$)	3.8–10.6	3.4–11.2
RBCs ($\times 10^6/mm^3$)	3.8–5.0	3.6–5.3
Hemoglobin (g/dL)	11.4–15.5	10.6–14.9
MCHC (g/dL)	32.7–35.3	31.9–35.0
Platelets ($\times 10^3/mm^3$)	188–438	193–485
MPV (μm^3)	7.7–11.5	7.7–11.6
Hematocrit (%)	34–45	31–44
MCV (μm^3)	78.0–98.0	72.9–97.5
MCH (pg)	25.9–33.8	23.7–33.1
RDW (%)	11.7–15.2	12.0–17.3
Three-part differential cell count	(n = 284)	(n = 375)
Lymphocytes ($\times 10^3/mm^3$)	1.14–3.19	1.28–3.29
Monocytes ($\times 10^3/mm^3$)	0.10–0.74	0.10–0.67
Granulocytes ($\times 10^3/mm^3$)	2.03–7.46	1.43–7.68
Manual differential cell count	(n = 216)	(n = 175)
Segmented neutrophils ($\times 10^3/mm^3$)	2.023–7.33	1.50–8.14
Band cells ($\times 10^3/mm^3$)	0.00–0.13	0.00–0.09
Lymphocytes ($\times 10^3/mm^3$)	1.01–3.38	1.05–3.48
Monocytes ($\times 10^3/mm^3$)	0.00–0.82	0.02–0.72
Eosinophils ($\times 10^3/mm^3$)	0.00–0.52	0.00–0.46
Basophils ($\times 10^3/mm^3$)	0.00–0.16	0.00–0.20

Abbreviations: MCHC = mean corpuscular hemoglobin concentration; MPV = mean platelet volume; MCV = mean cell volume; MCH = mean corpuscular hemoglobin; RDW = red cell distribution width.

[*]From Saxena S, Wong ET. Heterogeneity of common hematologic parameters among racial, ethnic, and gender subgroups. *Arch Pathol Lab Med.* 1990;114:715–719.

Range	
Latina	Asian
(n = 394)	(n = 175)
4.1–11.8	3.5–9.7
3.7–5.1	3.7–5.4
10.3–15.1	11.3–15.0
32.0–35.3	32.2–35.5
198–460	193–417
7.8–11.5	7.6–11.1
31–44	33–44
69.6–95.8	72.4–97.0
22.3–33.0	22.1–33.8
11.9–16.4	11.6–16.6
(n = 295)	(n = 130)
1.07–3.44	0.94–2.75
0.11–0.67	0.09–0.51
2.19–8.24	1.93–6.13
(n = 114)	(n = 50)
1.85–7.57	1.60–7.33
0.00–0.13	0.00–0.11
0.89–3.73	1.24–2.59
0.06–0.66	0.00–0.65
0.00–0.50	0.00–0.49
0.00–0.15	0.00–0.16

Table 8   Red Blood Cell Values at Various Ages: Mean and
Lower Limit of Normal (-2 SD)*†

Age	Hemoglobin (g/dL)		Hematocrit (%)	
	Mean	−2 SD	Mean	−2 SD
Birth (cord blood)	16.5	13.5	51	42
1–3 Days (capillary)	18.5	14.5	56	45
1 Week	17.5	13.5	54	42
2 Weeks	16.5	12.5	51	39
1 Month	14.0	10.0	43	31
2 Months	11.5	9.0	35	28
3–6 Months	11.5	9.5	35	29
0.5–2 Years	12.0	10.5	36	33
2–6 Years	12.5	11.5	37	34
6–12 Years	13.5	11.5	40	35
12–18 Years				
Female	14.0	12.0	41	36
Male	14.5	13.0	43	37
18–49 Years				
Female	14.0	12.0	41	36
Male	15.5	13.5	47	41

*From *Wintrobe's Clinical Hematology*. 9th ed. Philadelphia, Pa: Lea & Febiger; 1993.

†These data were compiled from several sources. Emphasis is on recent studies employing electronic counters and on the selection of populations that are likely to exclude individuals with iron deficiency. The mean ±2 SD can be expected to include 95% of the observations in a normal population. (From Dallman PR. In: Rudolph A, ed. *Pediatrics*. 16th ed. East Norwalk, Conn:

Table 9   Hematology Reference Values During the First Month
of Life in the Term Infant*

Value	Cord Blood	Day 1
Hemoglobin (g/dL)	16.8	18.4
Hematocrit (%)	53	58
RBCs ($\times 10^6$/mm^3)	5.25	5.8
MCV (μm^3)	107	108
MCH (pg)	34	35
MCHC (g/dL)	31.7	32.5
Reticulocytes (%)	3–7	3–7
Nucleated RBCs ($\times 10^3$/mm^3)	500	200
Platelets ($\times 10^3$/mm^3)	290	192

Abbreviations: MCV = mean corpuscular volume; MCH = mean corpuscular hemoglobin; MCHC = mean corpuscular hemoglobin concentration.

*From Oski F, Naiman JL. *Hematologic* Problems in the Newborn. 2nd ed. Philadelphia, Pa: Saunders Co; 1972.

RBCs ($\times 10^6$/mm³)		MCV (µm³)		MCH (pg)		MCHC (g/dL)	
Mean	–2 SD	Mean	–2 SD	Mean	–2 SD	Mean	–2 SD
4.7	3.9	108	98	34	31	33	30
5.3	4.0	108	95	34	31	33	29
5.1	3.9	107	88	34	28	33	28
4.9	3.6	105	86	34	28	33	28
4.2	3.0	104	85	34	28	33	29
3.8	2.7	96	77	30	26	33	29
3.8	3.1	91	74	30	25	33	30
4.5	3.7	78	70	27	23	33	30
4.6	3.9	81	75	27	24	34	31
4.6	4.0	86	77	29	25	34	31
4.6	4.1	90	78	30	25	34	31
4.9	4.5	88	78	30	25	34	31
4.6	4.0	90	80	30	26	34	31
5.2	4.5	90	80	30	26	34	31

Appleton-Century-Crofts; 1977. Lubin BH. Reference values in infancy and childhood. In: Nathan DG, Oski FA, eds. *Hematology of Infancy and Childhood*. 3rd ed. Philadelphia, Pa: Saunders Co; 1987.)

Day 3	Day 7	Day 14	Day 28
17.8	17.0	16.8	15.6
55	54	52	45
5.6	5.2	5.1	4.7
99	98	96	91
33	32.5	31.5	31
33	33	33	32
1–3	0–1	0–1	0–1
0–5	0	0	0
213	248	252	240

Table 10 Leukocyte Counts and Differential Counts: Reference Values in Children*†

Age	Total Leukocytes		Neutrophils		
	Mean	(Range)	Mean	(Range)	%
Birth	18.1	(9.0–30.0)	11.0	(6.0–26.0)	61
12 Hours	22.8	(13.0–38.0)	15.5	(6.0–28.0)	68
24 Hours	18.9	(9.4–34.0)	11.5	(5.0–21.0)	61
1 Week	12.2	(5.0–21.0)	5.5	(1.5–10.0)	45
2 Weeks	11.4	(5.0–20.0)	4.5	(1.0–9.5)	40
1 Month	10.8	(5.0–19.5)	3.8	(1.0–9.0)	35
Months	11.9	(6.0–17.5)	3.8	(1.0–8.5)	32
1 Year	11.4	(6.0–17.5)	3.5	(1.5–8.5)	31
2 Years	10.6	(6.0–17.0)	3.5	(1.5–8.5)	33
4 Years	9.1	(5.5–15.5)	3.8	(1.5–8.5)	42
6 Years	8.5	(5.0–14.5)	4.3	(1.5–8.0)	51
8 Years	8.3	(4.5–13.5)	4.4	(1.5–8.0)	53
10 Years	8.1	(4.5–13.5)	4.4	(1.8–8.0)	54
16 Years	7.8	(4.5–13.0)	4.4	(1.8–8.0)	57
21 Years	7.4	(4.5–11.0)	4.4	(1.8–7.7)	59

*From *Wintrobe's Clinical Hematology.* 9th ed. Philadelphia, Pa: Lea & Febiger; 1993.

†These data were compiled from several sources. Emphasis is on recent studies employing electronic counters and on the selection of populations that are likely to exclude individuals with iron deficiency. The mean ±2 SD can be expected to include 95% of the observations in a normal population. (From Dallman PR. In: Rudolph A, ed. *Pediatrics.* 16th ed. East Norwalk, Conn: Appleton-Century-Crofts; 1977. Lubin BH. Reference values in infancy and childhood. In: Nathan DG, Oski FA, eds. *Hematology of Infancy and Childhood.* 3rd ed. Philadelphia, Pa: Saunders Co; 1987.)

Table 11 Hematology Reference Values in Adults for Ancillary Tests*

	Men	
Test	Conventional Units	SI Units
Serum iron	70–201 μg/dL	12.7–35.9 μmol/L
Total iron-binding capacity	253–435 μg/dL	45.2–77.7 μmol/L
Ferritin	20–250 ng/mL	20–250 μg/L
Serum B_{12}	200–1000 pg/mL	150–750 pmol/L
Serum folate	2–10 ng/mL	4–22 nmol/L
Red cell folate	140–960 ng/mL	550–2200 nmol/L
Hemoglobin A_2	1.5%–3.5%	0.015–0.035
Hemoglobin F	<2%	<0.02

*Modified from: Wintrobe MM. *Clinical Hematology.* 8th ed. Philadelphia, Pa: Lea & Febiger; 1984. Henry JB. *Clinical Diagnosis and Management by Laboratory Methods.* 17th ed. Philadelphia, Pa: Saunders Co; 1984. Miale JB. *Laboratory Medicine: Hematology.* 6th ed. St Louis, Mo: CV Mosby; 1982. Williams WJ, Beutler E, Erslev AJ, Lichtman MA. *Hematology.* 3rd ed. New York, NY: McGraw-Hill Book Co; 1983.

| Lymphocytes | | | Monocytes | | Eosinophils | |
Mean	(Range)	%	Mean	%	Mean	%
5.5	(2.0–11.0)	31	1.1	6	0.4	2
5.5	(2.0–11.0)	24	1.2	5	0.5	2
5.8	(2.0–11.5)	31	1.1	6	0.5	2
5.0	(2.0–17.0)	41	1.1	9	0.5	4
5.5	(2.0–17.0)	48	1.0	9	0.4	3
6.0	(2.5–16.5)	56	0.7	7	0.3	6
7.3	(4.0–13.5)	61	0.6	5	0.3	3
7.0	(4.0–10.5)	61	0.6	5	0.3	3
6.3	(3.0–9.5)	59	0.5	5	0.3	3
4.5	(2.0–8.0)	50	0.5	5	0.3	3
3.5	(1.5–7.0)	42	0.4	5	0.2	3
3.3	(1.5–6.8)	39	0.4	4	0.2	2
3.1	(1.5–6.5)	38	0.4	4	0.2	2
2.8	(1.2–5.2)	35	0.4	5	0.2	3
2.5	(1.0–4.8)	34	0.3	4	0.2	3

| Women | |
Conventional Units	SI Units
62–173 µg/dL	11–30 µmol/L
253–435 µg/dL	45.2–77.7 µmol/L
10–200 ng/mL	10–200 µg/L
200–1000 pg/mL	150–750 pmol/L
2–10 ng/mL	4–22 nmol/L
140–960 ng/mL	550–2200 nmol/L
1.5%–3.5%	0.015–0.035
<2%	<0.02

Table 12 Age-Related Coagulation Reference Values[*]

Coagulation test	Age 5 d	90 d
Fibrinogen (g/L)	1.62–4.62	1.5–3.79
Prothrombin (U/mL)	0.33–0.93	0.45–1.05
Factor V (U/mL)	0.45–1.45	0.48–1.32
Factor VII (U/mL)	0.35–1.43	0.39–1.43
Factor VIII (U/mL)	0.5–1.54	0.5–1.25
Factor IX (U/mL)	0.15–0.91	0.21–1.13
Factor X (U/mL)	0.19–0.79	0.35–1.07
Factor XI (U/mL)	0.23–0.87	0.41–0.97
Factor XII (U/mL)	0.11–0.83	0.25–1.09
HMW-K (U/mL)	0.16–1.32	0.3–1.46
Prekallikrein (U/mL)	0.2–0.76	0.41–1.05
vWF antigen[†] (U/mL)	0.5–2.54	0.5–2.06
Ristocetin cofactor (U/mL)	—	—
Antithrombin III (U/mL)	0.41–0.93	0.73–1.21
Protein C (U/mL)	0.2–0.64	0.28–0.80
Protein S[†] (U/mL)	0.22–0.78	0.54–1.18
Plasminogen (U/mL)	—	—
t-PA (ng/mL)	—	—
PAI (U/mL)	—	—
α_2-Antiplasmin (U/mL)	—	—

Abbreviations: HMW-K = high molecular weight kininogen; vWF = von Willebrand's factor; t-PA = tissue plasminogen activator; PAI = plasminogen activator inhibitor.

[*]Prothrombin time and partial thromboplastin time values are not shown due to dependence of these values on reagent selection. Adult values represent those of the University of Utah Medical Center Hemostasis and Thrombosis Laboratory. Pediatric values are for healthy full-term infants (from Andrew M, et al. Maturation of the hemostatic system during childhood. *Blood.* 1992;80:1998; and Andrew M, et al. Development of the hemostatic system in the neonate and young infant. *Am J Pediatr Hematol Oncol.* 1990;12:95).

[†]Results are based on antigenic assays. All other results are based on functional assays. The adult fibrinolysis tests (t-PA, PAI) are based on reference range values drawn between 7 and 9 AM.

[‡]Adult α_2-antiplasmin values are listed in terms of mg/dL.

		Age	
1–5 y	6–10 y	11–16 y	Adult
1.7–4.05	1.57–4.0	1.54–4.48	1.5–3.50
0.71–1.16	0.67–1.07	0.61–1.04	0.79–1.31
0.79–1.27	0.63–1.16	0.55–0.99	0.62–1.39
0.55–1.16	0.52–1.2	0.58–1.15	0.50–1.29
0.59–1.42	0.58–1.32	0.53–1.31	0.50–1.50
0.47–1.04	0.63–0.89	0.59–1.22	0.65–1.50
0.58–1.16	0.55–1.01	0.5–1.17	0.77–1.31
0.56–1.5	0.52–1.2	0.5–0.97	0.65–1.50
0.64–1.29	0.6–1.4	0.34–1.37	0.50–1.50
0.64–1.32	0.6–1.3	0.63–1.19	0.60–1.46
0.65–1.3	0.66–1.31	0.53–1.45	0.60–1.46
0.6–1.2	0.44–1.44	0.46–1.53	0.43–1.50
—	—	—	0.52–1.60
0.82–1.39	0.9–1.31	0.77–1.32	0.85–1.22
0.4–0.92	0.45–0.93	0.55–1.11	0.78–2.32
0.54–1.18	0.41–1.14	0.52–0.92	0.62–1.25
0.78–1.18	0.75–1.08	0.68–1.03	0.74–1.24
1.0–4.5[†]	1.0–5.0[†]	1.0–4.0[†]	3.0–12.0
1.0–10.0	2.0–12.0	2.0–10.0	2.0–15.0
0.93–1.17	0.89–1.10	0.78–1.18	4.4–8.5 mg/dL[‡]

Table 13 Differential Counts of Bone Marrow Aspirates From 12 Healthy Men[*]

Cell Type	Mean (%)	Observed Range (%)	95% Confidence Limits (%)
Neutrophilic series (total)	53.6	49.2–65.0	33.6–73.6
Myeloblasts	0.9	0.2–1.5	0.1–1.7
Promyelocytes	3.3	2.1–4.1	1.9–4.7
Myelocytes	12.7	8.2–15.7	8.5–16.9
Metamyelocytes	15.9	9.6–24.6	7.1–24.7
Band	12.4	9.5–15.3	9.4–15.4
Segmented	7.4	6.0–12.0	3.8–11.0
Eosinophilic series (total)	3.1	1.2–5.3	1.1–5.2
Myelocytes	0.8	0.2–1.3	0.2–1.4
Metamyelocytes	1.2	0.4–2.2	0.2–2.2
Band	0.9	0.2–2.4	0–2.7
Segmented	0.5	0–1.3	0–1.1
Basophilic and mast cells	0.1	0–0.2	—
Erythrocytic series (total)	25.6	18.4–33.8	15.0–36.2
Pronormoblasts	0.6	0.2–1.3	0.1–1.1
Basophilic	1.4	0.5–2.4	0.4–2.4
Polychromatophilic	21.6	17.9–29.2	13.1–30.1
Orthochromatic	2.0	0.4–4.6	0.3–3.7
Lymphocytes	16.2	11.1–23.2	8.6–23.8
Plasma cells	1.3	0.4–3.9	0–3.5
Monocytes	0.3	0–0.8	0–0.6
Megakaryocytes	0.1	0–0.4	—
Reticulum cells	0.3	0–0.9	0–0.8
Myeloid:Erythroid ratio	2.3	1.5–3.3	1.1–3.5

[*]From Wintrobe MM. *Clinical Hematology.* 8th ed. Philadelphia, Pa: Lea & Febiger; 1984.

INDEX

Numbers in *italics* refer to pages on which Tables, Figures, or Images appear.
Numbers in **boldface** refer to pages on which Tests appear.

in drug-related hemolytic anemia, 212

in eosinophilia, 258

in essential thrombocythemia, 511, *514*

in extrinsic hemolytic anemia, 188

in granulocyte colony-stimulating factor therapy, 676, *681*

in granulocyte functional defects, 296–297

in hemoglobin synthesis disorders, 154

in hereditary erythrocyte membrane defects, 115

in Hodgkin's lymphoma, 652

in hypochromic anemia, 26, *28, 29*

in hypoplastic anemia, 60–61

indications for, 20, *21*

in iron deficiency anemia, *28, 29,* 103

in lymphadenopathy, 350

in lymphocytopenia, 338–339

in megaloblastic anemia, 80–81

in monoclonal gammopathy of undetermined significance, 710

in monocytosis, 273–274

in multiple myeloma, 688–689, *702–703*

in myelodysplastic syndromes, 371–372, *373, 393–395*

in myelofibrosis/myeloid metaplasia, 482–483, *488–489*

in neutropenia, 282–283, *287*

in neutrophilia, 244, 247

in non-Hodgkin's lymphoma, 605, 609, *640*

in paroxysmal nocturnal hemoglobinuria, 103, 175

in polycythemia, *488,* 498, *505–506*

in qualitative platelet disorders, 767

reference values for, 912

sampling sites, 19

in sideroblastic anemia, *28, 29*

in thalassemia, *28, 29*

in thrombocytopenia, 745

in Waldenström's macroglobulinemia, 697, *705*

Bone marrow replacement disorders
blood cell measurements in, 64–65

bone marrow examination in, 65

causes of, *64*

clinical findings in, 64

course of, 65–66

hematologic findings in, 64–65

pathophysiology of, 63–64

peripheral blood smear morphology in, 65

treatment of, 65–66

Bone marrow testing. *See* Stainable bone marrow iron

Bone marrow transplantation
for acute lymphoblastic leukemia, 466

for acute myeloid leukemia, 427

for aplastic anemia, 62–63

for Chédiak-Higashi syndrome, 308

for chronic myelogenous leukemia, 525

complications of. *See* Posttransplantation disorders

disorders treated with, *675*

granulocyte abnormalities after, 304, *305*

for granulocyte functional defects, 299

granulocyte functional defects in, *292*

for Hodgkin's lymphoma, 657

for multiple myeloma, 696

for myelodysplastic syndromes, 388

for non-Hodgkin's lymphoma, 626

for paroxysmal nocturnal hemoglobinuria, 180

for severe combined immunodeficiency disease, 341

Bone pain, in accelerated erythrocyte turnover, 98

Bone radiographs, in multiple myeloma, 688, 695

Breast cancer, *479*

Breast milk jaundice, 104

Brucellosis, *348*

BSAP. *See* B-cell lineage specific activator protein

Budd-Chiari syndrome, 174, 180

Burkitt's leukemia/lymphoma, 456

Burkitt's-like lymphoma, 462, 590, *605, 623*

Burkitt's lymphoma (BL), 448, *449,* 462, 560, *568, 570, 574,*

Corticosteroid therapy
for autoimmune hemolytic anemia, 233
for cryoglobulinemia, 713
neutrophil functional defects in, 292
neutrophilia in, *240, 242, 249*
for paroxysmal nocturnal hemoglobinuria, 180
for red cell aplasia, 62
Coulter Counter, 4
Coulter S+ STKR, *898, 900*
Coumadin. *See* Warfarin therapy
Creatinine testing. *See* Serum creatinine
Crigler-Najjar syndrome, 104
Cryoglobulin(s), 713
Cryoglobulinemia, 713, *714*
Cryoprecipitate, 807
Cryptococcus infection, *347, 674*
Crystal cells, of hemoglobin C disease, 164, *167*
CSF. *See* Colony-stimulating factor(s)
Cutaneous T-cell lymphoma, 594
Cyanine 5, 864, *866*
Cyclic AMP, 752
Cyclic neutropenia, 269, 278, *279–280*
Cyclin D-1, 868, *873*
Cyclooxygenase, 752
Cyclooxygenase deficiency, *758*
Cyclophosphamide, 696
Cyclosporine, 664–665
for aplastic anemia, 63
for red cell aplasia, 63
Cytochemical studies, **417–420,** *418*
in acute lymphoblastic leukemia, *418, 426,* 445, 450–452
in acute myeloid leukemia, 401, 417–420, *418*
in non-Hodgkin's lymphoma, 612
Cytogenetic analysis, **519–521, 885–890**
in acute lymphoblastic leukemia, 445, 459–462, *460–461, 473, 888*
in acute myeloid leukemia, 385, 401, 407, 421–422, *423, 426, 888*
in aplastic anemia, 62
chromosome metaphase spread analysis. *See* Chromosome metaphase spread analysis
in chronic lymphocytic leukemia, 535–536, 540–541, *888*

in chronic myelogenous leukemia, 515, 517, *517, 519–521, 526, 888*
in essential thrombocythemia, 512
fluorescent in situ hybridization. *See* Fluorescent in situ hybridization
in granulocytic disorders with abnormal morphology, 308
in Hodgkin's lymphoma, 656
in hypochromic anemia, 26
in hypoplastic anemia, 62
in lymphoma, *889*
in monocytosis, 273–274
in multiple myeloma, *889*
in myelodysplastic syndromes, 26, 370–371, 379, 383–385, *386, 888*
in myelofibrosis/myeloid metaplasia, 481, 483
in neutrophilia, 244, 247, 249
in non-Hodgkin's lymphoma, 560–562, *561,* 620
in paroxysmal nocturnal hemoglobinuria, 180
in persistent polyclonal B-cell lymphocytosis, 327
in polycythemia, *499*
in prolymphocytic leukemia, *888*
Cytokine receptor studies, in polycythemia, 501
Cytokine therapy, for aplastic anemia, 62
Cytomegalovirus infection, 223, 269, 315, *316,* 323–325, *324, 347,* 350, *354, 606, 674*
Cytoplasmic vacuolization, 241, *244, 251*

D
Dacrocytes, *6–7*
DAF. *See* Decay-accelerating factor
Danazol, for red cell aplasia, 63
D antigen, 196
DAT. *See* Direct antiglobulin test
Daunorubicin, 425
D-dimer, 795, 798, 802
D-dimer test, **803–805**
in acquired coagulation disorders, 803–805
in thrombotic disorders, 824
in venous thromboembolism, 824
Decay-accelerating factor (DAF), 172
Deep venous thrombosis, 805, 824, 847

Heparin cofactor II, 832
Heparin-induced thrombocytopenia, 849
Heparin-induced thrombocytopenia test, **746–747**
Heparin level, **856**
   anticoagulant therapy, 856
Heparinlike glycosaminoglycans, *820*
Heparin therapy, 732–733, 741, *755*, 821, 832, 846. *See also* Anticoagulant therapy; Heparin level
   administration methods, 847
   clinical indications for, 847
   in disseminated intravascular coagulation, 807
   heparin level, 856
   low-molecular-weight heparins, 846–849, 856
   monitoring of, *812,* 848–849
Hepatitis, viral, 58, *59, 316, 324, 334*
   hepatitis C, 713, *714*
Hepatocellular carcinoma, *493*
Hepatoma, 794
Hepatomegaly
   in accelerated erythrocyte turnover, 98
   in beta-thalassemia, 151
   in chronic myelogenous leukemia, 265
   in extrinsic hemolytic anemia, 186
   in granulocytic disorders with abnormal morphology, 306
Hepatosplenic γδ T-cell lymphoma, *561, 571, 574, 577,* 601
Hereditary elliptocytosis. *See also* Erythrocyte membrane defects, hereditary
   accelerated erythrocyte turnover in, *96*
   clinical findings in, 113
   pathophysiology of, 112
Hereditary giant neutrophils, *303, 308*
Hereditary hypersegmentation of neutrophils, *303, 308*
Hereditary methemoglobinemia, 149
Hereditary nonspherocytic hemolytic anemia (HNSHA)
   clinical findings in, 122–124
   course of, 129
   defects associated with, *125*
   diagnostic approach in, 125
   fluorescent screening test for

      pyruvate kinase deficiency in, 126–127
   in glucose-6-phosphate dehydrogenase deficiency, 135
   glucose-6-phosphate dehydrogenase test in, 125
   hematologic findings in, 125–126
   hemoglobin electrophoresis in, 125
   isopropanol stability test in, 125, 129
   molecular identification of red cell enzyme defects in, 128–129
   osmotic fragility test in, 125, 129
   pathophysiology of, 121–122, *123–124*
   pyruvate kinase test in, 125–127
   red cell enzyme activity assays in, 127–128
   treatment of, 129
Hereditary persistence of fetal hemoglobin (HPFH)
   acid elution test for fetal hemoglobin in RBCs in, 163
   alkali denaturation test for fetal hemoglobin in, 160–161
   beta-thalassemia vs, 151
   hemoglobin analysis in, *161*
Hereditary spherocytosis. *See also* Erythrocyte membrane defects, hereditary
   accelerated erythrocyte turnover in, *96*
   diagnostic approach in, 60
   hemoglobin F in, 161
   osmotic fragility test in, 115–117, *116–117*
   pathophysiology of, 112
   peripheral blood smear morphology in, *10,* 102
   workup of Coombs'-negative anemia, *17*
Hermansky-Pudlak syndrome, *758*
Herpes virus infection, *348, 606, 674, 680*
Heterophil antibody test, **319–320**
   in infectious mononucleosis, 317, 319–321, *322, 323*
   in lymphadenopathy, 351
Hexokinase deficiency, *123–124*
Hexose monophosphate (HMP) shunt, 122, *125,* 131, *132*
Hexose monophosphate (HMP) shunt disorders, 131–142. *See also*

cytogenetic analysis in, 481, 483
diagnostic approach in, 480–481, *509*
differential diagnosis of, *486–487*
hematologic findings in, 481–483
leukocyte alkaline phosphatase test in, 483
molecular analysis in, 481
pathophysiology of, 477–479
peripheral blood smear morphology in, 481–482, *488*
platelet aggregation studies in, 484
platelet dysfunction in, 765, *766*
radiographic studies in, 484
reticulin stain in, 482–483, *489*
serum alkaline phosphatase in, 484
thrombocytosis in, *508*
treatment of, 484–485
Myeloid metaplasia. *See* Myelofibrosis/myeloid metaplasia
Myeloid sarcoma, *412,* 416–417, *429*
Myelokathexis, *280, 303*
Myeloma. *See* Multiple myeloma
Myeloperoxidase, *615, 618, 867,* 868
Myeloperoxidase deficiency, *292*
Myeloperoxidase stain, **298**
in acute lymphoblastic leukemia, 451, *452*
in acute myeloid leukemia, 417–420, *418, 426–427, 440*
in granulocyte functional defects, 295, 298
Myelophthisis, *284*
Myeloproliferative disorders
chronic. *See* Chronic myeloproliferative disorders
common features of, *478*
diagnostic algorithm for, *496*
myelofibrosis/myeloid metaplasia. *See* Myelofibrosis/myeloid metaplasia
platelet dysfunction in, 765, *766*
polycythemia. *See* Polycythemia
reduced glutathione determination in, 142
stainable bone marrow iron in, 32
thrombocytosis. *See* Thrombocytosis

Myeloproliferative syndrome
atypical, 380, 485–486
differential characteristics of, *486–487*
undifferentiated, 485–486
Myocardial infarction, 326, 847, *853, 855*
Myoglobinuria, 193
MZBCL. *See* Marginal zone B-cell lymphoma

N

Nalidixic acid, *135, 209*
Naphthalene, *135, 209*
Naproxen, *755*
Nasopharyngeal carcinoma, *348, 641*
National Cancer Institute staging system, for non-Hodgkin's lymphoma, 564–565, *565*
Natural killer-cell lymphoma, 591–601
Near haploidy, *460*
Near tetraploidy, *460*
Necrotizing granulomatous lymphadenitis, *649*
Neonatal purpura fulminans, 833
Neonatal thrombocytopenia, 741
Nephrotic syndrome, *854*
Neuroblastoma, 465
Neurofibromatosis, 383, 399
Neurologic manifestations, of megaloblastic anemia, 78–79, 89
Neutralization studies, in hemolytic disease of the newborn, 198
Neutropenia
in acute lymphoblastic leukemia, 446
in acute myeloid leukemia, 402
age-related causes of, 278, *279*
in aplastic anemia, *279, 284*
autoimmune, 278, *278–279, 287*
blood cell measurements in, 283
bone marrow examination in, 282–283, *287*
causes of, 278, *278*
chronic, 270, *270*
clinical findings in, 280–281
constitutional, 278, *280*
course of, 284–285
cyclic. *See* Cyclic neutropenia
definition of, 277–278
diagnostic approach in, 282
drug-related, 278, 280, *283*
folate deficiency in, 283, *284*
hematologic findings in, 283

hypergranular promyelocytic
leukemia
disseminated intravascular coag-
ulation in, *795*
Pronormoblasts, 3
Propidium iodide, 864–865, *866*
Propranolol, *755*
Prostacyclin, 752, *820,* 823, 855
Prostaglandins, 271, 752
Prostate cancer, *479*
Prosthetic heart valve. *See* Heart valve
prosthesis
Protac functional protein C assay,
832–833
Protamine plasma paracoagulation
test, **803**
in acquired coagulation disor-
ders, 803
Protamine sulfate, 846
Protein C, 819, 821, *821,* 823, 846
activated. *See* Activated protein C
reference values for, *910–911*
Protein C deficiency, 794, 824, *825,*
830–831, 832–833
Protein C determination, **832–833**
in thrombotic disorders, 827,
832–833
Protein-calorie malnutrition, *334,* 335
Protein electrophoresis. *See* Serum
protein electrophoresis; Urine
protein electrophoresis
Protein-losing enteropathy, *334*
Protein S, *820,* 821, *821,* 823, 846
reference values for, *910–911*
Protein S deficiency, 794, 824, *825,*
828, 830–831, 834–835
Protein S determination, **834**
in thrombotic disorders, 827, 834
Prothrombin, 721–723, *722–723, 730,*
846
reference values for, *910–911*
Prothrombin abnormality, 729
Prothrombin antibodies, 793, *799*
Prothrombin assay, **784–785**
in inherited coagulation disorders, 784–786
Prothrombin deficiency, *777,* 778,
794, 800
Prothrombin inhibitor, 802
Prothrombin mutation, 824, *825,* 827,
829, 839
Prothrombin time (PT) assay,
728–731, *730*
in acquired coagulation disorders, *799, 801*

in bleeding disorders, 728–731,
730, 812
coagulation factors measured by,
730
in disseminated intravascular
coagulation, *801*
in hemophilia, *729*
in inherited coagulation disorders, 776, *777,* 778
monitoring warfarin therapy, 849
preoperative hemostasis screening, *816*
PT ratio, 850, *852*
in thrombocytopenia, *729,* 745
in vitamin K deficiency, *729,* 798
in von Willebrand's disease, *729*
Protoporphyrin testing. *See* Free erythrocyte protoporphyrin
Protozoal infections, 269
Pseudodiploidy, 460
Pseudo-Howell-Jolly bodies, 304, *305*
Pseudo-Pelger-Huët anomaly, 246,
304, *305, 311, 373, 393*
Pseudo-von Willebrand's disease. *See*
von Willebrand's disease,
platelet-type
Pseudoxanthoma imperfecta, *758*
PT assay. *See* Prothrombin time assay
PTLD. *See* Posttransplantation lym-
phoproliferative disorders
Pulmonary embolism, 805, 847, *853*
Pure red cell aplasia, 53, *54*
PV. *See* Polycythemia vera
Pyelonephritis, *41*
Pyridoxine, 36
Pyrimethamine, *78*
Pyrimidine-5¢-nucleotidase deficien-
cy, 126, 142
Pyruvate kinase deficiency, 121,
123–124, 124. *See also*
Hereditary nonspherocytic
hemolytic anemia
accelerated erythrocyte turnover
in, *96, 100*
fluorescent screening test for,
126–127
molecular identification of, 128
treatment of, 129

Q

5q- syndrome, *375, 378, 385, 888*
Qualitative platelet disorders,
734–735, 754–763, *755–762*
acquired conditions associated
with, *766*

RPI. *See* Reticulocyte production
index
Rubella, *316, 324,* 325, *348*

S
Salicylazosulfapyridine, *135, 209*
Sarcoidosis, *41, 254,* 259, *270, 334,*
336, 338, 347–348, 349–350,
354, 356
Sarcoma. *See also* specific types of
sarcoma
immunophenotyping in, *618*
Schilling test
in macrocytic anemia, *13*
in megaloblastic anemia, 87
Schistocytes, *6–7,* 744, 796, 802
SCID. *See* Severe combined immunodeficiency disease
Secondary granules
basophils, 264–265
eosinophils, 254–256
neutrophils, 242
Sedimentation rate, reference values
for, *896–897*
Segmented neutrophils, 241–242
reference values for, *900–905*
Serine endopeptidases, 721
Serologic tests for infectious agents,
350–352
in lymphadenopathy, 349–352
Serotonin, 721
Serous effusion cytology, in non-
Hodgkin's lymphoma, 611
Serum alkaline phosphatase
in essential thrombocythemia,
512
in myelofibrosis/myeloid metaplasia, 484
Serum antibody detection, **226–227**
in autoimmune hemolytic anemia, *221,* 226–227
Serum antibody screening, **188–189**
in accelerated erythrocyte
turnover, *101*
in extrinsic hemolytic anemia,
187
in transfusion reactions, 187–189
Serum antibody tests, **213–215**
in drug-related hemolytic anemia, 211, 213–215
Serum bilirubin, total and fractionated, **103–104**
in accelerated erythrocyte
turnover, 99, *99–100,*
103–104

in extrinsic hemolytic anemia,
187
in hemolytic disease of the newborn, 198
Serum calcium
in acute myeloid leukemia, 424
in lymphadenopathy, 349, 356
in monoclonal gammopathy of
undetermined significance,
709
in non-Hodgkin's lymphoma,
621
Serum chemistry
in acute myeloid leukemia, 401,
424
in non-Hodgkin's lymphoma,
621
Serum complement measurement,
230–231
in autoimmune hemolytic anemia, *221,* 230–231
Serum creatinine, in monoclonal gammopathy of undetermined significance, 709
Serum ferritin quantitation, **32–33**
in anemia of chronic disease, 42,
45–46
in hemochromatosis, 33
in hypochromic anemia, 32–33
in inflammatory disease, 33
in iron deficiency anemia, 33
in sideroblastic anemia, 33
Serum folate quantitation, **84–85**
in megaloblastic anemia, *82–83,*
84–85, 87
reference values for, *908–909*
Serum haptoglobin quantitation,
105–106
in accelerated erythrocyte
turnover, 99–100, *99,*
105–106
in autoimmune hemolytic anemia, 231
in extrinsic hemolytic anemia,
187, 191–192
in transfusion reactions, 191–192
Serum immunofixation, **693–694**
in amyloidosis, 699
in monoclonal gammopathy of
undetermined significance,
709, 711
in multiple myeloma, 688,
693–694, *694*
Serum immunoglobulin quantitation,
694–695

in chronic lymphocytic leukemia,
536, 540
in monoclonal gammopathy of
undetermined significance,
709, 711
multiple myeloma, 694–695
Serum iron quantitation, **29–31**
in anemia of chronic disease, *28,
30, 42, 44–45*
in hypochromic anemia, 26, *28,
29–31*
in iron deficiency anemia, *28,
29–31*
in macrocytic anemia, *13*
in polycythemia, *499*
reference values for, *908–909*
in sideroblastic anemia, *28,* 31
in thalassemia, *28,* 31
Serum lactate dehydrogenase
in megaloblastic anemia, *82–83*
in non-Hodgkin's lymphoma,
621
Serum lysozyme, in monocytosis, 274
Serum magnesium, in acute myeloid
leukemia, 424
Serum pigments, in accelerated erythrocyte turnover, 99, *100,*
107–108
Serum potassium, in essential thrombocythemia, 512
Serum protein electrophoresis,
691–692
in monoclonal gammopathy of
undetermined significance,
709–710
in multiple myeloma, 688,
691–692, 692
in non-Hodgkin's lymphoma, 621
in Waldenström's macroglobulinemia, 697–698
Serum sickness, *347*
Serum soluble transferrin receptor,
33–34
in anemia of chronic disease, *16,
28*
in folate deficiency, 34
in hemoglobinopathy, 34
in hemolytic anemia, 34
in hypochromic anemia, *28,*
33–34
in iron deficiency anemia, *28,*
33–34
in sideroblastic anemia, *28*
in thalassemia, *28*
in vitamin B$_{12}$ deficiency, 34

Serum viscosity, in multiple myeloma,
696
Serum vitamin B$_{12}$ quantitation,
81–84
in AIDS, 84
in megaloblastic anemia, 81–84,
82–83, 87
reference values for, *908–909*
Severe combined immunodeficiency
disease (SCID), 334–335,
334, 337, 340–341
Sézary cells, 547, *555,* 594, *637*
Sézary syndrome (SS), 534, 547, *555,
568, 571, 574, 576,* 594, *637,
872*
Shwachman-Diamond syndrome, 53,
54, 56–57, 280
Sickle cell(s), *6–7*
Sickle cell anemia. *See also*
Hemoglobin synthesis disorders
blood cell measurements in, *10,*
153
course and treatment of, 165
diagnostic approach in, 60
granulocyte functional defects in,
292
pathophysiology of, 146, 148
peripheral blood smear morphology in, 154, *168*
sickle cell test, 158
Sickle cell test, **158**
in hemoglobin synthesis disorders, 152, 159
Sickle cell trait, 146, 148, *156,* 158
Sideroblast(s), 25, *27,* 31–32, *38,* 50,
395
Sideroblast count, in iron deficiency
anemia, 32
Sideroblastic anemia, *14, 24, 766*
abnormal iron metabolism in,
24–25
bone marrow examination in, *28,*
29
free erythrocyte protoporphyrin
in, 35
hematologic findings in, 27–29,
27
hereditary, 387
percent transferrin saturation in,
28
peripheral blood smear morphology in, 29
serum ferritin quantitation in, 33
serum iron quantitation in, *28,* 31